Technical
Manual

AMERICAN ASSOCIATION OF BLOOD BANKS

Mention of specific commercial products or equipment by contributors to the American Association of Blood Banks' *Technical Manual* does not represent an endorsement of such products by the American Association of Blood Banks, nor does it necessarily indicate a preference for those products over other similar competitive products.

Efforts are made to have publications of the AABB consistent in regard to acceptable practices. However, as new developments in the practice and technology of blood banking occur, the Committee on Standards recommends changes when indicated from available information. It is not possible to revise each publication at the time each change is adopted. Thus, it is essential that the most recent edition of the *Standards for Blood Banks and Transfusion Services* be used as the ultimate reference in regard to current acceptable practices.

Technical Manual

of the
**AMERICAN ASSOCIATION
OF BLOOD BANKS**

NINTH EDITION

1985

AMERICAN ASSOCIATION OF BLOOD BANKS
1117 NORTH 19TH STREET   SUITE 600   ARLINGTON, VIRGINIA 22209

American Association of Blood Banks
1117 North 19th Street, Suite 600
Arlington, VA 22209

Library of Congress Cataloging in Publication Data

Technical manual of the American Association of Blood Banks.

Half-title: Technical manual.
Includes bibliographies and index.
1. Blood banks. 2. Blood banks—Quality control.
3. Blood—Collection and preservation. 4. Blood—Transportation. I. American Association of Blood Banks.
II. Title: Technical manual. [DNLM: 1. Blood Banks—laboratory manuals. WH 25 T255]
RM172.T43   1985   615′.65   85-1346
ISBN 0-915355-06-X

Distributed outside the
United States and Canada by:
S. Karger, AG
Medical and Scientific Publishers
P.O. Box CH-4009 Basel
Switzerland

Committee on Technical Manual

Editor
Frances K. Widmann, MD

Committee

Frances K. Widmann, MD, *Chairman*

Edward L. Snyder, MD, *Vice-Chairman*

Asa Barnes, Jr., MD

Leonard I. Boral, MD

John Case, FIMLS

Michelle D. Inkster, FAIMLS

W. John Judd, FIMLS, MI Biol

Arthur J. Silvergleid, MD

Susan M. Steane, MS, MT(ASCP)SBB

Joberta Wells, MT(ASCP)SBB

FDA Office of Biologics Research and Review Liaison

P. Ann Hoppe, MT(ASCP)SBB

Acknowledgments

The Committee on the Technical Manual extends special thanks to those who reviewed the manuscripts and made other special contributions:

Paul J. Schmidt, MD and the members of the AABB Committee on Standards

Harvey J. Alter, MD

Theresa A. Bolk, MT(ASCP)SBB

Hugh Chaplin, Jr., MD

Marie Crookston, BSc

Richard J. Davey, MD

Sandra S. Ellisor, MT(ASCP)SBB

Bruce A. Friedman, MD

Armand B. Glassman, MD

Alfred J. Grindon, MD

F. Carl Grumet, MD

L. Ruth Guy, PhD

Emanuel Hackel, PhD

Paul V. Holland, MD

Peter D. Issitt, FIMLS

Nancy L. Johnson, MT(ASCP)SBB

Louise J. Keating, MD

Melanie S. Kennedy, MD

Harvey G. Klein, MD

Robert E. Klein, MD

Donna Kostyu, PhD

Naomi L.C. Luban, MD

Delores M. Mallory, MT(ASCP)SBB

W.L. Marsh, FIMLS, FI Biol

Harold T. Meryman, MD

Jacqueline D. Miller, MD

William V. Miller, MD

Paul D. Mintz, MD

Phyllis A. Morel, MT(ASCP)SBB

Victor H. Muller, MD

Grace M. Neitzer, MT(ASCP)SBB

Thomas A. Noto, MD

Jacob Nusbacher, MD

Harold A. Oberman, MD

Malcolm O. Orr, MD

Lawrence D. Petz, MD

Steven R. Pierce, SBB(ASCP)

Patricia T. Pisciotto, MD

Susan D. Rolih, MT(ASCP)SBB

Ronald A. Sacher, MD

Page D. Sanchez, MT(ASCP)SBB

S. Gerald Sandler, MD

Elizabeth S. Sebring, MT(ASCP)SBB

Mary Ann Sharpe, MT(ASCP)SBB

Toby L. Simon, MD

Marcus B. Simpson, MD

David E. Smith, MD

Mary Jo Smith, MT(ASCP)SBB

Joel M. Solomon, PhD

E. Ann Steiner, MT(ASCP)SBB

Marjory Stroup, MT(ASCP)SBB

Edwin G. Taft, MD

Patricia A. Tippett, PhD

Peter A. Tomasulo, MD

Margaret E. Wallace, MHS, MT(ASCP)SBB

M. Jane Wilson, MT(ASCP)SBB

Special thanks are due to Kathryn Ennis of the American Red Cross and Joan Maher, Janet McGrath, Laurel Munk and Lorry Rose of the AABB National Office who provided invaluable editorial and administrative support to the Committee.

Introduction

The ninth edition of the *Technical Manual* continues the tradition of its predecessors in providing a conceptual background for the techniques of serologic practice as well as details of the techniques themselves. In the four years since the eighth edition was first published, there have been significant changes in our understanding of immunologic events, clinical interactions, biochemical phenomena and technical approaches. Along with these have come changes in clinical and financial concerns. The decisions blood bankers must make increasingly involve considerations beyond the strictly technical. The Committee on Technical Manual has attempted to provide sufficient theoretical and clinical information so that blood banking professionals can select procedures and strategies appropriate to specific needs.

A major difference between the ninth edition and its predecessors is that this *Technical Manual* does not address every area covered in the current edition of *Standards for Blood Banks and Transfusion Services*. It was the decision of the Committee that presenting theoretical and practical material necessary to fulfill the requirements of *Standards,* Section N, Histocompatibility Testing, would expand this volume beyond its appropriate and applicable size and scope. Although there is a chapter on the HLA system and a brief procedure given for lymphocytotoxicity testing, the reader looking for detailed information about histocompatibility testing should consult more extensive sources devoted exclusively to these techniques.

This volume entered final production phases in March, 1985, a few weeks after licensure of the first tests for antibodies to human T-cell lymphotropic virus, type III (HTLV-III). The techniques, the applications and the significance of these tests constitute an area so fluid that it seemed inappropriate to incorporate specific, and surely evanescent, details in a hard-back volume intended to stand without major revision for several years. Weekly publications from the FDA, the Centers for Disease Control, the AABB and other authoritative sources provide a far more suitable forum for this rapidly evolving field.

The material in the *Technical Manual* reflects the experience and opinions of the Committee on Technical Manual, augmented by advice and suggestions from the Committee on Standards, the National Committee on Inspection and Accreditation as well as a large number of expert reviewers. If there are errors, these should be laid at the feet of the Committee and the editor, not the reviewers. If there are areas in which readers' opinions differ with the ideas expressed, we will be happy to discuss other approaches and consider them for adoption in a subsequent edition.

Techniques and policies outlined in the *Technical Manual* are, to the best of the Committee's corporate ability, in conformance with *Standards*. They are not to be considered the only permissible way in which the requirements of *Standards* can be met. Other methods, not included, may give equally acceptable results. If discrepancy occurs between techniques or suggestions in the *Technical Manual* and the requirements of *Standards*, authority resides in *Standards*. The reader should not refer to the *Technical Manual* as an alternative authority, since it is intended as an adjunct publication of the Association.

FRANCES K. WIDMANN, MD
Editor

Contents

xi

Immunologic Principles

Blood Groups

Application of Serologic Principles to Transfusion Practice

Clinical Considerations in Transfusion Practices

Other Considerations

Components 469

Equipment 475

Hemolytic Disease of the Newborn 481

Miscellaneous 487

Normal Values 493

Index 497

Technical
Manual

1

Blood Collection

Blood Donors

Blood banks and transfusion services depend on voluntary donors to provide the blood necessary to meet the needs of the patients they serve. To attract volunteer donors initially and to encourage their continued participation, it is essential that conditions surrounding blood donation be as pleasant, safe and convenient as possible.

The donor area should be attractive, well-lighted, comfortably ventilated, clean and open at convenient hours for donors. Personnel should be interested, friendly and understanding, as well as professional and well-trained. Whether donors are drawn at the blood center or on mobile units, every effort should be made to make the donation a pleasant experience.

Each blood bank must prepare its own procedures manual, covering all phases of activity in the donor area. These procedures must meet the requirements of the AABB *Standards*[1] for AABB accreditation. The manual should contain any local or state, in addition to federal, regulations pertaining to blood bank operation. The procedures manual must be reviewed annually by the medical director of the blood bank, and should be available at all times to blood bank personnel.[2]

Registration

The information obtained from the donor during registration must make it possible to identify and, if necessary, recall that individual. Current information must be obtained and recorded for each donation; single-use or multiple-donation forms may be used. This record must be kept for at least 5 years or as required by local statutes, whichever is longer.

The following information must be included:

1. Date of donation
2. Name: Last, first and middle initial
3. Address: Residence and/or business
4. Telephone: Residence and/or business
5. Sex
6. Age and/or date of birth: Blood donors must be between the ages of 17 and 65 years (up to 66th birthday) with the following exceptions:
   a. Donors who are considered minors under applicable law may be accepted only if written consent to donate blood has been obtained in accordance with applicable law. Since these laws vary among jurisdictions, local legal opinion should be obtained and a copy of the state law should be readily available.
   b. After the 66th birthday, prospective donors may be accepted at the discretion of the blood bank physician. Many blood centers safely involve their senior citizen population in the donation process. The decision to accept donors above the

age of 66 may be made on a case-by-case basis or there may be general policy statements embodied in the procedures manual.

7. Written consent for the blood bank to take and use blood from the prospective donor: The consent form is part of the donor record, to be completed at the time of registration. The procedure must be explained in terms the donor can understand, and the donor must have an opportunity to ask questions and to decide whether or not to give consent by signing the form.

8. A record of reasons for previous deferrals, if any

The following information may also be useful:

1. Additional identification such as social security or driver's license number. This information may be necessary for information retrieval in some computerized systems and provides additional identifying information.

2. Name of patient or group to be credited, if a credit system is used. Even if the donor is deferred, a record of these donors may be useful to the patient or to others concerned with donor recruitment or credit accounts.

3. Race. This information may be particularly useful when blood of a specific phenotype is needed for patients, usually of the same race, with unexpected antibodies.

4. Unique characteristics of the donor. Certain information about the donor may enable the blood bank to make optimal use of the donation. For example, blood from donors who are seronegative for cytomegalovirus (CMV), or who are group O, Rh negative, is often designated for neonatal patients. The blood center may wish to specify that blood from these individuals be drawn routinely into special bags for pediatric transfusion. Individuals known to have circulating antibodies may be identified so that their blood can be processed into components that contain only minimal amounts of plasma and their red cells be made available to patients with the same antibodies.

Donor Selection

Donor selection is based on a limited physical examination and a medical history that determines whether giving blood will harm the donor or if transfusion of the unit will harm the recipient.[1-3] Careful donor selection contributes vitally to the safety of both donor and recipient.

Volunteer donors come to the collection site because they want to give blood. Deferring or rejecting the potential donor often leaves the individual with a negative feeling about himself as well as the system. Donor deferral rates should be closely monitored by the blood bank physician to ensure they are within a reasonable range—usually less than 12%.[4] Donors who are deferred should be given a full explanation and be informed whether and when they can return.

The medical history questions may be asked by a qualified interviewer or donors may complete their own record, which must then be reviewed and initialed by a knowledgeable individual responsible to the blood bank.

The interview and physical examination should be performed in a manner that ensures adequate auditory and visual privacy, allays apprehensions and allows time for any necessary discussion or explanation. Answers to questions must be recorded "yes" or "no" with details explaining answers added as indicated. Results of all tests must be recorded.

Medical History

During the medical history, some very specific questions will be necessary, but a great deal of pertinent information can be obtained by using some general or leading questions in simple language that the donor can understand. The examples given below include all requirements and are followed by suggested or required responses to information received.

1. Blood donation: Have you ever donated blood, platelets or plasma? Have you donated blood or plasma in the last 8 weeks?

   The interval between donations of whole blood must be 8 weeks except in unusual circumstances and with the written permission of the blood bank physician. After plasmapheresis or cytapheresis, at least 48 hours must elapse before whole blood donation.

2. Deferral as a donor: Have you ever been deferred as a blood donor? When? Why?

   Information regarding prior deferrals should be considered when evaluating current eligibility.

3. Pregnancy: Are you pregnant? Have you been pregnant during the last 6 weeks?

   Defer during pregnancy and for 6 weeks after third-trimester delivery. Exception may be made by the blood bank physician for autologous transfusion or if the woman's blood is needed for exchange transfusion of her infant. Donors who have recently had first-trimester abortions need not be deferred if they meet other donor criteria.

4. Surgical procedures or major illnesses: Have you had surgery or a major illness in the last 6 months? When, what type? Are you under the care of a doctor for any reason? Why?

   Donors who have undergone operations should be deferred for at least 6 months if they received blood or components during the procedure. Uncomplicated surgery is disqualifying only until healing is complete and full activity has been resumed. A distinction between "major" and "minor" surgery is unnecessary so long as blood was not transfused and the patient has resumed full activity.

   Questionable answers that might indicate the donor is not in good health should be referred to the blood bank physician for further evaluation.

5. Heart, lung and liver diseases: Have you ever had heart disease? When? What type? Do you ever suffer from chest pain? Shortness of breath? Explain. Have you had any serious lung disease? Explain. Have you had any type of liver disease? Explain.

   A history of coronary heart disease or rheumatic heart disease with known residual damage is cause for deferral unless evaluated and approved by the blood bank physician. A single episode of rheumatic fever or pericarditis, a heart murmur or successful repair of a congenital defect does not necessarily disqualify a donor.

   Active pulmonary tuberculosis, or any active pulmonary disease, is cause for deferral. Previous tuberculosis, successfully treated and no longer active, need not disqualify. Donors with a reactive tuberculin skin test but without other abnormalities may be accepted.

   An active inflammatory or degenerative disease of the liver or one that might impair organ function is cause for deferral of the donor. Chronic conditions must be evaluated by a physician.

6. Unexplained weight loss: Have you lost weight recently? How much? Why?

   Unexplained excessive weight loss, often defined as 10% or more of previous weight, could indicate undiagnosed serious illness, and should be investigated further and evaluated by a physician (see also 9).

7. Drugs and medications: Are you taking any drugs or medications? Why? What?

   In general, medications taken by a donor are not harmful to the recipient and most donors taking medications, even prescription medications, are acceptable blood donors.

   Deferral for most drugs is based on the nature of the disease process, not on properties of the drug itself. This is true of most donors requiring antibiotics, anticonvulsants, anticoagulants, digitalis, insulin, systemic corticosteroids, vasodilators, and antiarrhythmic or anti-inflammatory drugs.

Use of drugs and medication should be evaluated by the blood bank physician. Listed below are some drugs and medical conditions that are often permitted in blood donors, at the discretion of the individual facility's medical director.[5] The approval to draw these donors may be 1) a general approval included in the facility procedures manual or 2) an approval given individually as each problem arises, providing verbal approval is documented on the donor's record.

a. Tetracyclines and other antibiotics for acne. Use of Isoretinoin (Accutane®) disqualifies a donor, as it may be a teratogen.

b. Topical steroid preparations for skin lesions not at the venipuncture site.

c. Blood pressure medications, taken chronically and successfully so that pressure is at or below allowable limits. The prospective donor taking antihypertensives should be free from side effects of the drug, especially episodes of postural hypotension, and should be free of any cardiovascular symptoms.

d. Isoniazid given because the tuberculin skin test has converted but without evidence of active tuberculosis.

e. Over-the-counter bronchodilators and decongestants.

f. Oral hypoglycemic agents in well-controlled diabetics without any vascular complications of the disease.

g. Tranquilizers, under most conditions. A physician should evaluate the donor to distinguish between tranquilizers and antipsychotic medications.

h. Hypnotics used at bedtime.

i. Marijuana (unless currently under the influence), oral contraceptives, mild analgesics, vitamins, replacement hormones or weight reduction pills.

Aspirin or aspirin-containing compounds depress platelet function for 1-3 days. Since platelets from a donor who has taken these drugs within 2-3 days should not be the only source of platelets for a patient, platelet concentrates prepared from such donors should be so labeled.

8. Hepatitis: Have you ever had hepatitis or jaundice? Have you had a reactive test for hepatitis (HBsAg)? Have you had intimate contact with a person with hepatitis? When? Have you received injections of hepatitis B immune globulin (HBIG)? When? Have you been transfused with blood or blood components? When? Have you had a tattoo? When? Have you ever injected drugs into your veins or skin? If ear piercing and/or acupuncture are commonly performed in the area the donor should be questioned about these procedures to make sure that single-use equipment, or disposable or properly sterilized needles were used.

The possible presence of hepatitis virus cannot be detected with certainty by any presently available means including history, physical examination or laboratory tests, including those for HBsAg; therefore, strict regulations for donor acceptability must be established and followed[1-2] (see also Chapter 18). Defer permanently any prospective donor:

a. With a history of viral hepatitis at any time, regardless of the causative virus. However, liver inflammation associated with well-documented infectious mononucleosis or cytomegalovirus infection is not a cause for permanent deferral.

b. Who has ever had a positive test for HBsAg.

c. Who is or has been an intravenous drug abuser. Check both arms for evidence of sclerotic veins.

d. Who previously donated the only unit of blood, blood component or derivative administered to a recipient who, within 6 months, developed posttransfusion hepatitis.

e. Whose involvement in two or more posttransfusion hepatitis cases results in a cumulative probability value of greater than 0.4 (see page 354 for explanation and details of method).

Defer for at least 6 months:

a. Recipient of blood, blood components or derivatives such as Factors II, VII, IX, X complex or AHF (Factor VIII) concentrate. This includes donors who are in blood immunization programs.

b. Recipient of a skin allograft or tattoo. Ear piercing and acupuncture done under questionable conditions may also be reason for deferral.

c. Donor who has had close contact with a person with viral hepatitis.

The type of contact that hospital personnel and physicians encounter in their work is not considered close contact and is not cause for deferral. Personnel in dialysis units have high potential for especially intense exposure to blood from patients at high risk of HBsAg positivity. If the dialysis unit has many patients positive for HBsAg, it may be wise to defer personnel who work there. The medical director of the blood drawing facility should establish a policy for those dialysis units that provide significant numbers of potential donors.

d. Former inmates of penal or mental institutions. The likelihood of exposure to hepatitis is very high in these settings, and current inmates of penal or mental institutions should not be drawn as donors.

Defer for at least 12 months:

Prospective donors who have received HBIG, since this is given only to individuals with especially close contact with hepatitis B. HBIG may prolong the incubation period of hepatitis B beyond the 6-month period usually considered adequate to ensure absence of developing hepatitis B.

9. Malaria: Have you ever had malaria? When? Have you been out of the USA in the past 3 years? When? Where? Have you ever taken any medication to prevent malaria?

Travelers who have been in areas considered endemic for malaria by the Malaria Program, Centers for Disease Control, US Department of Health and Human Services, may be accepted as regular blood donors 6 months after return to the nonendemic area, providing they have been free of symptoms and have not taken antimalarial drugs in the interim. A recent World Health Organization list of endemic areas should be available to the interviewing personnel. Prospective donors who have had malaria must be deferred for 3 years after cessation of therapy, or after departure from the malarial area, if they have been asymptomatic in the interim. Donations to be used for the preparation of plasma, plasma components, or fractions devoid of intact red blood cells are exempt from these restrictions.

10. Acquired immune deficiency syndrome (AIDS):

Have you had, within the past 6 months, any of the following: night sweats; unexplained fever above 99F for more than 10 days; persistent cough or shortness of breath; lymph nodes swollen for more than a month;

blue or purple spots or lumps, on or under the skin or mucous membranes; white patches or unusual lesions in the mouth; persistent diarrhea; or unexpected weight loss? Are you a member of or a sexual partner of a member of a category considered at high risk of AIDS?

Individuals in categories at high risk for acquiring or transmitting AIDS, and their sexual partners, should not donate blood. These include[6] persons with AIDS; persons who have experienced the symptoms listed above; males who have had sex with, or whose male partners have had sex with, more than one male since 1979; past or present abusers of intravenous drugs; Haitian entrants to the US after 1977; hemophiliacs; and the sexual partners of individuals in these categories. Prospective donors should be given information describing these categories, with instruction that such individuals should abstain from donation. Donor room personnel must question all individuals who elect to donate about the signs and symptoms listed, and should be alert to abnormalities on physical examination, especially evidence of IV drug abuse, skin lesions, fever, or evidence of recent weight loss. At some centers, donors unwilling to discontinue the selection process are offered an opportunity to signify confidentially that their blood should not be used for transfusion.

11. Abnormal bleeding tendencies: Do you bleed a long time when you have a cut or a tooth pulled? After surgery? After childbirth?

An abnormal bleeding tendency may be cause for deferral, subject to evaluation by the blood bank physician. Individuals with such a history may experience excessive bleeding at the site of venipuncture, and plasma from a donor deficient in coagulation factors would not confer expected therapeutic benefits if given to a recipient who needed these factors.

12. Convulsions, fainting spells: Do you have epilepsy? Have you had convulsions or fainting spells? Last episode?

Donors who have epilepsy or have had fainting spells or convulsions, except for febrile convulsions in early childhood, may have a reaction or seizure if they donate. Individuals who are off medication and have been seizure-free for 2 or more years are thought by many to be acceptable donors. Policy about accepting such donors should be included in the facility's procedures manual.

13. Cancer: Have you ever had cancer? What type? Have you ever had any form of blood disease? What type?

Prospective donors who have had cancer, other than minor skin cancer, carcinoma-in-situ of the cervix and papillary thyroid carcinoma should be evaluated by a qualified physician before being accepted as a blood donor. Donors who have or have had leukemia or lymphoma must be permanently deferred. If the donor has another blood disease, it should be evaluated by the blood bank physician.

14. Vaccinations, inoculations: Have you been vaccinated or had any shots in the past 12 months? What? When?

Symptom-free donors who recently have been immunized need not be deferred, with the following exceptions:

a. Smallpox: Donors are acceptable either after the scab has fallen off or 2 weeks after an immune reaction.

b. Measles (rubeola), mumps, yellow fever, oral polio vaccine: Donors are acceptable 2 weeks after their last immunization.

c. German measles (rubella): Donors are acceptable four weeks after their last injection.
d. Rabies, if given following a bite by a rabid animal: Defer for 1 year.
e. Hepatitis B vaccine: Prospective donors are acceptable provided they would not otherwise be disqualified.

15. General health: Do you feel well now? Do you have other health problems?

    The donor should appear to be in good health. Pain, cough, sore throat, headache, nausea, dizziness, menstrual cramps or extreme nervousness may be cause for deferral, at the discretion of the blood bank physician.

Physical Examination

Exceptions to the following guidelines must be evaluated individually by the blood bank physician.

1. Weight: Donors weighing 50 kg (110 lb) or more may ordinarily give 450 ± 45 ml of blood as well as up to 30 ml for processing tubes. For donors weighing 45-50 kg (100-110 lb), as little as 405 ml may be drawn without reducing the amount of anticoagulant in the primary bag, but it is important that there be accurate measurement of the volume of blood withdrawn. If it is necessary to draw less than 405 ml, the amount of anticoagulant must be reduced proportionally by expressing the excess into an integrally attached satellite bag and sealing the tubing. The volume of blood drawn must be measured carefully and accurately. To determine the amount of anticoagulant to remove, the following formula may be used:

Amount of anticoagulant to remove =

$$63 \text{ ml} - \left[\frac{\text{donor's weight}}{50 \text{ kg } (110 \text{ lb})} \times 63 \text{ ml} \right]$$

Amount of blood to draw =
$$\frac{\text{donor's weight}}{50 \text{ kg } (110 \text{ lb})} \times 450 \text{ ml}$$

2. Temperature: The oral temperature must not exceed 37.5 C (99.6 F). Caution: If a glass thermometer is used, it should not be in the donor's mouth during puncture to obtain blood for hematocrit or hemoglobin determination.

3. Pulse: The pulse should be counted for at least 30 seconds. It should exhibit no pathologic irregularity, and should be between 50 and 100 beats per minute. If a prospective donor is an athlete with high exercise tolerance, a lower pulse rate may be acceptable. A blood bank physician should evaluate marked abnormalities of pulse and recommend acceptance, deferral or referral for additional evaluation.

4. Blood pressure: The systolic blood pressure should be 90-180 mm Hg and the diastolic blood pressure should be 50-100 mm Hg. Prospective donors whose blood pressure is outside these ranges should not be drawn without individual evaluation by a qualified physician.

5. Skin lesions: The skin at the site of venipuncture must be free of lesions. Both arms must be examined for signs of intravenous drug abuse, especially multiple needle puncture marks and/or sclerotic veins. Mild skin disorders such as acne, psoriasis or the rash of poison ivy should not be cause for deferral unless unusually extensive or present in the antecubital area. Donors with boils, purulent wounds or severe skin infections anywhere on the body should be deferred, as should anyone with purplish-red or hemorrhagic nodules or indurated plaques suggestive of Kaposi's sarcoma (see above).

6. General appearance: If the donor looks ill, appears to be under the influence of drugs or alcohol, or is excessively nervous, it is best to defer. This should, if possible, be done in a way that does not antagonize the donor and does encourage donation at a future time.

7. Hematocrit or hemoglobin: The hemoglobin value must be no less than 12.5 g/dl for female donors and no less than 13.5 g/dl for male donors. The hematocrit, if used instead of hemoglobin measurement, must be no less than 38% for female donors and no less than 41% for male donors. Hemoglobin concentration may be measured by spectrophotometric methods, or the presence of an acceptable minimum value may be estimated by using copper sulfate.

a. Copper sulfate method:

Principle This method is based on specific gravity. A drop of blood dropped into copper sulfate solution becomes encased in a sac of copper proteinate, which prevents any change in specific gravity for about 15 seconds. If the drop of blood has a higher specific gravity than the solution it will sink within 15 seconds. If not, the sinking drop will hesitate, remain suspended or rise to the top of the solution. This is not a quantitative test; it shows only whether the hemoglobin is below or above acceptable limits. Results indicating satisfactory hemoglobin levels are usually accurate; that is, false-positive reactions are rare. False-negative reactions occur fairly commonly and cause many inappropriate deferrals. Measuring hematocrit or hemoglobin by a different method often reveals that the prospective donor is, after all, acceptable.

Materials Use solution of copper sulfate with specific gravity of 1.053, equivalent to 12.5 g/dl hemoglobin, to test females. Use copper sulfate with specific gravity of 1.055, equivalent to 13.5 g/dl hemoglobin, to test males. The solutions should be stored at room temperature in tightly capped containers to prevent evaporation. For routine use, dispense 30 ml of solution into appropriately labeled, clean, dry tubes or bottles. Change solution daily or after 25 tests. Be sure the solution is adequately mixed before beginning each day's determinations.

Procedure Clean the site of skin puncture thoroughly with antiseptic solution and wipe dry with sterile gauze. Puncture the finger firmly, near the end but slightly to the side, with a sterile, disposable lancet, or spring-loaded disposable needle system. A good free flow of blood is important. Do not squeeze the finger repeatedly, as this may dilute the drop of blood with excess tissue fluid and give falsely low results. Note that since blood obtained from ear lobe puncture has a higher hemoglobin or hematocrit than blood from a fingerstick, ear lobe puncture may allow donors with unsuitably low levels to give blood.[7] This method is no longer acceptable.[1]

Collect blood in an anticoagulated capillary tube without allowing air to enter the tube. Let one drop of blood fall gently from the tube at a height of about 1 cm above the surface of the copper sulfate solution. Observe for 15 seconds. Record results as greater or less than 12.5 g/dl for females, and greater or less than 13.5 g/dl for males.

b. Spectrophotometric methods: Use standard techniques.[8]

c. Hematocrit measurement: Use standard techniques.[8]

The record of physical examination and medical history must be identified with the examiner by initials or signature. Any reasons for deferral must be recorded and explained to the donor or referred to a physician, if indicated. The donor should be informed of abnormal findings in the physical examination or medical history.

Donors who are accepted should be made aware that recipients experience risk from transfusion; they should be asked to report any illness developing within a few days of donation and especially to report hepatitis or AIDS that develops within 6 months.

The size, shape and recording sequence of the donor information form should be designed to fit the needs of the blood bank and facilitate filing and retrieval. The form, in addition, must include space in which the donor provides informed consent to the blood donation procedure.

Special Donor Categories

Exceptions to the usual requirements may be made for special donor categories:
1. Therapeutic bleedings: This term is used when phlebotomy is done for medical indications. The records must include the request of the patient's physician and specify the amount of blood to be drawn, the frequency of bleeding and/or a hemoglobin or hematocrit level at which the patient should be bled. The record may be a written request or documentation by blood bank personnel of a telephoned request. The blood bank physician must decide whether to accept responsibility for having these patients bled in the donor area. If the patient is seriously ill, phlebotomy should be performed in a hospital setting.

   If the patient's blood is unsuitable for homologous transfusion, it must be labeled "Not for Transfusion" and either discarded or used for research purposes. If the unit is suitable for homologous transfusion, as determined by the blood bank physician, it may be transfused after the usual processing, provided that the label indicates a therapeutic bleeding and specifies the donor's disease. The recipient's physician must agree to use the blood for transfusion and a record must be made of this agreement.
2. Autologous transfusion: The indications and procedures for autologous

transfusion are discussed in Chapter 19.
3. Plasmapheresis: Special requirements and recommendations for cytapheresis donors or for donors in a plasmapheresis program are detailed in Chapter 2.
4. Recipient-specific donations: Although generally discouraged because of the added expense and logistical problems, there are certain situations in which it may be appropriate for blood collection facilities to draw, process and store homologous blood intended for a specific recipient. One such situation is for the patient anticipating a kidney transplant from a living (usually related) donor. For these patients, protocols have been developed[9] whereby the intended recipient is repeatedly transfused prior to transplantation with blood from the intended donor. Donor-specific transfusions of this sort have been shown to improve graft survival, especially when lymphocytotoxicity testing after transfusion but before transplantation reveals absence of antibody formation.[10]

   In this situation, as in programs of autologous donation, donated blood must be processed according to *Standards*. Special tags identifying the donor and the intended recipient must be affixed to the blood or component bag, and all such units must be segregated from the normal inventory. A protocol for the handling of such units must be developed and made a part of the procedures manual.

Collection of Blood

Blood is to be collected only by trained personnel working under the direction of a qualified, licensed physician. Blood collection must be by aseptic methods, utilizing a sterile, closed system, and a single venipuncture. If more than one skin puncture is needed, a new container and donor set must be used for each additional venipuncture. The phlebotomist must sign or initial the donor record, whether or not the phlebotomy resulted in a transfusable unit.

Materials and Instruments

Many items used for phlebotomy are available in sterile, single-use, disposable form. If these leak or the paper envelope becomes wet, the contents must not be used. Items such as gauze, cotton balls, applicators, forceps and forceps holders may be adequately sterilized by steam under pressure for at least 30 minutes at 121.5 C, by dry heat for at least 2 hours at 170 C or by gas sterilization. Containers of bulk sterilized items should be labeled and dated as to when they were sterilized and when opened. Transfer forceps should have at least the lower third immersed in an effective antiseptic solution (eg, 70% alcohol) and should be resterilized after 1 week. Unopened sterilized containers may be stored for 2 or 3 weeks if the intact container closure ensures sterility of the contents. Open containers may be used for 1 week if the lids are replaced after removal of contents and contents are removed with aseptic technique.

Blood Containers

Blood must be collected into an FDA-approved container that is pyrogen-free, sterile, and contains sufficient anticoagulant for the quantity of blood to be collected. The container label must state the kind and amount of anticoagulant, the amount of blood collected and the required storage temperature. The name and address of the collecting facility must be on the container label and any numeric or alphanumeric identification code assigned to the facility. There must be a reference to the *Circular of Information* for further guidelines, and a caution to identify properly the intended recipient.

Blood bags may be supplied in containers holding 2-12 bags. Manufacturers' directions should be followed for the length of time unused bags may be stored in containers that have been opened and resealed.

Identification

Identification is important in each step from donor to final disposition. A numeric or alphanumeric system must be used to identify and relate the donor record, the processing tubes and the containers. Extreme caution is necessary to avoid any mix-up or duplication of numbers. All cards and labels should be checked for printing errors. Duplicate numbers must be discarded. It is good practice to record voided numbers.

Before starting the phlebotomy:
1. Identify donor record with the donor at least by name.
2. Attach identically numbered labels to donor record, blood collection container and test tubes for donor blood samples. Attaching the numbers at the donor chair, rather than during the examination procedures, helps reduce the likelihood of identification errors.
3. Be sure that the processing tubes are correctly numbered and that they accompany the container during the collection of blood. These may be attached in any convenient manner to the primary bag or integral tubing.
4. Recheck all numbers.

Preparing Venipuncture Site

Blood should be drawn from a large, firm vein in an area that is free of skin lesions. It is often helpful to inspect both arms and, to make the veins more prominent, use either a tourniquet or a blood pressure cuff inflated to 40-60 mm Hg. Having the donor open and close the hand a few times is also helpful. Once the vein is selected, the pressure should be released before the skin site is prepared.

There is no way to prepare a completely aseptic site for venipuncture, but surgical cleanliness can be achieved to provide maximum assurance of a sterile product. Two acceptable procedures follow but other satisfactory procedures exist.

Prepare an area of at least 1½ inches in all directions from intended site of venipuncture (ie, 3 inches in diameter). Use sterile materials and instruments. After the initial scrub, apply other solutions starting at the site of venipuncture and moving outward in a concentric spiral.

Method 1

1. Scrub vigorously with 15% aqueous (not alcoholic) soap or detergent solution for at least 30 seconds to clean away fat, oils, dirt, skin cells and other debris.
2. Remove soap and froth with 10% acetone in 70% isopropyl alcohol (1 part acetone and 9 parts isopropyl alcohol) and allow to dry.
3. Apply tincture of iodine (3 or 3½% in 70% ethyl alcohol) and allow to dry.

   Keep the tincture of iodine bottle tightly capped to prevent evaporation of alcohol. Higher concentrations of iodine may cause skin reactions.
4. Remove the iodine with 10% acetone in 70% isopropyl alcohol. The iodine serves its antiseptic purpose rapidly, and rarely causes skin reactions if properly removed. Allow the solution to dry.
5. Cover site with dry sterile gauze if venipuncture will not be done immediately.

Method 2

1. Scrub area for 30 seconds with 0.7% aqueous scrub solution of iodophor compound (eg, PVP-iodine or poloxamer-iodine complex). Excess foam must be removed, but the arm need not be dry before the next step.
2. Apply iodophor complex solution (eg, 10% PVP-iodine) and let stand for 30 seconds. This solution contains only 1% free iodine and need not be removed before completing venipuncture. It has the advantages of less odor and stain than tincture of iodine and seldom causes skin reactions even in iodine-sensitive individuals. Iodophor complexes may be substituted for tincture of iodine in method 1, step 3, above. Both iodophor "scrub" and iodophor "prep" solutions are available in pre-packaged single-use form.

3. Cover the area with dry sterile gauze if venipuncture will not be done immediately.

After the skin has been prepared, it must not be touched again. Do not repalpate the vein.

For donors sensitive to iodine (tincture or PVP), another method, such as green soap scrub followed by acetone-alcohol, should be designated by the blood bank physician.

Phlebotomy and Collection of Samples for Processing and Compatibility Tests

1. Inspect bag for any defects. Apply pressure to check for leaks. The anticoagulant solution must be clear.
2. Position bag carefully, being sure it is below the level of the donor's arm.
   a. If balance system is used, be sure counterbalance is level and adjusted for the amount of blood to be drawn. Unless metal clips and a hand sealer are used, make a very loose overhand knot in tubing. Hang the bag and route tubing through the pinch clamp.
   b. If balance system is not used, be sure there is some way to monitor the volume of blood drawn.
   c. If a vacuum-assist device is used, the manufacturer's instructions should be followed.
3. Reapply tourniquet or blood pressure cuff. Have donor open and close hand until previously selected vein is again prominent.
4. Uncover sterile needle and do venipuncture immediately. A clean, skillful venipuncture is essential for collection of a full, clot-free unit. Tape the tubing to hold needle in place and cover site with sterile gauze.
5. Open the temporary closure between the interior of the bag and the tubing, if present.
6. Have donor open and close hand, squeezing a rubber ball or other resil-

ient object slowly every 10-12 seconds during collection. Keep the donor under observation throughout phlebotomy. The donor should never be left unattended during or immediately after donation.

7. Mix the blood and anticoagulant gently and periodically (approximately every 30 seconds) during collection. Mixing may be done by hand, by placing bag on a mechanical agitator, or by using a rocking vacuum-assist device.

8. Be sure blood flow remains fairly brisk, so that coagulation activity is not triggered. Rigid time limits are not warranted if there is continuous, adequate blood flow and constant agitation, although units requiring more than 8 minutes to draw may not be suitable for preparation of platelet concentrates, fresh frozen plasma or cryoprecipitate.

9. Monitor volume of blood being drawn. If a balance or vacuum-assist device is used, blood flow will stop after the proper amount has been collected. One ml of blood weighs at least 1.053 g, the minimum allowable specific gravity for female donors. A convenient figure to use is 1.06 g; a unit containing 405-495 ml should weigh 425-520 g plus the weight of the container with its anticoagulant.

10. Clamp tubing temporarily using a hemostat, metal clip or other temporary clamp. Next, collect blood processing sample by a method that precludes contamination of the donor unit. There are several ways in which this may be accomplished. 1) If the blood collection bag contains an in-line needle ("sid connector"), make an additional seal with a hemostat, metal clip, hand sealer or a tight knot made from previously prepared loose knot just distal to the in-line needle. Open the connector by separating the needles. Insert the proximal needle into a processing test tube, remove the hemostat, allow the tube to fill and reclamp tubing. Carefully re-attach "sid connector." Donor needle is now ready for removal. 2) If the blood collection bag contains an in-line processing tube, be certain that the processing tube, or pouch, is full when the collection is complete and the original clamp is placed near the donor needle. Entire assembly may now be removed from donor. 3) If a straight-tubing assembly set is used there are two alternative procedures: In the first method, remove the needle from the donor's arm as soon as the tubing is clamped. Take bag and assembly to sealer area or collect processing tube at the donor chair by placing a hemostat close to where donor tubing enters the bag, leaving the tubing full of blood. Remove the clamp next to donor needle, empty contents of donor tubing into the processing test tube, reapply clamp or permanently seal next to donor needle, remove hemostat next to donor bag and allow the donor tubing to refill with blood, well-mixed, from donor bag. In the second method, place two hemostats or temporary seals on the tubing. Cut tubing between the seals, put cut end of the tubing into the processing test tube, remove the proximal hemostat, allow tube to fill and reclamp tubing.

11. Deflate and remove tourniquet. Remove needle from arm. Apply pressure over gauze and have donor raise arm (elbow straight) and hold gauze firmly over phlebotomy site with the other hand.

12. Discard needle assembly into special container designed to prevent accidental injury to and contamination of personnel.

13. Strip donor tubing as completely as possible into the bag, starting at seal. Work quickly, to avoid allowing the blood to clot in the tubing. Invert bag several times to mix thoroughly; then allow tubing to refill with anticoagu-

lated blood from the bag. Repeat this procedure a second time.

14. Seal the tubing left attached to the bags into segments on which the segment number is clearly and completely readable. Knots, metal clips or a dielectric sealer may be used to make segments suitable for crossmatching. It must be possible to separate segments from the container without breaking sterility of the container.

15. Reinspect container for defects.

16. Recheck numbers on container, processing tubes and donation record. Be sure the expiration date of the unit is on the container label.

17. Place blood at appropriate temperature. Unless platelets are to be removed, whole blood should be placed at 1-6 C immediately after collection. If platelets are to be harvested, blood should not be chilled but should be maintained at room temperature (about 20-24 C) until platelets are separated. Platelets should be separated within 6 hours after collection of the unit of whole blood.

Care of the donor after phlebotomy

1. Check arm and apply bandage after bleeding stops.

2. Have donor remain reclining on bed or in donor chair for a few moments under close observation by staff.

3. Allow donor to sit up when his/her condition appears satisfactory. Someone should remain with the donor as he/she assumes an upright position and walks to an observation area. The period of observation and provision of refreshment should be designated in the procedures manual.

4. Give donor instructions about postphlebotomy care. The medical director may wish to include some of the following suggestions:
   - Eat and drink something before leaving.
   - Do not leave until released by staff member.
   - Drink more fluids than usual in next 4 hours.
   - It is probably better not to have any alcohol until you have eaten.
   - Do not smoke for a half hour.
   - If there is bleeding from phlebotomy site, raise arm and apply pressure.
   - If you feel faint or dizzy, either lie down or sit down with your head between your knees.
   - If any symptoms persist, either return to blood bank or see a doctor.
   - You may resume all normal activities after about a half hour if you feel well.
   - Remove bandage after a few hours.
   - Your blood volume rapidly returns to the normal level, usually 4000-5500 ml or 8-11 pints, depending on size and weight. With adequate fluid intake, complete blood volume restoration should take less than 72 hours.

5. Thank the donor for an important contribution, encourage repeat donation after proper interval (56 days) and offer refreshments to the donor. The personnel on duty throughout the donor area should be friendly and qualified to observe for signs of impending reaction such as lack of concentration, pallor, rapid breathing or excessive perspiration. They should be competent to interpret instructions and answer questions, and to accept responsibility for releasing the donor in good condition.

6. Note on the donor record any adverse reations that occurred and, if the donor leaves the area before being released, note this on the record.

7. There must be a mechanism to notify donors of any clinically significant abnormalities detected in either predonation evaluation or in postdonation laboratory tests, especially a positive test for HBsAg. Predonation abnormalities may be explained verbally by qualified

personnel. Postdonation abnormalities may be reported by telephone or letter.

Adverse Donor Reactions

Most donors tolerate giving blood very well, but occasional adverse reactions may occur. Personnel must be trained to recognize reactions and treat some of them. In many blood banks, donor room personnel are required to have training in cardiopulmonary resuscitation (CPR).

Syncope (fainting or vasovagal syndrome) may be caused by the sight of blood, by watching others give blood, by individual or group excitement or for unexplained reasons. Whether caused by psychologic factors or by neurophysiologic response to blood donation, the symptoms may include weakness, sweating, dizziness, pallor, loss of consciousness, convulsions and involuntary passage of feces or urine. The skin feels cold and blood pressure falls, sometimes to systolic levels as low as 50 mm Hg or to inaudibility on auscultation. The pulse rate often slows significantly, occasionally a useful sign in distinguishing between vasovagal attack and severe cardiogenic or hypovolemic shock, in which pulse rates rise.[11] This distinction, although characteristic, is far from absolute. Deep breathing or hyperventilation may cause the anxious or excited donor to lose an excess of CO_2, resulting in alkalosis and hyperventilation tetany, characterized by spontaneous muscular contractions, or spasm.

The blood bank physician must provide written instructions for handling donor reactions. This must include a procedure for obtaining emergency medical help.

1. General
   a. Remove the tourniquet and withdraw the needle from the arm at the first sign of reaction during the phlebotomy.
   b. If possible, remove any donor who experiences an adverse reaction to an area where he/she can be attended to in privacy.
   c. Call the blood bank physician or the physician designated for such purposes if the measures given below do not lead to rapid recovery.
2. Fainting
   a. Place the donor on his/her back and raise the feet above the level of the donor's head.
   b. Loosen tight clothing.
   c. Be sure the donor has an adequate airway.
   d. Apply cold compresses to the donor's forehead or the back of the neck.
   e. Administer aromatic spirits of ammonia by inhalation. Test the ammonia on yourself before passing it under the donor's nose, as it may be too strong or too weak. Strong ammonia may injure the nasal membranes; weak ammonia is not effective. The donor should respond by coughing, which elevates the blood pressure.
   f. Check and record the blood pressure, pulse and respiration periodically until the donor recovers.
      Note: Some donors who experience prolonged hypotension may respond to an infusion of normal saline. The decision to initiate such therapy should be made by the blood bank physician either on a case-by-case basis or in a policy stated in the facility procedures manual.
3. Nausea and vomiting
   a. Make the donor as comfortable as possible.
   b. Instruct the donor who is nauseated to breathe slowly and deeply.
   c. Apply cold compresses to the donor's forehead.
   d. Turn donor's head to the side.
   e. Provide a suitable receptacle if the donor vomits, and have cleansing tissues or a damp towel ready. Be sure the donor's head is turned to the side because of the danger of aspiration.
   f. Give the donor water to rinse out his/her mouth.

4. Twitching or muscular spasms
The most common cause of twitching or muscular spasms occurs with loss of consciousness. Almost one-half of unconscious donors have brief, weak, convulsion-like movements of one or more extremities. Extremely nervous donors may hyperventilate, causing faint muscular twitching or tetanic spasm of their hands or face. Donor room personnel should watch closely for these symptoms during the phlebotomy. Diverting the donor's attention by engaging in conversation can interrupt the hyperventilation pattern. However, if symptoms are apparent, having the donor breathe into a paper bag will usually bring prompt relief. **Do not give oxygen.**

5. Hematoma
   a. Remove the tourniquet and the needle from the donor's arm.
   b. Place three or four sterile gauze squares over the hematoma and apply firm digital pressure for 7-10 minutes with the donor's arm held above the heart level.
   c. Apply ice to the area for 5 minutes, if desired.
   d. Should an arterial puncture be suspected, immediately withdraw needle and apply firm pressure for 10 minutes. Apply pressure dressing afterwards. Check for the presence of a radial pulse. If pulse is not palpable call blood bank physician.

6. True convulsions are rare.
   a. Call someone to help you immediately. Prevent the donor from injuring himself. During severe seizures, some people exhibit great muscular power and are difficult to restrain.
   • If possible, place tongue blades, well-padded and wrapped with adhesive tape, between the donor's back teeth to prevent the donor from chewing his tongue. Keep the blades in place until the donor recovers.
   • If possible, hold the donor on the chair or bed; if not possible, place the donor on the floor. Try to prevent injury to the donor or to yourself.
   b. Be sure the donor has an adequate airway.
   c. Notify the blood bank physician.

7. Serious cardiac difficulties are exceedingly rare, probably one in 10,000,000 donors.
   a. Call for medical aid and/or an emergency care unit immediately.
   b. If the donor is in cardiac arrest, begin CPR immediately and continue until medical aid and/or an emergency care unit arrives.

The nature and treatment of all reactions should be recorded on the donor record or a special incident report form. This should include a notation as to whether or not the donor should be accepted for future donations.

The medical director should decide what supplies and drugs should be in the donor bleeding area, readily available to personnel. The distance to the nearest emergency room or emergency care unit heavily influences decisions about necessary supplies and drugs. Most blood banks maintain some or all of the following:

1. Emesis basin or equivalent
2. Towels
3. Sterile needles, both 20-gauge, 2-inch, and 25-gauge, ¾-inch
4. Sterile hypodermic syringes, 1 or 2 ml
5. Administration sets
   a. Intravenous fluids
   b. Blood
6. Sodium chloride injection USP (normal saline)
7. Tongue blades, well-padded and wrapped with tape, kept covered for cleanliness.
8. Oropharyngeal airway, plastic or hard rubber
9. Oxygen and mask
10. Emergency drugs: Drugs are seldom required to treat a donor who has had a reaction. If the blood bank physician wishes to have any drugs available, the

kind and amount to be kept on hand must be specified in writing. In addition, the medical director must provide written policies as to when and by whom any of the above may be used.

Processing Donor Blood

All reagents used for required tests must meet or exceed appropriate FDA regulations. Cells and serum used in automated or microtiter procedures must have been tested in parallel with conventional methods and the results approved by the Office of Biologics before the procedures and reagents are adopted.

Previous records of a donor's ABO and Rh groups must not be used for labeling a unit of blood. Every unit must undergo complete testing. The results of all tests must be recorded immediately after observation, and the interpretation recorded upon completion of testing. The record system must be such that any unit of blood and any component can be traced from its source to its disposition. All laboratory records pertaining to an individual unit must be retrievable, including investigations of reported adverse reactions. For a drawing facility, the source would be the donor; for a transfusion service it could be the donor or another blood provider. Disposition could be transfusion to a named patient; shipment to a named receiving facility; or discarding in a manner specified by the local procedures manual. Records should be retained for 5 years or in accordance with local requirements.

Details of testing procedures, storage and shipping requirements and inspection criteria appear in subsequent chapters of this manual. The current edition of *Standards* should be consulted for requirements of preparation, testing and labeling. General considerations in processing donor blood are as follows:

1. Numbers on blood bag, processing tubes and donor record should be rechecked prior to processing.

2. ABO group must be determined by testing the red blood cells with anti-A and anti-B sera and by testing the serum or plasma with group A_1 and B cells. Blood must not be released until discrepancies, if any, are resolved. Accurate ABO testing and labeling assumes even greater importance in areas where the conventional crossmatch is abbreviated or eliminated.

3. The Rh group must be determined with anti-D serum. Units found to be D-negative in direct agglutination tests must be tested for the D^u phenotype. Units that are D-positive, including those reactive only by the D^u test, must be labeled Rh-positive. Routine testing for additional red blood cell antigens is not recommended or encouraged.

4. Blood from donors with a history of prior transfusion or pregnancy should be tested for unexpected antibodies before the crossmatch, preferably at the time of processing. Most blood banks test all donor blood for unexpected antibodies, because of the difficulty determining donor's past histories and/ or attempting to segregate those to be tested from those not to be tested.

   Methods for testing for unexpected antibodies must be those that will demonstrate clinically significant antibodies. Blood in which such antibodies are found should be processed into components that contain only minimal amounts of plasma. In processing donor blood, it is permissible to pool serum from several donors or to use pooled reagent red cells; pooled reagents must not be used in pretransfusion testing of patient blood samples.

5. All donor blood must be tested for HBsAg with reagents and techniques approved by the FDA, or proven to have equivalent sensitivity and specificity. The blood component or unit of whole blood must not be used for transfusion unless the test is nonreactive. In an emergency, blood may be transfused before HBsAg testing is

complete, but this fact must be conspicuous on the blood label. If the test is subsequently found to be reactive, the recipient's physician must be notified as well as the donor.

6. The facility performing the compatibility testing must do confirmatory tests on a sample obtained from the originally attached segment of all units of whole blood or red blood cells. This must include, for all units containing significant amounts of red cells, confirmation of ABO group on all units, and the Rh group of all D-negative units. Discrepancies must be reported to the collecting facility and must be resolved before issue of the blood for transfusion purposes. Routine repetition of other tests on donor units is not required or recommended.

7. A stoppered or sealed sample of each donor blood must be stored in the transfusion service at 1-6 C for at least 7 days after transfusion. Many workers prefer storage for longer periods, up to 14 days.

8. Blood collected from a donor later found to have, or to be at high risk of, AIDS should be quarantined immediately, and the Office of Biologics Research and Review (Division of Blood and Blood Products) should be notified. Each facility's procedures manual should make it clear that such blood, and all components, products or samples prepared from it, is potentially infectious and should be labeled, stored or shipped with standard precautions for infectious material. Such donor units may be held in quarantine pending clarification of the donor's diagnosis; used for investigative use related to AIDS; or disposed of by autoclaving or controlled incineration. Units should be overwrapped, to protect personnel in case of breakage.

References

1. Schmidt P, ed. Standards for blood banks and transfusion services. 11th ed. Arlington, VA: American Association of Blood Banks, 1984.

2. US Department of Health and Human Services, Food and Drug Administration. The code of federal regulations, 21 CFR 600.3, current edition. Washington, DC: US Government Printing Office.

3. Mollison PL. Blood donation: use of cell separators. In: Blood transfusion in clinical medicine. 7th ed. Oxford: Blackwell Scientific Publications, 1983.

4. Tomasulo PA, Anderson AJ, Paluso MB, Gutschenutter MA, Aster RH. A study of criteria for blood donor deferral. Transfusion 1980;20:511-518.

5. Widmann FK. Questions and answers. American Association of Blood Banks News Briefs 1978;8(4):41-43.

6. Public Health Service Memorandum: Revised recommendations to decrease the risk of transmitting acquired immunodeficiency syndrome (AIDS) from blood and plasma donors. Dec. 14, 1984.

7. Avoy DR, Canuel MD, Otton BM, Mileski EB. Hemoglobin screening in prospective blood donors: a comparison of methods. Transfusion 1977;17:261-264.

8. Nelson DA, Morris MW. Basic methodology. In: Henry JB, ed. Todd-Sanford-Davidsohn Clinical diagnosis and management by laboratory methods. 17th ed. Philadelphia: WB Saunders, 1984.

9. Carpenter CB. Deliberate transfusion of potential renal transplant recipients with specific donor blood. Am J Kidney Dis 1981;1:116-118.

10. Salvatierra O Jr, et al. Incidence, characteristics, and outcome of recipients sensitized after donor-specific blood transfusions. Transplantation 1981;32:528-531.

11. Roekel IE. Donor reactions. In: Donor room procedures. Washington, DC: American Association of Blood Banks, 1977.

2

Hemapheresis

Hemapheresis is the removal of whole blood from a donor or patient, separation into components, retention of the desired component and return of the recombined remaining elements to the donor or patient. Hemapheresis can be used to collect a component intended for transfusion or to remove a pathologic component in order to treat a patient's disease. This chapter devotes separate sections to component preparation and therapeutic applications. Cell separators that separate components by centrifugal force can be used for either application. New instruments that apply novel approaches to separation are being developed for sole use in therapeutic or plasma collection applications.

Cytapheresis, the collection of cells, requires an instrument capable of processing sufficiently large volumes for a satisfactory yield of platelets or granulocytes. Plasmapheresis, in contrast, can be accomplished using either a manual multiple-bag system or automated equipment. The manual system, which utilizes a refrigerated centrifuge and multiple bags joined by tubing, is simple and inexpensive, but time-consuming. It also carries a risk that red cells could be returned to the wrong donor. The manual apheresis technique is described in detail in the Special Methods section.

Both AABB *Standards* and the *Code of Federal Regulations* contain sections concerned with hemapheresis. All personnel involved in performing hemapheresis procedures should be thoroughly familiar with these regulations and qualified by training or experience to perform apheresis.

Component Preparation

Apheresis machines use centrifugal force and the differing densities of various blood components to achieve separation of the desired fraction. Red cells and plasma are returned to the donor by either intermittent or continuous flow. All such systems require prepackaged sets of sterile bags, tubing and centrifugal devices unique to the machine. Intermittent flow machines, in which the centrifuge bowl is alternately filled and emptied, require only a single venipuncture because drawing blood and returning it to the donor can be accomplished through the same line. Continuous flow equipment usually requires two venipunctures, one for removal and the other for return.

Citrate solution used for anticoagulation is added in a metered quantity to the whole blood as it enters the tubing. The blood is pumped into a spinning centrifugal container (bowls, chambers or tubular rotors) wherein separation of components occurs. This process is similar to the operation of a dairy cream separator, with less dense elements layered above the densest constituents, in this case, the red blood cells. After the desired components are harvested, red cells are recombined with remaining elements and returned to the donor. Donation requires about 2 hours. Each manufacturer supplies detailed information and operational protocols for the various apheresis machines. Each facility must have, in a manual readily available to nursing and technical personnel, detailed descriptions of all procedures performed, specific for each type of cell separator.

Donors

Donors of components prepared by apheresis must meet the criteria applicable to donors of whole blood. Donors who do not meet these requirements may sometimes be drawn if the component will be of special value to the intended recipient, such as HLA-matched platelets. A physician must certify in writing that the donor's health permits the donation, and, if the exception imposes an element of risk to the recipient, the recipient's physician should be notified.[1]

During thrombocytapheresis, the donor's platelet count decreases about 30%; although this usually has little clinical significance, the count may require up to 72 hours to return to normal. Since such a drop could harm a donor with a bleeding tendency, thrombocytapheresis donors should be carefully evaluated for a personal and family history of excessive bleeding. In addition, a drug history should be obtained. Donors who have taken aspirin or aspirin-containing medications within 3 days of donation should ordinarily be deferred, because the platelet concentrate obtained by apheresis is often the single source of platelets given to a patient.

Granulocytapheresis donors who will receive predonation steroid stimulation to increase granulocyte yields should be carefully questioned about hypertension, diabetes and ulcer history and/or symptoms. The signed informed consent must include specific permission for use of steroids and hydroxyethyl starch (HES).

Laboratory Monitoring

Before initiation of the procedure the hemoglobin and/or hematocrit must be measured. It is desirable to evaluate the platelet count, white blood cell count and differential. A platelet count below 150,000/mm^3 is usually a contraindication to platelet donation. The quantity of granulocytes harvested is directly related to the absolute granulocyte count in the peripheral blood. For satisfactory yields the donor's absolute granulocyte count should be greater than 4000/mm^3. Coagulation studies are indicated only if a careful medical history suggests a congenital or acquired bleeding tendency. If multiple donations are anticipated, serum protein concentration must be above 6.0 gm/dl and levels of IgG and IgM be shown to be normal. Other laboratory studies increase costs and are rarely indicated.

Frequency of Donation

Frequency of donation is limited by the following[1]:
1. Red blood cell loss incidental to the procedure should be no more than 25 ml per week.
2. Plasma loss, exclusive of anticoagulant, should be less than 1000 ml per week for donors weighing less than 80 kg (175 lbs); for donors weighing more than 80 kg, 1200 ml may be retained.
3. A serum protein electrophoresis or quantitative determination of IgG and IgM must be determined once every 4 months for donors undergoing frequent plasmapheresis and must be within normal limits.
4. At least 48 hours should elapse between successive procedures.
5. The total accumulation of hydroxyethyl starch (HES) in donors undergoing intensive leukapheresis should be kept to a minimum.

Records

There must be records of donor identification, anticoagulants given, drugs used, duration of the procedure, volumes of all products collected, and occurrence and treatment of any reaction. The average red cell loss for each type of procedure should be calculated. All adverse reactions during and following the procedure must be recorded on the donor's record. For donors undergoing repeated hemapheresis procedures, records of all laboratory findings and collection data must be reviewed by a knowledgeable physician at least once every 4 months.

Drugs Administered for Granulocytapheresis

Corticosteroids

Oral administration of the adrenal cortical steroids prednisone or dexamethasone is often used to increase the donor's granulocyte count. Since granulocyte yields depend upon the level of cells circulating at the time of leukapheresis, raising the circulating cell count increases the number of cells collected. Corticosteroids cause the granulocytes in the bone marrow storage pool to leave the marrow and also decrease egress of granulocytes from the peripheral blood. Corticosteroids can double the number of circulating granulocytes, but dosage, timing and route of administration affect the increment in granulocyte harvest. A protocol using 20 mg of oral prednisone at 15, 12 and 2 hours prior to donation gives superior granulocyte harvests with minimal systemic steroid activity.[2,3]

Hydroxyethyl Starch (HES)

Rouleaux-promoting agents are used in leukapheresis to produce aggregates of red cells which sediment in the centrifugation phase more effectively than single cells, producing a sharply defined interface between red cells and buffy coat. This enhances granulocyte harvest and minimizes red cell contamination of the product. HES is a synthetic analog of naturally occurring starch. Its intravascular half-life is 24 to 29 hours. Macrophages of the reticuloendothelial system clear some from the circulation, but residual colloid can be detected in blood for up to 17 weeks after injection.[4] For this reason leukapheresis donors are usually limited in number of donations and total quantity of HES given. Because HES is cleared only gradually, decreasing sequential doses may be utilized during intensive leukapheresis; for example, for three successive donations 48 hours apart, doses might be 500 ml, 300 ml and 200 ml of HES solution.

The erythrocyte sedimentation rate (ESR) correlates directly with residual HES and may be used as follows to estimate circulating levels in donors with initial ESR below 5 mm/hr[5]:

$$\text{Serum HES concentration} = 1.797 + (0.396 \times \text{postinfusion ESR}) \text{ mg/ml}$$

The optimal level of HES for component preparation is approximately 7.0 mg/ml. Since HES is a colloid, it acts as a volume expander. Leukapheresis donors who have received it may experience headaches or peripheral edema as a result of their expanded circulatory volume. Rare anaphylactic reactions have occurred with HES.[6]

Platelet Concentrates

Most thrombocytapheresis is performed to obtain single-donor platelets from a donor of known HLA phenotype. Some patients who are thrombocytopenic from bone marrow failure or suppression may become refractory to transfusions of pooled random-donor platelet concentrates. (See page 273.) Such patients often respond with better platelet count increments when transfused with platelets obtained by thrombocytapheresis from an HLA-matched donor.

Platelets obtained by hemapheresis may be stored for only 24 hours if the method of preparation utilizes an open collection system; 5 days is approved for platelets collected in a completely closed system.

Platelet Content

The commonly used cell separators consistently produce platelet harvests of at least 4×10^{11} platelets.[7] Some centers centrifuge the apheresis component to remove red cells and leukocytes at the expense of 20-30% of the final platelet yield.[8] This has been reported to decrease the rate of sensitization to HLA antigens and delay the onset of the refractory state in platelet recipients. *Standards* requires 3.0×10^{11} platelets in at least 75% of the units tested.

Platelet concentrates intended for transfusion to bone marrow transplant recipients or to immunodeficient or severely immunosuppressed patients may be irradiated to avoid the risk of graft vs. host disease (GVH). Since living lymphocytes, the cause of GVH, contaminate many other blood components, irradiating platelets makes sense only if all lymphocyte-containing components are similarly irradiated.

Laboratory Testing

ABO and Rh grouping, antibody screening and HBsAg testing must be done by the collecting facility in a manner similar to that for other blood components. A blood specimen tube may be attached to the primary container so that the transfusion service can perform indicated pretransfusion testing.

The donor plasma should be ABO-compatible with the recipient's red cells. Platelet or granulocyte concentrates prepared by hemapheresis need not be crossmatched if prepared by a method expected to cause contamination with less than 5 ml red blood cells.

If a cytapheresis concentrate contains more than 5 ml red blood cells, there should be compatibility with the recipient's serum. If the recipient has a negative antibody screening test, ABO compatibility must be demonstrated. If the recipient has a significant antibody, an antiglobulin crossmatch must be done.

When the recipient does not show expected platelet increments after transfusion and is thought to be alloimmunized to leukocyte antigens, or when febrile transfusion reactions are frequent, leukocytes may be removed by a soft spin technique described in Special Methods.

Storage

Platelets prepared as described should be stored at 20 to 24 C with continuous gentle agitation. Thrombocytapheresis concentrates that have been prepared in an open system may be stored for no longer than 24 hours. Those prepared in a closed system may be stored for 5 days. The pH must be 6.0 or higher at the end of allowable storage in all units tested.

Quality Assurance

During establishment of the procedure, it is advisable to test every thrombocytapheresis component for red blood cell content, volume and platelet count. This makes it possible to calculate the total number of platelets and red blood cells in the unit and to estimate loss of donor's erythrocytes. Once the procedure is operating satisfactorily, fewer concentrates need to be tested. A method for collecting a representative specimen is given on page 470.

Granulocyte Concentrates

The therapeutic efficacy of granulocyte transfusion is still debated.[9] Many controlled studies support the conclusion that, for properly selected patients, transfusions of concentrates containing adequate numbers of granulocytes is effective in clearing the blood stream of bacteria and achieving short-term control of infection.[10] Unless the patient subsequently experiences bone marrow recovery, granulocyte transfusions eventually become futile because of sensitization to leukocyte antigens or infection with virulent organisms. One reason for the continuing debate about therapeutic efficacy is that in many studies, suboptimal numbers of granulocytes were infused.[11] A daily dose of at least 10^{10} functional granulocytes seems to be an essential minimum to achieve a therapeutic effect.[12]

With most available equipment, consistent harvests of more than 10^{10} granulocytes requires corticosteroid treatment of donors.

Storage and Infusion

Granulocyte concentrates should be transfused as soon as possible after donation.[13] *Standards* requires storage at room temperature, for no longer than 24 hours. Agitation during storage is undesirable. Infusion through microaggregate filters may impair clinical efficacy.

Laboratory Testing

ABO and Rh grouping, antibody screen and HBsAg testing are required. If possible these should be accomplished before or during donation so that transfusion of the granulocyte concentrate is not delayed. Because red cell contamination in granulocyte concentrates is often significant, the red cells should be ABO-compatible with the recipient's plasma. If future immunization would present clinical problems, D-negative recipients should receive granulocyte concentrates from D-negative donors or receive RhIG immunoprophylaxis. If more than 5 ml of red blood cells contaminate the unit, the red cells must be compatible with the recipient's serum.

Quality Assurance

Concentrate volume, white blood cell count with leukocyte differential and calculation of total number of granulocytes harvested should be recorded. The donor's red cell loss and the amount of HES given at each donation should be documented in records both of the apheresis procedure and

of the individual donor. *Standards* requires 1×10^{10} granulocytes in 75% of the units tested.

Therapeutic Hemapheresis

Hemapheresis has been used to treat patients with many different diseases. Cells, plasma or plasma components may be removed from the circulation, to be replaced by normal plasma or inert solutions of electrolytes or albumin. The theoretical basis for benefit from hemapheresis is that the patient's blood contains a pathogenic substance that can be reduced by the apheresis procedure to levels that will favorably affect the course of the disease. Another indication is absence from plasma of an essential substance that is supplied in the replacement solution. See Table 2-1.

Physiology
Removal of Material

During plasma exchange, plasma that contains the pathogenic substance is continuously being removed while replacement fluid is infused. The removal of the pathogenic substance during a continuous exchange can be calculated using the following formula:[14]

$$X_t = X_o e^{\frac{-b}{v}t}$$

where X_o = concentration of the pathogenic substance in the patient's blood before exchange; X_t = concentration of the substance remaining in the patient's blood after time; t = the duration of the exchange; b = the volume of plasma exchanged; and v = the blood volume of the patient; e is a constant, 2.71828.

Use of this formula requires the following assumptions, which cannot always be documented: 1) the patient's blood volume does not change; 2) mixing occurs immediately; and 3) the pathogenic substance undergoes neither increased pro-

Table 2-1. Proposed Mechanisms of Benefit from Therapeutic Hemapheresis

Accepted Conditions	Diseases
To remove or reduce:	
1. Leukocytes	Hyperleukemic leukostasis with >100,000/μl blasts
2. Platelets	Thrombocytosis with >1 × 10⁶/μl platelets, if symptomatic
3. Abnormal red cells with replacement by normal red cells	Sickle cell disease with crisis
4. Immunoglobulins causing hyperviscosity	Waldenström's macroglobulinemia Multiple myeloma with hyperviscosity
5. Autoantibodies	Myasthenia gravis Goodpasture's syndrome Systemic lupus erythematosus Factor VIII antibodies
6. Lipoproteins	Hypercholesterolemia
Speculative Conditions	
To remove or reduce:	
7. Circulating immune complexes	Immune complex glomerulonephritis Systemic vasculitis Systemic lupus erythematosus (Many other "autoimmune" diseases)
8. Factors interfering with reticuloendothelial function	(Same as #7)
9. Serum factors aggravating tissue damage(such as complement and fibrinogen)	(Same as #7)
10. Factors interfering with cellular immunity	Disseminated cancer
11. Protein-bound substances and toxins	Thyroid storm *Amanita phalloides* toxins
Other Mechanisms	
12. Replacement of deficient serum factors	Thrombotic thrombocytopenic purpura
13. Normalization of T cell helper/ suppressor ratios	Rheumatoid arthritis

duction nor mobilization from the extravascular into the vascular compartment. As calculated from this formula, removal of material has the following efficiency during continuous exchange of one, two or three plasma volumes:

One plasma volume exchanged: 63.2% of pathologic substance removed
Two plasma volumes exchanged: 86.5% of pathologic substance removed

Three plasma volumes exchanged: 95% of pathologic substance removed

Efficiency of removal is greatest early in the procedure and diminishes progressively during the exchange. Plasma exchange procedures can be scheduled according to two alternative approaches. Exchanges may be limited to about one plasma volume, which minimizes time required for each procedure but may necessitate more frequent procedures.

Alternatively, two or three plasma volumes may be exchanged, resulting in greater initial diminution of the pathologic substance but requiring considerably more time to perform the procedure[15]; following removal of several plasma volumes, fresh frozen plasma may be required to maintain normal coagulation mechanisms. The acute phase of a life-threatening disease usually is treated with large volume plasma exchanges, while for maintenance therapy of chronic diseases, smaller volumes are appropriate. The optimal schedule has not been determined for most diseases.

Effects on Normal Constituents

Plasma volume of an average size adult is 2.5 to 3 liters. With currently available equipment, it is possible to exchange 2 liters of plasma in 1 hour and 4 liters in 2 hours. The rate of plasma exchange should be individualized for each patient; smaller patients may not tolerate exchanges of 2 liters per hour. When plasma exchange exceeds 1.5 times the plasma volume, various blood components manifest different rates of removal and restitution.[16] Depletion is more efficient than predicted for fibrinogen, the third component of complement (C3), and immune complexes, when present, with 75% to 85% actually removed. Immunoglobulins are removed as expected, about 65%. Electrolytes, uric acid and some proteins, including Factor VIII, are removed at less than expected rates. Erythrocyte loss is about 30 ml and platelet depletion is approximately 30%.

Three to 4 days are required for fibrinogen and C3 to return to normal levels. Platelets reach preexchange values in 2 to 4 days and coagulation factors (except fibrinogen) achieve preapheresis levels within hours. Recovery patterns for immunoglobulins vary, because IgM is predominately (75%) intravascular, but only about 45% of total body IgG is intravascular. Thus, IgG levels return to 40%

of the pretreatment level within 48 hours because of reequilibration. After this, the rate of synthesis becomes the rate-determining factor and 80% recovery requires about 2 weeks. These facts are important when considering frequency of therapeutic procedures. Weekly procedures permit recovery of normal plasma components, while daily procedures will deplete most normal, as well as abnormal, constituents.

The rate at which the pathologic substance is synthesized and its relative distribution between intravascular and extravascular fluid may determine success or failure in application of therapeutic plasmapheresis. For example, the abnormal IgM of Waldenström's macroglobulinemia is mostly intravascular and is synthesized slowly, making apheresis an effective mode of treatment. In contrast, anti-D antibody is IgG; efforts to prevent hydrops fetalis by lowering maternal IgG levels with intensive plasmapheresis have produced conflicting results.[17] When IgG antibody levels are rapidly and massively decreased by plasmapheresis, antibody synthesis increases rapidly. This rebound response complicates treatment of autoimmune diseases. Many protocols specify use of immunosuppressive drugs to blunt IgG rebound response to apheresis.

Evaluating Efficacy

Controlled Studies

Therapeutic hemapheresis has been applied to more than 50 different diseases. As many publications are reports of individual cases or small series with historical controls, these studies do not constitute reliable evidence of efficacy.[18] Controlled studies of therapeutic apheresis are few because, among other problems, they require use of sham treatments as a control. Sham procedures have two major drawbacks: they are expensive, because personnel and equipment costs are the same as for a therapeutic procedure, and they do carry some risk and morbidity without providing any benefit to the individual serving as a control.[19] Using sham treatment as a control process requires patients to be screened from view of the apheresis equipment. The separated plasma and cells are recombined before reinfusion to the sham group, while plasma is exchanged with 5% albumin or FFP for the treatment group. Evaluation before and after therapy must be performed by personnel blinded to mode of therapy. The complexity and problems of such controlled double blind investigations are illustrated by the ambiguous results of three studies of rheumatoid arthritis treated with hemapheresis.[20,21,22]

Placebo Effect

Most new therapies have been shown to have a 30 to 40% placebo effect.[23] The complicated apheresis machines and associated intensive attention from nursing and medical personnel may well amplify the placebo effect and bias evaluation of clinical improvement. For many of the diseases being treated, the etiology and pathogenesis are incompletely understood and changes in the measured variables, such as decrease in complement components, rheumatoid factor or immune complexes, cannot reliably be correlated with changes in disease activity. For example, the erythrocyte sedimentation rate (ESR) is a commonly used index of rheumatoid activity. The ESR invariably decreases during intensive plasmapheresis, but this reflects decreases in fibrinogen, not necessarily in disease activity.

Conclusions

In this climate of continuing inquiry, there is agreement among most physicians that hemapheresis is effective treatment for some conditions.[24,25,26,27,28,29] See Table 2-2. When the pathogenic substance is identifiable (for example, the IgM causing hyperviscosity in Waldenström's macroglobulinemia) and the treatment clearly reduces levels of known pathogenic agent, controlled trials are unnecessary. Unfortunately, this is not true for most diseases

Table 2-2. Classification of Treatment by Hemapheresis of Selected Diseases[24]

1. Hemapheresis is acceptable but not mandatory treatment in these diseases:
   Hyperviscosity syndrome
   Thrombotic thrombocytopenic purpura
   Myasthenic crisis
   Goodpasture's syndrome without renal insufficiency
   Crescentic glomerulonephritis with renal insufficiency
   a) Idiopathic (rapidly progressive)
   b) Wegener's granulomatosis
   c) Polyarteritis nodosa
   Posttransfusion purpura
   Thyroid storm
   Poisoning (protein-bound toxins)
   Refsum's disease
   Familial hypercholesterolemia

2. Hemapheresis should be reserved for patients in whom standard therapy has proved ineffective:
   Inflammatory polyradiculoneuropathy (Guillain-Barré syndrome)
   Progressive vasculitis with immune complexes
   Refractory progressive lupus erythematosus
   Hemophilia with inhibitors
   Renal allograft rejection
   Crescentic glomerulonephritis without renal insufficiency

3. Value of hemapheresis therapy not proven, or inadequately tested:
   Rheumatoid arthritis
   Multiple sclerosis
   Amyotrophic lateral sclerosis
   Dermatomyositis
   Juvenile and psoriatic arthritis
   Goodpasture's syndrome with renal insufficiency
   Immune thrombocytopenic purpura
   Maternal-fetal incompatibility
   Fabry's disease
   Autoimmune hemolytic anemia
   Pure erythrocyte aplasia
   Disseminated carcinomatosis

treated by therapeutic hemapheresis and controversy is likely to continue. Intense apheresis can induce rapid reduction in autoantibodies, circulating immune complexes and plasma proteins. For conditions being treated by cytotoxic or immunosuppressive therapy, reducing these plasma constituents and decreasing the number of circulating lymphocytes probably augments therapeutic benefits. Apheresis seems to be chiefly useful as adjunctive or palliative therapy. Its effects are usually short-term and not curative.[26]

Peer Review

A group of responsible physicians (possibly a Human Subjects Committee or the Hospital Transfusion Committee) should monitor all policies of the apheresis facility; review the indications for, and effectiveness of, each procedure or series of procedures; and maintain surveillance of all adverse effects. This committee should establish a list of conditions for which therapeutic apheresis is appropriate and evaluate all unusual requests. Approval for the latter should be obtained before apheresis is instituted. For a regional blood center a Medical Advisory Committee could serve the same function.

Patient Care Considerations

Informed Consent

Therapeutic hemapheresis procedures impose significant risk of morbidity and even mortality for the patient.[30,31,32] Fatalities have occurred.[32,33] Often vascular damage is so severe that shunts or fistulas must be surgically implanted. Extracorporeal circulation imposes risks of acute hypovolemic reactions, fluid shifts and electrolyte imbalances. Hemostatic defects may be precipitated, complement components may be activated and host defense against microorganisms may be prejudiced. Finally, there may be long-term adverse effects which are, as yet, unrecognized.

The informed consent of a prospective patient should be obtained in writing after a qualified person explains the procedure and possible alternative therapy if appropriate.[34] The patient or the legal guardian must have an opportunity to ask questions and to refuse consent. The patient's personal physician should certify in writing that the possible benefit warrants the risk.

The Patient's Condition

Evaluation of the patient's general condition is the responsibility of both the personal physician and the physician in charge of the apheresis facility. Close consultation between these two is important especially when the patient is small or elderly, or has circulatory problems or poor vascular access. The patient should be completely evaluated before making a commitment to perform the procedure. The physician in charge of the apheresis facility has final responsibility to determine that the procedure is indicated and the patient is a suitable candidate.[1,34] The therapeutic goals should be defined in terms of the patient's disease process and differentiated from his or her general condition. There should be understanding and agreement between physicians on all aspects of the patient's care: division of responsibility during the patient's course of treatment, provision of vascular access, expected side effects of apheresis such as decrements of plasma proteins and coagulation factors, responsibility for monitoring laboratory test results and objectives of treatment.

Laboratory Tests

Excessive and esoteric laboratory testing can significantly increase the cost of a series of therapeutic apheresis procedures. Some pretreatment studies are usually indicated to anticipate possible problems and permit evaluation of therapeutic effect. Serum protein electrophoresis, hemoglobin or hematocrit and platelet count are useful because hemapheresis will affect all these. Coagulation studies are indicated only if clinical history or observation suggest a congenital or acquired hemorrhagic tendency, or if procedures are done more frequently than three times a week. The patient should be weighed before each procedure. The results of tests do not ordinarily exclude patients from therapeutic apheresis, but medical judgement must be exercised when results are abnormal.

When specific tests are available and there are the explicit indications, the following may be employed to monitor the effect of therapy:

  Viscosity, for hyperviscosity syndromes
  Antinuclear antibody, for lupus erythematosus
  Antiacetylcholine receptor, for myasthenia gravis
  Antiglomerular basement membrane antibody, for glomerulonephritis
  Components of complement, for renal diseases
  Immune complex assay, for conditions associated with immune complexes.

Replacement Fluids

The choice of replacement fluids may vary. The responsible physician should prescribe fluids to be given, and the records must note the nature and volume of the replacement fluids as well as the volume of plasma or cells removed. The selection significantly affects the total cost of the procedure. The three alternative replacement solutions are: crystalloids, albumin solutions and fresh frozen plasma. There are advantages and disadvantages to each. See Table 2-3. A combination is usually used, the relative proportions being determined by the patient's physical condition, the disease, the planned frequency of procedures and cost.

Complications of Hemapheresis

Death

Patients undergoing therapeutic apheresis may be critically ill, having failed to improve on other, more traditional, therapies. Manipulation during apheresis of their intravascular fluid volumes and the associated movement of electrolytes, globulins and other substances from one physiologic compartment to another can stress the patient's already compromised homeostatic mechanisms. Worldwide, more than 50 deaths have been associated with therapeutic hemapheresis.[33] The estimated case fatality rate is about 3 in 10,000 procedures.[32] The two most common mechanisms of death are cardiovascular, characterized by cardiac arrhythmias or arrest during or shortly after the procedure; and respiratory, characterized by acute pulmonary edema or adult respiratory distress syndrome occurring during a procedure. Other fatal mechanisms are anaphylaxis, vascular perforation, hepatitis, sepsis, thrombosis and hemorrhage. Less severe examples of these conditions may seriously complicate a patient's clinical course without causing death.

Vascular Access

Patients referred for therapeutic apheresis often have received intensive medical care and their veins have suffered repeated punctures for laboratory samples and intravenous medications. As a result, vascular access usually is difficult, often requiring special venous access devices such as an indwelling double-lumen catheter. Usually requiring special surgical techniques for placement, these devices may produce more vascular damage or inflict infrequent, but severe, complications such as perforation of the great vessels or heart, thrombosis or septicemia.[30] Arterial puncture, dissecting deep hematomas and arteriovenous fistula formation have been reported.[35]

Alteration of Pharmacodynamics

Plasmapheresis can precipitously lower blood levels of drugs. Patients receiving anticonvulsant medications may develop convulsions unless supplemental doses are given. Plasma levels of antibiotics and digitalis are decreased by apheresis. Drugs that bind to albumin will be significantly decreased. The pharmacokinetics of all drugs used to treat patients undergoing apheresis should be considered before starting therapy, and dosage schedules adjusted appropriately.

Table 2-3. Comparison of Replacement Fluids

Replacement Solution	Advantages	Disadvantages
Crystalloids	Low cost Hypoallergenic No hepatitis risk	2–3 volumes required Hypo-oncotic No coagulation factors No immunoglobulins
Albumin	Iso-oncotic No contaminating "inflammatory mediators" No hepatitis risk	High cost No coagulation factors No immunoglobulins
Plasma Protein Fraction	Slightly less expensive than albumin	Possible induction of hypotensive reactions
Fresh Frozen Plasma	Maintains normal levels of: immunoglobulins fibrinogen complement antithrombin III other proteins	Hepatitis risk Citrate load ABO incompatibility Allergic reactions Sensitization

Effects of Citrate

Perioral paresthesias result from reduced serum levels of ionized calcium and are related to the rate at which citrate anticoagulant is returned to the patient. Use of FFP as a replacement solution may exacerbate citrate toxicity. Hyperventilation may also contribute to hypocalcemic reactions. Perioral paresthesia, when it occurs, can usually be controlled by reducing the proportion of citrate or slowing the reinfusion rate. One antacid pill, which contains 500 mg calcium, will often relieve symptoms. Symptoms can become more severe if untreated, progressing to twitching of muscles of the extremities, chills, pressure in the chest, nausea, vomiting and, finally, tetany. Asking the patient to report any vibrations or tingling sensations can help determine the correct reinfusion rate.

When central catheters are used for reinfusion, cardiac arrhythmias may result from direct perfusion of the sinoatrial node or the cardiac conduction system with citrated fluid. Electrocardiographic changes have been noted to remit upon partial withdrawal of central catheters.

Circulatory Effects

Intermittent-flow cell separators that require large extracorporeal volumes impose a risk of hypotensive reactions. Selection of an inappropriately large centrifuge bowl makes hypovolemia more likely. Such reactions occur frequently if the extracorporeal blood exceeds 15% of total blood volume. Hypotension is more common in children and the elderly. Hypotensive medications also aggravate hypovolemic reactions. Slow infusion and rapid withdrawal may produce hypovolemia in the patient and excessive volume in the cell separator. Some centers routinely use a double line setup to facilitate rapid infusion of fluids, should this become necessary, during therapeutic procedures. Hypovolemic reactions can occur with continuous-flow machines if return flow is inadvertently diverted to a waste collection bag, either through operator oversight or mechanical failure of a switch.

Mechanical Hemolysis

Kinked plastic tubing, malfunctioning pinch valves or improperly threaded pumps may damage the red cells in the extracorporeal circuit. In a survey reporting 12,658 therapeutic procedures, eight equipment-related hemolytic episodes were observed.[36] Although the patient is usually asymptomatic, in all apheresis procedures it is important for the operator to carefully observe the plasma collection lines for pink discoloration, the telltale sign of traumatic hemolysis.

Respiratory Distress

The differential diagnosis for respiratory embarrassment during or immediately following apheresis includes: pulmonary edema, massive pulmonary embolus, pulmonary microvascular obstruction and anaphylactic reactions. Pulmonary edema resulting from volume overload or cardiac failure is usually indicated by an increase of more than 50 mm of mercury in the diastolic blood pressure. Acute pulmonary edema, associated with use of FFP, has been attributed to an immunologic reaction that damages alveolar capillary membranes and allows fluid to leak across them.[37] Massive pulmonary embolus associated with apheresis could be due to inadequate anticoagulation of the withdrawn blood. Minor allergic reactions with urticaria and bronchospasm are fairly common during apheresis and usually respond to antihistamines and/or steroids.[38,39] Complement activation has been detected during some of these urticarial reactions when FFP was being used as the replacement solution.[38] However, one patient who died with bronchospasm and hypotension received only 5% albumin and had no evidence of complement activation. At autopsy this patient had microvascular occlusion by aggregates of platelets and leukocytes.[39] In a similar case proteinaceous embolic material was found in the pulmonary capillaries.[40]

Infections

Among the commonly used replacement solutions, only fresh frozen plasma may transmit hepatitis. Two deaths due to hepatitis communicated this way have been reported.[32] Other potential sources of contamination or infection could be leakage of the centrifuge seal or plastic harness, or defects in the prepackaged software.

Some apheresis procedures are undertaken to decrease immunoglobulin levels, especially in treating conditions associated with autoantibodies. The opsonic components of complement are simultaneously depleted, and, in addition, immunosuppressive drugs may prevent rebound increases in antibody levels after apheresis therapy. This induced immunocompromised state might be expected to result in increased susceptibility to infections. Indeed, high incidence of complicating infections has been reported in patients treated for glomerulonephritis.[41,42] Contrastingly, neurological patients treated with apheresis have a much lower frequency of infections.[43] This suggests the basic disease process is an important factor in determining susceptibility to infection. Some patients undergoing intensive therapeutic apheresis are routinely given prophylactic immune serum globulin.

Possible Long-Term Effects

Long-term adverse effects of hemapheresis are the subject of considerable speculation. Normal donors undergoing frequent cytapheresis procedures have been shown to have decreases in absolute numbers of both T and B lymphocytes, which persisted for at least 8 months.[44] The decrease in circulating B lymphocytes was proportionately greater. The normal ratio of T helper to T suppressor cells was maintained, although the absolute numbers of both subsets of immunoregulatory lymphocytes were decreased.[45] At present, there are no known complications of this induced lymphopenia, but much remains to be investigated. T lymphocyte subsets are of special interest because of the use of lymphoplasmapheresis to treat certain autoimmune diseases. In light of our incomplete understanding of both autoimmune diseases and therapy, the possibility exists that therapy could, over the long term, exacerbate the disease.

Future Developments

The cell separators currently used for therapeutic hemapheresis may be considered the "second generation" of instruments, much more sophisticated and reliable than the first instruments that were originally developed to collect platelets and granulocytes. Third generation instruments are presently undergoing field trials; these, designed specifically for therapeutic use, bear only slight resemblance to their progenitors and promise significant savings in replacement solutions and operator time.

Membrane Filtration

Instruments that filter plasma through a membrane are not suitable for cytapheresis.[46] Whole blood, containing all protein and cellular elements, flows across a membrane. Higher pressure in the blood phase than in the filtrate pushes particles smaller than the membrane pores through the membrane into the filtrate. Most such machines have the membranes arranged as hollow fibers, although there are several flat plate devices. As blood crosses the membrane in a laminar flow, repulsive forces intrinsic to the material of the wall keep cellular elements away from the membrane. Thus, platelets are not activated and red cell survival is not shortened. Plasma permeates the matrix of the membrane and escapes at right angles to the stream of flow. Varying membrane pore size allows specific proteins to be removed from plasma while the remainder are returned to the patient.

Absorbents

Membrane devices can readily be modified for selective removal of specific soluble plasma constituents. Sorbents such as charcoal, DNA-collodion, staphylococcal protein A and monoclonal antibodies have been incorporated into columns designed to remove bile acids, anti-DNA immunoglobulins, autoantibodies and specific antigens. As plasma filters through the membrane, contact with the sorbent in the column causes selective removal of the pathogenic substance. The treated plasma can be returned with the cellular components to the patient, eliminating the need for replacement fluids.

Cryofiltration

Cold temperatures cause polymerization of many macromolecular substances, including IgM autoantibodies, immune complexes and lipids. These polymers then precipitate or gel.[47] In a two-step hemapheresis process, plasma is filtered and then cooled so that the large molecular substances gel and can be removed by a second macromolecular filter. The plasma is then rewarmed, united with the cellular elements and returned to the patient. In pilot studies on patients with rheumatoid arthritis, this process effectively removed circulating immune complexes and rheumatoid factor, an IgM autoantibody.[48]

Selective apheresis techniques that remove specific plasma substances suspected of mediating specific diseases should enhance investigations into the pathogenesis of these conditions. Controlled studies are essential to prove the efficacy and safety of these techniques before they are generally applied.

References

1. Schmidt PJ ed. Standards for blood banks and transfusion services. 11th ed. Arlington, VA: American Association of Blood Banks, 1984.

2. Hinckley ME, Huestis DW. Premedication for optimal granulocyte collection. Plasma Therapy 1981;2:149–152.

3. Barnes A, DeRoos A. Increased granulocyte yields obtained with an oral three dose prednisone premedication schedule (abstract). Am J Clin Pathol 1982;78:267.

4. Mishler JM. Donor conditioning agents in leukocytapheresis and thrombocytapheresis: preliminary guidelines for use. Plasma Therapy 1982;3:5–26.

5. Mishler JM. New dosage regimens for HES during intensive leukapheresis. Transfusion 1978;18:126–127.

6. Ring J, Messmer K. Incidence and severity of anaphylactoid reactions of colloid volume substitutes. Lancet 1977;i:466–469.

7. Kurtz SR, McMican A, Carciero R, et al. Plateletpheresis experience with the Haemo-

netics Blood Processor 30, the IBM Blood Processor 2997 and the Fenwal CS 3000 Blood Processor. Vox Sang 1981;41:212–218.

8. Slichter SJ. Controversies in platelet transfusion therapy. Ann Rev Med 1980;31:509–540.

9. International Forum. Granulocyte transfusions—an established or still an experimental therapeutic procedure? Vox Sang 1980;38:40–56.

10. Higby DJ, Barnett D. Granulocyte transfusions: current status. Blood 1980;55:2–8.

11. Winston DJ, Ho WG, Gale RP. Therapeutic granulocyte transfusions for documented infections—a controlled trial in 95 infectious granulocytopenic episodes. Ann Intern Med 1982;97:509–515.

12. Higby DJ. Controlled prospective studies of granulocyte transfusion therapy. Exp Hematol 1977;5(Suppl 1):57–64.

13. Palm SL, Furcht LT, McCullough J. Effects of temperature and duration of storage on granulocyte adhesion, spreading and ultrastructure. Lab Invest 1981;45:82–88.

14. Collins JA. Problems associated with the massive transfusion of stored blood. Surgery 1974;75:274–295.

15. Nusbacher J. Therapeutic hemapheresis. In: Myhre BA ed. Clinics in laboratory medicine. Philadelphia: WB Saunders 1982 ;2:87–106.

16. Orlin JB, Berkman EM. Partial plasma replacement: removal and recovery of normal plasma constituents. Blood 1980;56:1055–1059.

17. Rock GA, Lafreniere I, Chan L, McCombie N. Plasma exchange in the treatment of hemolytic disease of the newborn. Transfusion 1981;21:546–551.

18. Klein HG. Therapeutic plasma exchange: a healthy dose of skepticism. West J Med 1983;138:92–94.

19. Berkman E. Issues in therapeutic apheresis. N Engl J Med 1982;306:1418–1420.

20. Karsh J, Klippel JH, Plotz PH, Decker JL, Wright DG, Flye MW. Lymphapheresis in rheumatoid arthritis: a randomized trial. Arthritis Rheum 1981;24:867–873.

21. Wallace D, Goldfinger D, Lowe C, et al. A double-blind, controlled study of lymhoplasmapheresis versus sham apheresis in rheumatoid arthritis. N Engl J Med 1982;306:1406–1410.

22. Dwosh IL, Giles AR, Ford PM, Pater JL, Anastassiades TP. Plasmapheresis therapy in rheumatoid arthritis, a controlled, double-blind, crossover trial. N Engl J Med 1983;308:1124–1129.

23. Beecher HK. The powerful placebo. JAMA 1955;159:1602–1606.

24. Advisory Panel to the Council on Scientific Affairs of the American Medical Association: Use of therapeutic apheresis. American Medical Association, Chicago, (to be published).

25. Shumak KH, Rock GA. Therapeutic plasma exchange. N Engl J Med 1984;310:762–771.

26. Taft EG. Therapeutic apheresis. Hum Pathol 1983;14:235–240.

27. Silvergleid AJ. Applications and limitations of hemapheresis. Ann Rev Med 1983;34:69–89.

28. Linker C. Plasmapheresis in clinical medicine. West J Med. 1983;183:60–69.

29. Kennedy MS, Domen RE. Therapeutic apheresis, applications and future directions. Vox Sang 1983;45:261–277.

30. Hazards of apheresis. Editorial. Lancet 1982;2:1025–1026.

31. Huestis DW. Hazards of therapeutic plasmapheresis (plasma exchange). Apheresis Bull (IBM# UK) 1983;1:76–83.

32. Huestis DW. Mortality in therapeutic haemapheresis. Lancet 1983;2:1025–1026.

33. Huestis DW. Personal communication; March, 1984.

34. AABB Committee on Hemapheresis: Guidelines for physician responsibility in therapeutic apheresis procedures. American Association of Blood Banks News Briefs, 1984;7:1–4.

35. Grindon AJ. Adverse reactions to whole blood donation and plasmapheresis. CRC Crit Rev Clin Lab Sci 1981;17:51–75.

36. Barnes A, Taft EG. Therapeutic apheresis activities of AABB members. American Association of Blood Banks News Briefs, 1983;6:5–6.

37. O'Connor PC, Erskine JG, Pringle TH. Pulmonary oedema after transfusion with fresh frozen plasma. Br Med J 1981;282:379–380.

38. Rosenkvist J, Berkowitz A, Holsoe E, Sorensen H, Taaning E. Plasma exchange in myasthenia gravis complicated with complement activation and urticarial reactions using fresh frozen plasma as replacement solution. Vox Sang 1984;46:13–18.

39. Rubenstein MD, Wall RT, Wood GS, Edwards MA. Complications of therapeutic apheresis, including a fatal case with pulmonary vascular occlusion. Am J Med 1983;75:171–174.

40. Brewer EJ, Nickeson RW, Rossen RD. Plasma exchange in selected patients with juvenile rheumatoid arthritis. J Pediatr 1981;98:194–200.

41. Wing EJ, Bruns FJ, Fraley DC, Segel DP, Adler S. Infectious complications with plasmapheresis in rapidly progressive glomerulonephritis. JAMA 1980;244:2423–2426.

42. Lockwood CM, Peters DK. Plasma exchange in glomerulonephritis and related vasculitides. Ann Rev Med 1980;31:167–179.

43. Rodnitzky RL, Goeken JA. Complications of plasma exchange in neurological patients. Arch Neurol 1982;39:350–354.

44. Senhauser DA, Westphal RG, Bohman JE, Neff JC. Immune system changes in cytapheresis donors. Transfusion 1982;22:302–304.

45. Heal JM, Horan PK, Schmitt TC, Bailey G, Nusbacher J. Long-term followup of donors cytapheresed more than 50 times. Vox Sang 1983;45:14–24.

46. Wenz B. Automated blood cell separators. J Clin Lab Autom 1982;2:403–407.

47. Malchesky PS, Asanuma Y, Zawicki T, et al. On-line separation of macro-molecules by membrane filtration with cryogelation. In: Gurland JH, Heinze U, Lee HA eds. Plasma exchange. New York: Springer Verlag, 1980:20.

48. Malchesky PS, Smith JW, Kayashima K, Asanuma Y, Nose Y. Membrane plasmapheresis with cryofiltration in rheumatoid arthritis. Cleve Clin Q, 1983;50:11–18.

3

Blood and Blood Components: Preparation, Storage and Shipment

The primary goals of procedures for collection, preparation, storage, and shipment of blood and blood components are to: 1) maintain viability and function of each relevant constituent; 2) prevent physical changes detrimental to the constituents; and 3) minimize bacterial proliferation. The anticoagulant-preservative solution prevents clotting and provides proper nutrients for continued metabolism of cells during storage. As with other living systems, blood cells depend for their integrity during storage on a delicate biochemical balance of many materials, especially glucose, hydrogen ion (pH) and adenosine triphosphate (ATP). For whole blood and red blood cells, this balance is best preserved by storing and shipping at temperatures between 1 and 6 C, whereas platelets and granulocytes retain better function when stored at room temperature. Labile coagulation factors in plasma are best maintained at temperatures of − 18 C or lower. Refrigeration or freezing additionally minimizes proliferation of bacteria that might have entered the unit during venipuncture.

Anticoagulation and Preservation

CPD and CPDA-1

CPD (citrate phosphate dextrose) is an anticoagulant-preservative approved by the FDA for 21-day storage of red blood cells maintained at 1 to 6 C.[1-4] Blood collected in CPDA-1 may be stored for up to 35 days at 1 to 6 C. Maintenance of ATP levels correlates with viability during storage. The low storage temperature, 1 to 6 C, slows glycolytic activity enough that the dextrose substrate is not rapidly consumed, and intermediary metabolites that may inhibit glycolysis are not generated excessively. CPD contains enough dextrose to support continuing ATP generation by glycolytic pathways. The added adenine in CPDA-1 provides a substrate from which red cells can synthesize ATP during storage, resulting in improved viability when compared with CPD without adenine.

The quantity of citrate in CPD and CPDA-1 solutions is more than sufficient to bind the ionized calcium present in the volume of whole blood for which the bag is designed. Citrate prevents coagulation by inhibiting the several calcium-dependent steps of the coagulation cascade. Additionally, it retards glycolysis. The amount of anticoagulant-preservative in commercially available containers is suitable for 450 ml ± 10% of blood (ie, 405 to 495 ml).

Additive Systems

Currently approved by the FDA for extended storage of red blood cells are

35

two systems in which a second preservative solution is added for red cell storage in addition to the anticoagulant solution used for whole blood collection. Both require that the plasma be separated from the red cells before additional preservative solution is combined with the red cells. This combination should take place as soon as possible but no later than 24 hours after phlebotomy.

One system consists of a primary collection bag containing CPD. To this bag are attached satellite bags, one of which contains 100 ml of additive solution consisting of saline, dextrose, mannitol and adenine.

The second system consists of a primary collection bag containing citrate phosphate double dextrose (CP2D), a CPD solution with additional dextrose. A satellite bag contains contains 100 ml of additive solution consisting of saline, dextrose and adenine.

Shelf-Life

Maximum allowable storage time, referred to as shelf-life, is defined by the requirement for 70% recovery at 24 hours, ie, at least 70% of the transfused cells remain in the recipient's circulation 24 hours after transfusion. Transfused red blood cells that circulate after 24 hours will have a normal survival curve in the recipient.[5] Blood collected in CPD may be stored for 21 days, although 24-hour recovery of cells is usually well over 70% at 21 days.[2,6] Blood collected in CPDA-1 may be stored up to 35 days. The additive solution systems, approved only for red cell storage and not whole blood, permit a 49-day and a 35-day dating period respectively.

The auxiliary preservative solutions in the additive systems are not approved for whole blood, plasma components, platelets or for use in plasmapheresis procedures. The anticoagulant CP2D has been approved for the preparation of routine blood components including single donor plasma, cryoprecipitated antihemophilic factor and platelet concentrate.

Certain measurable biochemical changes occur when blood is stored at 1 to 6 C. These changes, some of which are reversible, are known as the "storage lesion" of blood. These changes are tabulated for CPD and CPDA-1 stored blood in Table 3-1 and additive systems in Table 3-2. Except for oxygen-transporting functions, discussed below, these rarely have clinical significance because transfusion volumes are small and the recipient's compensatory homeostatic mechanisms reverse these changes. Even in massive transfusion, the adverse effects of the red cell storage lesion are usually inconsequential unless the recipient is already severely compromised.

Oxygen Dissociation

The primary function of red blood cells is to deliver oxygen from the lungs to the tissues. This function is mediated by a reversible hemoglobin-oxygen equilibrium. In the lungs, where oxygen partial pressure (PO_2) is high, hemoglobin takes up oxygen to form oxyhemoglobin. In the tissues, where PO_2 is lower, hemoglobin releases oxygen. Hemoglobin may achieve 100% oxygen saturation in the lungs, and characteristically releases only some of the oxygen at the lower PO_2 of normal tissues. Oxygen saturation of hemoglobin varies at various PO_2 levels, a relationship that can be plotted as the oxygen dissociation curve. (See Figure 3-1.) Although the shape remains fixed, the position may shift to the right or left, depending on such variables as the presence or absence of red cell 2,3-diphosphoglycerate (2,3-DPG), tissue pH and other factors. The degree of shift to the right or left is embodied by the P_{50} value, which is the partial pressure of oxygen at which hemoglobin is 50% saturated. A high P_{50} value means the curve has shifted to the right and more oxygen can be released at any given PO_2. A left shift means that the P_{50} is lower and less oxygen than normal is released at any given PO_2.[7]

Table 3-1. Biochemical Changes of Blood Stored in CPD and CPDA-1

| | | CPD Whole Blood | | CPDA-1 | | | |
| | | | | Whole Blood | Red Blood Cells | Whole Blood | Red Blood Cells |
Variable	Days of Storage:	0	21	0	0	35	35
% viable cells (24-hour posttransfusion)		100.0	80.0	100.0	100.0	79.0	71.0
pH (measured at 37 C)		7.20	6.84	7.6	7.55	6.98	6.71
ATP (% of initial value)		100.0	86.0	100.0	100.0	56.0 ($\pm$16)	45.0 ($\pm$12)
2,3-DPG (% of initial value)		100.0	44.0	100.0	100.0	<10.0	<10.0
Plasma K^+ (mEq/l)		3.9	21.0	4.2	5.1	27.3	78.5*
Plasma Na^+ (mEq/l)		168.0	156.0	169.0	169.0	155.0	111.0
Plasma hemoglobin (mg/dl)		1.7	19.1	8.2	7.8	46.1	658*

*Values for plasma hemoglobin and potassium concentrations may appear somewhat high in 35-day stored red blood cell units; the total plasma in these units is only about 70 ml.

Table 3-2. Biochemical Changes of Red Cells Stored in Additive Systems (AS) for 35 Days

Variable	AS-1 Adsol*	AS-2 Nutricel**
% viable cells (24-hour posttransfusion)	88.0($\pm$7)	78.6($\pm$7.6)
ATP (% of initial value)	76.0	65.0($\pm$15)
2,3-DPG (% of initial value)	<10.0	<10.0
RBC lysis (%)	0.33	0.5($\pm$0.25)
Plasma K^+ load (mEq per unit of RBCs)	5.0	5.7($\pm$0.3)

Moore GL. A longer life for stored red cells. Diagnostic Medicine, 1983;6:33-43.

*Fenwal Laboratories
**Cutter Laboratories

Effect of pH and 2,3-DPG

In red cell storage and preservation it is important to maintain oxygen-carrying and oxygen-releasing capacities of hemoglobin. The concentration of red cell 2,3-DPG influences the release of oxygen to the tissues. If 2,3-DPG levels are high, more oxygen is released at a given PO_2. Lower red cell levels of 2,3-DPG cause greater affinity of hemoglobin for oxygen so that less oxygen is released at the same PO_2.

Concentrations of 2,3-DPG are affected by pH. The initial pH of blood collected in CPD and measured at the temperature of storage is approximately 7.4 to 7.5. As stored red blood cells metabolize glucose to lactate, hydrogen ions accumulate, plasma pH falls and 2,3-DPG declines. Table 3-1 tabulates these changes for CPD and CPDA-1. During the second week of storage, the pH of CPD-stored blood falls below 7.0. As pH drops, there is a fall in red cell 2,3-DPG. Concentrations of 2,3-DPG are normal in CPD-stored blood for about 10 days. When blood is stored in CPDA-1, 2,3-DPG levels initially fall slightly more rapidly than in CPD, but near normal levels are maintained for 12 to 14 days.[8,9]

Restoration of Function

Following transfusion, stored red blood cells regenerate ATP and 2,3-DPG,

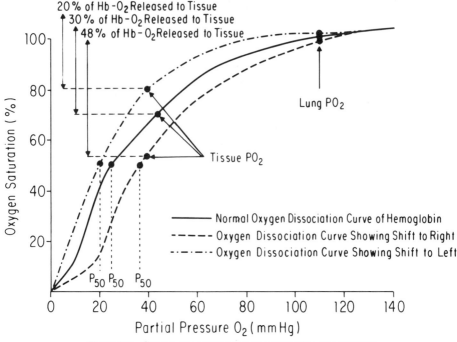

Figure 3-1. Oxygen dissociation curves under different conditions.

resuming normal energy metabolism and hemoglobin function as they circulate in the recipient. It usually takes from 3 to 8 hours for severely depleted cells to regenerate half of their 2,3-DPG levels and approximately 24 hours for complete restoration of 2,3-DPG and normal hemoglobin function.[10] In red cell storage, maintaining cell viability is clearly a critical consideration, but the importance of maintaining levels of 2,3-DPG is unclear. On theoretical grounds, recipients likely to be most affected by low 2,3-DPG levels in transfused blood are those receiving massive quantities of stored blood in a short time, and those particularly vulnerable to the effects of tissue hypoxia; examples include newborns undergoing exchange transfusion, patients with small blood volume who receive large volumes of blood and patients undergoing coronary artery bypass surgery. Such patients usually receive blood less than 7 to 10 days old.

Stored red cells, even those at the end of their allowable shelf-life, can be rejuvenated with FDA-approved solutions containing pyruvate, inosine, phosphate, adenine and, in some cases, glucose. The rejuvenated red cells have increased levels of 2,3-DPG and ATP.[11] Rejuvenated red cells can be frozen and stored in the same manner as fresh red cells and demonstrate normal oxygen transport when transfused.[11] (See page 41 for further discussion.)

Heparin

Heparin exerts its anticoagulant effect by potentiating the action of the endogenous plasma protein, antithrombin III (AT III). Synthesized in the liver, AT III is an inhibitor of most serine esterase clotting factors. Because it lacks dextrose, heparin serves only as an anticoagulant, not as a preservative. Heparinized blood must be transfused within 48 hours, preferably within

24 hours. Heparin is not recommended for routine blood collection.

Plastic Bags

The availability of plastic bags with integral tubing and technologic advances in high-speed centrifugation make it possible to prepare components from whole blood. Donor blood can be processed to yield the following single-donor components: red blood cells, platelets, leukocytes, plasma and cryoprecipitate. Multi-donor pools of plasma harvested from whole blood or obtained by apheresis can be processed industrially to yield derivatives such as albumin, plasma protein fraction, Factor VIII concentrate, immune serum globulin preparations and concentrates of Factors II, VII, IX and X. Appropriate blood component therapy expands the number of patients who can achieve therapeutic benefits from what is still a limited resource—human blood.

Preparation of Components

Table 3-3 lists the proper names and commonly used terms for blood and components commonly used in transfusion practice.

Blood Collection

To prevent partial activation of the coagulation system during collection, blood must be collected rapidly and with minimal trauma to tissues. There should be a single venipuncture and frequent, gentle mixing of the blood with the anticoagulant. Blood collection lasting longer than 10 minutes usually results from a poor venipuncture and slow blood flow.

When possible, blood destined for component preparation should be drawn into bags with integrally attached satellite bags (closed system) to avoid breaking the hermetic seal when removing components. If it is necessary to break the hermetic seal (open system), aseptic techniques and pyrogen-free equipment must be used. Breaking the hermetic seal is sometimes unavoidable, for example, in pooling platelets or cryoprecipitates prior to transfusion. When the hermetic seal has been broken, the resulting components must be used within 24 hours if stored at 1 to 6 C or within 6 hours if stored at 20 to 24 C. Components to be stored frozen must be prepared within 6 hours if an open system has been used.

When the final container is not the container used for collection, the final container must be accurately identified as coming from the original unit. This applies to plasma components and platelets as well as red cells transferred to washing or freezing containers. Records must indicate that the transfer has been made. Secondary containers must be labeled while still attached to the primary container, either with the original unit number or by another means to relate it to the original unit number.

Centrifugation

Using large centrifuges requires caution. At high speeds, heavy rotor heads and cups develop a gravity force (g) of thousands of pounds. Contents in opposing cups must be equal in weight; eccentric loads cause impaired efficiency in centrifugation and irregular wear on the rotor. Swinging cups offer better cell-liquid interfaces for maximal removal of plasma than do fixed-angle cups. Blood bags sometimes have imperfections through which centrifuge pressures may force blood. Occasionally bags may rupture or the seals between tubing segments may leak during centrifugation. Overwrapping the bags with plastic prevents leakage if the blood or component bag breaks. The bag should be placed so that a broad side faces the outside wall of the centrifuge to reduce centrifugal force on the sealed margins.

Balancing material should be dry. Weighted rubber discs and large rubber bands are excellent, and are available in several thicknesses to provide flexibility in balancing without the need to cut discs.

Table 3-3. Blood and Blood Components

Proper Name*	Commonly Used Names
Whole Blood	Whole Blood
Red Blood Cells	Red Blood Cells, Packed Cells, Red Cell Concentrate
Red Blood Cells Frozen	Frozen Red Blood Cells
Red Blood Cells Deglycerolized	Deglycerolized Red Blood Cells, Thawed Red Blood Cells
Red Blood Cells Leukocytes Removed by Centrifugation	Leukocyte-Poor Red Blood Cells
Red Blood Cells Leukocytes Removed by Washing	Washed Red Blood Cells
Red Blood Cells Leukocytes Removed by Filtration	Leukocyte-Poor Red Blood Cells
Plasma	Single-Donor Plasma
Liquid Plasma	Single-Donor Plasma
Fresh Frozen Plasma	Fresh Frozen Plasma
Cryoprecipitated AHF	Cryoprecipitate
Whole Blood Cryoprecipitate Removed	Modified Whole Blood
Platelet Rich Plasma	Platelet Rich Plasma
Platelets	Platelet Concentrate
Platelets Apheresis	Single-Donor Platelets, Apheresis Platelet Concentrates
Granulocytes** Apheresis	Granulocyte Concentrate
Granulocytes-Platelets** Apheresis	Granulocyte-Platelet Concentrate

*Designated by FDA
**These products are not recognized by the FDA. Names are as proposed for Uniform Labeling.

Rotor speed and duration of spin are the critical variables in preparing components by centrifugation. The Special Methods section contains a guide for centrifugation (page 469), but these *g* values and times of spin are approximations. Each centrifuge should be calibrated for optimal speeds and times of spin for each component prepared. The times listed include only the time of acceleration and "at speed," not the deceleration time. The automatic electronic braking devices of some centrifuges can decrease the deceleration time with minimal resuspension of centrifuged elements. Manual braking causes unacceptable resuspension. The cover must never be opened until the machine has stopped.

Quality Assurance

Optimal conditions of speed and time for component preparation should be determined for each centrifuge in each laboratory and should be checked periodically. The most practical way to evaluate centrifugation is to scrutinize quality assurance data on components prepared in each centrifuge. For example, see page 477 for calculating platelet yield in preparing platelet concentrates. If platelet concentrates give inconsistent yields, variables to examine include calibration of the centrifuge;

the initial platelet count in the donors; storage time and conditions between blood collection and platelet preparation; or other investigations appropriate to local circumstances. Records should be maintained that identify the individuals processing components. This can also be useful in evaluating erratic yields.

Red Blood Cells

Preparation

For the preparation of Red Blood Cells, colloquially referred to as "packed cells," it is desirable to use blood-collection units with integrally attached transfer container(s). Red Blood Cells may be allowed to sediment during refrigerated storage of the Whole Blood, or cells and plasma may be separated by centrifugation at any time up to the date of expiration of the whole blood. A procedure for the preparation of Red Blood Cells is found on page 53.

Expiration Date

After the plasma has been harvested, Red Blood Cells must be refrigerated at 1 to 6 C. Unmodified red cells, separated in a closed system and properly refrigerated, have the same expiration date as the Whole Blood from which they were separated, provided the hematocrit does not exceed 80%. A red cell preparation with less than 20% plasma and anticoagulant-preservative solution undergoes accelerated aging during storage and survives poorly when transfused.[12] It is important to verify that the method of preparing packed red cells does not usually result in a hematocrit above 80%. This can be done by measuring the hematocrit of units that have outdated. If the hermetic seal was broken during processing, the Red Blood Cells must be transfused within 24 hours, and the new date and time of expiration must be noted on the label and in the records. If additive solutions are used, the appropriate expi-

ration date and the volume and nature of the additive must be noted on the label.

Rejuvenation: Red blood cells show a significant decrease in 2,3-DPG and ATP after storage at 1 to 6 C. These depleted substances can be restored to normal levels by incubating the stored red cells with a rejuvenating solution. Rejuvenated red cells regain normal characteristics of oxygen transport and delivery and improved posttransfusion survival.[11]

Rejuvenation may be performed up to 2 to 3 days after the red cells expire, provided they have been stored continuously at 1 to 6 C. After rejuvenation, the red cells may be either 1) washed, re-concentrated and transfused within 24 hours, or 2) glycerolized and frozen.

Leukocyte-Poor Red Blood Cells

Patients with severe and/or repeated febrile, nonhemolytic transfusion reactions often do better when transfused with leukocyte-depleted red blood cells.[13] The designation "Leukocyte-Poor Red Blood Cells" implies removal of at least 70% of the original white cells and retention of at least 70% of the original red cells. Several methods that remove leukocytes from whole blood also remove plasma, to which patients may additionally be immunized.

Methods for separating and removing the majority of leukocytes from donor red cells include centrifugation with or without saline washing, microaggregate blood filtration, and deglycerolization of frozen red cells. Whole Blood stored for 6 to 10 days appears to be optimal for removal of leukocytes by most methods.[14] None of the techniques to prepare Leukocyte-Poor Red Blood Cells removes all leukocytes.

Prepared by Centrifugation: Inverted centrifugation is a simple and moderately effective method to reduce the leukocyte count of donor blood. The resulting red cell preparation may be tolerated quite well by patients with antibodies to leukocytes. This simple centrifugation method can be improved by following it with sufficient saline washes that residual buffy coat is discarded with the supernatant fluid. This open system of preparation shortens the red cell shelf-life to 24 hours. A procedure for the preparation of leukocyte-poor red cells by inverted centrifugation appears on page 54.

Prepared by Double Centrifugation: A modification of the centrifugation technique allows harvesting fresh frozen plasma and platelet concentrates[15] if performed in a closed system, and results in a unit of Leukocyte-Poor Red Blood Cells with no reduction of allowable storage. The procedure for double centrifugation appears on page 54.

Prepared by Saline Dilution and Centrifugation: One of the most efficient methods of preparing leukocyte-poor red cells is saline dilution with centrifugation.[14] Using this procedure to process Red Blood Cells 6 to 10 days old gives excellent removal of leukocytes. The procedure for saline dilution and centrifugation appears on pages 54–55.

Transfusion Through Microaggregate Blood Filters: It is possible to reduce the number of leukocytes in units of Red Blood Cells by transfusing them through microaggregate blood filters[16] after centrifugation with a "heavy" spin (eg, 5000 g for 20 minutes). The microaggregate filter is simply used during administration. This method has the advantage that it is highly effective with blood close to its expiration date.[16] Centrifuging the blood before passage through the microaggregate blood filter increases the size of the microaggregates, although centrifugation may not be necessary with units of blood stored over one week. (See Chapter 17.)

Prepared by Freezing and Deglycerolizing: Previously frozen Deglycerolized Red Blood Cells are leukocyte-poor. See Chapter 4 for preparation of this leukocyte-depleted component, which has lower levels of residual leukocytes, platelets and plasma constituents than any other leukocyte-poor red cell component. *Standards*[17]

requires that at least 80% of the original red cells be recovered.

Washed Red Blood Cells

Washing red cells is not the most efficient way to remove leukocytes [14,15,16] but it does, additionally, remove plasma. Febrile, non-hemolytic transfusion reactions may occur with transfusion of any component containing leukocytes. Urticarial reactions complicate some transfusions, probably due to allergenic substances in donor plasma. Patients who are IgA-deficient and have anti-IgA antibodies may have anaphylactic reactions following transfusion of blood or blood components containing IgA. Transfusing washed red cells reduces the incidence of febrile, urticarial and, possibly, anaphylactic reactions.[18] Patients with anti-IgA may require blood from IgA-deficient donors, but red blood cells washed at least five times with saline or Deglycerolized Red Cells may be satisfactory.

Washed red cells are prepared with the same kind of automated or semi-automated equipment used to deglycerolize frozen red cells. Automated cell washers are more efficient than manual centrifugation techniques but they are more expensive. The washing process removes most of the plasma proteins, microaggregates, platelets and leukocytes. Red cells stored in CPDA-1 up to 35 days as Whole Blood or Red Blood Cells have been shown to have a normal survival after washing. Washed cells must be used within 24 hours because preparation must necessarily be in an open system.

For a procedure for the manual preparation of washed red cells, see page 55.

Neocytes

Neocytes are relatively young red cells which may be desirable for transfusion to patients with thalassemia major or other conditions requiring chronic transfusion that may lead to transfusion-induced hemochromatosis.[19] Red cell senescence releases into tissue stores approximately 1.08 mg of iron per 1 ml of red cells.

Transfused red cells have, theoretically, a mean cell age of 60 days, but in practice generally survive less than that length of time.[20] Isolation and transfusion of red cells with a mean cell age of 30 days and a potential survival of 90 days could possibly halve a patient's chronic transfusion requirement and iron deposition.

A technique for isolating younger red cells exploits the fact that, on an automated cell processor, the larger, less dense red cells are expressed earlier than the older, heavier cells during deglycerolization and/or washing.[21] Collecting the first half unit processed provides a uniformly younger cell population. The remaining half unit of older red cells may be transfused to patients for whom chronic red cell transfusion therapy is not indicated. This technique can be used for units of whole blood, liquid-stored red cells or frozen/deglycerolized red cells.

A hemapheresis technique has been developed to separate young red cells using continuous-flow blood cell separators.[20,21] This approach is expensive and requires four hours of the donor's time. The automated cell processor technique, described above, can be used in almost any blood bank; its cost is comparable to that of a unit of deglycerolized red blood cells, and the time involved is little more than that required to deglycerolize a unit of frozen red blood cells.

Plasma

Along with water and electrolytes, plasma contains proteins, principally albumin, globulin and coagulation factors. Although widely used for temporary volume replacement in patients depleted of whole blood or colloid, plasma is uniquely appropriate for replacement of coagulation factors. Most of the coagulation factors are stable at refrigerator temperatures except for Factor VIII and, to a lesser extent, Factor V. To maintain adequate levels of Factors V and VIII, plasma must be stored frozen. (For further discussion of coagulation factors, see Chapter 15, Blood Transfusion Practice.)

Plasma is usually prepared from Whole Blood during the preparation of other components, such as Red Blood Cells and Platelet Concentrates. As a byproduct of component preparation, plasma is separated according to the techniques described for these components (see below).

Plasma should be frozen in a manner that makes thawing and subsequent refreezing apparent. Some methods to accomplish this are:
1. Press a tube into the bag during freezing to leave an impression that disappears if the unit thaws.
2. Freeze plasma flat (horizontally) in the freezer but store it upright (vertically). An air bubble formed on the side of the bag during freezing will move to the top of the bag if thawing has occurred.
3. Place a rubber band around the middle of the bag of plasma prior to freezing, but cut it off after the unit is frozen, leaving an indentation that disappears with thawing.

Fresh Frozen Plasma

To be labeled "Fresh Frozen Plasma," plasma must be separated from the red cells and placed at −18 C or below within 6 hours after collection. *Standards* requires that Fresh Frozen Plasma, usually referred to as FFP, be stored at −18 C or lower. Optimal storage is at −30 C or colder. Stored at or below these temperatures, FFP has a dating period of 12 months after donation of the original unit of blood. Beyond this period, the Factor VIII may have decreased in some units to such an extent that the plasma is not optimal for treating patients deficient in this labile coagulation factor.

If many units of liquid plasma are placed in a mechanical freezer at the same time, freezing may be delayed. Rapid freezing can be accomplished by placing units in a dry ice-ethanol or dry ice-antifreeze bath; in layers between blocks of dry ice; in a blast freezer; or in a mechanical freezer maintained at −65 C or lower. If plasma is frozen in a liquid freezing bath, the plasma container must be overwrapped for protection from chemical alteration.

A procedure for the preparation of fresh frozen plasma appears on page 55.

Single Donor Plasma

Single Donor Plasma may be prepared by separation from the red blood cells on or before the fifth day after the expiration date of the whole blood. If not frozen, Single Donor Plasma must be stored at 1 to 6 C and may be kept for no more than 26 days from phlebotomy for CPD anticoagulant or 40 days for CPDA-1. When stored frozen at −18 C or lower, Single Donor Plasma may be kept up to 5 years. The separation technique for Single Donor Plasma is the same as for FFP.

If Fresh Frozen Plasma has not been used after 1 year of storage at −18 C or colder, it may be redesignated and relabeled "Single Donor Plasma." Thus redesignated, the plasma has 4 more years of shelf-life at −18 C or colder. A unit of Fresh Frozen Plasma thawed at 30 to 37 C and not transfused after storage at 1 to 6 C for 24 hours may also be relabeled and redesignated "Single Donor Plasma." Records must include these changes.

Plasma prepared from outdated Whole Blood is somewhat different from plasma originally prepared as Fresh Frozen Plasma, the major changes being high levels of potassium and ammonia in plasma prepared after long contact with red cells. See Tables 3-1 and 3-2 for storage changes in refrigerated blood.

If cryoprecipitate has been removed from whole blood or plasma, this must be stated on the plasma label. Plasma from which cryoprecipitate has been removed must not be designated as Fresh Frozen Plasma because it has been depleted of Factor VIII and fibrinogen.

Cryoprecipitated AHF

Cryoprecipitated antihemophilic factor (AHF) is the cold-insoluble portion of plasma remaining after fresh frozen plasma has been thawed between 1 and 6 C. It contains approximately 50% of the Factor VIII (AHF), 20-40% of the fibrinogen, and some of the Factor XIII originally present in the fresh plasma.

Standards requires that at least 75% of the bags of Cryoprecipitate tested contain a minimum of 80 International Units of Factor VIII. *The Code of Federal Regulations* (21 CFR 640.56) requires that there be an average of 80 IU of Factor VIII per final container and that at least four Cryoprecipitates be tested per month from units collected within the previous 30 days to determine the average. Each unit contains approximately 150 mg of fibrinogen but testing is not required.

Use for von Willebrand's Disease or Hypofibrinogenemia

No components are available specifically for treating either von Willebrand's disease or hypofibrinogenemia. Although Fresh Frozen Plasma can be used for temporary replacement therapy in both conditions, Cryoprecipitate is a more suitable component because of its smaller volume. The cryoprecipitation process concentrates not only Factor VIII but also fibrinogen (Factor I) and von Willebrand's Factor.[22,23] In von Willebrand's disease, there is abnormal platelet function as well as deficiency of Factor VIII coagulation activity. Commercial Factor VIII concentrates have coagulation activity but do not reliably contain von Willebrand's Factor needed for normal platelet function.[23] The average bag of Cryoprecipitate usually contains at least 150 mg of fibrinogen but may contain as much as 250 mg.[24]

Fibronectin, an opsonic protein believed to participate in phagocytosis, is present in Cryoprecipitate and other plasma components.[25] Because of its small volume, Cryoprecipitate would be the component of choice should fibronectin therapy prove to be clinically useful.

Preparation

CPDA-1, CPD and sodium citrate are suitable anticoagulants. The plasma may be obtained by apheresis or from Whole Blood units. A procedure for preparation of Cryoprecipitate appears on page 56.

Cryoprecipitate Pooled

Units of Cryoprecipitate can be pooled into groups of two to six units prior to labeling and storage. They should be pooled promptly after preparation, using an aseptic technique, and then be refrozen immediately to prevent possible bacterial growth and loss of labile coagulation factors.

Quality control procedures should ensure a minimum of 80 × "X" ("X" equals number of cryoprecipitates in the pool) units of Factor VIII in the final pool container.

The component is to be labeled "Cryoprecipitate Pooled" and the number of units pooled stated on the label. If saline has been added to facilitate pooling, the volume must appear on the label. The instruction "Use Within 4 Hours After Thawing" must be included on the label unless uniform labeling is used. In this case, the statement should appear in the circular of information rather than on the container label.

Whole Blood Cryoprecipitate Removed

With component separation, a single donor unit can yield red cells; platelets; cryoprecipitate; and cryoprecipitate-poor plasma, which still contains albumin, and most globulins and coagulation proteins. If whole blood is the desired end product it is still possible to harvest cryoprecipitate or platelets, using special storage and separation techniques.

A procedure for preparing Whole Blood Cryoprecipitate Removed appears on page 56.

Whole blood may be reconstituted after removal of platelets as well as cryoprecipitate. For aseptic removal of both the platelets and cryoprecipitate, the blood must be collected in a triple-unit collecting system. Starting with a platelet separation technique (see page 57) and following it with removal of cryoprecipitate, as described on page 56, permits harvest of either whole blood or packed red cells plus other therapeutically useful components. The blood must be labeled "Whole Blood Cryoprecipitate Removed"; platelet removal need not be noted on the label. Since whole blood stored more than 48 hours has few functional platelets and an unpredictably reduced level of Factor VIII, whole blood modified by removing platelets and cryoprecipitate is functionally the same as stored Whole Blood.

Platelets

The platelet concentrate prepared from a single unit of whole blood can temporarily elevate the platelet count by 10,000 to 12,000/mm^3/M^2 body surface area in patients whose thrombocytopenia is not due to increased destruction. Platelet transfusions are used to prevent spontaneous bleeding or stop established bleeding in patients with hypoplastic anemia or marrow failure due to replacement with malignant cells or to chemotherapy.

Platelet-rich plasma must be separated from whole blood by centrifugation within 6 hours after phlebotomy. The platelets may then be concentrated by additional centrifugation and removal of most of the supernatant plasma. A procedure for preparation of Platelet Concentrates from single units of Whole Blood appears on page 57. (See page 469, Special Methods, for calculation of g force and relative centrifugal force. A method for calibrating a centrifuge for optimal platelet yield is detailed on pages 476 to 477, Special Methods.)

Platelet Concentrates prepared by hemapheresis are discussed in Chapter 2.

Aspirin in Donors

Aspirin may affect platelet function for as long as 3 days after ingestion. A donor who has taken aspirin during this time should not be the sole source of platelets for a single patient.[26] Since most adults receive multiple units, this becomes a consideration only when large numbers of platelets are collected from a single donor by apheresis or when the patient is an infant or small child who requires only one unit of platelets. Units of platelets prepared from donors who have ingested aspirin within 3 days of blood donation should be labeled so that the transfusion facility is aware that the donor has ingested aspirin and that platelet function may be impaired.

Evaluating Platelet Concentrates

Evaluating the clinical response to platelet transfusions can help maintain quality assurance, but does not replace quantitative evaluation of the prepared concentrates. There must be at least 5.5×10^{10} platelets per bag and the pH must be 6.0 or higher in at least 75% of the units tested at the end of the allowable storage period. Standard practice is to test four units per month.

Granulocyte Concentrates

Granulocyte concentrates are prepared by leukapheresis, as described in Chapter 2.

Granulocytes may be stored at 20 to 24 C without agitation for up to 24 hours. However, recent studies have shown that after 8 hours of storage granulocytes have reduced ability to circulate and migrate to a site of inflammation.[28] Although granulocytes may be stored for up to 24 hours, it is best to transfuse them as soon as possible after collection.

Storage of Blood and Components

It is permissible to store, in refrigerator compartments used for storing blood, blood components, blood derivatives, blood samples from patients and donors, and reagents for blood bank tests other than HBsAg testing. The temperature in all areas of the refrigerator must be maintained between 1 and 6 C. The refrigerator must have a fan or be of capacity and design to ensure that the designated temperature is maintained. The interior should be clean and adequately lighted, and there should be clearly apparent organization of storage areas labeled or designated for: 1) unprocessed blood; 2) labeled blood; 3) crossmatched blood; and 4) rejected, outdated or quarantined blood. Blood of different blood groups may be stored on labeled separate shelves or areas.

Blood kept in sites outside the blood bank, such as surgical or obstetric suites, must be stored in refrigerators that meet the same standards. Temperature records are required for such refrigerators during periods of blood storage. Blood must never be stored in unmonitored refrigerators. It is best for the blood bank to assume responsibility for monitoring these refrigerators in the same way that blood bank refrigerators are monitored.

Monitoring Temperature

Recording thermometers and audible alarms are required for all blood storage refrigerators. The sensor for these systems should be on a high shelf and must be in a liquid-filled container. Glass bottles or standard blood bags are generally used. These should contain water or other fluids to a volume no greater than the volume of the smallest component stored. Red Blood Cells usually have 200 to 250 ml volume, but if split units or pediatric units are stored, the sensors should be kept in a smaller volume. The alarm signal must be activated at a temperature that allows personnel to take proper action before the stored blood reaches undesirable temperatures. An acceptable range is 1 to 6 C. The electrical source for the alarm system must be separate from that of the refrigerator; either a continuously rechargeable battery or an independent electrical circuit served by an emergency generator is suitable.

In large refrigerators it is advisable to have at least two independent thermometers, one immersed with the recorder sensor and the other in a similar container on the lowest shelf on which blood is stored. The temperatures of both these thermometers must be between 1 and 6 C at all times. These thermometers should be checked and the temperatures recorded periodically, usually daily. If the thermometer immersed with the recorder sensor does not agree within 1 C of that shown on the automatic recorder, both should be checked against an NBS thermometer, and suitable adjustments be made in the recorder. It is desirable to record the temperatures from the two independent thermometers on the recorder chart when it is changed regularly. In large walk-in refrigerators, several thermometers should be used, placed in areas determined to reflect the possible range of temperature fluctuations.

Sophisticated automated monitoring systems are increasingly in use. Some refrigerators have automatic temperature monitor and digital readout systems as well as automatic alarms, with continuous temperature surveillance at various pre-set areas within the refrigerator. Another system is a central monitor and alarm system capable of monitoring numerous refrigerators simultaneously. The temperature must be recorded at least once every 4 hours.

At the end of each time period, temperature charts from mechanical recording devices should be changed, dated inclusively and labeled to identify the refrigerator and the person changing the charts. Any departure from normal temperature should be explained in writing on the chart beside the tracing. A chart that habitually traces a perfect circle suggests that the recorder is not functioning properly, because slight variations occur in any refrigerator that is actively used.

Temperature records are retained as part of the blood bank records for at least 1 year.

Refrigerator and Freezer Alarms

Refrigerator and freezer thermometers and alarms should be checked periodically to ascertain that they are functioning properly. The temperatures of activation in refrigerators may be checked following the procedure in Special Methods, page 479. Before electronically monitored alarm systems are accepted for routine use, there should be a period of simultaneous monitoring, in which temperatures of activation are determined directly and compared with the figures generated electronically.

Freezers must be equipped with a continuously recording thermometer and an audible alarm. The alarm should be checked periodically. Ideally the alarm sensor should be accessible near the door of the freezer, but in some older units it is placed between the inner and outer freezer walls and its location is not apparent or accessible. In these cases, the site of the sensor can be determined from the manufacturer and a permanent mark placed on the wall at that location. The temperature of activation can be tested approximately by placing a flexible container (ie, water bottle) filled with cold tap water against the inner freezer wall where the sensor is located. When the alarm goes off, usually in a short time, the recording chart should be checked immediately to determine the temperature of activation. More details about checking freezer alarms are in Special Methods, page 479.

Freezers and refrigerators must have a source of electricity that operates independently of standard house circuits in case of a power failure, and it is extremely important that the alarms have a continuous power source. This should be tested periodically to ensure proper function. There must be written instructions for personnel to follow when the alarm sounds. These should include steps to determine the immediate cause of the temperature change and ways to handle temporary malfunctions, as well as steps to take in the event of prolonged power failure. It is important to list the names of key people to be notified and what steps should be taken to ensure that proper storage temperature is maintained for all blood, components and reagents.

Storing Platelets

Platelet Concentrates are to be stored either at 1 to 6 C or at 20 to 24 C. Shelf-life and storage conditions differ with intended storage temperature and with the type of plastic bag used to store the platelets. Refrigerated platelets do not maintain either function or viability as well as platelets stored at room temperature.[28]

Platelets may be stored at 1 to 6 C without agitation for 48 hours if prepared in a closed system. If storage is at 20 to 24 C, continuous gentle agitation is essential. Elliptical, circular and flat-bed agitators are available. The type of agitator and the type of plastic used for storing the platelets affect preservation of platelet function. The types of platelet storage bags and the agitators giving best in vitro results[29,30] are:

1. Polyvinyl chloride with 2-diethylhexyl phthalate plasticizer for 3-day platelet storage on an elliptical rotator.
2. Polyolefin without plastizer for 5- or 7-day platelet storage on a circular rotator or flat-bed agitator. Elliptical rotators are not recommended.
3. Polyvinyl chloride with tri(2-ethyl-hexyl)trimellitate plasticizer for 5- or 7-day platelet storage on circular or elliptical agitators. Flat-bed agitators are not recommended.

Platelets stored in polyvinyl chloride bags at 20 to 24 C may be stored for as long as 72 hours before transfusion if prepared in a closed system. If stored in the newer plastics that allow more gas diffusion, they may be stored at 20 to 24 C for up to 7 days before transfusion. If the hermetic seal of any bag is broken, the platelets should be used as soon as possible but must be transfused within 24 hours if stored between 1 and 6 C or within 6 hours if stored between 20 and 24 C.

Platelets collected using open-system apheresis procedures may be stored up to 24 hours at 20 to 24 C; those collected using closed-system apheresis procedures may be stored up to 5 days. Both must be stored using gentle agitation. As with platelets prepared from single units of whole blood, the type of agitation depends on the type of plastic used for the storage bag.

The temperature in the immediate vicinity of the platelet storage area must be monitored and recorded to ensure that storage temperatures are within the proper range.

Donor Blood Inspection

It is desirable to examine all stored whole blood and red cell units periodically, and it is required that each unit be inspected immediately before issue for transfusion or shipment to other facilities. Preissue inspections must be recorded and include the date, donor number and description of any abnormal units, the action taken and the identity of personnel involved. Blood with abnormal color or other appearance should be rejected for transfusion. Contamination should be suspected if the red blood cell mass looks purple, if a zone of hemolysis is observed just above the cell mass, if clots are visible or if the plasma is murky. Other obvious features that can make blood unsuitable for transfusion are purple, brown or red plasma. A green hue in plasma may be seen if donors use oral contraceptives and need not cause the unit to be rejected. The presence of blood or plasma at sealing sites in the tubing or in the ports may indicate inadequate sealing or closure, and renders the unit suspect and possibly unsuitable for transfusion.

Disposition

Blood units that are questionable for any reason should be quarantined until a responsible person decides their disposition. Evaluation of a questionable unit should include inverting it gently a few times to mix the cells and plasma. A great deal of undetected hemolysis, clotting or other alterations may have occurred in the undisturbed red blood cell mass. If, after sedimentation, the blood no longer appears abnormal, it may be returned to the available blood supply. Appropriate records should be completed by the responsible person.

Abnormal blood that cannot be released for transfusion should either be returned to the provider or investigated to delineate the problem. Results of the investigation should be reported to the blood supplier. The findings may require notification of the donor or local health department or both, or may indicate the need for improvement in donor techniques, screening of donors or handling of blood units during processing. Disposal procedures must conform to the local public health codes. Autoclaving and/or incineration is recommended.

Bacteriologic Examination

Routine sterility testing of blood or components is not required by the FDA unless the hermetic seal of the bag is broken during preparation. Culturing may be desirable if inspection reveals abnormal appearance of blood or components, or if a patient has any adverse reaction possibly related to contaminated donor blood. A good blood culture technique follows (21 CFR 640.2):

1. Perform the test with a total sample of no less than 10 ml of blood and a total volume of fluid thioglycollate or thioglycollate broth medium 10 times the volume of the sample of blood.
2. Inoculate the test sample into one or more test vessels in a 1:10 ratio of blood to medium for each vessel.
3. Mix thoroughly and incubate for 7 to 9 days at a temperature of 30 to 32 C.

4. Examine for evidence of growth of microorganisms every workday through the test period.
5. On the third, fourth or fifth day, remove for subculturing at least 1 ml of material from each test vessel. Add this to additional test vessels containing the same culture medium in a 1:10 ratio of diluted blood to medium. This proportion will facilitate visual inspection.
6. Mix thoroughly and incubate subcultures for 7 to 9 days at 30 to 32 C.
7. Examine for evidence of growth of microorganisms every workday throughout the test period. Turbidity is the earliest indication of bacterial growth. Subcultures are important because the original culture has a high concentration of blood and is usually slightly turbid, but the subculture is normally clear.

If the sterility studies are done in another laboratory or institution, the director of the blood bank must ascertain that they have been done properly and reported to the blood bank adequately. Positive cultures should arouse suspicion of poor donor arm preparation or pooling technique. If growth is observed in any test vessel, additional cultures can be made to rule out faulty culturing procedures. Culture results should be recorded and blood with positive cultures destroyed.

Reissuing Blood

Blood that has been returned to the blood bank must not be reissued for transfusion until the following conditions have been met:

1. The container closure must not have been penetrated or entered in any manner. This is to be certain that sterility is maintained.
2. The blood must have been maintained continuously between 1 and 10 C, preferably 1 and 6 C. Warming the blood beyond these limits, even with subsequent cooling, tends to accelerate red cell metabolism, produce hemolysis and

may permit bacterial growth in the unit. Most transfusion services will not reissue a unit of blood that has remained out of a monitored refrigerator longer than 30 minutes.

3. At least one sealed segment of integral donor tubing must remain attached to the container if the blood has left the premises of the issuing facility.
4. Records must indicate that the blood has been reissued and has been inspected prior to reissue.

Transportation of Blood and Blood Components

Whole Blood and Red Cell Components

The temperature of blood and red blood cell components must be kept between 1 and 10 C during transport. Sturdy, well-insulated cardboard and/or styrofoam shipping containers maintain these temperatures if they contain adequate cooling material. The refrigerant recommended for most shipments is wet ice in leakproof containers such as plastic bags. Wet ice from commercial ice-making machines is satisfactory. Super-cooled cubed ice or canned ice and dry ice should not be used for shipping or storing Whole Blood or Red Blood Cells because they can cause local temperatures low enough that red cells in their immediate vicinity may undergo hemolysis. Blood shipped by air may freeze if transported in an unpressurized storage compartment. The cargo compartments of buses and trucks often reach temperatures above 100 F. Temperature of the blood or components should be monitored closely during shipment and upon receipt.

Ice should be placed above the blood because cool air moves downward. During long hot trips, the ice and the blood should be in direct contact; a layer of cardboard or an air space between ice and blood may act as internal insulation, preventing the ice from adequately protecting the blood

from high environmental temperatures. In very hot weather and during trips of several hours, placing wet ice under as well as above the blood is necessary. Cubed wet ice may be better than chipped or broken ice for long distance shipments of blood because it melts slowly. In boxes shipped long distances or at high environmental temperatures, the volume of ice should at least equal that of the blood. In an insulated container, the temperature can be considered to be in the 1 to 6 C range as long as unmelted ice remains in the box and is in contact with the blood.

Monitoring Temperature

Some form of temperature indicator or monitoring is desirable when shipping blood over a regular route. An easy method to ascertain the temperature of the contents of a shipping box upon receipt is as follows:

1. Remove two bags of blood or components.
2. Place the sensing end of a mercury-in-glass or electronic thermometer between the bags (labels facing out) and secure the "sandwich" with two rubber bands.
3. After a few minutes, read the temperature.
4. If the temperature exceeds 10 C, quarantine the blood until appropriate disposition is determined.

Other suitable methods for monitoring shipments are:

1. Use time/temperature tags that indicate whether, at anytime during the shipping process, the temperature has exceeded 10 C.
2. Place a "high-low" mercury thermometer in the shipping box. These simple, reusable thermometers record the highest and lowest temperatures achieved during a time period.
3. Use a temperature indicator in which the location of glass beads in an ampule filled with wax-like material indicates whether or not the wax has reached its 10 C melting point.

4. Use other monitoring devices shown to be satisfactory. The accuracy of any temperature-indicating device should be checked before it is placed in routine use and periodically thereafter.

Monitoring shipping temperatures of blood and red cells may uncover a need for better insulated containers or larger amounts of ice. Record forms, periodically placed in shipping cartons for completion and return by blood bank personnel receiving blood shipments, provide written evidence of sufficient ice and insulation. It is the responsibility of the shipping or issuing facility to ascertain that shipping practices satisfactorily maintain the temperature of blood or red cells below 10 C during transportation.

Follow-up Actions

The disposition of blood exposed to temperatures above 10 C is best decided by experienced technical personnel. Factors such as the length of time in shipment, mode of transportation, magnitude of variance over 10 C, presence of residual ice in the shipping box and the presence of hemolysis should be taken into account. The shipping facility should be notified whenever unacceptably high temperatures are noted.

Mobile Collection Facilities

When blood is shipped from a mobile collection facility to the component preparation laboratory for processing, cooling must be as outlined above except that those units destined for platelet separation must not be chilled below 20 C because platelets are best separated from whole blood at room temperature. Such units should be transported from collection site to component preparation laboratory as soon as possible, but elapsed time between collection and centrifugation for platelet harvest must not exceed 6 hours.

In-house Transport

Issue of blood or red cells from the blood bank to other parts of the hospital must

be controlled so that unused blood is returned within a set period of time. Because blood at 1 to 6 C warms to 10 C or above in approximately 30 minutes at room temperature, blood or red cells should either be used or returned to the blood bank within 30 minutes. If a slightly longer time must elapse before transfusion, individual units may be placed in an insulated paper bag precooled to 1 to 6 C. Picnic chests or insulated plastic buckets with lids are useful for issuing blood to operating rooms. The insulated container maintains the appropriate temperature and conveniently segregates blood for the individual patient in the operating room.

Frozen Components

During transport, frozen components must be maintained at or below the required storage temperature. This can be achieved with a suitable quantity of dry ice in well-insulated containers or standard shipping cartons lined with insulating material such as plastic air bubble packaging or dry packaging fragments. The dry ice, obtained as sheets, should be layered at the bottom of the container, between each layer of frozen components, and on top. The use of dry ice "snow" (delivered by spray from a CO_2 tank) is useful for filling the nooks and crannies between components. This not only provides some physical cushioning that helps prevent breakage, but it also rapidly establishes a freezing temperature. Each shipping facility must determine optimum conditions for shipping frozen components depending on the temperature requirements of the component, the distance to be shipped, the shipping container used and the ambient temperature encountered.

Platelet and Granulocyte Concentrates

Every reasonable effort must be made to ensure that platelets and granulocyte concentrates are maintained at temperatures about 20 and 24 C during shipment. A well-insulated container without added ice is often sufficient. If outdoor temperatures are extreme and the distance is great, these components should not be shipped in luggage or freight compartments without heating or air conditioning (depending on the time of year). If outdoor temperatures are extremely high, special chemical coolant pouches are available that may be shipped with the components and will maintain temperatures of approximately 20 to 24 C for up to 12 hours. Also available are containers with a power source that maintain temperatures between 20 and 24 C.

Special Considerations

Thawing Fresh Frozen Plasma for Transfusion

Fresh Frozen Plasma must be thawed with agitation in a waterbath at temperatures between 30 and 37 C. It is important to prevent water from contaminating the entry port.[31] This can be accomplished by wrapping the container in a plastic overwrap, or by maintaining the container in an upright position with entry ports above the water level. *Standards* requires that thawed Fresh Frozen Plasma used for correction of labile coagulation factor deficiencies be stored at 1 to 6 C and be infused within 24 hours after thawing. The FDA requires infusion within 6 hours after thawing, if intended for correction of these deficiencies. Fresh Frozen Plasma unused within the allowable time after thawing should not be used to correct deficiencies of labile coagulation factors, but may be stored and infused as Single Donor Plasma.

Reconstituting and Pooling Cryoprecipitate

Cryoprecipitate should be rapidly thawed at 30 to 37 C.

1. Cover the container with a plastic overwrap to prevent contaminating the ports with unsterile water, or use a device to keep the containers upright with the ports above water. Specially designed dry air heat equipment may be used.
2. Resuspend the thawed precipitate carefully and completely, either by kneading it into the residual 10 to 15 ml of plasma, or by adding approximately 10 ml of 0.9% sodium chloride USP and gently resuspending.
3. Pool the cryoprecipitates by inserting a medication injection site into a port of each bag. Aspirate contents of one bag into a syringe and inject into the next bag. Use the ever-increasing volume to flush each subsequent bag of as much dissolved cryoprecipitate as possible until all contents are in final bag.
4. Maintain reconstituted cryoprecipitate at room temperature until transfusion. Storage in the refrigerator may cause reprecipitation of the concentrated Factor VIII. Cryoprecipitate must be administered within 6 hours of thawing and 4 hours of pooling. Pools made from thawed individual units may not be refrozen.

Handling Donor Units

Blood should not remain at room temperature unnecessarily. It is desirable to monitor routine handling procedures to ensure that personnel do not keep blood out of the refrigerator too long. When units are removed from the refrigerator for testing or labeling, a fluid-filled container with a thermometer may be removed from the blood refrigerator along with the units to be labeled. The temperature in this container should be observed, and if it rises to near 6 C, the blood should be returned to the refrigerator without delay.

When blood is issued for transfusion, it should not be allowed to remain unnecessarily at room temperature. Delayed delivery to the patient, delayed arrival of equipment or personnel to begin transfusion and delays during infusion are all undesirable. Transfusion therapy teams trained in handling and infusing blood and components have been effective in reducing mishandling of donor blood.

Labels

The following information is required in clear, readable letters on a label firmly attached to all blood and blood component containers:

1. The proper name of the component, in a prominent position
2. The identification of the blood bank that collected the blood and/or prepared the component; if FDA-licensed, its license number. For components, the label must include the identification of all facilities performing any part of component preparation.
3. The unit number relating the unit to the donor
4. The expiration date, including the date and year, and where applicable, the hour
5. Recommended storage temperature
6. Reference to an instruction circular that shall be available for distribution, containing dosage information, adequate directions for use, route of administration, contraindications and other directions if component is not intended for further manufacturing
7. For platelet concentrate, plasma and components prepared by hemapheresis, quantity of component in container, which shall be accurate within ±10%, except that the quantity of cryoprecipitate need not be stated on the label
8. The amount of blood collected and the kind and quantity of anticoagulant, except for components prepared by hemapheresis.
9. Additives and cryoprotective agents added to the component that may still be present in the component
10. Results of all tests performed when necessary for safe and effective use
11. A reminder to identify properly the intended recipient
12. The appropriate donor classification statement, "paid donor," or "volunteer donor," in no less prominence than the proper name of the compo-

nent, is required by the FDA (CFR 606.120b). This is not required by the AABB.

Records

Records must be made concurrently with each step of component preparation, must be legible and indelible, must identify the person immediately responsible, must include dates of various steps and must be as detailed as necessary for clear understanding. For specific records to be kept for each component, see Chapter 21.

Component Preparation Procedures

Red Blood Cells

1. Collect blood in a collection unit with integrally attached transfer container(s).
2. Centrifuge at "heavy" spin, with a temperature setting of 5 C. If red cells have sedimented, centrifugation is not necessary.
3. Place the primary bag containing centrifuged or sedimented blood on a plasma expressor, and release the spring, allowing the plate of the expressor to contact the bag.
4. Clamp the tubing between the primary and satellite bags with a hemostat, or, if a mechanical sealer will not be used, make a loose overhand knot in the tubing.
5. If two or more satellite bags are attached, apply the hemostat to allow plasma to flow into only one of the satellite bags. Penetrate the closure of the primary bag. A scale, such as a dietary scale, may be used to measure the expressed plasma. The removal of 232-258 g (225-250 ml) of plasma will generally result in residual red cells with a hematocrit between 70 and 80%.
6. Reapply the hemostat when the desired amount of supernatant plasma has entered the satellite bag. Seal the tub-

ing between the primary bag and the satellite bag in two places.

7. Check that the satellite bag has the same donor number as that on the primary bag and cut the tubing between the two seals.

If blood is collected in a single bag, modify the above directions as follows: after placing the bag on the expressor, apply a hemostat to the tubing of a sterile transfer bag, aseptically insert the cannula of the transfer bag into the outlet port of the bag of blood, release the hemostat and continue as outlined above.

Leukocyte-Poor Red Blood Cells

Inverted Centrifugation

1. Collect blood in a collection unit with integrally attached transfer containers.
2. Centrifuge the blood bag upside down in a refrigerated centrifuge at 5 C using a "heavy" spin. (See Special Methods, page 469.)
3. Hang the centrifuged, inverted bag on a ring stand or inverted plasma expressor. Allow the bag to hang undisturbed for several minutes.
4. Affix the donor number to the transfer bag and place the transfer bag on a scale below the blood bag. Adjust the scale to zero to obtain the tare weight of the final product.
5. Penetrate the closure of the primary bag, avoiding agitation of the contents and allow red cells to flow to the transfer bag.

Note: At least 70% of the red cells must be transferred to the transfer bag. Calculate the amount of red cells to be expressed by multiplying the amount of blood (excluding anticoagulant) in the bag by the donor's hematocrit (assume 40% for females and 43% for males) and ignore the weight of the plasma that may be trapped with the red cells.

Example:

450 ml of blood in bag × 0.40 (hematocrit of donor) = 180 ml RBC

180 ml of RBC in bag × 0.70 (minimum % of RBC to be transferred) = 126 ml

126 ml of RBC to be transferred × 1.08 (weight in g of 1 ml RBC) = 136 g

136 g = minimum weight of RBC to be transferred

6. Label the separated component "Red Blood Cells Leukocytes Removed by Centrifugation." If the hermetic seal was broken the unit expires in 24 hours; if prepared in a closed system, the component has the same expiration date as the Whole Blood from which it was prepared. Since the hematocrit is higher than in Red Blood Cells prepared by simple upright centrifugation, sufficient plasma should be returned to the red cells to achieve an 80% or lower hematocrit if the unit will be stored. If plasma is not added, it is desirable to transfuse this component as soon as possible.
7. Write on the transfer bag the volume in ml. Seal the tubing in two places. Cut between the two seals.

Double Centrifugation

1. Collect blood in a quadruple-collection unit. The blood must not be refrigerated if platelets are to be harvested.
2. Affix donor number to each transfer bag. Remove the platelet-rich plasma by an initial "light" spin (see Special Methods section, page 469); platelet-rich plasma can be further processed to a platelet concentrate and single donor plasma or fresh frozen plasma (see pages 55 and 57).
3. Detach bag containing platelet-rich plasma and one satellite bag from the collection bag, leaving one satellite bag attached.
4. Centrifuge the red cells in the inverted position (see previous procedure), using a "heavy" spin.
5. Harvest the lower 70-80% of the inverted-spun red cells as a leukocyte-poor unit.

Saline Dilution and Centrifugation

1. Dilute the red blood cells by allowing approximately 300 ml of 0.9% saline

USP to run from a collapsible plastic bag into the blood bag. Do not detach the now-empty saline bag.

2. Mix the red cells and saline, and centrifuge upright at approximately 5000 g for 5 minutes.

3. Express the supernatant fluid, the buffy coat and the top 10-20 ml of red cells back into the saline bag.

4. Seal the transfer tubing and discard the contents of the saline wash bag.

5. Refrigerate the leukocyte-poor red cells at 1 to 6 C until they are transfused; as they have been prepared in an open system, they must be transfused within 24 hours.

Washed Red Blood Cells, Manual Method

1. Collect blood in a collection unit with integrally attached transfer container(s).

2. Centrifuge the blood in a refrigerated centrifuge at 1 to 6 C using a "light" spin (see Special Methods section, page 469).

3. Express the plasma and buffy coat into the transfer bag. Seal the tubing and remove transfer bag. Salvage the plasma as fresh frozen or single donor plasma.

4. Place a temporary clamp on a plasma-transfer set. Insert one end of the set into the injection site of a 250-ml container of sterile, cold (1 to 6 C) 0.9% saline USP. Insert the other end into one of the outlet ports of the primary blood bag.

5. Drain the saline to the blood bag. Place a temporary clamp on the tubing. Remove the cannula from the saline container; replace the cannula's original plastic cover. Cover the exposed injection site of the saline container with sterile gauze. Bind the transfer set tubing to the outside of the primary bag with tape; be sure the cannula is in a vertical position at the top of the bag to prevent leakage or damage to the bag.

6. Resuspend the red cells in the saline and mix thoroughly. Centrifuge again at 1 to 6 C, this time using a "heavy" spin.

7. Place the blood bag on the expressor and carefully release the taped cannula. Insert the cannula of the transfer tubing into the injection site of the empty saline bag. Express the saline and residual buffy coat into the empty container.

8. Remove the cannula from the used saline container when only red cells remain in the blood bag and insert it into another 250-ml container of cold, sterile saline. Discard the first saline container.

9. Repeat steps 4 through 8 until the red cells have been washed a total of three times. Do not remove the cannula from the primary bag after the last wash.

10. Seal the tubing close to the blood bag, separate and discard the saline container.

11. Change the expiration date on the red cell container to 24 hours from the time the unit was entered. Store the washed red cells at 1 to 6 C until transfused.

Fresh Frozen Plasma

1. Collect blood in a collection unit with integrally attached transfer container(s).

2. Centrifuge blood at 1 to 6 C using a "heavy" spin within 6 hours after collection.

3. Place primary bag containing centrifuged blood on a plasma expressor and place the attached satellite bag on a dietary scale adjusted to zero. Express the plasma into the satellite bag and weigh the plasma.

4. Seal the transfer tubing with a dielectric sealer or metal clips, but do not obliterate the segment numbers of the tubing. Place another seal nearer the transfer bag.

5. Label the transfer bag with the unit number prior to separation from the

original container and record volume of plasma on the label.

6. Cut the tubing between the two seals. The tubing may be coiled and taped against the plasma container; the segments are then available for reverse grouping or other tests, if desired.

7. Place plasma at −18 C or lower within 6 hours of collection of the unit of whole blood.

Cryoprecipitated AHF

1. Collect blood in a collection unit with two integrally attached transfer containers.

2. Centrifuge blood at 1 to 6 C using a "heavy" spin. Separate plasma from the red blood cells within 6 hours of phlebotomy. Collect at least 200 ml (206 g) of cell-free plasma for processing into cryoprecipitate.

3. Place plasma at −18 C or lower within 6 hours of phlebotomy. The plasma should become solidly frozen within 1 hour of the time freezing was initiated. Suitable freezing devices include blast freezers or mechanical freezers capable of maintaining temperatures of −65 C or below, dry ice or an ethanol-dry ice bath. In a bath of 95% ethanol and chipped dry ice, freezing will be complete in about 15 minutes. Plasma containers immersed in liquid must be protected with a plastic overwrap. Frozen plasma for cryoprecipitate preparation may be stored for up to 12 months at −18 C or lower, preferably −30 C or lower. The cryoprecipitate may be prepared at any time during these 12 months, but the expiration date of the cryoprecipitate is 12 months from the date the whole blood was collected.

4. Allow the plasma to thaw at 1 to 6 C by placing the bag in a 4 C shaking waterbath[32] or in a refrigerator. If thawed in a waterbath, use a plastic overwrap (or other means) to keep container ports dry.

5. When the plasma has a slushy consistency, follow either step below:

a. Centrifuge the plasma at 1 to 6 C using a "heavy" spin. Hang the bag in an inverted position and allow the supernatant plasma to flow rapidly into the transfer bag, leaving the cryoprecipitate adhering to the sides of the primary bag. Ten to 15 ml of supernatant plasma may be left in the bag to resuspend the cryoprecipitate after thawing. Separate promptly to prevent the cryoprecipitate from redissolving and flowing out of the bag, and then refreeze immediately.

b. Place the thawing plasma in a plasma expressor when approximately one tenth of the contents is still frozen. With the bag in an upright position, allow the supernatant plasma to flow slowly into the transfer bag, using the ice crystals at the top as a filter. The cryoprecipitate paste will adhere to the sides of the bag or to the ice. Seal the bag when about 90% of the cryoprecipitate-poor plasma has been removed and refreeze the cryoprecipitate immediately.

6. Store cryoprecipitate at −18 C or lower, preferably −30 C or lower, for up to 12 months from the date of blood collection.

Whole Blood Cryoprecipitate Removed

1. Collect blood in a collection unit with integrally attached transfer container(s) and centrifuge the freshly drawn whole blood to prepare fresh frozen plasma as outlined on page 55.

2. Express the plasma into the transfer bag and temporarily clamp the tubing between the transfer bag and the primary bag.

3. Freeze the plasma so that the frozen plasma unit does not come into contact with the red cells, which must be kept at 1 to 6 C.

4. Thaw the plasma at 4 C in a shaking waterbath or in a 1 to 6 C refrigerator.

5. Centrifuge both bags using a "heavy" spin to separate cryoprecipitate from plasma. Open the temporary closure between the bags and express the supernatant plasma back into the red cells in the primary container.
6. Seal the tubing twice and cut between the seals to separate the two bags.
7. Immediately refreeze the cryoprecipitate and refrigerate the whole blood at 1 to 6 C.

Platelets

1. Collect blood in a collection unit with two integrally attached transfer container(s). The transfer containers may be polyvinyl chloride bags for 72-hour platelet storage or the plastics approved for 5- or 7-day platelet storage. Keep blood at room temperature (about 20 to 24 C) before separating the platelet-rich plasma from the red blood cells. This separation must take place within 6 hours after collection of the whole blood.
2. Do not chill the blood at any time before or during platelet separation. If the temperature of the centrifuge is at 1 to 6 C, set the temperature control of the refrigerated centrifuge at 20 C and allow the temperature to rise to approximately 20 C. Centrifuge the blood using a "light" spin (see Special Methods, page 469).
3. Express the supernatant platelet-rich plasma into the transfer bag intended for platelet storage. Seal the tubing twice between the primary bag and Y connector of the two satellite bags and cut between the two seals. Refrigerate the red cells at 1 to 6 C.
4. Centrifuge the platelet-rich plasma at 20 C using a "heavy" spin.
5. Express the supernatant platelet-poor plasma into the second transfer bag and seal the tubing. Some plasma should remain on the platelet button for storage, but the exact volume is not specified. *Standards* requires that sufficient plasma remain with the platelet con-

centrate to maintain the pH at 6.0 or higher for the entire storage period, in all the units tested. This usually requires a minimum of 30 ml of plasma when storage is at 20 to 24 C, but 50 to 70 ml may be preferable. The platelet-poor plasma may be frozen promptly and stored as Fresh Frozen Plasma, if the separation is completed and freezing initiated with 6 hours of collection of the blood. The volume of Fresh Frozen Plasma prepared after platelet preparation will be substantially less than that prepared from Whole Blood or after preparing Cryoprecipitated AHF.

Resuspension of Platelet Concentrates

At no time should the Platelet Concentrate be roughly agitated because this may cause platelets to aggregate irreversibly. The container should be left stationary at room temperature (20 to 24 C) for approximately 1 hour. The platelet button may then be resuspended in either of two ways:
1. Manipulate the platelet container gently by hand to allow uniform resuspension.
2. Place the container on a rotator at 20 to 24 C, permitting gentle agitation until the platelets are uniformly resuspended. This may take up to 2 hours.

References

1. Gibson JG, Gregory CB, Button LN. Citrate-phosphate-dextrose solutions for preservation of human blood: a further report. Transfusion 1961;1:280-287.
2. Gibson JG, Rees SB, McManus TJ, Scheitlin WA. A citrate-phosphate-dextrose solution for preservation of human blood. Am J Clin Pathol 1957;28:569-578.
3. Bailey DN, Bove JR. Chemical and hematological changes in stored CPD blood. Transfusion 1975;15:244-249.
4. Dawson RB, Kocholaty WF, Gray JL. Hemoglobin function and 2,3-DPG levels of blood stored at 4 C in ACD and CPD, pH effect. Transfusion 1970;10:299-304.
5. Valeri CR. Viability and function of preserved red cells. N Engl J Med 1971;284:81-88.

6. Bowman HS. Red cell preservation in citrate-phosphate-dextrose and in acid-citrate-dextrose. Transfusion 1963;3:364-367.

7. Huestis DW, Bove JR, Busch S. Practical blood transfusion. 3rd edition. Little, Brown and Company, 1981.

8. Simon ER. Adenine in blood banking. Transfusion 1977;17:317-325.

9. Akerblom OCH, Kreuger A. Studies on citrate-phosphate-dextrose (CPD) blood supplemented with adenine. Vox Sang 1975;29:90-100.

10. Beutler E, Wood L. The in vivo regeneration of red cell 2,3-diphosphoglyceric acid (DPG) after transfusion of stored blood. J Lab Clin Med 1969;74:300-304.

11. Valeri CR, Zaroulis CG, Vecchione JJ, et al. Therapeutic effectiveness and safety of outdated human red blood cells rejuvenated to restore oxygen transport function to normal, frozen for 3 to 4 years at −80 C, washed, and stored at 4 C for 24 hours prior to rapid infusion. Transfusion 1980;20:159-170.

12. Beutler E, West C. The storage of hard-packed red blood cells in citrate-phosphate-dextrose (CPD) and CPD-adenine (CPDA-1). Blood 1979;54:280-284.

13. Perkins HA, Payne R, Ferguson J, Wood M. Nonhemolytic febrile transfusion reactions: quantitative effects of blood components with emphasis on isoantigenic incompatibility of leukocytes. Vox Sang 1966;11:578-600.

14. Meryman H, Bross J, Lebovits R. The preparation of leukocyte-poor red blood cells: a comparative study. Transfusion 1980;20:285-292.

15. Miller WV, Wilson MJ, Kalb HJ. Simple methods for production of HL-A antigen poor red blood cells. Transfusion 1973;13:189-193.

16. Wenz B, Gurtlinger K, O'Toole A, Dugan E. Leukocyte-poor red blood cells prepared by microaggregate blood filtration (MABF), (abstract). Transfusion 1979;19:645.

17. Schmidt PJ, ed. Standards for blood banks and transfusion services. 11th ed. Arlington, VA: American Association of Blood Banks, 1984.

18. Goldfinger D, Lowe C. Prevention of adverse reactions to blood transfusion by the administration of saline-washed red blood cells. Transfusion 1981; 21:277-280.

19. Propper RD, Button LN, Nathan DG. New approaches to the transfusion management of thalassemia. Blood 1980;55:55-60.

20. Corash L, Klein H, Deisseroth A, et al. Selective isolation of young erythrocytes for transfusion support of thalassemia major patients. Blood 1981;57:599-606.

21. Graziano JH, Piomelli S, Seaman C, et al. A simple technique for preparation of young red cells for transfusion from ordinary blood units. Blood 1982;59:865-868.

22. Burka ER, Harker LA, Kasper CK, Kevy SV, Ness PM. A protocol for cryoprecipitate production. Transfusion 1975;15:307-311.

23. Weinstein M, Deykin D. Comparison of Factor VIII-related von Willebrand Factor proteins prepared from human cryoprecipitate and Factor VIII concentrate. Blood 1979;53:1095-1105.

24. Ness PM, Perkins HA. Cryoprecipitate as a reliable source of fibrinogen replacement. JAMA 1979;241:1690-1691.

25. Snyder EL, Ferri PM, Mosher DF. Fibronectin in liquid and frozen stored blood components. Transfusion 1984;24:53-56.

26. Stuart MJ, Murphy S, Oski FA, Evans AE, Donaldson MH, Gardner FH. Platelet function in recipients of platelets from donors ingesting aspirin. N Engl J Med 1972;287:1105-1109.

27. McCullough J, Weiblen BJ, Fine D. Effects of storage of granulocytes on their fate in vivo. Transfusion 1983;23:20-24.

28. Slichter SJ. Controversies in platelet transfusion therapy. Ann Rev Med 1980;31:509-540.

29. Snyder EL, Koerner TAW Jr, Kakaiya R, Moore P, Kiraly T. Effect of mode of agitation on storage of platelet concentrates in PL-732 containers for 5 days. Vox Sang 1983;44:300-304.

30. Snyder EL, Bookbinder M, Kakaiya R, Ferri P, Kiraly T. 5-Day storage of platelet concentrates in CLX containers: effect of type of agitation. Vox Sang 1983;45:432-437.

31. Rhame FS, McCullough J. Hospital Infections Br, Bacterial Diseases Div, Bur of Epidemiology, CDC. Nocosomial *Pseudomonas cepacia* infection. Morbidity and Mortality Weekly Report. Center for Disease Control 1979; Vol 28-No 25.

32. Slichter SJ, Counts RB, Henderson R, Harker LA. Preparation of cryoprecipitated Factor VIII concentrates. Transfusion 1976;16:616-625.

Suggested Reading

- A seminar on blood components: E unum pluribus. Washington, DC: American Association of Blood Banks, 1977.
- Blood, blood components and derivatives in transfusion therapy. Washington, DC: American Association of Blood Banks, 1980.
- Blood storage and preservation. Arlington, VA: American Association of Blood Banks, 1982.

4

Cryopreservation of Blood and Tissue

Cryobiology is the study of the effects of subfreezing temperatures on biological systems. The application of this scientific discipline to cellular preservation began in 1949 with the freezing and recovery of live fowl sperm, using glycerol as a cryoprotectant.[1] In 1950, glycerol techniques were applied to the freezing of red blood cells.[2]

Cold Injury and Cryoprotective Agents

Meryman has suggested[3] that cell injury occurring during the freeze-thaw process results from: 1) cellular dehydration and 2) mechanical trauma caused by the formation and growth of intracellular ice crystals. As shown in Fig 4-1, extracellular water freezes earlier than intracellular water, at rates of freezing slower than 10 C/min, causing an osmotic gradient such that water diffuses from inside the cell to outside the cell. The cell loses volume and becomes dehydrated. Moderate to severe dehydration causes significant cell injury.

At more rapid rates of freezing, more than 10 C/min, extracellular and intracellular ice formation occur at a comparable pace. Since the osmotic gradient has almost no time to develop, there is minimal dehydration and volume reduction. The problem with rapid freezing is spontaneous intracellular formation of ice crystals, which

damage the cells from within. With slower rates of freezing, the intracellular environment is hypertonic and ice crystals do not form.

The ideal is to find a cooling rate just less than that which causes intracellular freezing. At this ideal cooling rate, enough water leaves the cell to produce mild intracellular hypertonicity and retard intracellular ice formation, but not so much as to cause significant dehydration. Cryoprotective agents prevent severe freezing injury by altering the tonicity of the cell and, therefore, its freezing rate. Only two cryoprotective agents are in current clinical use—glycerol and dimethylsulfoxide (DMSO).[4]

Glycerol, a trihydric alcohol, is a clear, colorless, syrup-like fluid with a sweet taste. It is miscible with both water and alcohol. Pharmacologically, glycerol is relatively inert, and systemic effects from infusion are negligible except for the shifts in intracellular fluid that occur if improperly deglycerolized cells are exposed to circulating plasma. Dimethylsulfoxide (DMSO), a byproduct of petroleum distillation, is a colorless liquid with a sulfur-like smell. It is highly polar and dissolves many water- and lipid-soluble substances. DMSO given intravenously may cause nausea, vomiting, local vasospasm and an objectionable garlic-like odor and taste.

4

59

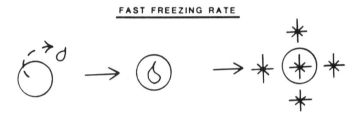

Large amounts of water leave cell, causing dehydration injury.

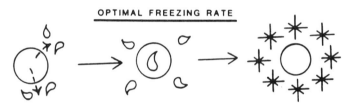

Little water leaves cell allowing for intracellular ice formation.

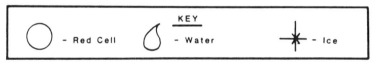

Only part of water leaves cell resulting in minimal dehydration injury and retarded intracellular ice formation.

Figure 4-1. Illustration of effects of varied freezing rates. (Modified from Meryman.[3])

Freezing Red Cells

Previously frozen deglycerolized red cells were first successfully transfused in 1951.[5] Frozen cells did not become clinically useful until the 1960s, after the development of effective techniques for removing glycerol. Several mechanical devices for deglycerolization are now available.[6] Preparation of frozen cells fits easily into component preparation programs. It is possible to obtain both platelets and fresh plasma from a donor unit, and then freeze the red cells. Frozen preservation of red cells is particularly advantageous for stockpiling rare blood types and for autologous transfusion. It is less useful in inventory management because the cost is

high and because the thawed, deglycerolized red blood cells have only a 24 hour
shelf-life.

Processing Methods

There are three basic methods that have
been used to freeze red blood cells, as
shown in Table 4-1. This chapter will discuss in detail only the high-concentration
glycerol technique, which is used by the
great majority of centers that freeze red
cells. The manufacturer of each instrument provides detailed instructions for
using the instrument. Because so many
technical variations exist, it is inappropriate to give step-by-step directions, so
only general comments about glycerolizing, freezing, storing, thawing and deglycerolizing will be given. For a detailed discussion of additional techniques of red cell
freezing, the reader should consult these
American Association of Blood Banks

publications: *Red Cell Freezing* (1973) and
*Clinical and Practical Aspects of the Use of
Frozen Blood* (1977).

Preparing Red Cells for Glycerolization

Blood for subsequent freezing can be collected in CPD or CPDA-1 and stored as
whole blood or red blood cells for up to 6
days before glycerolizing.[11] Following
rejuvenation (see page 41), red cells can
be frozen at a time several days after their
expiration date.

Glycerol is used for freezing in concentrations hypertonic to blood, and its rapid
introduction can cause damage to red blood
cells. This damage becomes manifest as
hemolysis only after thawing. Glycerol and
red blood cells should be well mixed as
they are transferred into the storage container. The 6.2M glycerol should be added

Table 4-1. Comparison of the Three Basic Methods of Red Blood Cell Freezing

Consideration	High Glycerol	Agglomeration[7]	Low Glycerol[8,9,10]
Final glycerol concentration (w/v)	Approx. 40%	Approx. 40%	Approx. 20%
Initial freezing temperature	−80 C	−80 C	−196 C
Freezing rate	Slow	Slow	Rapid
Freezing rate control	No	No	Yes
Type of freezer	Mechanical	Mechanical	Liquid nitrogen
Storage temperature (maximum)	−65 C	−65 C	−120 C
Change in storage temperature	Can be thawed and refrozen	Cannot be refrozen	Critical
Type of storage container	Polyvinyl chloride; polyolefin	Polyvinyl chloride	Polyolefin
Shipping	Dry ice	Dry ice	Liquid nitrogen
Special deglycerolizing equipment required	Yes	No	No
Deglycerolizing time (minutes)	20–40	35	30
Hematocrit (%)	55–70	85	50–70
WBC removed (%)	94–99	70	95

in two stages to allow full equilibration[12,13]; in the widely used high glycerol technique, the final glycerol concentration of 40% w/v. For standard units of red cells, approximately 100 ml of glycerol is added while the red blood cells are agitated. After at least five minutes for equilibration, the remaining 300 ml of glycerol is added.[11,12,13] Smaller volumes of glycerol should be used for smaller volumes of red blood cells.[11] Low temperatures delay diffusion of glycerol into the cells; the glycerol solution and red blood cells should be at room temperature or warmed to 30 or 32 C. Maintenance of these temperatures, careful mixing and slow stepwise addition of glycerol permit glycerolization without red cell damage or excessive hemolysis after storage and thawing.

Freezing and Storage
Storage Containers

There is some evidence that the composition of the storage container may be important in minimizing hemolysis.[11] For reasons not clearly understood, less hemolysis occurs with freezing in polyolefin containers than in polyvinyl chloride.[9] Red cells in contact with the container surface seem to sustain some injury that does not affect cells in the central portions. These differences in hemolysis are not large. Although polyvinyl chloride containers have given satisfactory results for freezing red cells in a high concentration of glycerol, polyolefin bags are currently more popular for the high glycerol method, since they are less brittle at − 80 C and can be handled and shipped with less likelihood of breakage.

Freezing Conditions

Red cells with a final glycerol concentration of 40% may be stored at temperatures of − 65 C or colder, in containers made of either polyvinyl chloride or polyolefin. Either kind of container may crack if bumped or handled roughly when frozen, and glycerolized red cells are usually placed

in cardboard or metal canisters for protection during freezing, storage and thawing. Up to 18 hours can elapse between glycerolizing and freezing without increased postthaw hemolysis,[9] and the rate at which freezing occurs is not critical.

No controlled studies exist that establish a maximum storage time for red cells kept at − 65 C or colder. Many units stored 10 years or longer have been transfused successfully.[6] The Office of Biologics and AABB *Standards* limit frozen storage of blood for routine use to 3 years. For blood of rare phenotypes, a facility's medical director may wish to extend the storage period. The medical director should document and record the unusual nature of such units and the reason for retaining them past the 3-year storage period prescribed for routine use.

Thawing and Deglycerolizing

Frozen red cells, in their protective canister, may be placed in either a 37 C waterbath or 37 C dry warmer. Gentle agitation in the waterbath may be used to speed thawing. The thawing process takes at least 10 minutes. Glycerol must be properly removed from thawed cells to avoid in vivo and/or in vitro hemolysis. The intracellular environment of glycerolized cells is hypertonic relative to plasma and the first solution used for deglycerolization must also be somewhat hypertonic. This allows the glycerol to begin diffusing out of the red cell while the intracellular environment remains hypertonic.

The three basic deglycerolization procedures—high glycerol, low glycerol, and agglomeration—use different hypertonic solutions and wash protocols, but the principle is the same: equilibration of the thawed red cells with a hypertonic solution, followed by washing with solutions progressively less hypertonic and final suspension of red cells in an isotonic electrolyte solution containing glucose.

Any of the commercially available instruments for semiautomated or batch washing can be used to deglycerolize cells frozen in high concentration glycerol. The thawed unit is first diluted with a quantity of 12% sodium chloride solution appropriate for the size of the unit and is allowed to equilibrate for approximately 5 minutes. This initial dilution is followed by washing with less hypertonic sodium chloride until deglycerolization is complete. Approximately 3 liters of wash solution are required. The cells are finally suspended in an isotonic solution of 0.9% NaCl with 0.2% dextrose. The dextrose provides nutrition for the cells, which have been reported to retain satisfactory posttransfusion viability and slightly increased oxygen affinity when stored for as long as 4 days at 1 to 6 C.[13]

Because there are so many small but potentially important variations in deglycerolization protocols for each instrument, the reader should follow individual manufacturers' specific recommendations.

Red Cells with Hemoglobin S

Red blood cells from persons with sickle trait tolerate glycerolizing, freezing and thawing normally but form a jelly-like mass and hemolyze during deglycerolization. In many cryopreservation programs, cells are screened for the presence of hemoglobin S before freezing is undertaken, but there may be occasions when cells from sickle trait donors must be frozen, especially for autologous transfusions. The hypertonic deglycerolizing solutions appear to cause sedimentation of the abnormal red cells, such that glycerol is not adequately removed from the packed red cells which then hemolyze when suspended in normal saline. Satisfactory deglycerolization can be achieved if the thawed red cells are massively diluted with 0.2% dextrose in 0.9% sodium chloride after equilibration with 12% sodium chloride and the hypertonic washing solution is omitted.[19] Deglycerolizing a unit of frozen sickle trait cells requires intensive technical attendance and the manual operation of the cell washer, with more washes than are necessary for normal cells.

Storing Deglycerolized Red Cells

Because deglycerolizing requires entering the container, it is considered an "open" system. Deglycerolized red blood cells can be stored for only 24 hours at 1 to 6 C. A longer postthaw shelf-life would make frozen red blood cells more useful for inventory management. Efforts are being made to develop sterile connector devices so that tubing connections can be made without bacterial contamination. Even with presently available systems, however, bacterial growth in deglycerolized red blood cells is very rare.[14] The deglycerolizing process reduces the number of organisms present, and those remaining grow very slowly during refrigerated storage for up to 72 hours. When deglycerolized red cells are stored up to 5 days, the most important change that occurs is increased concentration of potassium and hemoglobin in the supernatant fluid, which can easily be removed just before transfusion.

Refreezing Deglycerolized Red Cells

It may occasionally be desirable to refreeze thawed units of red cells, either after unintentional thawing or after deglycerolization of units that are not used. One study of cells frozen with the high glycerol method showed there was no loss of ATP, 2,3-DPG, or in vivo survival in units deglycerolized, stored 20 hours at refrigerator temperature, and then reglycerolized and refrozen.[15] In a different study,[16] units of red cells subjected three times to glycerolizing, freezing and thawing exhibited 27% loss of total hemoglobin. *Standards* does not address refreezing thawed units, since this should not be considered routinely desirable practice. To avoid losing units of high-priority blood, a responsible physician in a blood bank who decides to refreeze thawed units should document the valuable nature of such units and the reasons for refreezing them.

Transportability

Red cells that are freeze-preserved with high concentrations of glycerol tolerate fluctuations in temperature from -85 to -65 C without any significant effects on in vitro recovery or 24-hour posttransfusion survival.[6] These red blood cells can be transported on dry ice.

Quality Assurance

Freezers

All centrifuges, freezers, refrigerators and waterbaths involved in freeze-preservation should be part of the regular laboratory quality assurance program. The freezer for storing the red blood cells must have a continuous temperature recorder and at least an audible alarm. Placing the sensors for the recorder and the alarm near the door gives the greatest sensitivity in registering temperature fluctuations. Placement of thermometers in freezers is important. Mechanical freezers are designed to maintain the temperature at -85 C near the wall, but temperatures near the top may be much warmer. Small variations are not dangerous,[6] but the temperature throughout the freezer must be no warmer than -65 C. In addition to the sensor for the continuous recorder, there should be visual thermometers near the top and middle of the freezer.

Deglycerolized Cells

AABB *Standards* requires that methods used for freezing and deglycerolizing red cells be sufficient to ensure ". . . recovery of at least 80% of the original red blood cells following the deglycerolization process, [and] viability of at least 70% of the transfused cells 24 hours after transfusion. . . " If accepted methods are followed, individual centers need not repeat these tests. In centers where locally modified procedures are used, there must be documentation that these standards are met. It is especially cumbersome for each blood bank to determine posttransfusion

survival, since ^{51}Cr labeled red cell studies would be the optimum method to use.

Red Cell Recovery

Quality assurance programs should include regularly scheduled monitoring of red cell recovery and acceptable glycerol removal. The percent of red cell recovery can be calculated by using the following formula:

% red cell recovery =

$$\frac{\text{weight (g) of deglycerolized RBC}}{\text{weight (g) of RBC to be frozen}}$$

To determine the weight of red blood cells to be frozen, the weight of the red blood cell container is subtracted from the gross weight of the bag plus the red cell component before glycerolization. This net weight is then multiplied by the measured hematocrit of the red cell component. In order to prevent glycerol dilution, many technologists prefer to "hyperpack" the red cells prior to freezing, yielding a hematocrit of approximately 90%. To determine the weight of the deglycerolized red blood cells, the weight of the red blood cell container is subtracted from the gross weight of the bag plus the cells. This net weight is then multiplied by the measured hematocrit of the cells in the bag.

Glycerol Removal

Although adequate glycerol removal is important for satisfactory posttransfusion survival, it is not customary to measure directly the glycerol in deglycerolized red cell preparations. The adequacy of deglycerolization can be determined by: 1) measuring the osmolality of the deglycerolized unit, since glycerol is hyperosmolar; 2) carrying out a "simulated transfusion"; or 3) using a refractometer.

Osmolality of the deglycerolized unit can be measured with an osmometer. Normal serum osmolality is 280 mOsm. A glycerol content of 1% produces osmolality of approximately 420 mOsm.[17] Deglycerolized units with osmolality up to 500 mOsm apparently can be transfused without hemolysis,[18] and the maximum permissible osmolality for deglycerolized red blood cells should be 420 to 500 mOsm. If the osmolality is greater than 500 mOsm, a new specimen from the deglycerolized unit should be centrifuged and the osmolality of the supernatant measured. If the osmolality is again greater than 500 mOsm, the red cells should be washed with an additional liter of the final wash solution.

Glycerol removal can also be evaluated by a simulated transfusion[17] as follows:

1. Add 0.5 ml of deglycerolized red cells to 10 ml of normal saline.
2. Mix well and centrifuge for 1 minute at 1000 rcf.
3. Estimate level of hemolysis by comparing the specimen with a known control or by comparison with a commercially available color comparator. There should be no more than 3% hemolysis.

A screening method for osmolality uses a refractometer. Readings up to 28 correlate with glycerol levels below 1%. Readings above 28 indicate the need for more accurate measurement of osmolality, using an osmometer.[18]

Hemolysis

Hemolysis in the deglycerolized cell suspension indicates red cell damage someplace in the process. If extensive cell damage has occurred during freezing, thawing or deglycerolization, free hemoglobin will be visible in the last wash solution or in the supernatant of the resuspended cells. After deglycerolization of every unit, the color of the last wash or the supernatant should be inspected. If measured, the free hemoglobin in the last wash should be less than 200 mg/dl. Measuring supernatant hemoglobin is not an index of glycerol removal. It is an optional procedure less significant than determining osmolality or performing the simulated transfusion. However, the presence of excessive free hemoglobin occasionally indicates that the donor cells had some biologic abnormality, such as spherocytosis or abnormal hemoglobin.

Summary

A practical quality assurance program for deglycerolized red blood cells might include surveillance of all units by:

1. Measurement of volume of the deglycerolized unit
2. Observation of last wash solution for visible free hemoglobin
3. Observation of supernatant fluid for visible free hemoglobin, or measurement of free hemoglobin

For selected units the following should be determined and recorded:

1. Hematocrit of the deglycerolized unit
2. Calculation of red cell mass of the deglycerolized unit
3. Measurement of osmolality or performance of a simulated transfusion

Determination of hematocrit, calculation of red cell mass and measurement of osmolality or simulated transfusion need not be done on every unit. The number of units tested more extensively should be based on the total number of units deglycerolized. For example, 1% of all units might be tested. If more than one type of instrument is used for deglycerolization, units selected for more extensive testing should be representative of all methods and instruments in use.

Clinical Considerations

Deglycerolized red cells are comparable in volume and hematocrit to a standard unit of red cells. Since virtually all the plasma and anticoagulant and most of the leukocytes and platelets have been removed, the deglycerolized unit consists essentially of red cells in an electrolyte solution. In vivo survival and function are comparable to freshly drawn, liquid-stored red cells because 2,3-DPG levels and oxygen dissociation curves are normal.

Biological Composition

The long storage life of frozen red cells is, in some circumstances, a significant advantage over liquid-stored red cells; their unique composition makes them potentially advantageous in certain clinical situations. Deglycerolized red blood cells have very little plasma protein and can be used for IgA-deficient patients with anti-IgA antibodies, or others with severe immune reactions to transfused plasma proteins. Most hematologists use deglycerolized red blood cells for patients with paroxysmal nocturnal hemoglobinuria because there is no complement in the resuspended deglycerolized cells. Since red cells are frozen either within 6 days of collection or after appropriate rejuvenation, 2,3-DPG levels are nearly normal in deglycerolized red cells. This may be advantageous when transfusing newborns.

Glycerolizing and deglycerolizing red cells removes granulocytes and platelets, but some lymphocytes survive. Transfusing deglycerolized red cells prevents reactions in patients with granulocyte or platelet antibodies, but other less costly blood products may be equally effective. Since some viable lymphocytes are present,[20] deglycerolized red blood cells could theoretically cause graft-versus-host disease in immunodeficient patients.

Disease Transmission

Many blood banking texts written before 1978 list decreased incidence of posttransfusion hepatitis as an advantage of frozen red cells. Alter et al[21] demonstrated in 1978 that human blood in which the plasma was seeded before freezing with hepatitis B virus could transmit the virus to chimpanzees after processing, freezing and deglycerolization. Deglycerolized red cells have also been shown[22] to transmit hepatitis B to human recipients.

Hepatitis B virus exists in plasma. Cytomegalovirus (CMV) is usually found in white cells. The use of frozen cells to prevent CMV transmission is under investigation. Most workers believe that potential CMV transmission is not a problem for most blood recipients,[23,24] but deglycerolized red cells may prove to have the same transfusion effects as units seronegative for CMV, when given to severely immunosuppressed recipients or low-birth-weight neonates.

Immunization to HLA Antigens

Deglycerolized red cells contain reduced numbers of elements that express HLA antigens—granulocytes, lymphocytes and platelets. Transfusing deglycerolized cells instead of whole blood reduces immunization to HLA antigens.[25] Frozen cells were initially indicated to reduce the risk of HLA immunization in dialysis patients awaiting a cadaveric kidney transplant, but transfusion of blood components that contain HLA-active material has now been shown to improve survival of transplanted kidneys.[26] Potential recipients of kidney transplants now receive unmodified red cells as the transfusion product of choice. Candidates for bone marrow transplants do not do well if immunization occurs, and should, preferably, receive no pretransplantation transfusions. If transfusion is absolutely necessary, frozen red cells would be the product of choice. Since lymphocytes responsive to phytohemagglutinin stimulation have been found in deglycerolized frozen red cells,[20] irradiation should be considered to prevent graft-versus-host disease in the severely immunosuppressed patient.

Freezing Other Cells

Platelets

For patients with diseases whose therapy will cause bone marrow ablation, alloimmunized patients in remission and patients with expected episodic needs for platelets, frozen storage of autologous platelets is highly desirable. Routine frozen storage of allogeneic platelets has not been considered practical.

Several cryoprotectants have been used to freeze platelets, but dimethylsulfoxide (DMSO) is the only agent in current use.[27] Transfusion of frozen-stored platelets is still considered experimental, but use of DMSO no longer requires filing for investigational new drug (IND) approval, and several medical centers have developed protocols for collecting, storing and transfusing cryopreserved autologous platelets.

Technique

Schiffer has reported[28,29] a technique in which platelets are frozen with DMSO at a final concentration of 5%. Platelets are collected by hemapheresis and then concentrated by centrifugation and resuspended in 50 ml of plasma. To this is added, slowly and at room temperature, 50 ml of autologous plasma containing 10% DMSO. The polyolefin bag containing the DMSO-platelet mixture is placed between two metal plates and put in the vapor phase of liquid nitrogen (-120 C), giving a freezing rate of about 10 C/min. The platelets remain viable for at least 3 years.[30]

Thawing is accomplished by placing the frozen platelets in a 37 C waterbath with agitation. A mixture of 10 ml of ACD and 100 ml of autologous plasma is added to the thawed platelets over 10-15 minutes. The suspension is centrifuged and the DMSO-containing supernatant is removed. The platelet button is resuspended in 50-100 ml of autologous plasma for infusion. This protocol causes platelet loss of between 15 and 22% and gives posttransfusion increments approximately 60% of those expected with fresh platelets.[28,29]

Granulocytes

Treating the severely granulocytopenic, septic patient with single-donor granulocyte concentrate is difficult for two reasons. Granulocytes rapidly lose function upon storage at room temperature and, once infused, granulocytes have only an 8-hour half-life. Prolonging the shelf-life of autologous or allogeneic granulocytes would benefit many patients, but cryopreservation of granulocytes has met with poor results. Granulocytes are much more sensitive to freezing, thawing and hyperosmotic stress than are red cells, lymphocytes or platelets.[31]

Human granulocyte cryopreservation was first reported in 1963.[32] Since then, a variety of cryoprotectants, freezing rates, storage temperatures and isolation procedures have been tried, with questionable success.[33,34] It is difficult to monitor the safety and therapeutic effectiveness of transfused cryopreserved granulocytes in part because infusion of freshly drawn granulocytes causes little measurable increase in peripheral count and efficacy can only be inferred by clinical response. Labeling granulocytes with [111]Indium may prove helpful in studying both freshly drawn and cryopreserved granulocytes. In vivo migration of these tagged cells to sites of infection can be observed directly, allowing more immediate inferences about function than are obtained by counting circulating white cells or observing changes in body temperature.[35]

Lymphocytes

Frozen with a final concentration of 10% DMSO and kept in the vapor phase of liquid nitrogen, lymphocytes maintain their cellular immune reactivity when thawed.[36,37] Lymphocyte freezing is used primarily for preserving cells used in laboratory tests. The HLA reactivity of a patient's cells can be tested against previously frozen cells of known antigenic composition. Homozygous cells used to define HLA-D loci can be stored frozen, and cells, either reagent cells or patient's cells, can be frozen to maintain viability during shipping.

Bone Marrow

Many treatment protocols utilize high-dose chemotherapy and radiotherapy to induce cure or long-term remission in malignant disease.[38] Such treatment not only kills tumor cells but also acts on rapidly dividing bone marrow cells to induce severe myelosuppression and even marrow ablation. After such extreme cytoreductive therapy, intravenous infusion of previously frozen autologous marrow can lead to repopulation of the bone marrow within about 4 weeks, producing enough hematopoiesis to sustain normal life.[39,40]

Clinical Considerations

Autologous, frozen-thawed marrow was first used to reestablish marrow function in 1958.[41] Autologous marrow protocols are used experimentally in conjunction with high-dose anticancer therapy when other forms of antineoplastic treatment have not helped and when an HLA-matched compatible sibling is not available. When frozen autologous marrow is engrafted, there is no risk of graft-versus-host disease and the dose of antitumor therapy can be based solely on characteristics of the neoplasm without concern for posttransplant immuno- and myelosuppression.

Disadvantages to the use of frozen autologous marrow are: 1) there is no adequate in vitro assay for viability of hematopoietic precursor cells[39]; 2) it may be necessary to manipulate the marrow to remove malignant cells, for example, by using monoclonal antibody to the common acute lymphocytic leukemia antigen (CALLA) for removal of leukemic blasts[42]; and 3) if the tumor is one for which no specific monoclonal antibody is available, the marrow must be obtained early enough in the course of the disease that there is no chance of marrow infiltration by malignant cells.[40,43]

Technique

Marrow extraction is performed with the patient under general or regional anesthesia. Multiple 3-5 ml aliquots are aspirated from the posterior iliac crests to obtain about 750 ml of marrow from a normal-sized adult. The marrow is anticoagulated and filtered, and the hematopoietic stem cells obtained by differential centrifugation. The stem cells, suspended in plasma with DMSO, are frozen to -196 C in a commercially available controlled-rate freezer. Marrow has been successfully used after storage in the liquid phase of liquid nitrogen for 3 years.[38] Thawing is performed rapidly in a 40 C waterbath at the bedside, and the marrow is usually infused immediately. Dilution or wash steps to decrease the minimal effects of DMSO are apparently unnecessary and cause undesirable loss of stem cells.[43]

Freezing of Non-Blood Cells, Tissues and Organs

Single cells and more complex tissues have been made available for clinical use after freezing and storing for long periods: sperm,[44] skin,[45] corneas,[46] bone, cartilage, tendons[47,48] and parathyroid glands.[49]

Histocompatibility tests used to provide improved transplant survival require time between removing the organ from the cadaver donor and transplantation into the recipient. Serological studies of HLA antigens take 6 to 8 hours, and investigating the cellular immune response takes several days. The ability to store organs for a week or more would be an important step to increasing organ survival after transplantation and to making more organs available. Human organs such as the heart and kidney have not been successfully cryopreserved for long periods of time. There are obviously problems with organ cryopreservation: 1) the presence of different cells requires heterogeneous freezing conditions; 2) organ geometry is such that heat transfer is impossible to maintain evenly throughout; 3) extracellular architectural disruption by ice can destroy an organ even without evidence of cellular damage; and 4) freezing of the vasculature often leads to permanent damage.[50]

References

1. Polge C, Smith AU, Parkes AS. Revival of spermatozoa after vitrification and dehydration at low temperature. Nature 1949;164:666.

2. Smith AU. Prevention of haemolysis during freezing and thawing of red blood cells. Lancet 1950;2:910–911.

3. Meryman HT. Cryopreservation of blood and marrow cells: basic biological and biophysical considerations. In: Petz LD, Swisher SN, eds. Clinical practice of blood transfusion. New York: Churchill, Livingstone; 1981:313–331.

4. Meryman HT. Cryoprotective agents. Cryobiology 1971;8:173–183.

5. Mollison PL, Sloviter HA. Successful transfusion of previously frozen human red cells. Lancet 1951;2:862–864.

6. Meryman HT. The cryopreservation of blood cells for clinical use. Prog Hematol 1979; Vol XI:193–227.

7. Huggins CE. Practical preservation of blood by freezing. In: Red cell freezing. Washington, DC: American Association of Blood Banks; 1973:31–53.

8. Rowe AW, Eyster E, Kellner A. Liquid nitrogen preservation of red blood cells for transfusion. A low glycerol-rapid freeze procedure. Cryobiology 1968;5:119–128.

9. Hornblower M, Meryman HT. Influence of the container material on the hemolysis of glycerolized red cells after freezing and thawing. Cryobiology 1974;11:317–323.

10. Rowe AW. Preservation of blood by the low glycerol-rapid freeze process. In: Red cell freezing. Washington, DC: American Association of Blood Banks; 1973:55–71.

11. Valeri CR. Factors influencing the 24 hour post-transfusion survival and the oxygen transport function of previously frozen red cells preserved with 40% w/v glycerol and frozen at −80 C. Transfusion 1974;14:1–15.

12. Meryman HT, Hornblower M. A method for freezing and washing red blood cells using a high glycerol concentration. Transfusion 1972;12:145–156.

13. Valeri CR. Simplification of the methods for adding and removing glycerol during freeze-preservation of human red blood cells with high or low glycerol methods: biochemical modification prior to freezing. Transfusion 1975;15:195–218.

14. Simpson MB, Radcliffe JH. Bacteriological safety of cryopreserved erythrocytes. In: Dawson RB, Barnes A Jr, eds. Clinical and practical aspects of the use of frozen blood. Washington, DC: American Association of Blood Banks; 1977:37–59.

15. Kahn RA, Auster M, Miller WV. The effect of refreezing previously frozen deglycerolized red blood cells. Transfusion 1978;18:204–205.

16. Myhre BA, Nakasako YY, Schott R. Studies on 4 C stored frozen reconstituted red blood cells III. Changes occurring in units which have been repeatedly frozen and thawed. Transfusion 1978;18:199–203.

17. Roberts S, Franks ML. Quality control for cryopreserved red blood cells. A blood banker's approach. In: Dawson RB, Barnes A Jr, eds. Clinical and practical aspects of the use of frozen blood. Washington, DC: American Association of Blood Banks; 1977:23–26.

18. Meryman HT, Hornblower M. Quality control for deglycerolizing red blood cells. Transfusion 1982;21:235–240.

19. Meryman HT, Hornblower M. Freezing and deglycerolizing sickle-trait red blood cells. Transfusion 1976;16:627–632.

20. Kurtz SR, Van Deinse WH, Valeri CR. The immunocompetence of residual leukocytes at various stages of red cell cryopreservation with 40% w/v glycerol in an ionic medium at −80 C. Transfusion 1978;18:441–447.

21. Alter HJ, Tabor E, Meryman HT, et al. Transmission of hepatitis B virus infection by transfusion of frozen-deglycerolized red blood cells. N Engl J Med 1978;298:637–642.

22. Haugen RK. Hepatitis after the transfusion of frozen red cells and washed red cells. N Engl J Med 1979;301:393–395.

23. Bayer WL. The effect of blood on the relationship of cytomegalovirus and hepatitis virus to infection and disease. In: Dawson RB, Barnes A Jr, eds. Clinical and practical aspects of the use of frozen blood. Washington, DC: American Association of Blood Banks; 1977:133–147.

24. Kumar A, Nankervis GA, Cooper AR, et al. Acquisition of cytomegalovirus infection in infants following exchange transfusion: a prospective study. Transfusion 1980;20:327–332.

25. Polesky HF. Frozen deglycerolized versus washed red blood cells in transplantation and HLA-sensitization. In: Dawson RB, Barnes A Jr, eds. Clinical and practical aspects of the use of frozen blood. Washington, DC: American Association of Blood Banks; 1977:113–123.

26. Opelz G, Terasaki PI. Improvement of kidney-graft survival with increased numbers of blood transfusions. N Engl J Med 1978;299:799–803.

27. Meryman HT, Burton JL. Cryopreservation of platelets. In: Greenwalt TJ, Jamieson GA, eds. The blood platelet in transfusion ther-

apy. New York: Alan R. Liss, Inc.; 1978:153–165.

28. Schiffer CA, Aisner J, Dutcher JP, et al. Clinical program of platelet cryopreservation. In: Vogler WR, ed. Cytopheresis and plasma exchange: clinical indications. New York: Alan R. Liss, Inc.; 1982:165–180.

29. Schiffer CA. Platelet cryopreservation. In: Glassman AB, Umlas J, eds. Cryopreservation of tissue and solid organs for transplantation. Arlington, VA: American Association of Blood Banks; 1983:65–77.

30. Daly P, Schiffer CA, Aisner J, et al. Successful transfusion of platelets cryopreserved for more than 3 years. Blood 1979;54:1023-1027.

31. Meryman HT. Cryopreservation of blood cells for clinical use. In: Brown EB, ed. Progress in hematology. Volume XI. New York: Grune and Stratton, Inc.; 1979:193–228.

32. Rowe AW, Kaczmarek CS, Cohen E. Low temperature preservation of leukocytes in dimethyl sulfoxide. Fed Proc 1963;22:170.

33. Bank H. Granulocyte preservation circa 1980. Cryobiology 1980;17:187–197.

34. Valeri CR. Current state of platelet and granulocyte cryopreservation. CRC Crit Rev Clin Lab Sci 1981;14:21–74.

35. McCullough J, Weiblen BJ, Clay ME, Forstrom L. Effect of leukocyte antibodies on the fate in vivo of Indium-lll-labeled granulocytes. Blood 1981;58:164–170.

36. Strong DM, Sell KW. Frozen cell banking in immunology. In: Simatos D, Strong DM, Turc JM, eds. Cryobiology. Paris: INSERM; 1977:101–105.

37. Glassman AB, Bennett CE. Cryopreservation of human lymphocytes: a brief review and evaluation of an automated liquid nitrogen freezer. Transfusion 1979;19:178–181.

38. Zaroulis CG. Cryopreservation of bone marrow and its clinical application. In: Glassman AB, Umlas J, eds. Cryopreservation of tissue and solid organs for transplantation. Arlington, VA: American Association of Blood Banks; 1983:79–90.

39. Herzig GP. Autologous marrow transplantation in cancer therapy. In: Brown EB, ed. Progress in hematology. Volume XII. New York: Grune and Stratton, Inc.; 1981:1–24.

40. Gale RP. Autologous bone marrow transplantation in patients with cancer. JAMA 1980;243:540–542.

41. Kurnick NB, Montano A, Gerdes JC, et al. Preliminary observations on treatment of postirradiation hematopoietic depression in man by infusion of stored autogenous bone marrow. Ann Int Med 1958;49:973–986.

42. Neudorf SML, Filipovich AH, Kersey JH. Recent advances in bone marrow transplantation. In: Weiner RS, Hackel E, Schiffer CA, eds. Bone marrow transplantation. Arlington, VA: American Association of Blood Banks; 1983:147–160.

43. Herzig RH. Autologous bone marrow transplantation. In: Weiner RS, Hackel E, Schiffer CA, eds. Bone marrow transplantation. Arlington, VA: American Association of Blood Banks, 1983:123–146.

44. Olson JH. Cryopreservation of human spermatazoa and its clinical application. In: Glassman AB, Umlas J, eds. Cryopreservation of tissue and solid organs for transplantation. Arlington, VA: American Association of Blood Banks; 1983:91–106.

45. DeClement FA, May SR. Procurement, cryopreservation and clinical application of skin. In: Glassman AB, Umlas J, eds. Cryopreservation of tissue and solid organs for transplantation. Arlington, VA: American Association of Blood Banks; 1983:29–56.

46. Graham CR Jr, Leslie JM. Trends in organ procurement and corneal preservation. In: Glassman AB, Umlas J, eds. Cryopreservation of tissue and solid organs for transplantation. Arlington, VA: American Association of Blood Banks; 1983:57–64.

47. Bright RW, Friedlaender GE, Sell KW. Tissue banking: the United States Navy Tissue Bank. Milit Med 1977;142:503–510.

48. Friedlaender GE, Sell KW, Bond JC. The impact of tissue banking on treatment of musculoskeletal system trauma. Milit Med 1977;142:858–860.

49. Wells SA, Ross AJ, Dale JK, et al. Transplantation of parathyroid glands: current status. Surg Clin North Am 1979;59:167–177.

50. Pegg DE. Mechanism of cryoinjury in organs (abstract). Cryobiology 1981;18:617.

5

Antigens, Antibodies, Complement and the Immune Response

Introductory Definitions

The ability to mount an immune response resides in a system of interrelated cells, tissues and organs that collectively constitute the immune system. The ability to discriminate between "self" and "nonself" is established early in embryogenesis but how this discrimination is achieved is not understood. The human fetus has the ability to distinguish between normal constituents of the body and those that are foreign. Whatever is encountered before this mechanism is established will be regarded as self. Substances or molecules encountered after that time will be regarded as foreign.

Humoral and Cell-Mediated Responses

The response to foreign substances can be either production of antibodies, called the *humoral response*; or a *cell-mediated response*, which reflects actions of the T cell subset of lymphocytes. Immunohematology, the science of blood transfusion, is concerned primarily with the causes and the effects of humoral immunity, but should be understood in the broader context of immunology.

Antigens

An *antigen* is a substance that elicits a specific immune response when introduced into the tissues of an immunocompetent individual, often referred to as the *host*. Antigens must normally be foreign to the host, of a molecular weight greater than 1000 daltons and be protein or polysaccharide in nature.[1] Substances that have molecular weights below 1000 daltons can sometimes elicit an antibody response if they are complexed to a larger molecule called a *carrier*. The small molecule is referred to as a *hapten* and the complex, a *hapten-carrier complex*. Antigens capable of eliciting an immune response without prior coupling to a second molecule are called *immunogens*. The degree to which a substance is likely to elicit an immune response in a given category of hosts is called its *immunogenicity* or *antigenicity*.

Antibodies

Polypeptide Chains

Antibodies belong to a group of proteins, called *immunoglobulins*, that have a common structure of two pairs of chains arranged symmetrically along the long axis. All antibodies are capable of specific combination with antigens.[2] The basic immunoglobulin unit consists of two identical light (L) chains, each containing about 220 amino acids, and two identical heavy (H) chains, each containing about 440 amino

5

71

acids (see Fig 5-1). Distinctive amino acid sequences that characterize chains of individual classes are called *isotypes*. Two isotypes of light chains exist, called kappa (κ) and lambda (λ); there are five isotypes of heavy chains, alpha (α), delta (δ), epsilon (ε), gamma (γ) and mu (μ).

Heavy and light chains have subunits called *domains*, each consisting of about 110 amino acids. Serologic and biologic actions of antibodies result from the amino acid sequences within these domains. The amino acid sequence in the amino-terminal domain of both heavy and light chains varies from one antibody to another. This is called the *variable (V) domain*; the variable sequences of amino acids determine the ability to combine with specific antigens. Within the variable domain are amino acid sequences that are hypervariable, called the *complementarity-determining regions (CDR)*. These appear to contain the amino acids that constitute the antibody's combining site. The regions on either side of the CDRs are less variable and are called *framework regions (FR)*. Light chains consist of the variable domain and a single *constant (C) domain*, located at the carboxy-terminal end of the chain, in which the amino acid sequence is essentially identical

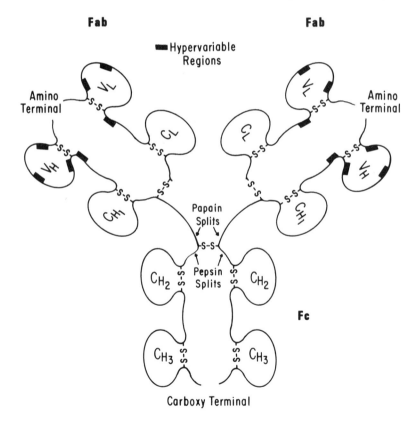

Figure 5-1. The basic four-chain immunoglobulin unit. Specificity of antibody activity derives from amino acid sequences in the hypervariable regions of the variable domains of heavy and light chains (V_H and V_L). Class-specific characteristics derive from amino acid sequences in the constant domains of the heavy chains (C_{H1}, C_{H2}, C_{H3}).

for all chains of a given isotype. Heavy chains consist of one variable domain and either three or four constant domains.

Immunoglobulin Classes

An assembled immunoglobulin molecule consists of two identical H and two identical L chains. The isotype of the heavy chain determines the immunoglobulin class of the molecule; IgA, IgD, IgE, IgG and IgM molecules have, respectively, alpha, delta, epsilon, gamma and mu heavy chains. The amino acid sequence in the constant domains are comparable or identical within each isotype. Many H chains have a region between the first and second C domain called the *hinge region*, which is flexible and allows the two combining sites of the molecule to move in relationship to each other.

Within immunoglobulin classes, the light chains may be either kappa or lambda. About 60% of immunoglobulin molecules have kappa chains and 40% have lambda. In any one molecule, the light chains are always of the same isotype. Different isotypes, for both heavy and light chains, characterize different species, ie, the mu chains of human IgM molecules are all very similar, and differ somewhat from the mu chains of rabbit IgM. Table 5-1 gives salient characteristics of human immunoglobulin molecules.

IgG

IgG, characterized by gamma (γ) heavy chains, is the preponderant class of immunoglobulins in the blood and is also found in extravascular fluid. It exists only as the single basic immunoglobulin unit of 2 H chains and 2 L chains. It is the only antibody that crosses the placenta from the mother to the fetus. Pronounced IgG production occurs during a secondary immune response (see page 77). IgG molecules can be divided into subclasses, *IgG1, IgG2, IgG3* and *IgG4*, which differ in the amino acid sequence of the H chain. These differences confer somewhat different serologic properties; for example, IgG1 and IgG3

molecules bind complement well, IgG2 poorly and IgG4 only under certain conditions. The quantitative distribution of IgG subclasses in blood is IgG1 > IgG2 > IgG3 > IgG4, but the biologic significance of the subclasses is only beginning to emerge.

IgM

IgM, defined by mu (μ) heavy chains, characteristically exists as a pentamer consisting of five basic immunoglobulin units and a short additional polypeptide chain called the J (for joining) *chain*. Although the pentameric molecule has 10 combining sites, the antibody combines with only five examples of antigen, and is described as having a *valence* of 5. Any one combining site of IgM usually has low binding affinity but this is balanced by the presence in the entire molecule of multiple antibody-binding sites.

IgM is the first class of immunoglobulin produced as the fetal immune system matures, and is the major class of antibody produced in the early stages of a primary antibody response. Blood is the only body fluid that contains significant amounts of IgM. IgM antibodies are highly effective agglutinins, and they fix complement very efficiently. A single molecule bound to the surface of a red cell can initiate complement-mediated lysis of that cell. Gentle reduction of IgM with 2-mercaptoethanol or dithiothreitol (see page 232) separates the five subunits and also releases the J chain. Both hemolyzing and agglutinating activity are destroyed by this treatment.

IgA

IgA, characterized by alpha (α) heavy chains, exists both as single immunoglobulin units and as polymers. Most serum IgA is the monomer, although a small proportion has the J chain and exists as multiples of the basic unit. In the epithelial secretions of the body, such as saliva, tears and the fluid that coats the respiratory and gastrointestinal tracts, IgA exists princi-

Table 5-1. Human Immunoglobulins

Class	IgG	IgA	IgM	IgD	IgE
Structure					
H-chain isotype	γ	α	μ	δ	ε
Number subclasses	4	2	1	?	?
L-chain, types	κ,λ	κ,λ	κ,λ	κ,λ	κ,λ
Molecular weight (daltons)	150,000	180,000– 500,000	900,000	180,000	200,000
Exists as polymer	no	yes	yes	no	no
Electrophoretic mobility	γ	γ	between γ and β	between γ and β	fast γ
Sedimentation constant (in Svedberg units)	6–7S	7–15S	19S	7S	8S
Gm allotypes (H chain)	+	0	0	0	0
Km allotypes (Kappa L chain; formerly Inv)	+	+	+	?	?
Serum concentration (mg/dl)	1000– 1500	200– 350	85– 205	3	0.01– 0.07
Present in epithelial secretions	no	yes	no	no	no
Antibody activity	yes	yes	yes	probably no	yes
Serologic characteristics	Usually nonagglu- tinating	Usually nonagglu- tinating	Usually agglu- tinating	?	?
Fixes complement	yes	no	yes	no	no
Crosses placenta	yes	no	no	no	no

pally as a dimer, including not only the J chain but also a polypeptide chain of epithelial origin called the *secretory component*. IgA antibodies are not agglutinins and do not bind complement. In humans two antigenically distinct subclasses have been described, designated IgA1 and IgA2.

IgD

IgD, characterized by delta (δ) heavy chains, exists as the single molecular unit. Most IgD is present as a membrane immunoglobulin on B lymphocytes, where it may serve as a receptor for antigen. Its concentration in serum is very low and no blood group antibodies have been found to belong to this class.

IgE

IgE, characterized by epsilon (ε) heavy chains, exists as a single immunoglobulin unit, present at extremely low concentrations in serum. Virtually all the body's IgE molecules are bound to basophilic granulocytes, both circulating basophils and their tissue equivalent, mast cells. Binding results from interactions between a receptor on the granulocyte membrane and a portion of the epsilon heavy chain. The combining sites of the antibody remain free to bind to antigen. Combination of the IgE molecule with its specific antigen triggers the underlying granulocyte to release histamine and other vasoactive substances from its granules. The clinical effects of these substances may include edema from increased vascular permeability, skin rashes, respiratory tract constriction and increased secretions from epithelial surfaces, depending upon the site involved.

Allotypes

The amino acid sequence in certain segments in the constant regions of immunoglobulin chains varies to produce heritable traits called *allotypes*, determined by allelic genes. At least 24 different allotypic sequences have been described in human gamma chains; these are called *Gm allotypes*. Three different sequences, called *Km allotypes*, have been identified in the constant region of human kappa chains. Km allotypes were formerly called Inv. Allotypic sequences on the alpha chain of IgA$_2$ molecules are *Am allotypes*. In any one individual, all the gamma chains will have the same Gm allotype, all alpha chains of subclass 2 will have the same Am allotype and all kappa chains will have the same Km allotype, because the immunoglobulin chain structure reflects the allelic genes present in that individual.

Idiotypes

Antibody molecules of any individual specificity have a unique amino acid sequence in the variable domains that comprise the antigen-binding portion of the molecule. The amino acid sequence confers the three-dimensional configuration that allows the antibody to interact with its specific antigen. The amino acid sequence characteristic of the antibody's specificity can, itself, serve as an antigen and elicit a corresponding antibody if suitably introduced into a susceptible host. The antigenically unique features of an antibody molecule are called its *idiotype*; antibodies that react with the combining site of an antibody molecule of any given specificity are called *anti-idiotype* antibodies. For example, IgG antibodies from a single individual, directed against different antigens, would have the same isotype and allotype but different idiotypes.

Cleavage by Enzymes

Antibody molecules can be cleaved into different characteristic fragments by proteolytic enzymes (see Fig 5-2). Papain cleaves the immunoglobulin unit at a heavy chain site just above the disulfide bonds that link them. The light chain remains attached to half the heavy chain, leaving intact the antigen binding site on each of the two identical fragments. These two identical fragments are called *Fab (fragment antigen binding) fragments*. The linked portions of the heavy chains, containing the constant-region domains that confer biologic activities, are called the *Fc fragment*, because the protein crystallizes readily. Pepsin cleaves the molecule below the site linking the two sides, producing a single fragment containing both antigen binding sites, the *F(ab')$_2$ fragment*. Individual Fab fragments can combine with individual examples of antigen. A F(ab')$_2$ fragment can crosslink two examples of antigen. Neither Fab nor F(ab')$_2$ fragments have the biological properties of intact antibody molecules because they lack the Fc portion.

Cells of the Immune Response

The cells principally involved in the immune response are macrophages, B lymphocytes and T lymphocytes. Since the 1960's it has been apparent that the T cell is responsible for cell-mediated immunity while the B cell is the major effector cell for humoral immunity, ie, production of antibody. The actions of T cells affect, in most cases, the activity of B cells. The macrophage plays an important role in many aspects of the immune response.

Macrophages

Monocytes are produced in the bone marrow, circulate in the peripheral blood and migrate to the tissues, where they become macrophages. As phagocytic cells, they engulf particulate and soluble materials, subjecting them to the effects of numerous enzymes and other proteins. Among the roles that macrophages play in the immune response are[3]: 1) degrading or altering antigenic material partially or completely; 2) presenting the antigen to

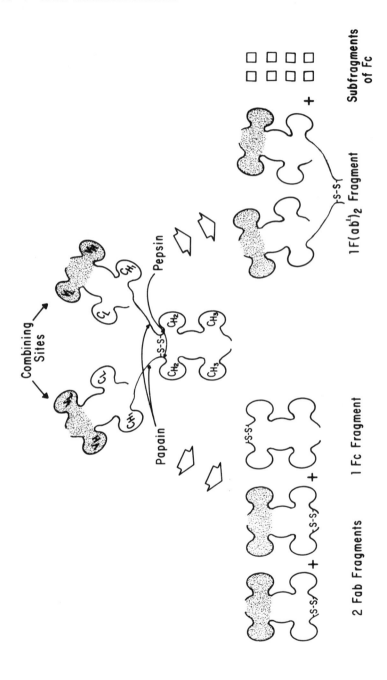

Figure 5-2. The different sites at which papain and pepsin cleave the immunoglobulin heavy chains.

responsive T cells and B cells, thereby initiating the immune response; and 3) releasing soluble substances, called *monokines*, that modulate activities of other cells. Macrophages have on their membranes receptors for complement and for the Fc portion of IgG molecules.

Lymphocytes

Lymphocytes are heterogeneous in size and function. They are capable of very precise recognition of foreign molecules and cells and of responding to successive contacts with previously encountered foreign materials in a manner called *memory*. All hematopoietic cells, ie, erythrocytes, granulocytes, monocytes, platelets and lymphocytes, are thought to evolve from a common precursor cell that gives rise first to pluripotent cells and then to stem cells committed to differentiation along a specific path. The pluripotent cells that appear in the yolk sac, liver, bone marrow and spleen of the fetus differentiate, at some still-unknown point, into precursors for the two broad categories of lymphocytes involved in the immune response, T and B cells.

B Lymphocytes

B lymphocytes have the capacity to synthesize the heavy and light chains described above and to assemble them into immunoglobulin molecules. B lymphocytes differentiate into the cells that actually produce antibodies, the *plasma cell*. In the adult, B cells constitute about 25% of lymphocytes in the circulating blood, and are found predominantly in the bone marrow and spleen.

B cells appear to perform fewer different functions than T cells. Most studies of B cells have concentrated on their ability to secrete immunoglobulin. B cells have immunoglobulin molecules, usually IgD and IgM, on their surface membrane, a feature that makes them easy to identify in tissue or in mixed cell populations. They also have receptors for complement and they express DR antigens (see page 182).

Primary Immunization

Before producing antibody, B cells must interact directly with antigen and, in most cases, with T cells. T cells are thought to present the B cell with antigen that has been processed by a macrophage and to initiate signals that promote B cell activity. Some large molecules, especially those with multiple repeating polysaccharide antigenic determinants, can induce antibody production without intervention from T cells and are called *T-cell-independent* antigens.

In a *primary immune response*, when the host first encounters a particular antigen, several days to several weeks elapse before detectable antibody is found; this is called the *lag period*. During the lag period the B cell undergoes reorganization of genetic material, assembly of ribosomes, initiation of DNA synthesis and, ultimately, mitosis. This is a key aspect of the immune response because if DNA synthesis and mitosis are disturbed the amount of antibody produced is drastically reduced.

Suitably stimulated by contact with antigen, B cells undergo clonal expansion and produce daughter cells that are genetically identical. The daughter cell may either develop into a *plasma cell*, the cell that actually secretes antibody, or become a *memory B cell*, which enters the circulating lymphocyte pool and persists for months or years. Antibody produced in the primary response is predominantly IgM.

Secondary Immunization

It is the memory B cell that responds to subsequent contact with antigens to produce the secondary response. The *secondary*, or *anamnestic, response* occurs very rapidly and results in greater antibody production than the primary response. This is because the memory B cells have already been exposed to antigen and have produced daughter cells that will recognize that antigen. On a subsequent encounter with the same antigen, therefore, more cells are able to respond. IgG is the major class of antibody produced in a secondary response. IgG production occurs in the same cells that originally produced IgM, through an imperfectly understood switching mechanism that permits synthesis of IgG antibody with specificity for the same antigen.

T Lymphocytes

T cells also arise from the bone marrow but migrate to the thymus where they mature and acquire an array of surface antigens that reflects both maturational phase and functional capacity.[4] Functionally and antigenically distinct subpopulations of T cells include helper cells (Th), suppressor cells (Ts) and cytotoxic effector cells (Tc). Helper cells promote the effector activities of both T and B cells, and stimulate macrophage activities. Suppressor cells inhibit B and T cell activities. Cytotoxic cells can, by their direct actions, kill foreign or altered cells.

T cells have the same capacity as B cells to recognize, with exquisite sensitivity, individual antigens but T cells do not have immunoglobulin receptors on their surface as B cells do. Some form of receptor molecule is present on the cell surface, apparently composed of chains with both constant and variable regions, but its complete nature is still under investigation.[5] Like B cells, T cells that have interacted with their specific antigen generate daughter cells that either carry out effector activities or enter the circulating lymphocyte pool as memory cells.

Regulation of the Immune Response

Once an immune response has been initiated it is important that there be mechanisms to regulate its magnitude or terminate it. The following mechanisms are involved in limiting antibody production: 1) individual plasma cells survive only a few days, and unless new plasma cells evolve, disappearance of plasma cells causes antibody production to cease; 2) antibody produced in the immune response may react with macrophage-bound antigen, coating it so that it no longer stimulates clonal expansion; 3) suppressor T cells are activated, causing them to inhibit stimulation of other lymphocytes; and 4) the antigen that initially elicited the response is often degraded or eliminated from the body.

Complement

General Concepts

The two major functions of complement are to promote the inflammatory response and to alter biological membranes so as to cause direct cell lysis or enhanced susceptibility to phagocytosis. Cell lysis occurs when antibody-mediated complement activation leads to sequential interaction of the entire complement cascade. Intermediary products in the complement sequence attract phagocytic cells, promote the efficiency of phagocytic activity, and alter vascular permeability and the stability of cell membranes, notably those of platelets and granulocytes.

Complement consists of at least 20 different glycoproteins with varying electrophoretic mobilities, most of which circulate in an inactive precursor form and develop proteolytic activity upon activation. Together they constitute approximately 3-4% of the total serum protein. Complement proteins are designated by C, followed by identifying numbers and letters. Many components are present in small or trace quantities although C4, C3, Factor B and C1 INH are each present in concentrations greater than 10 mg/100 ml.[6] Complement proteins undergo activation either by attaching to or associating with other proteins or, more often, by undergoing proteolytic cleavage, such that removal of part of the molecule leaves the residual portion enzymatically or biologically active. The sequence whereby each component undergoes activation and then activates the next component is often described as a cascade or waterfall-type reaction.

Sequential Interactions

Cleavage of many components generates a small fragment which enters the surrounding milieu, and a larger residual molecule which attaches to the cell surface and continues the reaction sequence. The complement cascade, like the coagulation cascade, requires the presence of cations; both calcium and magnesium are necessary for the classical pathway initiated by antibody activity but only magnesium ions are needed for the alternative pathway (see below). The major controls on the system are: 1) inhibitory proteins acting at the critical C1 and C3 activation steps; 2) spontaneous decay of the enzymatically active states produced during the cascade sequence; and 3) rapid clearance of active fragments.

There are two sequences whereby complement undergoes activation, called the classical and the alternative pathways (see Fig 5-3). The classical pathway follows occurrence of specific antigen-antibody reactions, and is the primary amplifier of the biologic effects of humoral immunity. The alternative pathway amplifies non-immune defense against microbial infection and other biologic alterations. By convention, individual complement components are designated C1, C4, C2 etc; cleavage fragments of complement components are designated C4a, C3d, etc; capital letters are used for components of the alternative pathway, eg, Factors B and D.

Classical Pathway
Attachment

The first component of complement, C1, interacts directly with the Fc portion of those immunoglobulin molecules that have the appropriate binding site in the C_{H2} domain of the heavy chain. All mu chains have this site, and most gamma chains. C1 is composed of three subunits, C1q, C1r

and C1s, which are held together by calcium ions. C1q consists of 18 polypeptide chains wound together into six subunits; each subunit can bind to one Fc region. C1q attaches only to those antibody molecules that have bound their corresponding antigen. The reaction of antibody with antigen may cause some conformational change in the antibody, exposing or altering the site where C1q attaches, or it may simply bring several Fc segments with their binding sites close enough together that a C1q molecule can interact with them. At least 2 of the 6 C1q subunits must bind to an Fc region. A single IgM pentamer attached to a cell surface antigen can provide sufficient binding sites, but 2 separate IgG molecules are required, and these must be close enough together on the cell surface that one C1q molecule can bind to them simultaneously. Individual IgG molecules attached to antigen sites widely separated on a cell surface are ineffective in activating complement regardless of the number of IgG molecules actually present.[6] Because the binding site resides in the C_{H2} region of the Fc fragment, $F(ab')_2$ fragments are unable to bind complement, even though they may crosslink nearby antigen sites.

Activation

Bound C1q undergoes a conformational change that activates C1r. This in turn activates C1s, the part of the molecule that propagates the complement sequence by cleaving C4 into C4a and C4b, and cleaving C2 to uncover a labile binding site. C4b contains a binding site through which it attaches to the cell membrane. C4a is released into the body fluid where it has a number of biologic actions collectively described as *anaphylatoxic* activity. *Anaphylatoxins* stimulate mast cell degranulation and histamine release, thereby increasing vascular permeability, and also induce contraction of smooth muscle and release of lysosomal enzymes from neutrophils.

Once C4b is bound to the cell membrane, activated C2 can attach to it or closely

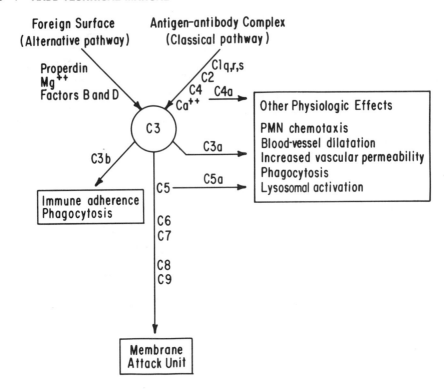

Figure 5-3. A schematic representation of the activation and physiologic effects of complement. Cleavage of C3 is pivotal for both classical and alternative pathways.

adjacent. The larger fragment, C2a, combines with C4b to produce activated C4b2a, which has enzymatic activity. Each site of C1q attachment to an Fc chain can generate 100-200 activated C4b2a complexes attached to the cell membrane.

Amplification

Activated C4b2a is called *C3 convertase*, because it cleaves the inactive C3 molecule into C3a and C3b. One C4b2a site can cleave hundreds of C3 molecules. The smaller fragment, C3a, is released into body fluids, where it acts as a potent anaphylatoxin. The larger fragment, C3b, either binds promptly to the cell membrane or decays in solution. C3b fragments by themselves are not active catalytically and do not promote cell lysis, but the presence

of C3b on a cell membrane greatly increases the susceptibility of that cell to phagocytosis, because macrophages and neutrophils have receptors for C3b. A material whose presence on the cell surface enhances susceptibility to phagocytosis is called an *opsonin*. C3b and the Fc portion of IgG molecules are powerful opsonins.

Some C3b fragments join activated C4b2a to form the next catalytic unit, activated C4b2a3b, which is called *C5 convertase* and has proteolytic activity against C5. Activated C4b2a3b splits C5 into C5a and C5b. C5a, like C4a and C3a, is released into the plasma where it is a potent anaphylatoxin and also acts as an attractant for polymorphonuclear leukocytes and as a stimulant to intracellular processes involved in inflammation.

Attack

C5b attaches to the cell membrane and initiates nonenzymatic assembly of other complement components. In the presence of C5b, molecules of C6, C7, C8 and a variable number of C9 molecules assemble themselves into aggregates called the *membrane attack unit*. This molecular complex causes an acute change in membrane permeability, allowing water to enter the cell such that it swells and bursts. It is not clear whether the membrane attack unit produces a pore in the red cell membrane or whether its presence causes a rearrangement of the phospholipid bilayer that alters permeability, or both. The membrane attack unit remains active for only a very short time, after which it loses its affinity for the cell membrane.

Alternative Pathway

In the alternative pathway, cleavage of C3 and activation of the remainder of the complement cascade occur independently of complement-fixing antibodies. Triggers for the alternative pathway include particulate polysaccharides and lipopolysaccharides such as those on the surfaces of some microorganisms; trypsin-like enzymes; and antigen-antibody complexes involving antibodies, such as IgA and IgG of the subclass IgG4, that do not activate C1.

Molecules of C3 undergo cleavage, at a continuous low level, in normal serum and other body fluids, apparently due to interaction with factor B in the fluid phase. Normally the resulting C3b, which is in fluid and not bound to any surface, is rapidly degraded by control proteins in plasma. If, however, the C3b comes in contact with particulate activators of the alternative pathway, the surface provides protection from the control proteins in fluid and acts as a sheltered environment in which C3b and factor B can associate. The bound C3b-factor B complex interacts with an active serum protease, factor D, which cleaves factor B to produce a C3bBb complex. C3bBb is an effective C3 convertase, generating additional C3b, which attaches itself to the complex and amplifies its activities. The association, on the surface of a microorganism or an aggregate of protein, of numerous C3b units, factor Bb and a stabilizing protein called *properdin* (P), has potent activity as a C5 convertase. With cleavage of C5, the remainder of the complement cascade continues as in the classical pathway. The action of C3bBb or C3bBbP on C3 generates C3a as well as C3b, and the C5 convertase activity of C3bBbP generates C5a as well as C5b, so the alternative pathway produces the anaphylatoxic effects of complement activation as well as the lytic effects.

Inactivation of C3b

In both the classical and the alternative pathway C3b binds to the surfaces of cells through a thioester bond. Several serum proteins may act on the C3b molecule to abolish its enzymic effects. Factor H (formerly called C3 binding protein or β-1-H) attaches to C3b and renders it susceptible to the proteolytic effects of factor I (formerly called C3b inactivator). Factor I cleaves C3b into C3c, which escapes into the fluid phase, and C3d, which remains permanently bound to the membrane. C3d has no activating effect on the complement sequence and does not interact with receptors on phagocytic cells. Factors H and I often exert this inhibitory effect when there is in vivo complement activation; coating of cells with C3d is frequently seen as the residual effect of antibodies acting in vivo against blood cells, and consequently the most important anticomplement aspect of antihuman globulin reagents is anti-C3d. Factor I may also cleave cell-bound C4b, to leave enzymically inert C4d attached to the cells. This occurs especially after in vitro attachment of complement to red cells, such as occurs at low temperatures or in a medium of low ionic strength.

In Vitro Detection of Antigen-Antibody Reactions

Once antibody has been formed in vivo there are various ways in which it can be detected in vitro. These include but are not limited to:

Agglutination

Agglutination is clumping of particles that have antigen on their surface by antibody molecules forming bridges between antigenic determinants on adjacent cells. Agglutination, the end point for most tests involving red cells and blood group antibodies, can be observed either through direct techniques, such as ABO testing, or indirect techniques such as those that use antihuman globulin. Agglutination is discussed in more detail in a later section.

Precipitation

Precipitation is the formation of a visible, insoluble complex when soluble antibody reacts with soluble antigen. Such complexes are detected in test tubes as a sediment and in agar gels as a white line appearing where the antigen and antibody interact. Precipitation is the basis of procedures such as immunodiffusion and immunoelectrophoresis.

Precipitation does not always occur, even though soluble antigen and its specific antibody are present. It depends on the formation of a lattice structure that requires the presence of equivalent amounts of antigen and antibody. If antibody is present in excess, there are too few antigen sites with which the molecules can cross-link, and the lattice structure is not formed. This is called a *prozone phenomenon*. The prozone phenomenon can occur in agglutination tests, if antibody is in very high concentration and there are few antigen-bearing particles, or if the antigen is in very low concentration on the surface of cells or particles.

Hemolysis

Hemolysis is rupture of red blood cells, with release of intracellular hemoglobin.

Cells of other types may undergo lysis, due to disruption of the membrane from a variety of causes. Antibody-mediated hemolysis requires activation of complement and does not occur if the antigen and antibody interact in the absence of complement or in plasma that contains an agent that chelates calcium and magnesium ions. Hemolysis constitutes a positive result in tests for red cell antibodies, because it indicates the activity of a complement-activating antibody. Pink supernatant fluid after incubation of antibody with red cells is an important observation, because antibodies that are lytic in vitro are likely to cause intravascular hemolysis.

Inhibition of Agglutination

In agglutination inhibition tests, the presence of antigen or antibody is detected by inhibition of previously documented agglutination. For example, the saliva of individuals who are secretors (see page 120) normally contains soluble blood group antigens. Their presence can be detected by incubating boiled saliva with a preparation of anti-A or anti-B known to cause agglutination at a certain dilution, and then adding A and B red cells. If the saliva contains blood group substance it will complex with the antibody and neutralize its agglutinating properties so that subsequently added red cells will not be agglutinated. Inhibition of agglutination indicates that the corresponding antigen is present in the test material. Conversely, agglutination of the indicator cells denotes the absence of the corresponding antigen.

Another important example of inhibition of agglutination is unwanted inactivation of antihuman globulin serum. Unbound globulin combines with antiglobulin molecules before they can react with cell-bound globulins. If red cells used in either direct or indirect antiglobulin testing are not thoroughly washed free of serum, residual globulin can inhibit the antihuman globulin reagent and cause a false-negative result (see page 95).

Immunofluorescence

Immunofluorescence allows identification and localization of antigens on cell surfaces and in cells. A fluorochrome such as fluorescein or rhodamine can be attached to an antibody molecule, rendering it intensely fluorescent without destroying its specificity. After a fluorescent-labeled antibody reacts with cellular antigens, the antibody-coated cell appears sharply visible and yellow-green when examined with a fluorescence microscope. This technique can be used as either a direct or an indirect procedure, analogous to direct and indirect antiglobulin testing and is also used in flow cytometry. In a direct test a specific antibody is fluorescent-labeled and reacted with tissues or cells. In an indirect test a fluorescent-labeled antiglobulin serum is added to cells that have been incubated with unlabeled antibody. Immunofluorescence is used in tests for surface antigens of T lymphocytes, and to identify the immunoglobulins present in and on B lymphocytes.

Radioimmunoassay

Radioimmunoassay procedures use a suitable radionuclide as marker for either antigen or antibody, and are suitable for either direct or indirect tests. In a direct test antibody is radiolabeled without destroying its specificity; following exposure to the antigen, the quantity of antibody bound can be very accurately measured. Tests for hepatitis B surface antigen (HBsAg) use an indirect technique, based on localization of the antigen upon fixed, unlabeled antibody. Unlabeled anti-HBs is coupled to a solid material and test material added. If HBsAg is present it combines with the fixed antibody and remains capable of reacting with radiolabeled anti-HBs added subsequently. A gamma counter quantifies very precisely the amount of radiolabeled anti-HBs that has attached to the previously bound antigen.

Radiolabeling is also used in competitive binding procedures, which employ the principle that labeled and unlabeled antibody of the same specificity have the same reactivity with the corresponding antigen. Calculating the proportion of a known dose of labeled material bound in a test system permits calculation of the amount of unlabeled material that must have been present.

ELISA (Enzyme-Linked Immunosorbent Assay)

Enzyme-linked assays are used to measure either antigen or antibody. Enzymes such as alkaline phosphatase can be linked to antibody without destroying either the antibody specificity or the enzyme activity. The enzyme acts as a quantifiable label, similar to radiolabeling. Enzyme labels are far more stable than radioactive labels, are cheaper and simpler to measure, and, in many cases, provide results that are comparably sensitive. A number of tests for hepatitis A and B markers use this principle.

Factors Affecting Agglutination

Red blood cell agglutination is thought to occur in two stages: 1) physical attachment of antibody to red cells, called *sensitization*; and 2) formation of bridges between the sensitized red cells to form the lattice that constitutes agglutination. A number of variables affect each stage.

The First Stage

The association of antigen with antibody is reversible. The amount of antibody attached to antigen at equilibrium is affected by the equilibrium constant, or affinity constant, of the antibody. In general, the higher the equilibrium constant, the higher the rate of association and the slower the rate of dissociation. The association of antigen with antibody is affected by the concentration of antigen and antibody and by various physical conditions such as pH, ionic strength and temperature. Altering the physical conditions of agglutination tests often increases their sensitivity.

Temperature

Most blood group antibodies show reactivity over a restricted temperature range; some, such as anti-P_1, react optimally at 18 C and some, such as anti-Fy^a, react optimally at 37 C. Generally, IgM antibodies are more reactive at temperatures ranging from 4 C to 27 C,[7] whereas IgG antibodies are detected better at temperatures ranging from 30 C to 37 C.[8] Methods for antibody detection often cover a range of temperatures (eg 22 to 37 C or 30 to 37 C). Antibodies that react in vitro only at temperatures below 30 C are considered to have little clinical significance. Antibodies that do not agglutinate red cells or activate complement above 30 C virtually never cause destruction of transfused cells.[8] Some cold-reactive IgM antibodies may activate complement at temperatures above 30 C but cause only minimally shortened survival of transfused incompatible red cells. Identification of these antibodies is discussed on page 206. Clinically significant antibodies are those that are active in vivo, at temperatures in the vicinity of 37 C. It may not be necessary to perform in vitro tests at 37 C to document their presence; antibodies with in vivo activity may be demonstrable by in vitro tests that do not involve warming the cells and serum.

pH

The optimum pH for antibodies of most blood group systems has not been determined. Some antibodies such as anti-M react best at low pH. Hughes-Jones et al[9] reported an optimum of between 6.5 and 7.0 for anti-D. Practically, a pH of around 7.0 is used for routine work.

Incubation Time

The time needed to reach equilibrium differs for different blood group antibodies. Significant variables include the class of immunoglobulin involved and how tightly it attaches to its specific antigen. Studies with serum and saline-suspended red cells have shown that, of the total amount of antibody ultimately bound, approximately 25% will be taken up in the first 15 minutes and 75% within the first hour.[10] The addition of various enhancing agents can increase the amount of antibody taken up in the first 15 minutes and therefore decrease the incubation time needed to demonstrate antibody presence.

Ionic Strength

In normal saline, Na^+ and Cl^- ions cluster around and partially neutralize opposite charges on antigen and antibody molecules. This shielding effect, which hinders the association of antibody with antigen, is reduced by lowering the ionic strength of the reaction medium. In general, antibody uptake is enhanced by lowering the salt concentration of the reaction medium.

Antigen-Antibody Ratio

The speed with which antigen and antibody bind is affected by the number of antibody molecules in the medium and the number of antigen sites per cell. Increasing the quantity of antibody present can increase the sensitivity of the test. Raising the serum-to-cell ratio (see page 231) provides more molecules of antibody relative to the number of antigen sites available.

The Second Stage
Distance Between Cells

There are several theories about the mechanism whereby sensitized red cells are linked into a lattice. Pollack and colleagues[11] suggest that the size of the IgG molecule is too small to span the distance between red cells separated from one another by repulsion of like charges. Red cells have a net negative charge at their surface; interaction with ions in the suspending medium alters this surface charge, resulting in a net charge they call the *zeta potential*. The distance between red cells is proportional to the zeta potential. Reducing the effective charge separating red cells allows them to come closer together and may permit agglutination by IgG molecules which can then effect crosslinking across the shorter distance.

Steane and Greenwalt[12] favor the water of hydration theory. Water tightly bound at the surface of the red cells keeps them separated in solution by maintaining a hydration shell around them, much like bubbles of water insulating the surface. They suggest that antibody binding to an antigen on the surface decreases the hydration layer and increases the tendency to agglutinate.

Effects of Enzymes

Proteolytic enzymes (eg papain, ficin) used in serologic tests reduce the surface charge of the red cell by cleaving sialoglycoproteins from the cell surface. Neuraminidase reduces the charge on the cell surface by cleaving N-acetylneuraminic acid molecules from polysaccharide chains. If it is the net charge that keeps cells apart, any mechanism that reduces the net charge on the cell surface should therefore enhance agglutination. Cells pretreated with proteolytic enzymes often show enhanced agglutination by IgG molecules, but cells pretreated with neuraminidase demonstrate no comparable increase in agglutinability. Steane and Greenwalt[12] postulate that each type of enzyme removes a different amount of water or insulation from the polypeptides that are cleaved by these enzymes and that this accounts for different effects observed when cells are treated with different enzymes.

Effect of Positively Charged Molecules

The behavior of cells polyagglutinable because of T or Tn reactivity with macromolecules such as Polybrene® gives additional information on the physical aspects of agglutination. Polybrene,® a positively charged polymer, causes nor-

mal red cells to aggregate spontaneously, an effect many workers believe results from neutralizing the negative surface charge contributed by sialic acid. T and Tn cells, which have intrinsically reduced levels of sialic acid, do not aggregate in Polybrene.® Steane and Greenwalt[12] postulate that hydration is again the important factor, that water is extruded from the cell surface as the macromolecules bind to oppositely charged groups, and the insulating shell of water molecules is removed.

Other Considerations

Stratton and colleagues[13] suggest that proteolytic enzymes affect the first stage of agglutination. They postulate that polypeptides protruding from the cell surface cause steric interference in antibody binding, and that enzyme-mediated removal of these polypeptide chains and of sialic acid facilitates antibody attachment. Van Oss and colleagues[14,15] emphasize that erythrocyte shape seems to be important in the agglutination reaction. They postulate that cells of abnormal shape can come into closer contact than normal cells and thus overcome the electrostatic repulsion normally present.

It is also possible that antigen mobility, antigen clustering and membrane flexibility play a role in the agglutination reaction. The exact mechanisms have yet to be determined.

Applied Concepts

Immunologically Mediated Diseases

The actions of the immune system are essential for healthy existence but in many circumstances immune responses cause unpleasant, dangerous or even fatal effects in the host. The harmful effects of immunity are often collectively described as *hypersensitivity*; *allergy* and *anaphylaxis* are terms applied to certain restricted immune-mediated disorders. Hypersensitivity reactions may cause illness or tissue damage through a variety of mechanisms.

Gell and Coombs[16] have proposed four mechanisms of hypersensitivity (see Table 5-2). Types I, II and III depend on interaction between antigen and humoral antibody, with or without complement or other mediators. Type IV involves the cell-mediated immune response and has a protracted course. The systemic anaphylactic reactions to IgA that occur in IgA-deficient individuals are probably an example of Type I. Transfusion reactions due to blood group antibodies are considered Type II, as are autoimmune hemolytic anemia and hemolytic disease of the newborn. Hemolytic conditions resulting from drug-antidrug immune complexes can be considered Type III reactions. Graft-versus-host disease, such as that seen in some bone marrow recipients, is an example of Type IV.

Transfer of Immunoglobulin from Mother to Fetus

The transfer of immunoglobulin and other proteins from the mother to the fetus is independent of molecular size; IgG, with a molecular weight of 150,000 daltons, is transferred much more readily than albumin, with a molecular weight of 64,000 daltons. Selective distribution must occur because IgG enters primarily the fetal blood while albumin enters primarily the amniotic fluid.[17] In humans, IgM does not reach the fetus and IgA is not readily transferred, although low levels have been found in the newborn infant.

Table 5-2. Classification of Immune-Mediated Tissue Damage (Modified from Gell and Coombs[16])

Type	Descriptive Terms	Ig Class	Effectors	Time Course at Onset	Examples of Pathologic Conditions
I	Reaginic Atopic Anaphylactic	E, ?IgG4	Histamine and other substances from basophil granules	Minutes	Anaphylaxis Some asthma Urticaria Hay fever
II	Membrane-reactive	G, M	Complement Phagocytic cells Proteolytic enzymes	Minutes to hours	Transfusion reactions Autoimmune hemolysis Hemolytic disease of the newborn Some types of glomerulonephritis Myaesthenia gravis
III	Immune complex Serum sickness	G, M	Complement Neutrophils	Minutes to hours	Some drug-induced hemolysis Post-streptococcal glomerulonephritis Many manifestations of lupus erythematosus Some pulmonary allergies Arthus reaction
IV	Cell-mediated	None	T lymphocytes Macrophages Lymphokines	Days to weeks	Allograft rejection Graft-vs-host disease Lung changes in tuberculosis Some chronic hepatitis

All four subclasses of IgG are transported but the rate varies between individual mother-fetus pairs. Early in pregnancy IgG probably passes from mother to fetus by diffusion, and concentration in fetal serum is low for all subgroups. Between 20 and 33 weeks gestation fetal IgG levels rise markedly, apparently due to maturation of a selective transport system. IgG1, the predominant subclass in maternal blood, is transported in greatest quantity. Part of the placental transport system seems to involve specific protein receptors on the membrane of placental cells,[18] but other mechanisms are also involved.

Hybridomas, a New Source of Antibody

In 1975 Köhler and Milstein[19] showed that antibody-secreting cells from immunized animals could be fused with cultured myeloma cells capable of indefinite reproduction. The resulting hybrid cells grow continuously in culture and secrete the antibody characteristic of the parent cell. This technique is called *somatic cell hybridization* and the multiplying hybrid cell culture a *hybridoma*.

The standard technique for selecting successful hybrid cells uses a myeloma cell that has lost the ability to secrete hypoxanthine - guanine - phosphoribosyl - transferase (HGPRT), an enzyme needed to synthesize nucleotides, the coding elements of nucleic acids essential for preservation and transfer of genetic information. Absence of HGPRT is not a problem for the myeloma cell in standard culture medium because it has an alternative metabolic pathway for producing nucleotides. Growing the cell fusion mixture in a medium that blocks the other pathway makes the cells dependent on HGPRT. Normal lymphocytes possess HGPRT. In hybrid cells, the lymphocyte provides HGPRT and the ability to produce antibody; the myeloma cell provides the ability to reproduce indefinitely. In the selective medium, unfused myeloma cells die out because they lack HGPRT and normal lymphocytes die out because they cannot reproduce themselves through many generations. Only successful hybrid cells will remain and reproduce.

The supernatant fluid above a successful culture of hybrid cells must be tested to determine the presence and the specificity of antibody. With appropriate selection and culture conditions, large numbers of antibody-producing cells can be isolated. Antibody can be harvested from the culture supernatant, but much higher concentrations are obtained if the cells are injected into the peritoneal cavity of mice where they multiply and secrete antibody into the resulting ascitic fluid. A practical approach is to inject some of the cultured cells into mice, and store the remaining cells frozen until more ascitic fluid is required. This also ensures that the original antibody specificity can be maintained for long periods of time, since hybrid cells become unstable if maintained in tissue culture conditions indefinitely.

There is careful enthusiasm at this time as to the use of hybridoma antibodies, also called monoclonal antibodies, in blood grouping serology. It is difficult to define the optimum characteristics desired in reagent antibodies of any derivation. Monoclonal antibodies embody a single specificity, as compared with the range of antibody molecules present in serum from even a single immunized individual. Most reagent antisera contain antibodies pooled from several or many immunized individuals, so there is substantial heterogeneity of antibodies now used as diagnostic agents. A monoclonal antibody is directed against the single example of antigen used to immunize the host, and contains only one of the immunoglobulin molecules that the host produces after exposure to what may be a complex antigen.

Lymphocyte Subsets

The human immune system contains discrete subsets of T cells named for the functions they perform in interactions with other cells, but identified by their reactions with carefully selected monoclonal antibodies. Three major subpopulations exist, helper (or inducer) T cells (Th), suppressor T cells (Ts) and cytotoxic T cells (Tc).[20] Helper and suppressor cells are collectively designated regulatory T cells because they function by regulating activities of B cells, macrophages and other T cells. Cytotoxic cells engage in lethal direct interaction with altered or foreign cells. They are responsible for defense against many viral infections and have an important role in the body's response to tumor cells. This cytotoxic activity depends upon recognition of antigens on the surface of the target cell, and is independent of both antibody and complement.

Suppressor T cells inhibit the effector activities of antibody-producing cells and of cell-mediated immunity. They modulate or terminate established immune responses and are also involved in induction and maintenance of immune tolerance.

Helper T cells are required for induction of cell-mediated immune responses, for production of antibodies against most antigens, and for activation of many suppressor-cell activities. Communication among the various subgroup populations requires recognition by the T cells of specific antigenic determinants and of self determinants encoded by the major histocompatibility complex (MHC, see Chapter 11), and appears to involve either formation of cell-to-cell bridges or elaboration of messenger molecules or both. The subpopulation of helper T cells is probably heterogeneous, with differing capabilities for, at the very least, B cells and T cells.

Different surface antigens characterize different maturational phases of T cell development, and different functional populations. These antigens are identified with monoclonal antibodies that have been given various designations. Table 5-3 depicts the acquisition, loss and preserva-

Table 5-3. Antigenic Markers of T Cell Maturation

Stage	Surface Antigens
Early cortical thymocytes	T11, T10, T9
Late cortical thymocytes	T11, T10, T8, T6, T4, T1
Medullary thymocytes	
All cells	T11, T10, T3, T1
T4 population	T4
T8 population	T5, T8
Peripheral T cells	
Helper cells, effectors of delayed hypersensitivity	T11, T4, T3, T1
Suppressor cells, effectors of cytotoxicity	T11, T8, T3, T1

tion of these surface characteristics.[21] Table 5-4 depicts some attributes of these antigenic markers.[21]

Lymphokines

Lymphokines are substances produced by T lymphocytes that regulate interactions among macrophages, T cells and B cells.[22] There are certain parallels between the current knowledge of lymphokines and the classification of antibodies before the structure of immunoglobulins was determined. Antibodies used to be called precipitins, hemolysins, opsonins and agglutinins, names chosen to describe the functions demonstrated by in vitro testing. Lymphokines have also been named from their effects on in vitro tests, resulting in names such as lymphocyte-activating factor, soluble immune response suppressor and T cell growth factor. While little is known about the biochemistry and structure of most lymphokines it is apparent that they function at much lower concentrations than immunoglobulins, and maintain functional abilities for only very short time periods.

Table 5-4. T Cell Antigens

Antigen	Monoclonal Antibody*	Characteristics
T1	OKT1 Leu 1	Pan-T; found on peripheral T-cells and cortical thymocytes
T3	OKT 3 Leu 4	Pan-T; associated with receptor for antigen on cells in periphery and thymic medulla
T4	OKT 4 Leu 3	Present on helper/delayed hypersensitivity cells, in periphery and thymic medulla
T6	OKT 6 Leu 6	Early differentiation antigen, present on cells in thymic cortex. Present on Langerhans cells (epidermal macrophages)
T8	OKT 8 Leu 2	Present on suppressor/cytotoxic cells, in periphery and thymic medulla
T11	OKT 11 Leu 5	Pan-T; responsible for sheep cell rosette formation

* OKT series is produced by Ortho Diagnostic Systems, Inc; Leu series is produced by Becton-Dickinson FACS Systems

References

1. Eisen HN. Immunology. 2nd ed. Hagerstown, MD: Harper and Row; 1980.

2. Kimball JW. Introduction to immunology. New York: MacMillan; 1983.

3. Unanue ER. The regulation of lymphocyte functions by the macrophage. Immunological Reviews 1978;40:227–255.

4. Alberts B, Bray D, Lewis J, Raff M, Roberts K, Watson JD. Molecular biology of the cell. New York: Garland; 1983.

5. Williams AF. The T-lymphocyte antigen receptor—elusive no more. Nature 1984;308:108–109.

6. Cooper NR. The complement system. In: Stites DP, et al, eds. Basic and clinical immunology. 5th ed. Los Altos, CA: Lange; 1984.

7. Issitt PD. Antibodies reactive at 30 centigrade, room temperature, and below. In: Butch SH, Beck M, eds. Clinically significant and insignificant antibodies. Washington, DC: American Association of Blood Banks; 1979.

8. Garratty G. Clinical significance of antibodies reacting optimally at 37 C. In: Butch SH, Beck M, eds. Clinically significant and insignificant antibodies. Washington DC: American Association of Blood Banks; 1979.

9. Hughes-Jones NC, Gardner B, Telford R. Studies on the reaction between the bloodgroup antibody anti-D and erythrocytes. Biochem J 1963;88:435–440.

10. Elliot M, Bossom E, Dupuy ME, Masouredis SP. Effect of ionic strength on the serologic behavior of red cell isoantibodies. Vox Sang 1964;9:396-414.

11. Pollack W, Hager HJ, Reckel R, Toren DA, Singher HO. A study of the forces involved in the second stage of hemagglutination. Transfusion 1965;5:158–183.

12. Steane EA, Greenwalt TJ. Erythrocyte agglutination. In: Sandler SG, Nusbacher J, Schanfield MS, eds. Immunobiology of the erythrocyte. (Volume 43 of Progress in clinical and biological research). New York: Alan R. Liss; 1979.

13. Stratton F, Rawlinson VI, Gunson HH, Phillips PK. The role of zeta potential in Rh agglutination. Vox Sang 1973;24:273–279.

14. van Oss CJ, Mohn JF, Cunningham RK. Influence of various physicochemical factors on hemagglutination. Vox Sang 1978;34:351–361.

15. van Oss CJ, Mohn JF, Cunningham RK. Physicochemical aspects of hemagglutination. In: Mohn JF, et al, eds. Human blood groups. (5th International convocation on immunology, Buffalo, NY, 1976) Basel: S Karger; 1977.

16. Gell PGH, Coombs RRA, Lachman PJ, eds. Clinical aspects of immunology. 3rd ed. Oxford: Blackwell; 1975.

17. Wild AE. Transport of immunoglobulins and other proteins from mother to young. In: Dingle JT, ed. Lysosomes in biology and pathology, Vol. 3. New York: American Elsevier; 1973.

18. Gitlin JD, Gitlin D. Protein binding by specific receptors on human placenta, murine pla-

centa, and suckling murine intestine in relation to protein transport across these tissues. J Clin Invest 1974;54:1155–1166.

19. Köhler G, Milstein C. Derivation of specific antibody-producing tissue culture and tumor lines by cell fusion. Eur J Immunol 1976;6:511–519.

20. Reinherz EL, Schlossman SF. The characterization and function of human immunoregulatory T-lymphocyte subsets. In: Masou-

redis SP, ed. Hybridomas and monoclonal antibodies. Washington, DC: American Association of Blood Banks; 1981.

21. Stobo JD. T cells. In: Stites DP, Stobo JD, Fudenberg HH, Wells JV, eds. Basic and clinical immunology. 5th ed. Los Altos, CA: Lange, 1984.

22. Smith KA. Lymphokine regulation of T cell and B cell function. In: Paul WE, ed. Fundamental immunology. New York: Raven Press, 1984.

6

The Antiglobulin Test

In 1945, Coombs, Mourant and Race[1] described a test for detecting nonagglutinating (coating) Rh antibodies in serum. Later, the same test was used to demonstrate in vivo coating of red cells with antibody,[2] and with complement components.[3] This test is now known as the antiglobulin test.

Two forms of antiglobulin testing are used in immunohematology, the direct antiglobulin test (DAT) and an indirect antiglobulin technique. The DAT is used to demonstrate in vivo coating of red cells with antibody or complement; it is used in investigating autoimmune hemolytic anemia, drug-induced hemolysis, hemolytic disease of the newborn and alloimmune reactions to recently transfused red cells. The indirect antiglobulin technique is used to demonstrate in vitro reactions between red cells and coating antibodies, as in antibody detection, antibody identification, blood grouping and compatibility tests.

Principles of the Antiglobulin Test

The antiglobulin test is based on the following simple principles:
1. Antibody molecules and complement components are globulins.
2. Injecting an animal with human globulin, either purified or in whole human serum, stimulates the animal to produce antibody to the foreign protein, ie, antihuman globulin (AHG). The animal serum, after suitable preparation, will react specifically with human globulins. Hybridoma technology is used to prepare some AHG reagents. Serologic tests employ a variety of AHG reagents reactive with various human globulins, including anti-IgG, antibody to the C3d component of human complement and polyspecific reagents that contain both anti-IgG and anti-C3d activity.
3. AHG will react with human globulin molecules either bound to red cells or free in serum. Unbound globulins may react with and neutralize AHG added to a system containing both coated red cells and free globulin molecules. Unless red cells are washed free of unbound globulin prior to AHG testing, unbound globulins may neutralize AHG and cause a false-negative result.
4. Washed red cells coated with human globulin are agglutinated by AHG, as shown in Fig 6-1. The Fab portion of the AHG molecule reacts with the Fc portion of the human antibody molecules attached to each of two separate cells. Uncoated red cells are not agglutinated. The strength of the observed agglutination reaction is proportional to the amount of globulin coating the red cells.

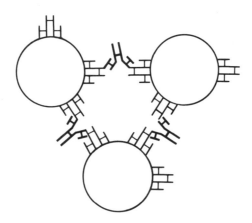

Figure 6-1. The antiglobulin reaction. A rabbit IgG molecule with antihuman globulin specificity is shown reacting with the Fc portion of human IgG molecules coating adjacent red cells (ie, anti-D coating D + red cells).

Antihuman Globulin Reagents

The Center for Drugs and Biologics has established definitions for a variety of AHG reagents, as shown in Table 6-1. The properties and applications of these reagents are discussed below.

Polyspecific AHG

Polyspecific AHG reagents are used for routine compatibility tests, alloantibody detection and the DAT. They contain antibody to human IgG and to the C3d component of human complement. Other anticomplement antibodies are often present, including anti-C3b, anti-C4b and anti-C4d. Commercially prepared polyspecific AHG contains little, if any, activity against IgA and IgM heavy chains; it may react with IgA or IgM molecules, however, since it may contain antibodies to kappa and lambda light chains common to all immunoglobulin classes.

Since most clinically significant antibodies are IgG, the most important function of polyspecific AHG is to detect the presence of IgG. These reagents are prepared and standardized to detect a wide variety of IgG antibodies, including especially those with Rh and Duffy specificities. In addition, the Center for Drugs and Biologics requires that reagents marketed as poly-

Table 6-1. Antihuman Globulin Reagents

Reagent	Definition*
Polyspecific	Contains anti-IgG and anti-C3d; may contain other anticomplement and anti-immunoglobulin antibodies
Anti-IgG	Contains anti-IgG with no anticomplement activity
Anti-IgG (Heavy Chains)	Contains only antibodies reactive against human gamma chains
Anti-C3d and Anti-C3b, Anti-C3d	Contain only antibodies reactive against the designated complement component(s), with no anti-immunoglobulin activity

*As defined by the Center for Drugs and Biologics: *Code of Federal Regulations 21 CFR 660* specific AHG contain anti-C3d activity at a level that equals or exceeds the Center's Anti-C3d Reference Serum.

The importance of anticomplement activity in reagents used for antibody detection and compatibility tests is debatable, since antibodies detectable only by their ability to bind complement are quite rare.[4-9] Anti-C3d activity is, however, extremely important if polyspecific AHG is used for the direct antiglobulin test, as in the investigation of autoimmune hemolytic anemia,[4,7,10,11] because C3d may be the only globulin detectable on red cells in autoimmune hemolytic anemia (see Chapter 14).

Anti-IgG

Reagents labeled "anti-IgG" contain no anticomplement activity. Their major component is antibody to human gamma chains, but unless labeled as "heavy chain specific," they may react with light chains common to all immunoglobulin classes. Anti-IgG is largely used as an alternative to polyspecific AHG in antibody detection and compatibility tests. Some workers prefer anti-IgG over polyspecific AHG, because it does not react with complement bound to cells by clinically insignificant cold-reactive autoantibodies such as anti-I (see Chapter 13).

Anti-IgG not designated "heavy chain specific" must be considered capable of reacting with light chains of IgA or IgM. A positive DAT with anti-IgG not specific for gamma chains does not prove IgG is present, but it is rare for cells to be coated, in vivo, with IgA or IgM without IgG. In a 10-year study of 347 patients with immune hemolytic anemia, Petz and Garratty[11] detected no cases of exclusively IgM coating, and only two cases of exclusively IgA coating.

Monospecific AHG Reagents

Monospecific antibodies to human globulins are prepared by either injecting animals with highly purified immunogens such as IgG, IgA, IgM, C3 or C4, or by harvesting from immunosecreting cell lines (hybridomas). Absorption of unwanted antibodies from multispecific sera was formerly used to obtain monospecific serum.

Two types of monospecific AHG reagents are licensed by the Center for Drugs and Biologics: 1) anti-IgG (heavy chains), containing only antibody against human gamma chains, and 2) anti-C3d, containing no anti-immunoglobulin or anti-C4 activity. The Center for Drugs and Biologics has established labeling requirements for other anticomplement reagents, including anti-C3b, anti-C4b and anti-C4d, but these products are not generally available.

Monospecific AHG reagents are used to determine the proteins responsible for a positive DAT with polyspecific AHG. (See Chapter 14.) Anti-IgG (heavy chains) and anti-C3d are also used in indirect antiglobulin techniques to distinguish patterns of reactivity produced when a single serum contains both complement-binding and non-complement-binding antibodies, for example, anti-Le[a] and anti-E.

Anti-C3b, Anti-C3d

Anti-C3b, anti-C3d reagents prepared by animal immunization contain no activity against human immunoglobulins, and are used in the situations described for anti-C3d. Animal anti-C3d serum characteristically reacts with C3b present on C3-coated cell surfaces, whereas monoclonal anti-C3d reacts almost exclusively with the C3d. (See page 81.)

Antiglobulin Techniques

Direct Antiglobulin Test (DAT)

The direct antiglobulin test is used to demonstrate in vivo coating of red cells with globulins, in particular IgG and C3d. Washed red cells from a patient or donor are tested directly with antihuman globulin (AHG) reagents. The following procedure is for direct testing with polyspecific AHG, but all AHG reagents are used in this manner:

1. Place 1 drop of a 2-5% suspension of red cells in a labeled 10 or 12 × 75-mm test tube. Red cells should be from a blood sample anticoagulated with EDTA, to avoid the in vitro uptake of complement that may occur on red cells exposed to their own serum (see page 81).

2. Wash the red cells three or four times with saline. Completely decant the final supernatant wash solution, and immediately add 1 or 2 drops of polyspecific AHG, as specified by the manufacturer.

3. Mix, centrifuge and examine the red cells for agglutination using an optical aid. Grade and record the reaction. The manner in which red cells are dislodged from the bottom of the test tube is critical. The tube should first be shaken gently, to dislodge the cell button completely, and then be tilted back and forth until an even suspension of red cells or agglutinates is observed.

4. Leave an apparently nonreactive test at room temperature for 5 minutes, recentrifuge and read again. This step is optional, but all manufacturers recommend performing this additional reading when maximal sensitivity for complement detection is desired, as in the investigation of immune hemolysis (see Chapter 15). This additional reading should never be substituted for an immediate reading because reactions due to IgG coating may become weaker after incubation.

5. Add 1 drop of IgG-coated red cells to any tests that are nonreactive. If monospecific anticomplement reagents are used, complement-coated red cells should be substituted for IgG-coated red cells. Centrifuge, examine the red cells for agglutination and grade and record the results. If red cells were not adequately washed, residual unbound globulins from the original serum will neutralize AHG reagents. This important test is the only way to monitor the efficacy of the washing process and demonstrate that reactive AHG was added.

Interpretation

The DAT is positive when agglutination is observed either after immediate centrifugation or after centrifugation following room temperature incubation. Immediate reactions are seen with IgG-coated red cells, but complement or IgA coating may only be demonstrable after incubation.[12] This distinction cannot be used for reliable determination of immunoglobulin type. Monospecific AHG reagents are needed to confirm the types of globulins present.

The DAT is negative when no agglutination is observed at either test phase, providing the IgG-coated red cells added in step 5 above are reactive. If the globulin-coated red cells are not agglutinated, the negative DAT result is considered invalid and the test must be repeated. A negative DAT does not necessarily mean absence of coating globulins. Polyspecific and anti-IgG reagents detect approximately 500 molecules of IgG per red cell,[13] but autoimmune hemolytic anemia has been reported with IgG coating below this level.[11]

Indirect Antiglobulin Testing

Indirect antiglobulin testing is used to demonstrate in vitro coating of red cells with antibody or complement, achieved by incubating serum with red cells, which are then washed to remove unbound globulins. Agglutination after the addition of AHG indicates that the serum contains antibody reactive with antigens present on the red cells. The antibody specificity may be known, as in blood grouping tests with coating antibodies such as anti-Fy^a, or the antigenic composition of the red cells may be known, as in antibody detection and identification tests. In the antiglobulin crossmatch, neither is known; the test is used to determine whether an antigen-antibody interaction occurs. Individual uses of indirect antiglobulin testing are detailed in other chapters, where specific procedures are described.

Factors Affecting the Sensitivity of Indirect Antiglobulin Tests

The following variables affect the in vitro attachment of antibody molecules to red cells, and are not relevant to the direct antiglobulin test.

Temperature

Red cells and serum are normally incubated at 37 C, since most clinically significant coating antibodies react optimally at this temperature. Incubation at lower temperatures decreases the rate of association between antigen and antibody, while incubation at higher temperatures may damage red cells or antibody molecules.

Ionic Strength

Red cells may be suspended in various media, including normal saline, albumin solutions and low ionic strength salt (LISS) reagents. In normal saline, Na^+ and Cl^- ions cluster around and partially neutralize oppositely charged sites on antigen and antibody molecules. This shielding effect, which hinders the association of antibody with antigen, is reduced by lowering the ionic strength of the reaction medium.[14] Consequently, lowering the salt concentration of the reaction medium enhances antibody uptake.[15-17] Albumin solutions, unless used under low ionic conditions, do little to promote antibody uptake.[18] Rather, albumin influences the second stage of hemagglutination (see pages 204–205).

Proportion of Serum to Cells

Increasing the ratio of serum to red cells increases the degree of antibody coating. A commonly used ratio is 2 drops of serum to 1 drop of a 2-5% red cell suspension. By increasing the ratio of serum to red cells, Mollison[13] detected weakly reactive antibodies that were not demonstrable under standard test conditions. It is sometimes useful to increase the volume of serum to 10 or even 20 drops, particularly when investigating a hemolytic transfusion reaction in which routine testing reveals no antibody.

In LISS techniques one volume of serum is used with one or two volumes of LISS solution or additive.[18-23] Increasing the serum volume without increasing the volume of LISS solution or additive increases the ionic strength of the reaction medium. It is important to use the specified volumes when performing LISS tests, especially when incubation time is 15 minutes or less.

Incubation Time

For saline or albumin techniques, 30 minutes incubation at 37 C is adequate to detect most clinically significant coating antibodies. With some weakly-reactive antibodies, however, antigen-antibody association may not reach equilibrium at 30 minutes, and extended incubation is necessary to demonstrate their presence. Extending incubation times beyond 30 minutes has few disadvantages, except for the extra time involved. In LISS tests, equilibrium for most antigen-antibody reactions is attained within 10 to 15 minutes,[19-23] due to the increased rate of association that occurs under low-ionic test conditions.[15-17]

Sources of Error

False-Negative Results

Direct and Indirect Tests

The following considerations apply to tests using either direct or indirect antiglobulin techniques.

1. Failure to wash red cells adequately is a major cause of false-negative antiglobulin tests, since globulins not bound to red cells will neutralize AHG. One volume of human serum diluted as much as 1 to 4000 in saline will neutralize an equal volume of AHG. The washing process must ensure adequate removal of unbound globulins. Cor-

rectly functioning automated cell washers achieve this objective,[24] as do three or four manual washes, providing the test tubes are filled at least three-quarters full with saline. Washing removes unbound globulins by dilution, so it is important to decant the maximum practical volume of supernatant saline from each wash phase. Red cells must be completely resuspended with each new addition of saline; the red cell button should be shaken briskly, and saline added in a forceful stream. The tube should not be inverted against finger or palm, partly because this endangers the worker's health and partly because it can introduce globulins into the wash solution if the hands are contaminated with blood or reagent serum.

2. False-negative reactions can occur if testing is interrupted or delayed. The entire washing process must be undertaken as quickly as possible, to minimize loss of bound antibody by elution from the cells. AHG must be added immediately after washing is completed; otherwise, bound globulins could elute and neutralize AHG when it is eventually added. Once AHG has been added, tests should be centrifuged and read immediately, since reactions due to IgG coating usually become weaker after incubation.

3. AHG reagents can lose activity following improper storage, bacterial contamination or contamination with human serum. AHG reagents are usually stored between 2 C and 8 C. They should never be frozen since this may impair antibody reactivity. AHG reagents, like all blood bank reagents, should be visually inspected with each use and should not be used if they appear turbid or discolored. The entire contents of a vial of AHG will be neutralized if contaminated with whole human serum or with another reagent such as anti-D grouping serum. This will not be apparent visually, and will

only be detected when globulin-coated cells are not agglutinated.

4. AHG may not be present in the test. Omission of AHG sometimes occurs when multiple tests are performed simultaneously.

5. Improper centrifugation influences the sensitivity of antiglobulin tests. Undercentrifugation provides suboptimal conditions for agglutination, while overcentrifugation packs red cells so tightly that the agitation required to resuspend them may break up fragile agglutinates.

6. The number of red cells present in an individual test influences reactivity. Weak reactions occur if too many red cells are present, while too few red cells make it difficult to read agglutination reactions accurately.

7. Prozone reactions are sometimes cited as a possible cause of nonreactive antiglobulin tests (see page 82). Prozones are rarely a problem with licensed AHG reagents which are standardized by the manufacturer. The manufacturer's directions must, however, be followed.

Note: Adding IgG-coated red cells to nonreactive tests will demonstrate false-negative reactions for reasons cited in items 1 through 4, but will not detect other causes of false-negative antiglobulin tests. AABB *Standards*[25] requires use of IgG-coated red cells to check negative results on antiglobulin tests performed in antibody screening and crossmatching procedures on patient samples.

Direct Antiglobulin Tests

The following additional consideration applies only to direct tests:

Complement coating may not be apparent as agglutination upon immediate reading. All manufacturers recommend that the test be incubated at room temperature and examined after recentrifugation when maximal sensitivity for complement detection is desired. This incubation can convert a negative DAT into a positive DAT when red cells are coated with complement or IgA.[12] IgG-coated red cells react more weakly after incubation than at immediate reading, so incubation and rereading should never replace an immediate reading.

Indirect Antiglobulin Tests

The following additional considerations apply only to indirect tests:

1. Red cells and serum lose reactivity if improperly stored. Exposure to excessive heat or repeated freezing and thawing impairs antibody reactivity. Red cells may be damaged at temperatures above 37 C, but some antigens undergo more subtle changes above 6 C.

2. Occasional examples of anti-Jk^a and anti-Jk^b may be detected only in the presence of active complement.[9] Most anticoagulants chelate calcium and magnesium ions that are essential for complement binding; the use of plasma instead of serum can lead to false-negative results. Old or improperly stored serum also has impaired complement activity.

3. Temperature and incubation time affect attachment of antibody or complement to red cells. For most clinically significant coating antibodies, the optimal temperature is 37 C. Incubation for 30 minutes is satisfactory for saline or albumin tests, but 10 to 15 minutes is adequate for LISS techniques.

4. An optimal proportion of serum to red cells should be achieved. If the usual 2 or 3 drops of serum are used, one drop of a 2-5% cell suspension is adequate for routine tests. Too heavy a cell suspension will result in inadequate coating, and too weak a suspension will provide insufficient red cells to read agglutination reactions accurately. Specified volumes of serum and red cells are required when using LISS techniques (see page 205).

False-Positive Results

Direct and Indirect Tests

The following considerations apply to both direct and indirect tests:

1. Red cells may be agglutinated before they are washed. If the prior presence of agglutination is not noted, agglutination observed after adding AHG may be incorrectly interpreted as the result of IgG or complement coating. Red cells from patients with potent cold-reactive autoantibodies may agglutinate in whole blood samples unless maintained at 37 C. This can be recognized by centrifuging washed red cells suspended in 6% bovine albumin, inert serum or AHG reagent diluent. In indirect procedures, some antibodies cause direct agglutination of red cells prior to the addition of AHG. This constitutes an antigen-antibody reaction, but the seemingly positive AHG result should not be interpreted as indicating coating with IgG or complement components.

2. Saline stored in glass bottles may contain colloidal silica particles, leached from the container, that can cause false-positive antiglobulin tests.[13] Saline stored in metal containers, or used in equipment with metal parts, may contain metallic ions that mediate nonspecific attachment of proteins to red cells.[13] The problems are both defined and solved by demonstrating nonreactive tests using saline from a different container, eg, plastic.

3. Improperly cleansed glassware may be contaminated with dust, detergent or other matter that causes red cells to aggregate. It is worthwhile to use test tubes from another source when all tests on different blood samples are weakly reactive.

4. Overcentrifugation packs red cells so tightly that they cannot be dispersed completely. This leads to red cell aggregation which can be mistaken for agglutination.

5. Improperly prepared AHG reagent may contain trace amounts of antihuman species antibodies and agglutinate uncoated red cells. This should not be a problem in tests with licensed AHG reagents and untreated red cells. Enzyme-treated red cells have enhanced reactivity with antispecies antibodies, and may react directly with those AHG reagents containing this contaminating activity. When enzyme-treated red cells are to be used in antiglobulin tests, it is advisable to evaluate AHG reagents for such reactivity prior to testing.[26] Problems due to antispecies should be suspected when all tests on different blood samples react with a particular AHG preparation.

Direct Antiglobulin Tests

The following additional considerations apply only to the DAT:

1. Complement components, primarily C4, may bind to red cells from clotted blood samples kept at 4 C, and occasionally those kept at room temperature.[4,27] This results from the activity of naturally occurring cold-reactive autoagglutinins often present in human serum,[13] and accounts for false-positive antiglobulin tests observed with potent anticomplement reagents.[4,10] Red cells from blood anticoagulated with EDTA, ACD or CPD should be used for the DAT. These anticoagulants chelate calcium and magnesium ions that are essential for in vitro complement activation, but do not affect complement components already bound to red cells following an immune reaction in vivo.

2. False-positive DAT results may occur with blood samples collected into tubes containing silicone gel. Geisland and Milam[28] found eight of 60 (13%) blood samples collected into such tubes had a spuriously positive DAT. Complement coating alone was demonstrable in all eight cases.

3. Blood samples collected from intravenous fluid lines used to administer low-ionic-strength solutions, such as 5% or 10% dextrose in distilled water, may have complement present on the red cells.[29] The gauge of the needle used in the intravenous line and the volume of blood obtained influence the strength of the DAT; strongest reactions are observed when large bore needles are used or when the sample volume obtained is less than 0.5 ml.

4. Septicemia in a patient or bacterial contamination of stored specimens may cause a positive DAT. Microbial agents can cause red cells to become T-activated, resulting in agglutination by anti-T that is present in some AHG reagents.[26]

Note: Extreme reticulocytosis has, in the past, been cited as a cause for false-positive DAT results, because reticulocytes have transferrin on their surface and AHG reagents used to contain antitransferrin. Modern AHG reagents are sufficiently specific for immunoglobulins and complement that this is not a present-day problem.[10]

Indirect Antiglobulin Tests

The following additional consideration applies only to indirect tests:

Red cells with a positive DAT will produce postive indirect antiglobulin tests with all sera. Red cells coated with IgG cannot be straightforwardly tested with antisera that react only by indirect antiglobulin techniques, such as anti-Fy[a]. Procedures for removing IgG from in vivo coated red cells are given on pages 417–418. With these procedures, sufficient IgG can often be removed from red cells to render them suitable for typing with antisera that react solely by indirect antiglobulin techniques.[30] Some antigens may undergo alteration if cells are chemically treated, and tests with reagent antisera may give discrepant results. Antigens of the Kell system are the most frequently affected.

Role of Complement in the Antiglobulin Reaction

Complement components may coat red cells, either in vivo or in vitro, through either of two mechanisms:

1. Complement-binding antibodies attach complement to the cell surface when they react with red cell antigens.
2. Immune complexes present in plasma activate complement components which may adsorb to red cells in a nonspecific manner. The antigen-antibody reaction does not involve specific red cell antigens and the red cells to which complement adsorbs are often described as "innocent bystanders."

Whichever mechanism is involved, red cells become coated with elements of the complement cascade, which may or may not proceed to hemolysis. If the cells do not undergo hemolysis, the presence of bound complement can be detected by AHG reagents containing anticomplement activity. C3 is the complement component most readily detected, since activity of only a few antibody molecules can bind several hundred C3 molecules to the red cell. C4 coating can also be detected, but C3 coating has more clinical significance.

Anticomplement Activity of AHG

C3b is bound to red cells following the action of C4b2a (see page 80). If the complement cascade does not proceed to hemolysis, C3b inactivator (Factor I) cleaves most of the C3b into C3c and C3d. Only C3d remains firmly attached to red cells. To detect complement coating, AHG reagents must contain adequate anti-C3d activity.

Human C3b molecules have receptors that interact with animal antibodies to C3d. Some reagent anti-C3d, notably those prepared in animals, react not only with residual C3d but also with C3b that has not been cleaved by Factor I. Such reagents are called anti-C3b, anti-C3d (see Table 6-1). In contrast, monoclonal anti-C3d reagents react weakly, if at all, with intact C3b. This may be due to the fact that the receptors for monoclonal anti-C3d are not well exposed on intact C3b molecules.

Antibody-Mediated Complement Binding

Some blood group antibodies bind complement to red cell membranes.[3–10,24,27] Most examples of anti-A, -B and -Tj[a] (-PP₁P[k]), and some examples of anti-Vel, -Jk[a] and -Le[a], do this very effectively, and may cause lysis of red cells both in vivo and in vitro. Other examples of anti-Le[a], and some examples of anti-Le[b], -Jk[b] and -P₁, coat red cells with complement components either in vivo or in vitro, but do not hemolyze normal red cells in vitro unless they have been pretreated with a proteolytic enzyme. Yet other examples of these antibodies, and some examples of anti-K, -Fy[a], -Fy[b], -S, -s, -I, -i and -HI, cause in vivo or in vitro coating with complement components but do not cause in vitro hemolysis. The clinical significance of these complement-binding antibodies is also variable. It is not understood why some blood group antibodies coat red cells with sufficient C3 to give strongly reactive antiglobulin tests without causing hemolysis.

Most complement-binding antibodies also coat red cells with immunoglobulins. Some, including anti-A, -B, -I, -i, -HI and -Le[a], are IgM, and cause agglutination as well as complement coating. Other rare IgM antibodies do not cause agglutination under normal conditions, but coat red cells with sufficient complement that their presence is demonstrable using the antiglobulin test. Still others, including most examples of anti-Jk[a] and anti-Jk[b], are IgG antibodies that also bind complement. With these antibodies, the antiglobulin test detects both IgG and complement coating. In a few instances the IgG coating is weak and the complement coating is strong.[4–10,13,24,27] This has been noted especially with anti-Jk^a and anti-Jk^b, both in vivo and vitro.[4,7,8,13,24]

Complement as the Only Coating Globulin

Complement alone, without immunoglobulin, may be present on washed red cells in certain situations described below.

1. IgM antibodies reacting in vitro occasionally coat the cells without causing direct agglutination. IgM coating is difficult to demonstrate in antiglobulin tests because IgM molecules tend to dissociate during the washing process, and polyspecific AHG contains little, if any, anti-IgM activity. Since IgM antibodies often bind complement, the reaction of antibody with antigen can best be recognized by reactivity with the anticomplement components of AHG, since one IgM molecule binds several hundred C3 molecules to red cells (see pages 79–80).

2. About 10% to 20% of patients with warm autoimmune hemolytic anemia have red cells with a positive DAT due to C3 coating alone. No IgG, IgA or IgM coating is demonstrable using routine procedures. Some of these patients have low levels of IgG on their red cells, but in amounts below the threshold of sensitivity for the standard DAT.[11]

3. In cold hemagglutinin disease the cold-reactive autoantibody reacts at temperatures up to 32 C. Skin temperature is at this level, so red cells become coated with autoantibody. The autoantibody then binds complement to red cells, which may or may not proceed to hemolysis. If red cells escape hemolysis, they return to the central circulation where the temperature is 37 C. Autoantibody elutes from the red cells, but complement components remain firmly bound and their presence can be detected with anticomplement reagents. The complement components present on the red cells are C3d

and C4d, since red cell-bound C3b and C4b are both cleaved by C3b inactivator (Factor I, see page 81).

4. Red cells may become coated with complement components that have been activated by immune complexes that form in the plasma and bind weakly and nonspecifically to red cells. The activated complement remains firmly bound to the red cell surface but the immune complex dissociates from the cells. C3 remains as the only surface globulin and can be detected by the antiglobulin test. An example of this mechanism is the positive DAT that sometimes occurs in patients with antibodies to phenacetin or quinidine.[11,31]

References

1. Coombs RRA, Mourant AE, Race RR. A new test for the detection of weak and incomplete Rh agglutinins. Br J Exp Pathol 1945;26:255–266.

2. Coombs RRA, Mourant AE, Race RR. In vivo sensitization of red cells in babies with haemolytic disease. Lancet 1946;1:264–266.

3. Dacie JC, Crookston JH, Christenson WN. "Incomplete" cold antibodies: role of complement in sensitization of antiglobulin serum by potentially haemolytic antibodies. Br J Haematol 1957;3:77–87.

4. Garratty G, Petz LD. The significance of red cell bound complement components in the development of standards and quality control for the anticomplement components of antiglobulin sera. Transfusion 1976;16:297–306.

5. Garratty G, Petz LD. An evaluation of commercial antiglobulin sera with particular reference to their anticomplement properties. Transfusion 1971;11:79–88.

6. Issitt PD, Issitt CH, Wilkinson SL. Evaluation of commercial antiglobulin sera over a two-year period. Transfusion 1974;14:93–102.

7. Petz LD, Garratty G. Anticomplement and the indirect antiglobulin test. Transfusion 1978;18:257–268.

8. Wright MS, Issitt PD. Anticomplement and the indirect antiglobulin test. Transfusion 1979;19:688–694.

9. Howard JE, Winn LC, Gottlieb CF, Grumet FC, Garratty G, Petz LD. Clinical significance of the anticomplement component of

antiglobulin antisera. Transfusion 1982;22:269–272.

10. Chaplin H. Clinical usefulness of specific antiglobulin reagents in autoimmune hemolytic anemia. In: Progress in hematology. New York: Grune and Stratton; 1973;8:25–49.

11. Petz LD, Garratty G. Acquired immune hemolytic anemia. New York: Churchill-Livingstone; 1980.

12. Sturgeon P, Smith LE, Chun HMT, Hurvitz CH, Garratty G, Goldfinger D. Autoimmune hemolytic anemia associated with IgA of Rh specificity. Transfusion 1979;19:324–328.

13. Mollison PL. Blood transfusion in clinical medicine. 7th ed. Oxford: Blackwell Scientific Publications; 1983.

14. Moore BPL. Antibody uptake: the first stage of the hemagglutination reaction. In: Bell CA, ed. Seminar on antigen-antibody reactions revisited. Arlington, VA: American Association of Blood Banks; 1982;47–66.

15. Hughes-Jones NC, Gardner B, Telford R. The effect of pH and ionic strength on the reaction between anti-D and erythrocytes. Immunology 1964;7:72–81.

16. Hughes-Jones NC, Polley MJ, Telford R, Gardner B, Kleinschmidt G. Optimal conditions for detecting blood group antibodies by the antiglobulin test. Vox Sang 1964;9:385–395.

17. Elliot M, Bossom E, Dupuy ME, Masouredis SP. Effect of ionic strength on the serologic behavior of red cell isoantibodies. Vox Sang 1964;9:396–414.

18. Case J. Potentiators of agglutination. In: Bell CA, ed. Seminar on antigen-antibody reactions revisited. Arlington, VA: American Association of Blood Banks; 1982:99–132.

19. Löw B, Messeter L. Antiglobulin test in low-ionic-strength salt solution for rapid anti-body screening and crossmatching. Vox Sang 1974;26:53–61.

20. Moore HC, Mollison PL. Use of a low-ionic-strength medium in normal tests for antibody detection. Transfusion 1976;16:291–296.

21. Wicker B, Wallas CH. A comparison of low-ionic-strength saline medium with routine methods for antibody detection. Transfusion 1976;16:469–472.

22. Rock G, Baxter A, Charron M, Jhaveri J. LISS-an effective way to increase blood utilization. Transfusion 1978;18:228–232.

23. Fitzsimmons JM, Morel PA. The effects of red blood cell suspending media on hemagglutination and the antiglobulin test. Transfusion 1979;19:81–85.

24. Issitt PD, Issitt CH. Applied blood group serology, 2nd ed. Oxnard, CA: Spectra Biologicals, 1975.

25. Standards for blood banks and transfusion services. 11th edition. Arlington, VA: American Association of Blood Banks; 1984.

26. Beck ML, Hicklin B, Pierce SR. Unexpected limitations in the use of commercial antiglobulin reagents. Transfusion 1976; 16:71–75.

27. Gilliland BC, Leddy JP, Baughn JH. The detection of cell-bound antibody on complement coated human red cells. J Clin Invest 1970;49:898–906.

28. Geisland JR, Milam JD. Spuriously positive direct antiglobulin tests caused by silicone gel. Transfusion 1980;20:711–713.

29. Grindon AJ, Wilson MJ. False-positive DAT caused by variables in sample procurement. Transfusion 1981;21:313–314.

30. Edwards JM, Moulds JJ, Judd WJ. Chloroquine dissociation of antigen-antibody complexes: a new technique for typing red cells with a positive direct antiglobulin test. Transfusion 1982;22:59–61.

31. Garratty G, Petz LD. Drug-induced hemolytic anemia. Am J Med 1957;58:398–407.

7

Genetics

The information necessary to determine specific biologic structures and processes resides in specific genes, which are present on chromosomes. In human beings there are 46 chromosomes, 23 pairs. One pair, *XX* in females and *XY* in males, carries the genes associated with sex determination. The other 22 pairs are called *autosomes*.

Terminology

For our purpose it is acceptable to think of a particular gene as occupying a specific position or *locus* on a given chromosome. Loci present on the same chromosome are said to be *syntenic* with one another, regardless of the distance between loci. Two other terms used in describing the relationship of genes to each other are *cis* and *trans*. When the loci that the genes occupy are on the same chromosome, they are in *cis* position; when they are on opposite chromosomes, they are in *trans* position. In Fig. 7-1a, the loci where *A* and *B* reside are in the *cis* relationship whereas those occupied by *A* and *b* are in *trans*.

Alternative genes that may occupy a single locus are called *alleles*; for example, the Kell blood group system includes a pair of alleles *K* and *k*. An individual who inherits identical genes at that locus on both chromosomes, eg, *KK* or *kk*, is *homozygous* for either *K* or *k*, respectively. In the *heterozygous* condition, *Kk*, the genes

present at that locus on each chromosome are nonidentical.

Red cells from a person whose genotype is *KK* are said to have a double dose of K antigen while those from a *Kk* individual have a single dose. It appears that, in some blood group systems, persons with two identical genes have more antigen on their cells than those with two nonidentical genes. The difference in dose of antigen on red cells from two such individuals may be detected serologically. For example, some anti-K sera may give the following pattern of reactivity:

	Genotype of RBC donor	
	KK	*Kk*
Anti-K	3 +	2 +

This variation in strength of antibody reactivity is called *dosage* effect. Dosage effects are not seen with all blood group antigens and antibodies.

Gene Transmission

All genes on a single chromosome are not transmitted as a unit to a gamete, either sperm or egg. During the reductive division of meiosis there is exchange of material between paired chromosomes. This process is called *crossing over*. For example, a parent who is heterozygous at two loci on the same chromosome (*Aa* at one locus and *Bb* at the second locus) may transmit

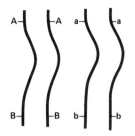

During meiosis, chromo-
somes are duplicated.

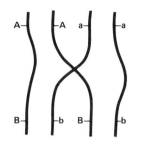

Portions of the paired chromosomes can "cross over";
genetic material is exchanged
between homologous chro-
mosomes.

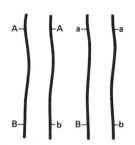

When the chromosomes sep-
arate, they are not exact copies of the original chromosomes. The new chromo-
somes are recombinants.

Figure 7-1. How crossing-over causes recombination of genetic material

any one of four different gametes to a child, *AB*, *Ab*, *aB*, *ab*. See Fig 7-1. The chance of inheriting any one of these combinations is influenced by the distance between the loci. Alleles at loci far apart on the same chromosome (as shown in Fig 7-1) or alleles at loci on different chromosomes are said to *segregate independently*. In the example shown (Fig 7-1) one fourth of the children would inherit *AB*; one fourth, *Ab*; etc. In the general population, however, the frequencies of the combinations *AB*, *Ab*, *aB* and *ab* would be determined by the frequency in the population of each allele, *A* and *a*, *B* and *b*. For example, if the genes are in the population with frequencies:

A	0.4	*B*	0.3
a	0.6	*b*	0.7

then the frequencies of the combinations should be the product of the frequency of each gene:

AB	0.12
Ab	0.28
aB	0.18
ab	0.42

In such a case the loci are said to be in *equilibrium*.

Linkage

An important exception to the rule of independent segregation is *linkage*. Linked loci do not segregate independently but are transmitted to the gametes in a non-random fashion. The closer the linkage (ie, the less distance between the loci) the less likely it is that a crossover will occur between them and the more likely that the genes occupying those loci will be inherited together. For example, Js^a and Js^b are antigens that are part of the Kell blood group system. As shown in Fig 7-2, Js^a and Js^b are alleles at a locus situated very close to the *K/k* locus and the alleles occupying these loci are characteristically transmitted together. These loci are, however, not closely linked to the hypothetical *Z/z* locus which, since it is on the same chromosome, is syntenic with both Js^a/Js^b and *K/k*.

Linkage Disequilibrium

When loci are closely linked, independent segregation does not occur and the loci are not in equilibrium. For example, in the MN blood group system the locus controlling expression of M and N determinants is very closely linked to the locus controlling expression of S and s. The approximate frequencies of the genes are:

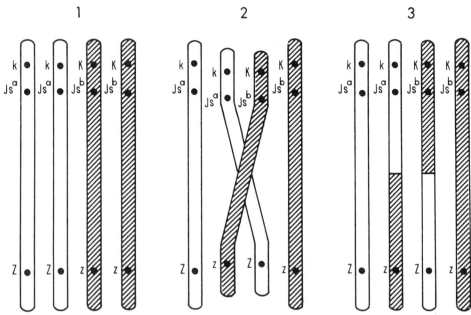

Figure 7-2. Crossing over is a random event that occurs between chromatids during meiosis, resulting in segregation of genes. Very closely linked genes (k and Js^a, K and Js^b in the example shown) are rarely affected by crossing over, whereas genes on the same chromosome that are not closely linked (the Js^aJs^b locus and the Z/z locus shown) manifest crossing over at a rate determined by chance and by the distance between them.

$$M = 0.53 \qquad S = 0.33$$
$$N = 0.47 \qquad s = 0.67$$

If the genes segregated independently, the expected frequencies of the gene complexes would be the product of the frequencies of the individual genes:

$$MS = 0.17$$
$$Ms = 0.36$$
$$NS = 0.16$$
$$Ns = 0.31$$

The observed frequencies are, however:

$$MS = 0.24$$
$$Ms = 0.28$$
$$NS = 0.08$$
$$Ns = 0.39$$

This is an example of *linkage disequilibrium*.

Another commonly cited example of linkage disequilibrium occurs in the HLA system. The HLA-A1,B8 haplotype occurs approximately five time more frequently than would be expected on the basis of frequencies of the individual genes.[1]

Gene Action

The genetic message is carried on chromosomes as a sequence of deoxyribonucleic acid (DNA). The sequence of DNA is transcribed into messenger ribonucleic acid (mRNA), which participates in a number of events that result in a sequence of amino acids. The direct product of a gene is a sequence of RNA; proteins are products of gene action.

Blood group antigens are inherited characteristics, but they are not all protein structures. The early work of Morgan and Watkins[2] showed that carbohydrates determine ABO blood group specificity. The structures of A and B determinants differ only by a single hexose. In the A determinant, N-acetyl-D-galactosamine (GalNAc) is the immunodominant sugar; the group B determinant has a different sugar, D-galactose (Gal), at the same location in the oligosaccharide chain. The corresponding substance from a group O source lacks both of these terminal sugars.[3] Since products of gene action are proteins, how are genetically determined carbohydrate antigens synthesized?

Enzyme Effects

A and B determinants on the red cell membrane consist of a lipid portion or a protein portion to which sugars are sequentially added. The attachment of a sugar occurs only when the enzyme specific for that sugar is present and active. The enzymes, *glycosyltransferases*, that are responsible for adding sugars to precursor molecules, are the protein products of gene action. The *A* gene codes for a transferase specific for GalNAc; the *B* gene, for a transferase specific for Gal.

The transferases must have available a specific acceptor for their respective sugars. For A and B activity, the acceptor is H substance, which, itself, derives from the action of the transferase produced by the *H* gene. The H immunodominant sugar, L-fucose (Fuc), is added to its oligosaccharide acceptor by the action of the fucosyltransferase determined by the *H* gene. If the *H* gene is absent, there will be no fucosyltransferase, no H substance produced, and no acceptor for the A and B immunodominant sugars. Individuals whose genotype is *hh* have no H, A or B antigens on the red cell membrane, a condition called the Bombay phenotype.[3] (See Fig 8-2.)

The *O* gene, once considered an *amorph* or silent gene, has now been shown to direct production of a protein,[4] but one that appears to have no transferase activity. In the group O individual neither

GalNAc nor Gal is attached to the H acceptor, which remains unchanged.

The specficity of certain other blood group antigens also resides in carbohydrate portions of related molecules, eg, those of the Lewis[3,5] and P[6] blood group systems. In other blood group systems, eg, the MNSs system, differences in antigen specificity result from differences in amino acid sequence.[7] (See page 158 and Fig 10-1.)

Dominant and Recessive Traits

Traits are the observed expressions of genes. A trait that is manifested when the determining allele is present in a single dose is called *dominant*; the individual may be heterozygous at that locus and still reveal the trait. A *recessive trait* is revealed only when the allele is present in double dose. It is important to note that these terms are properly used to describe traits; they should not be applied to genes or alleles. In an A^1A^2 individual the presence of the A^2 gene cannot be demonstrated by testing the red cells and A_1 is said to be dominant to A_2. In the A^2O individual, however, the A_2 trait is dominant to that determined by the *O* gene. In these examples the genetic formulae A^1A^2 and A^2O represent the genotypes of the individuals. The observable traits that they determine, A_1 and A_2, are called phenotypes.

Describing traits as dominant and recessive depends on the method used to detect gene products. For example, consider again the A_1 and A_2 traits. Based on red cell testing, the A_1 trait is dominant to A_2 in an A^1A^2 heterozygote. Techniques that detect the specific gene products, the transferases, reveal that the A^1A^2 heterozygote manifests the products of both genes, ie, both A_1 transferase and A_2 transferase.[8] Similarly the *O*-determined protein can be demonstrated in the serum of an A^2O heterozygote.[4] In terms of protein production, A_1, A_2 and O traits are *codominant*.

Blood group antigens are, as a rule, codominant traits; heterozygotes manifest the products of both alleles present. For example, the red cells of an Fy^aFy^b individual have Fy^a and Fy^b antigens, a red cell phenotype of Fy(a+b+).

Patterns of Inheritance

The genetic loci for most blood groups are located on one of the 22 pairs of autosomes. For example, Rh and Duffy genes are on chromosome 1.[9,10] ABO genes are on chromosome 9.[11] No blood group genes have been discovered on the Y chromosome; the *Xg* and *Xk* loci are the only blood group loci ascribed to the X chromosome.[12,13] The known chromosome assignments of the blood group loci are given in Table 7-1.

Autosomal Dominant or Codominant Inheritance

An autosomal dominant trait shows a characteristic pattern of inheritance that is easy to recognize. The trait appears in every generation and occurs with equal frequency in males and females. Most blood group and histocompatibility antigens fit into this category. Figure 7-3(a) presents a pedigree showing the pattern of autosomal dominant inheritance.

Autosomal Recessive Trait

Traits inherited in autosomal recessive fashion also occur with equal frequency in males and females. Individuals who manifest the trait are homozygous for the allele.

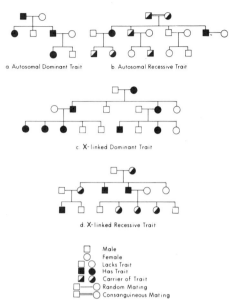

Figure 7-3. Pedigrees showing four different patterns of inheritance.

Their parents may either have or lack the trait. Parents who lack the trait must necessarily be *carriers*, ie, heterozygotes for a gene whose presence is not phenotypically apparent.

If a recessive trait is rare it characteristically occurs only in members of one generation and not in the preceding or successive generations, and related individuals are more likely to carry the same rare gene than unrelated individuals. When offspring are homozygous for a rare gene and display the trait, the parents are usually blood relatives (a consanguineous mating). See Fig 7-3(b).

Sex-Linked Dominant or Codominant Inheritance

A male always gets his single X chromosome from his mother. Therefore the predominant characteristic of X-linked inheritance, both dominant and recessive, is absence of male-to-male (father-to-son) transmission. A male passes his single X chromosome to all of his daughters.

Table 7-1. Blood Group Locus Assignments to Chromosomes[14]

Chromosome	Locus
1	Rh
	Fy
	Sc
	Rd
2	Jk
4	MNSs
6	Ch
	Rg
9	ABO
X	Xg
	Xk

Therefore all daughters of a man possessing a dominant X-linked trait also express the trait. If a woman expresses a dominant trait but is heterozygous, each child, male or female, has a 50% chance of possessing that trait. If the mother is homozygous, all her children will express the trait. A sex-linked dominant trait of interest in blood group genetics is the Xg^a blood group. Figure 7-3(c) demonstrates inheritance of an X-linked dominant trait.

Sex-Linked Recessive Trait

Hemophilia A provides a classic example of X-linked recessive inheritance. See Fig 7-3(d). Among the children of an affected male and a female who lacks the gene, all sons are normal and all daughters are carriers. Males inherit the trait from carrier mothers or, very rarely, from an affected mother homozygous for the gene. In the mating of a normal male and a carrier female, one-half of the male offspring are affected and one-half of the females are carriers. If the gene is rare, males are affected almost exclusively. If the gene is not rare, affected females will be seen, since the chances of an affected male mating with a carrier female increase with the frequency of the gene in the population.

Gene Interaction

Quite often a detectable trait results from interaction among the products of genes occupying unrelated loci. Among the blood groups, the best example of gene interaction involves the action of the *H* and *Le* transferases and the effects of the *Se* gene, which gives rise to the three red cell phenotypes of the Lewis blood group system.[15]

Terms such as *suppressor* and *modifier* are used to describe genes that affect the expression of other genes, but exact mechanisms of these postulated gene interactions are unknown. Some phenomena in blood group serology that have been explained by gene interaction are weakening of the D antigen when the C-determining gene is in *trans* position, and

suppression of Lutheran antigenic expression by the dominant modifier gene, *In(Lu)*. The reader is referred to *Blood Groups in Man*[16] for a discussion of other examples of gene interaction.

Blood Group Nomenclature

Only lately have there been concerted attempts to establish rational, uniform criteria on which to base the phenotype, genotype and gene notations used in blood group genetics. Nomenclature for the hemoglobins, immunoglobulin allotypes, histocompatibility antigens and certain other serum protein systems now often follow generally accepted principles. Similar attempts to standardize blood group notations have met with notably less success. Some examples are:

1. Codominance has been signified by different capital letters, as A and B of the ABO system, both of which are considered dominant to O, also capitalized. Without prior knowledge, it would be impossible to recognize any kinship of these traits to one another.

2. Mendel and other geneticists designated dominant traits with a capital letter, recessive traits with a lower case letter. Unfortunately, some codominants have also been so designated, for example, K and k of the Kell blood group system and C and c of the Rh system.

3. Some codominant traits have contrasting superscript symbols but identical base symbols such as Fy^a and Fy^b (Duffy system) and Lu^a and Lu^b (Lutheran system).

4. Sometimes authors have denoted absence of a serological specificity with a symbol devoid of superscripts or other adornments. Thus, in the Lutheran system, the assumed amorphic gene is not called *lu* (as it strictly should be) but rather *Lu*.

5. More recently, a system of numbers has been used in the Kell, Lutheran, Rh, Duffy and Kidd systems. Numbers

are given to the antibodies, the antigens and the genes that determine presence of the antigens. The numbers do not signify a genetic relationship among genes involved in a single blood group system. The following example demonstrates the proper way to use the numbering system: K1 is the symbol for the K antigen; anti-K1 is the antibody; K^1 denotes the gene. K:1 represents a phenotype; it indicates that the red cells have been tested with anti-K1 and are positive. K:-1, another phenotype, indicates that the red cells have been tested with anti-K1 and do not react. Absence of a number from a phenotype means that the red cells have not been tested for that antigen.

The currently accepted conventions in blood group serology have been reviewed by Issitt and Crookston.[17]

Parentage Testing

Since many of the blood group antigens are expressions of codominant traits with a straightforward mode of inheritance, they are useful in determining exclusion of paternity and probability of paternity. If one assumes that the mother is truly the mother and that the testing was properly done, there are two types of exclusions:

1. *Direct* exclusion is established when a character is present in the child that is absent from the mother and the alleged father. An example is given in the following case:

Child	Mother	Alleged Father
B	O	O

Provided that neither the mother nor the father is of the rare O^h phenotype, the child has inherited a *B* gene, which could not come from either the mother or the alleged father. The *B* gene, based on the phenotypes of mother and child, must have been contributed by the biologic father and is therefore called an *obligatory* gene.

2. In an *indirect* exclusion, genes are absent from the child that should be transmitted by the alleged father, given his observed phenotype. For example, in the following case:

Child	Mother	Alleged Father
Jk(a+b−)	Jk(a+b−)	Jk(a−b+)

the alleged father is presumably homozygous for Jk^b and should have given Jk^b to the child. Since the child is Jk(b−), there is an indirect exclusion.

Direct exclusions provide more convincing evidence that the alleged father is not the biologic father than indirect exclusions because only rarely can the test results be explained by established mechanisms, eg, suppressor genes. Apparent indirect exclusions, however, can sometimes result from the presence of a silent allele. In the example above, the alleged father could have passed the silent allele *Jk* to the child, and the child's genotype could be Jk^aJk. As this example demonstrates, the individual who interprets the results of serological testing must be thoroughly familiar with the inheritance of blood group genes and the factors that influence manifestation of blood group antigens.

In many paternity testing laboratories the probability of paternity is calculated when the alleged father cannot be excluded as the biologic father. These calculations are based on established gene frequencies (see below). The probability that the alleged father is the biologic father is compared with the probability that a random man is the biologic father. The result is expressed as an odds ratio (paternity index) or as a percentage (relative chance of paternity). The reader is referred to the AABB workshop manuals on paternity testing for additional information.[18,19]

Mathematical Genetics

Basic understanding of mathematical genetics is important not only in parentage testing but also in such clinical situations as predicting the likelihood of finding blood compatible with a serum that contains multiple antibodies. Such calculations derive from observations of phenotype frequencies.

Phenotype Frequencies

Phenotype frequencies are determined by testing red cells from a large number of randomly chosen individuals, then calculating the percentage of positive or negative reactions with a given antiserum. The frequency may also be expressed as a decimal. All the possible phenotype frequencies for a given blood group system should equal 100% or 1.00. For example, if red cells from a large number of Caucasian donors are tested with anti-Jk^a, the frequency should be 77% Jk(a+) and 23% Jk(a−). If blood is needed for a patient with anti-Jk^a, 23% or approximately one in four ABO-compatible units of blood should be compatible.

Calculations for Multiple Antibodies

If a patient has multiple blood group antibodies, it may be useful to estimate the number of units that will have to be screened with the patient's serum (or reagent antisera) to find units of blood negative for the appropriate antigens. For example, if a patient has anti-c, anti-K and anti-Jk^a, how many ABO-compatible units of blood will have to be tested to find four units of the appropriate phenotype?

	Phenotype Frequency %
c −	20
K −	91
Jk(a−)	23

To calculate the frequency of the combined phenotype, multiply the individual frequencies.

$$0.2 \times 0.91 \times 0.23 = 0.04$$

Approximately 100 units would have to be tested to find four. If there are only 20 ABO-compatible units available, it is most

unlikely that blood will be found for the patient without the assistance of the local blood supplier or reference laboratory.

Gene Frequencies

Gene frequency, which is calculated from phenotype frequencies, is the fraction that each allele contributes to the total gene pool. The sum of gene frequencies for alleles at a given locus must equal 1.00. To determine the frequency of genes Jk^a and Jk^b from the observation that 77% of bloods are Jk(a+), the Hardy-Weinberg formula for a two allele system can be used:

$$p^2 + 2pq + q^2 = 1.$$

In the equation

$$
\begin{aligned}
p &= \text{frequency of } Jk^a \\
q &= \text{frequency of } Jk^b \\
p^2 &= \text{frequency of } Jk^aJk^a \\
2pq &= \text{frequency of } Jk^aJk^b \\
q^2 &= \text{frequency of } Jk^bJk^b
\end{aligned}
$$

Then

$$
\begin{aligned}
p^2 + 2pq &= \text{frequency of Jk(a+)} \\
&= 0.77 \\
q^2 = 1 - (p^2 + 2pq) &= \text{frequency of } Jk^bJk^b \\
q^2 = 1 - 0.77 &= 0.23 \\
q &= \sqrt{0.23} \\
&= 0.48
\end{aligned}
$$

Since the frequency of all allelic genes must equal 1.00,

$$
\begin{aligned}
p + q &= 1 \\
p &= 1 - q \\
&= 1 - 0.48 \\
&= 0.52
\end{aligned}
$$

Once the gene frequencies have been calculated, the number of Jk(b+) individuals can be calculated as:

$$
\begin{aligned}
2pq + q^2 &= \text{frequency of Jk(b+)} \\
&= 2 (0.52 \times 0.48) + (0.48)^2 \\
&= 0.72
\end{aligned}
$$

If both anti-Jk^a and anti-Jk^b sera are available, gene frequencies can be deter-

Table 7-2. Gene Frequency in the Kidd Blood Group System Calculated Using Direct Counting

	Individuals	Kidd Genes	*Jkᵃ*	*Jkᵇ*
Jk(a + b −)	28	56	56	0
Jk(a + b +)	49	98	49	49
Jk(a − b +)	23	46	0	46
Totals	100	200	105	95

mined more easily by the direct count method. As shown in Table 7-2, the 100 individuals tested for Jkᵃ and Jkᵇ antigens possess 200 genes in the Kidd blood group system, one from each parent (2 × 100). The frequency of Jk^a = 0.52 and Jk^b = 0.48.

For more information on mathematical genetics the reader should see reviews by Walker[19] or Steane.[20]

References

1. Miller WV. The HLA system. In: Petz LD, Swisher SN, eds. Clinical practice of blood transfusion. New York: Churchill Livingstone, 1981:151.

2. Watkins WM, Morgan WTG. Inhibition by simple sugars of enzymes which decompose the blood-group substances. Nature 1955;175:676–677.

3. Watkins WM. Blood group substances. Science 1966;152:172–181.

4. Yoshida A, Yamaguchi YF, Dave V. Immunologic homology of human blood group glycosyltransferases and genetic background of blood group (ABO) determination. Blood 1979;54:344–350.

5. Marcus DM, Cass LE. Glycosphingolipids with Lewis blood group activity: uptake by human erythrocytes. Science 1969;164:553–554.

6. Naiki M, Marcus DM. An immunochemical study of the human blood group P₁, P and Pᵏ glycosphingolipid antigens. Biochemistry 1975;14:4837–4841.

7. Dahr W, Uhlenbruck G, Janssen E, Schmalisch R. Different N-terminal amino acids in the MN-glycoprotein from MM and NN erythrocytes. Hum Genet 1977;35:335–343.

8. Schacter H, Michaels MA, Tilley CA, Crookston MC, Crookston JH. Qualitative diffferences in the N-acetyl-D-galactosaminyltransferases produced by A¹ and A² genes. Proc Natl Acad Sci USA 1973;70:220–224.

9. Ruddle F, Ricciuti F, McMorris FA, et al. Somatic cell genetic assignment of peptidase C and the Rh linkage group to chromosome A-1 in man. Science 1972;176:1429–1431.

10. Donahue RP, Bias WB, Renwick JH, McKusick VA. Probable assignment of the Duffy blood group locus to chromosome 1 in man. Proc Natl Acad Sci USA 1968;61:949-955.

11. Van Cong N, Weil D, Finaz C, et al. Assignment of the ABO-Np-Ak₁ linkage group to chromosome 9 in man-hamster hybrids. Cytogenet Cell Genet 1976;16:241–243.

12. Mann JD, Cahan A, Gelb AG, et al. A sex-linked blood group. Lancet 1962;i:8–10.

13. Marsh WL, Øyen R, Nichols ME, Allen FH. Chronic granulomatous disease and Kell blood groups. Br J Haematol 1975;29:247–262.

14. Lewis M. Recent advances in blood groups. Clin Lab Med 1982;2:137–154.

15. Mollison PL. Blood transfusion in clinical medicine. 7th ed. Oxford: Blackwell Scientific Publications, 1983:323.

16. Race RR, Sanger R. Blood groups in man. 6th ed. Oxford: Blackwell Scientific Publications, 1975.

17. Issitt PD, Crookston MC. Blood group terminology: current conventions. Transfusion 1984;24:2–7.

18. Silver H, ed. Probability of inclusion in paternity testing. Arlington, VA: American Association of Blood Banks, 1982.

19. Walker R. Mathematical genetics. In: Wilson JK, ed. Genetics for blood bankers. Washington, DC: American Association of Blood Banks, 1979:55–100.

20. Steane EA. Basic genetics. In: Pittiglio DH, ed. Modern blood banking and transfusion practices. Philadelphia: FA Davis Co, 1983:23–53.

8

The ABO System

Introduction

In 1900, Karl Landsteiner studied blood samples from his colleagues by mixing each person's serum with suspensions of each person's cells. Noting agglutination in some mixtures but not in others, he was able to classify blood samples into three categories, now named A, B and O. The fourth group, AB, was discovered by Landsteiner's pupils, von Decastello and Sturli, in 1902. Landsteiner recognized that the presence or absence of only two antigens, A and B, was sufficient to explain the four blood groups. He also showed that serum contained an antibody directed against the antigen absent from that person's red blood cells.

Significance

The ABO blood group system is the only system in which the antibodies are consistently and predictably present in the serum of normal individuals whose red cells lack the antigen(s) (see Table 8-1). The first blood group system to be discovered, the ABO system remains by far the most significant for transfusion practice. ABO compatibility between donor and patient is the essential foundation on which all other pretransfusion testing rests.

The ABO system includes many phenotypes and several antibody specificities. A blood group system is a group of anti-

gens produced by allelic genes located at a single locus and inherited independently of any other genes. Since several different sets of genes, each at different loci, affect the phenotypes associated with the ABO system, it is perhaps not strictly correct to refer to all the antigens and antibodies as belonging to a single system. Nonetheless, it is appropriate to discuss the phenotypic observations in a broadly inclusive context.

Antigens of the ABO System

Although A, B, and the associated precursor H antigens can be detected on red cells in embryos 5 to 6 weeks old, the antigens are not fully developed at birth.[1] Reagent sera may give weaker reactions with red cells from neonates than with red cells from adults. By the time an individual is 2 to 4 years old the red blood cell antigens are fully developed and remain constant throughout life.[2]

A_1 and A_2

The two principal subgroups of A are A_1 and A_2. Serologic distinction between A_1 and A_2 is based on reactivity of the cells with human anti-A_1 serum or with lectin anti-A_1 prepared from *Dolichos biflorus* seeds; reagent anti-A sera very seldom differentiate between A_1 and A_2. Both human anti-A_1 and lectin anti-A_1 agglutinate A_1

113

Table 8-1. Routine ABO Grouping

Reaction of Cells Tested With		Reaction of Serum Tested Against			Interpre- tation	Frequency (%) in U.S. Population			
Anti-A	Anti-B	A Cells	B Cells	O Cells	ABO Group	Whites	Blacks	American Indians*	Orientals*
0	0	+	+	0	O	45	49	79	40
+	0	0	+	0	A	40	27	16	28
0	+	+	0	0	B	11	20	4	27
+	+	0	0	0	AB	4	4	<1	5

+ = agglutination; 0 = no agglutination
*Composite figures, calculated from Mourant, et al.[14]

cells but not, under prescribed test conditions, A_2 cells. Red cells from approximately 80% of persons with A antigen are agglutinated by anti-A_1; those persons are classified as A_1 or A_1B. The remaining 20%, whose red cells are agglutinated by anti-A but not by anti-A_1, are called A_2 or A_2B.

It is not necessary to classify group A patients or donors as A_1 or A_2 except when working with an A_2 or A_2B individual whose serum contains anti-A_1. Anti-A_1 occurs in the serum of 1 to 8% of A_2 persons and 22 to 35% of A_2B persons.[3] Anti-A_1 causes discrepancies between ABO cell and serum tests and may also cause crossmatch incompatibilities, but is considered to be clinically insignificant unless it reacts at 37 C.[1]

Weak Subgroups of A

Subgroups weaker than A_2 occur infrequently and, in general, are characterized by declining numbers of A antigen sites on the red cells and reciprocal increase in H reactivity. (See Genetic and Biochemical Considerations, below). The genes responsible contribute less than 1% of the total pool of A genes. Classification of weak A subgroups is generally based on[4]:
1. Degree of red cell agglutination by anti-A and anti-A_1.
2. Degree of red cell agglutination by anti-A,B.
3. Degree of H reactivity on the red cells.

4. Presence or absence of anti-A_1 in the serum.
5. Presence of A and H substances in saliva of secretors.

See Table 8-2 for the serologic characteristics of A phenotypes.

Use of Anti-A,B

Anti-A,B does not agglutinate red cells of the less common A or B subgroups. A_x cells are those most reliably identified by anti-A,B but the immediate spin technique does not usually uncover this activity. The antiserum and red cells must be incubated at least 10 minutes at room temperature before centrifugation. If the manufacturer's package insert recommends using the anti-A,B for detection of weak subgroups, it means that reactivity against A_x cells has been demonstrated with that reagent.[5]

A_3 Phenotype

Of the rare subgroups of A, the most common is A_3. When tested with anti-A, A_3 red cells characteristically show a mixed-field pattern of small agglutinates among many free cells. A_3 cells are agglutinated by anti-A,B but not by lectin anti-A_1 or by human anti-A_1. With anti-H, A_3 cells react more strongly than A_1 cells. Occasionally, A_3 persons have anti-A_1 in their serum. Secretors who are A_3 have A substance in their saliva in addition to H substance.

Table 8-2. Serologic Reactions of A and B Phenotypes*

Red Blood Cell Phenotype	Reaction of Cells with Known Antiserum to					Reaction of Serum Against Reagent Red Blood Cells				Saliva of Secretors Contains
	A	B	A,B	H	A₁	A₁	A₂	B	O	
A_1	++++	0	++++	0	++++	0	0	++++	0	A & H
A_{int}	++++	0	++++	+++	++	0	0	++++	0	A & H
A_2	++++	0	++++	++	0	†	0	++++	0	A & H
A_3	+ +^{mf}	0	+ +^{mf}	+++	0	†	0	++++	0	A & H
A_m	0/±	0	0/±	++++	0	0	0	++++	0	A & H
A_x	0/±0	0	+/++	++++	0	++	0/+	++++	0	H
B	0	++++	++++	0		++++	++++	0	0	B & H
B_3	0	+^{mf}	+ +^{mf}	++++		++++	++++	0	0	B & H
B_m	0	0	0/±	++++		++++	++++	0	0	B & H
B_x	0	0/±	0/++	++++		++++	++++	0	0	H

+ to + + + +, agglutination of increasing strength; ±, weak agglutination; mf, mixed-field pattern of agglutination; 0, no agglutination.
*Adapted from Beattie[4]
†The occurrence of anti-A_1 is variable in these phenotypes. A_x persons frequently have anti-A_1; A_3 persons usually do not, but a few A_3 individuals with anti-A_1 in the serum have been found.

Weak Subgroups of B

Subgroups of B are even less common than subgroups of A. Criteria for their differentiation resemble those for subgroups of A (see Table 8-2).

"Bombay" or O_h Phenotype

Individuals homozygous for the rare gene *h* have red cells devoid of A, B or H antigens. On initial testing the cells appear to be group O, and the phenotype is called O_h. The O_h phenotype is popularly called "Bombay" because it was first discovered in Bombay and seems to occur more often in India than elsewhere.[6] In routine testing, O_h bloods may appear to be group O since the red cells are not agglutinated by anti-A or anti-B and the serum agglutinates both A and B red cells. Because O_h persons lack H substance on their red cells, their serum contains anti-H that is as strong as the anti-A and anti-B.

The presence of the phenotype quickly becomes apparent when the serum reacts strongly with all group O red blood cells. Existence of O_h blood type is confirmed by testing the red cells with a saline extract of *Ulex europaeus* (anti-H) and demonstrat-ing absence of H. If O_h cells from a person known to have the "Bombay" phenotype are available, the serum can be tested against these cells and will be compatible.

Antibodies of the ABO System

Ordinarily, individuals possess antibodies directed against those ABH antigens absent from their own cells. (See Table 8-1.) This predictable complementary relationship permits using both serum and cell tests in ABO blood grouping. (See page 120.)

Development of Anti-A and Anti-B

The immunoreactive configurations that confer A, B and H specificity on molecules of the red cell membrane (see page 119) also exist in other biologic entities, notably bacterial cell walls. Bacteria are widespread in the environment and it appears that their presence in dust, food and other widely distributed agents ensures constant exposure of all persons to A, B and H-like antigens. Immunocompetent persons react to these stimuli by producing antibodies against those ABH antigens foreign to their own systems. Thus, anti-A occurs in the sera of group O and group B persons and anti-B in the sera of group O and group A individuals. Group AB persons, having both antigens, make neither antibody. The serum of persons of the O_h phenotype routinely contains anti-H; occasional A_1 or A_1B persons have very little H antigen on their cells and may form a weakly reactive anti-H.

Anti-A_1

The anti-A in group O and group B sera appears, from simple studies, to contain separable anti-A and anti-A_1. Absorbing the serum with A_2 cells leaves reactivity against A_1 but not A_2 cells. The difference, however, is quantitative and not qualitative. The apparent anti-A_1, made by absorption of group B serum with A_2 cells is, in fact, a weakened form of anti-A. It reacts with A_1 cells because those cells have more A antigen sites than do A_2 cells. Weakened anti-A obtained by absorbing group B serum can be used, at the practical level, to identify A_1 cells, but further absorption with A_2 cells can remove all anti-A activity.

Time of Appearance

Since production of blood group antibodies normally begins only after birth,[7] tests on serum from newborns and infants up to about 4 to 6 months of age are unreliable. Serum from newborns may contain IgG antibodies passively acquired by placental transfer from the mother if she has IgG anti-A or anti-B. Anti-A and anti-B production begins during the first few months of life, increases for the first 5 or 6 years and then remains fairly constant until late in adult life. In elderly people, the level of anti-A and anti-B is often significantly lower than in young adults.[1]

Antibody Behavior

Anti-A and anti-B consistently agglutinate saline-suspended red blood cells. Other effects can and do occur under appropriate test conditions. If complement is present, the red cells may be lysed. In serum (reverse grouping) tests (see page 121),

hemolysis becomes apparent by pink discoloration of the supernatant fluid and, sometimes, total destruction of the red cells after centrifugation. Because hemolysis of this sort requires complement, it will not occur if A and B reagent red cells are suspended in solutions containing EDTA or other anticoagulants.

ABH antibodies sometimes coat red cells without causing agglutination. When a serum contains both coating and agglutinating antibodies of the same specificity, agglutination is the only detectible end point unless the agglutinating antibodies are neutralized or inactivated. Coating antibodies are usually IgG. Small amounts of IgG anti-A or anti-B can be found in all group B or group A sera and larger amounts are frequent in group O serum. Since IgG antibodies readily cross the placenta, they frequently coat the red cells of infants born to mothers with high antibody levels.

"Immune" and "Naturally Occurring" Antibodies

Agglutinating anti-A and anti-B develop so regularly after environmental exposure that they are considered to be "naturally occurring," ie, not stimulated by foreign red cells. Some kinds of exposure to A and B antigens result in production of antibodies with the same specificity but different biologic behavior. These are sometimes called "immune" antibodies. Immunization may follow pregnancy with an ABO-incompatible fetus, transfusion of incompatible red blood cells or of plasma containing blood group substance, injection of purified blood group substances or inoculation with viral or bacterial products that contain blood group-active materials.

After the immunizing stimulus, the anti-A or anti-B may increase in titer or avidity, develop powerful hemolytic properties, become more difficult to inhibit with soluble blood group substances or become more active at 37 C. These changes are more common in group O persons but may occur in group A or group B persons. Although the distinction is not always clear, non-red-cell-stimulated antibodies in group A and B individuals tend to be IgM, and those produced in response to an immunogenic stimulus are more often IgG.

Both IgM and IgG classes of anti-A and anti-B agglutinate saline-suspended red cells, react at room temperature and cause in vitro hemolysis. Group O persons regularly have in their serum anti-A and anti-B of both immunoglobulin classes in addition to anti-A,B. The distinguishing features of IgM and IgG anti-A and anti-B are shown in Table 8-3.

Anti-A,B (Group O Serum)

Serum from group O individuals contains an antibody designated anti-A,B. It reacts with A cells and B cells and the anti-A and anti-B activities cannot be separated by differential absorption (see page 234). When A cells are used to absorb anti-A from group O serum, the eluate contains anti-A and also an antibody that reacts with both A cells and B cells. Similar reactions are observed when B cells are used for absorption. Saliva from group A or group B secretors inhibits the reaction of this antibody with either A or B red cells. Anti-A,B from group O serum reacts more strongly than anti-A or anti-B with red cells of some A and B subgroups.

Some workers routinely use reagent anti-A,B as a check in ABO grouping tests to avoid mistakenly designating weakly reactive cells as group O. *Standards* does not require the use of anti-A,B or of any procedure to detect weak A or B phenotypes, many of which distinguish themselves from group O by failing to give expected serum grouping results (see Table 8-2). Anti-A,B can be used alone as the required procedure to confirm the ABO labelling of group O cells prior to transfusion.

Anti-H

There are two kinds of human anti-H. One occurs as a cold-reactive agglutinin in the serum of individuals with relatively little H on their cells, usually group A_1 or A_1B individuals; the other is produced by the rare O_h individuals whose cells have no H.

Cold-reactive anti-H agglutinins are relatively rare because individuals of all blood groups have some H substance on their red cells. The amount of H on red cells is, in order of dimishing quantity, $O > A_2 > A_2B > B > A_1 > A_1B$. Occasional group A_1, A_1B or, less commonly, B, individuals have red cells on which there is so little unconverted H substance that they are able to produce anti-H. The anti-H in such sera is weak, never reaching the agglutinating strength of the anti-H in O_h individuals or reacting at 37 C.

Because O_h individuals completely lack the H antigen, anti-H is regularly present in the serum. Anti-A and anti-B are also present. This form of anti-H reacts over a wide thermal range between 4 and 37 C with all cells other than O_h. This antibody binds complement and causes hemolysis. O_h persons must be transfused only with O_h blood[8] because their anti-H rapidly destroys group O red cells and their anti-A and anti-B destroy A or B cells.

Table 8-3. Distinguishing Characteristics of IgM and IgG Anti-A and Anti-B

	IgM	IgG
Reactions enhanced		
—by enzyme-treating cells	yes	yes
—by lowering temperatures	yes	no
Readily inhibited by soluble A or B antigens	yes	no
Inactivated by 2-ME or dithiothreitol (DTT)	yes	no
Predominant in non-immunized group A and B donors	yes	no

Genetic and Biochemical Considerations

Nature of A, B and H Antigens

A, B, and H antigenic activity resides in sugar linkages on short chains of sugars (oligosaccharides) present on either of two types of molecules: glycoproteins, in which the oligosaccharide chains are linked via galactosamine to a polypeptide backbone; and glycosphingolipids (glycolipids), in which they are linked via glucose to a lipid, primarily ceramide. Oligosaccharide chains range from relatively short simple chains to complex branching structures. No matter what the underlying molecule on which the oligosaccharide chain is located, the sugar linkages that determine A, B and H activity are unvarying.

Glycosphingolipids form part of the red cell membrane, and also occur in membranes of most endothelial and epithelial cells. Glycosphingolipids in soluble form are present in plasma, but not in secreted body fluids. Soluble glycoproteins with ABH activity exist in the body's serous and mucous secretions and membrane-associated glycoproteins are present in red cells and other body cells. Oligosaccharide chains unattached to a protein or lipid moiety are found in milk and urine.

Type 1 and Type 2 Chains

The terminal sugar linkages of the oligosaccharide chain exist in two different configurations, called type 1 and type 2 (see Fig 8-1), differing in the manner in which the terminal β-galactose (Gal) joins the subterminal β-N-acetylglucosamine (GlcNAc). The carbon 1 of the 6-carbon sugar galactose can be attached to either carbon 3 or carbon 4 of GlcNAc. The oligosaccharide chain with the 1→3 linkage is called the type 1 chain and the chain with 1→4 linkage is called type 2. Blood group-active glycoproteins present on cell surfaces or in fluids have both type 1 and type 2 chains. Glycosphingolipids present in plasma and those on membranes of

TYPE 1

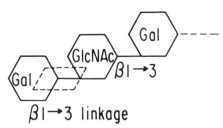

$\beta 1 \rightarrow 3$ linkage

TYPE 2

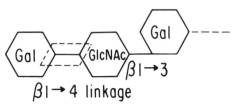

$\beta 1 \rightarrow 4$ linkage

Gal = Galactose
GlcNAc = N-acetylglucosamine

Figure 8-1. Type 1 and type 2 oligosaccharide chains differ only in the linkage between the N-acetylglucosamine and the terminal galactose.

most glandular and parenchymatous cells have either type 1 or type 2 chains, but the glycolipid chains synthesized on the red cell membrane are exclusively type 2.

Immunodominant Sugars

ABH antigenic activity depends on the attachment of specific individual sugars to the terminal portions of the oligosaccharide chains. The sugar whose presence determines the activity of a specific antigen is called the immunodominant sugar for that antigen. Attachment of the immunodominant sugars depends on the action of sugar-transferring enzymes, collectively called glycosyl transferases. An individual's genes determine the presence or absence of specific transferases,[9] hence the presence or absence of specific sugars on the oligosaccharide chain, and thus the presence or absence of specific antigens.

ABO blood groups are genetically determined but the antigens are not the direct products of the blood group genes; the genes control the enzymes that attach the sugars that confer antigen specificity.

The Genes Involved

Genes at three separate loci (ABO, Hh and Sese) determine the occurrence and location of the A, B and H antigens. At the ABO locus on chromosome 9 are three common alleles—A, B and O—and numerous rare alleles. Family studies have shown[10] that the H and Se (secretor) loci are closely linked but the chromosome on which they are located has not been identified. There are only two recognized alleles at the H locus—the active form H and the very rare h. No product has been demonstrated for h, which is often designated an amorph. At another locus on the same chromosome is the Se gene or its allele se. The Se gene is necessary for the expression of A, B and H antigenic activity on the glycoproteins in epithelial secretions. The se gene, having no demonstrable product, is also an amorph.

Interactions at the Phenotypic Level

Studies of antigens present in the secretions of persons with the O_h phenotype suggest the possibility that two types of H antigen exist. Persons who lack the H gene and also lack the Se gene have no A, B or H antigens present on red cells or in their secretions. ABH antigens are, however, found in the secretions of O_h persons who possess the Se gene. It has been suggested that H and Se genes each code for a different α-L-fucosyl transferase[10]: the one produced by the Se gene reacting preferentially with type 1 oligosaccharide chains and acting primarily in secretory glands; and the one produced by the H gene reacting preferentially with type 2 chains and manifesting activity primarily in membrane-associated molecules of vascular endothelium and red cells.

The transferase produced by the H gene is essential for the subsequent expression of ABH antigens on red blood cells. It attaches L-fucose, the immunodominant sugar for H, to the terminal galactose of type 2 oligosaccharide chains. Only if there is a fucose moiety on the 2 carbon of that galactose can additional sugars be added. The A-specified transferase (α-N-acetylgalactosaminyl transferase) and the B-specified transferase (α-galactosyl transferase) attach the immunodominant sugars necessary for A and B activity (N-acetyl-galactosamine and D-galactose, respectively) to carbon 3 of the terminal galactose of the H-active chain. If the individual is group O, there are no A- or B-specified transferases and the H activity remains unmodified (see Fig 8-2). The O gene is a silent allele which may control production of a protein that can be detected immunologically but has no detectable transferase activity.[11]

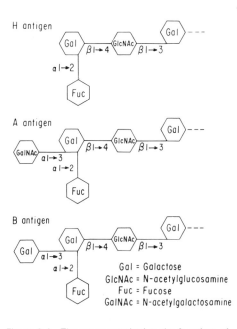

Figure 8-2. The sugar attached to the 3 carbon of galactose determines antigenic activity. N-acetyl-galactosamine confers A activity; galactose confers B activity. Unless the fucose moiety that determines H activity is attached to the 2 carbon, galactose does not accept either sugar on the 3 carbon.

The Se Gene

Secretors, those persons possessing the *Se* gene, comprise approximately 80% of the population. They have in their epithelial secretions H, A, and/or B-active glycoproteins, depending upon their ABO phenotype. The *Se* gene is essential for the expression of the ABH antigens in secretions. The suggested role for the *Se*-specified transferase[10] is to attach L-fucose to the terminal galactose of type 1 chains, thus forming H substance in the secreted material. *A* or *B*-specified transferases then attach the A or B immunodominant sugar to the H substance. Nonsecretors, those lacking the *Se* gene (*sese*), secrete type 1 and type 2 glycoproteins with no H, A or B activity.

Rare individuals exist who are homozygous for the amorphic *h* gene (the O$_h$ or "Bombay" phenotype). In the absence of fucosyl transferase produced by the *H* gene, fucose is not attached to the type 2 oligosaccharide chains. These *hh* individuals have normal levels of the *A*- or *B*-specified transferases if they have the *A* or *B* gene, but there is no substrate on which they can act.[12,13] As a result, the red cells of these individuals lack A, B and H substance, the O$_h$ or "Bombay" phenotype described on page 115.

Subgroups of A

Different alleles at the *ABO* locus determine transferases with differing properties and efficiency in converting H, but the vast majority of transferases fall into a few simple categories. The two commonest forms of the *A* gene are A^1, comprising 80% of the *A* gene pool, and A^2, comprising nearly 20%. A$_3$ and some of the rarer subgroups result from the activity of rare genes whose α-GalNAc transferases are biologically much less effective. Most group B persons have a galactosyl transferase of fairly uniform properties.

Routine Testing for ABO

For both donors and patients, routine ABO grouping must include both red cell testing and serum testing; each test serves as a check on the other. To confirm the ABO group of units of donor blood already labeled, it is permissible to test either cells or serum or plasma. ABO tests are performed at room temperature or lower. Incubation at 37 C weakens the reactions, so a lighted or otherwise warmed viewbox must not be used in ABO testing.

Red cells are tested with anti-A and anti-B for the presence or absence of agglutination. Reagent antisera are usually prepared from sera of individuals stimulated with A or B blood group substances to produce high antibody titers. These antisera contain potent antibodies that agglutinate most red cells on direct contact, without centrifugation. Testing cells for ABO, sometimes called *direct* or *forward* grouping, can be performed on a slide, in tubes or in microplates (see Special Methods, page 435).

Testing serum against known A and B cells is sometimes called *reverse* or *serum* grouping. Serum grouping cannot reliably be performed on slides because unstimulated anti-A and/or anti-B are not always strong enough to agglutinate red cells without enhancement by centrifugation.

Considerations Common to All Tests

Each manufacturer provides, with each package of antiserum, detailed instructions for the use of anti-A and anti-B. Manufacturers' instructions vary in details of testing; it is important to follow the directions for the specific antiserum in use. Instructions that apply to all tests for ABO grouping are:

1. Label all tubes, slides or microplates. Do not rely on the color of dyes to identify reagent antiserum.
2. Perform tests at temperatures no higher than room temperature (20 to 24 C).
3. Inspect for agglutination against a well-lighted background, but not on a warm viewbox.
4. Record results immediately after observation.

Slide Tests for A and B Antigens

Slide tests should be performed according to the manufacturer's directions for the antiserum used. Some manufacturers recommend using whole blood, while others specify a certain concentration of cells suspended in serum, plasma or saline.

Instructions that apply to all slide tests are:

1. Label the sections of the slide to identify the antisera used.
2. Use a separate, clean stick to mix cells with each antiserum.
3. Mix cells and antiserum gently but thoroughly over an area about 2 cm in diameter.
4. Do not place slide on or over a warmed viewbox or other heat source.
5. Keep cell-serum mixture in continuous, gentle motion and observe for 2 minutes before concluding that agglutination is absent.
6. Do not confuse clumps due to drying around the edges with agglutination.
7. Avoid touching the cell-serum mixture with fingers to reduce risk of hepatitis transmission.
8. Record results immediately after observation.

Tube Tests for Anti-A and Anti-B

Most sera have anti-A and/or anti-B strong enough to agglutinate A_1 or B cells promptly upon centrifugation. A_1 and B cells used for serum testing may be prepared locally or purchased as reagent red cells. If prepared locally, the cells should be prepared fresh each day of use, as a 2 to 5% suspension of cells washed and resuspended in saline. The cells may be from single individuals known to be group A_1 and group B.

1. Place 2 drops of serum into each of two properly labeled tubes.
2. Add 1 drop of A_1 cells to the A tube, and 1 drop of B cells to the B tube.
3. Mix by gentle shaking. To enhance agglutination, tubes may be incubated 5 minutes or more at room temperature.

4. Centrifuge at speed and time determined to be optimal.
5. Observe supernatant fluid against a well-lighted white background for evidence of hemolysis, if cells are in a suspending medium that permits complement activity.
6. Gently disperse cell button and inspect for agglutination, against a well-lighted background.
7. Record results immediately after observation.

Interpretation of Routine ABO Tests

Table 8-1 gives the results and interpretations of routine ABO cell and serum testing. Note that the ABO groups have different frequencies in different segments of the U.S. population.[14]

Discrepancies may occur between the results of cell and serum tests, causing difficulty in interpreting the ABO group. If this happens the results should be recorded, but the report of interpretations must be delayed until the discrepancy is resolved. (See section below.)

Discrepancies Between Cell and Serum Results

When results of cell and serum tests for ABO do not agree, the discrepancy must be investigated. If the blood is from a donor unit, the unit must not be released for transfusion until the discrepancy is resolved. When the blood is from a potential recipient, it may be necessary to administer group O red cells of the appropriate Rh group before investigations are complete. It is important to obtain enough of the patient's blood before transfusion that testing can be continued on a sample free of transfused cells.

Discrepancies in ABO testing may result from technical errors, from intrinsic properties of the red cells, or from intrinsic properties of the serum.

Technical Errors

Errors in technique cause unpredictable inaccuracies. Most such problems occur sporadically, although continuing problems with equipment, reagents or interpretation may affect tests on many different specimens.

1. Incorrect identification of specimens or materials or incorrect recording of results or interpretations cause false-positives or false-negatives.
2. Failure to add patient's or donor's serum to the test causes a false-negative.
3. Contamination of antisera or reagent red cells may cause false-positives or negatives.
4. Inappropriate ratio of cells to serum may cause a false-positive or false-negative.
5. Overcentrifugation may cause a false-positive and undercentrifugation may cause a false-negative.
6. Failure to identify hemolysis as a positive reaction causes a false-negative.
7. Warming cell-serum mixture may cause a false-negative.
8. Dirty glassware may cause false-positive reactions.

Problems in Testing Red Cells

1. If the cells are suspended in their own serum, rouleaux formation may simulate agglutination. This can result from abnormal concentrations of serum proteins, the presence of other macromolecules, or, in cord blood samples from newborns, the presence of Wharton's jelly. Unwashed cells suspended in saline may carry enough serum to mimic the reactions of cells suspended in serum.
2. The patient may have recently been transfused or received a bone marrow transplant, so the sample may be a mixture of cell types.
3. The cells may have inherited or acquired surface abnormalities that render them polyagglutinable.[15]

4. The A or B antigens may be weakly expressed because of an unusual genotype.
5. There may be acquired "B-like" activity, usually resulting from action of gram-negative organisms.[16]
6. The A or B antigens on red cells may be weakened in patients with leukemia.[1]
7. There may be such high concentrations of A or B blood group substances in the serum that, if serum-suspended cells are used, the reagent antibody may be inhibited from reacting with antigens on the red cells.[8]

Problems in Testing Serum

1. Altered protein proportions, abnormal proteins or high concentrations of fibrinogen may cause rouleaux formation that resembles agglutination.
2. The patient may have received agents whose presence in serum causes rouleaux, such as plasma expanders of high molecular weight, intravenously injected contrast materials, or various drugs.
3. There may be an unexpected antibody in the serum that reacts with other antigens on the A_1 or B cells used for serum grouping. Autoanti-I is the antibody most commonly encountered in reverse grouping. Anti-A_1 in serum from A_2 or A_2B persons may agglutinate A_1 cells fairly strongly. Anti-H in serum from A_1 or A_1B persons rarely causes a problem in reverse grouping because A_1 and B cells used for serum grouping have relatively little H.
4. The patient may be an infant who has not begun producing antibodies or who has antibodies acquired in utero from the mother. Reverse grouping is not routinely done on serum from newborn infants.
5. The patient may be an elderly person whose antibody levels have declined markedly.
6. The patient may have antibodies against constituents of the preservatives, sus-

pending media, or reagent solutions used in testing.[17]

7. The patient may have an immunodeficiency due to disease or therapy and thus lack expected antibodies.
8. The patient may have received a bone marrow transplant from a donor of a different ABO group.
9. The patient may have undergone therapeutic plasma exchange or received transfusions of perfluorocarbons. The expected antibodies may be so diluted during the procedure that they become difficult or impossible to detect.

Resolving ABO Discrepancies

When there is an apparent ABO discrepancy, it is advisable simply to repeat the cell and serum tests as the first step before undertaking extensive investigation. Strict adherence to proper technique, use of quality-controlled reagents and careful observation and interpretation of test results resolve many apparent problems. A discrepancy that persists must be investigated.

Preliminary Procedures

1. Obtain a new blood specimen from the donor unit or patient. This step identifies discrepancies due to contaminated or misidentified samples.
2. Wash the red cells several times and repeat tests on a 2-5% saline suspension of washed cells.
3. Perform a direct antiglobulin test on the cells. (See Chapter 15 for details of testing cells heavily coated with antibody.)
4. Test the cells with anti-A,B, anti-A_1 or anti-H, as appropriate for the individual problem.
5. Test the serum against appropriate A_1, A_2 and B cells. Group O cells and autologous cells should be used as controls. It may be helpful to test group O (or ABO-compatible) cord cells if anti-I is suspected. If necessary, incubate cell and serum tests at least 30 minutes at room temperature and at 4 C before concluding that the results are negative. Group O and autologous control cells are especially important for tests incubated at 4C, to prevent misinterpretation of positive test results due to autoagglutinins or alloagglutinins reactive at these temperatures.

Anomalies Involving Red Cells
Missing or Weak Antigens

Weak or missing A (or B) should be suspected when the serum contains anti-A (or anti-B) but the red cells are not agglutinated as expected by complementary reagent anti-B (or anti-A). This can occur in individuals with rare alleles of *A* or *B* that code for A or B antigens of diminished reactivity, or in patients in whom leukemia has decreased antigen reactivity. If, for example, anti-B is the only antibody present in the serum but the red cells do not react with anti-A:

1. Retest washed red cells with anti-A, anti-A_1, anti-A,B and anti-H; incubate the tests and the group O and autologous control cells at least 30 minutes at room temperature and at 4 C.
2. If agglutination does not occur and the presence of A is still suspected, incubate cells with anti-A to adsorb antibody onto the cells. (Do not use anti-A_1 lectin.) After cells and serum have been incubated, prepare an eluate and test it against group A_1 cells. If the cells had A antigen that adsorbed anti-A, the eluate will agglutinate A_1 cells. (See page 458 for details of adsorption and elution procedures).
3. Test the saliva for the presence of A and H substances. (See page 459 for hemagglutination-inhibition tests for salivary antigens.) This test is helpful only if the individual is a secretor.

Acquired B Antigen

Acquired B antigen should be considered when the red cell group appears to be AB and the serum contains anti-B. A_1 cells are the only group that exhibits acquired B activity in vivo.[3] To identify an acquired B antigen:

1. Observe the strength of red cell agglutination with anti-A and anti-B. The reactions with anti-A are usually much stronger than with anti-B. This difference is often more conspicuous when the test is performed on a slide.
2. Test the patient's serum against his own cells. Anti-B in the patient's serum does not agglutinate red cells with acquired B antigen.
3. Test saliva for the presence of A and B substance. If the patient is a secretor, A substance is present but B is not.
4. Check the patient's diagnosis. Acquired B antigens tend to be associated with carcinoma of the colon or rectum, infection with gram-negative organisms and intestinal obstructions.[3,15]

Polyagglutinable Red Cells

Polyagglutinability should be considered when the red cells are agglutinated by all reagent antisera, giving ABO results at variance with alloantibodies present in the serum. ABO discrepancies caused by polyagglutination are resolved in different ways. See Special Methods, page 428, for the reactions that polyagglutinable cells exhibit when tested with various lectins. See also the discussion by Beck[15] of ways to distinguish the causes of this phenomenon.

Mixed-Field Agglutination

Two distinct, separable populations of red cells may be present in a blood sample, usually following transfusion of group O red cells to a group A or B patient, but also in patients who have received bone marrow transplants of an ABO group different from their own. Much less frequently, the two cell populations are constitutional, a condition called *chimerism*, that can result from intrauterine exchange of erythropoietic tissue by fraternal twins or from mosaicism caused by dispermy. In all such circumstances, cell typing tests may give a mixed-field pattern of agglutination.

Following transfusion and bone marrow transplants, the mixture of cell populations lasts only for the life of the transfused cells or, in the case of the bone marrow transplant, the original red cells, whereas genetic chimerism is present throughout the life of the individual. The two cell populations can be separated by procedures involving agglutination or hemolysis or both. A more detailed discussion of chimerism and separation of cell populations is given by Beattie.[4]

Mixed-field agglutination is the characteristic pattern seen when A_3 cells are tested with anti-A. If the agglutinated cells are removed and the remaining cells are again tested with anti-A, mixed-field agglutination occurs in the residual population as well. Mixed-field agglutination may also be seen with the weakened A antigens that sometimes accompany leukemia.[1]

Antibody-Coated Red Cells

Red cells may be heavily coated with antibody in hemolytic disease of the newborn, in autoimmune hemolytic anemia, or following incompatible transfusions. Such cells may agglutinate spontaneously in the presence of any high-protein medium, including ABO typing reagents. It is often possible to remove much of the antibody by gentle elution (see page 417), after which anti-A and anti-B can be used to test the red cells reliably.

Anomalies Involving Serum
Rouleaux

Serum with rouleaux-producing properties causes most red cells tested to appear agglutinated. Rouleaux are easily recognized microscopically if the aggregates form the characteristic "coin-like" stacks, but often the aggregates are irregularly shaped and closely resemble antibody-mediated agglutinates. Reverse grouping results can usually be clarified by one of the following procedures:

1. Add 1-3 drops of saline to the tube after gently resuspending the centrifuged cells. Adding saline usually disperses rouleaux but does not alter agglutination due to anti-A and/or anti-B.
2. Use the saline replacement technique as described on page 452.
3. Make doubling dilutions of the serum and test the diluted serum against autologous cells. Determine the dilution at which rouleaux are no longer seen, and test serum diluted to this level against A₁, B and O cells. A or B alloantibodies nearly always have a higher titer than the rouleaux-forming properties[4] and can be easily detected by this method.

Autoanti-I

Autoanti-I in serum agglutinates all red cell samples from adult donors, including the patient's own and those used in serum grouping tests.[4] Except in fulminant cold hemagglutinin disease (CHD, see section in Chapter 15) in which the anti-I is the most avid antibody present, the agglutination caused by anti-I is usually weaker than that caused by anti-A and anti-B. Cord cells, which exhibit less I reactivity than adult cells, are generally not agglutinated. If autoanti-I is suspected, serum grouping can be done as follows:
1. Absorb the anti-I from the serum using a cold autoabsorption method as described on page 466.
2. Test the absorbed serum against A₁ and B cells.
3. Use as a negative control either group O cells or autologous cells that are not coated with anti-I.

Another procedure is to treat the serum with the reducing agents 2-mercaptoethanol (2-ME) or dithiothreitol and test the treated serum for the presence of IgG anti-A and anti-B.

Anti-A₁

Anti-A₁ in the serum of A₂ or A₂B individuals usually agglutinates the A₁ cells used for serum grouping tests. To identify anti-A₁ as the cause of an ABO discrepancy:
1. Test the serum against several examples, preferably three each, of A₁, A₂ and O red cells. The group O cells used for the antibody screen may be used. The antibody can be considered to be anti-A₁ if it agglutinates all the A₁ cells and none of the A₂ or O cells.
2. Test the cells with anti-A₁. Cells of A₂ or weaker subgroups will not be agglutinated by anti-A₁.

Anti-A₁ sometimes causes incompatibility on crossmatches. If, on carefully temperature-controlled tests, the antibody is reactive at 37 C, it should be considered clinically significant, and only A₂ or O cells be used for transfusion.

Unexpected Alloantibodies

Unexpected alloantibodies that react at room temperature, such as anti-P₁ or anti-M, may agglutinate the cells used for reverse grouping if the A₁ or B reverse grouping cells happen to have the corresponding antigens. This should be suspected as the cause of the ABO discrepancy if the antibody detection test is positive at room temperature. Rarely, the serum may react with an antigen on the reverse grouping cells that is absent from the antibody screening cells. To determine the serum group:
1. Identify the alloantibody, as described in Chapter 13.
2. Test the reverse grouping cells for the presence of the corresponding antigen.
3. Test the serum against examples of A₁ and B cells lacking the antigen corresponding to the identified antibody. For instance, if anti-M is identified, use A₁ and B cells that are M-negative.
4. If the antibody screening test is negative, repeat the serum tests on several other examples of A₁ and B cells. If the antibody reacts with an antigen so uncommon that the antibody detection cells do not possess it, randomly selected

A_1 and B cells can be expected to lack the antigen also.

Expected Antibody Not Present

Expected alloantibodies may be absent from serum of patients with immunodeficiency diseases such as agammaglobulinemia or hypogammaglobulinemia. Newborns are not expected to have ABO alloantibodies. Very elderly people may have low or undetectable levels. In these instances, the ABO blood group can be determined only by cell testing. If the individual has normal levels of other antibodies and serum globulins, the possibility of a very weak antigen should be considered. (See "Missing or Weak Antigens," page 123.)

References

1. Mollison PL. Blood transfusion in clinical medicine. 7th ed. Oxford: Blackwell Scientific Publications, 1983.

2. Grundbacher FJ. Changes in the human A antigen of erythrocytes with the individual's age. Nature 1964;204:192-194.

3. Issitt PD, Issitt CH. Applied blood group serology. 2nd ed. Oxnard, CA: Spectra Biologicals, 1975.

4. Beattie KM. Discrepancies in ABO blood grouping. In: A seminar on problems encountered in pretransfusion tests. Washington, DC: American Association of Blood Banks, 1972:129-165.

5. Code of federal regulations (21 CFR), part 660.26. Washington, DC: US Govt Printing Office, 1982.

6. Bhatia HM, Sathe MS. Incidence of "Bombay" (O_h) phenotype and weaker variants of A and B antigens in Bombay (India). Vox Sang 1974;27:524-532.

7. Toivanen P, Hirvonen T. Iso- and heteroagglutinins in human fetal and neonatal sera. Scand J Haematol 1969;6:42-48.

8. Davey RJ, Tourault MA, Holland PV. The clinical significance of anti-H in an individual with the O_h (Bombay) phenotype. Transfusion 1978;18:738-742.

9. Watkins WM. The glycosyltransferase products of the A, B, H, and Le genes and their relationship to the structure of the blood group antigens. In: Mohn JF, Plunkett RW, Cunningham RK, Lambert RM, eds. Human blood groups. Basel: S Karger, 1977:134-142.

10. Oriol R, Danilovs J, Hawkins BR. A new genetic model proposing that the Se gene is a structural gene closely linked to the H gene. Am J Hum Genet 1981;33:421-431.

11. Yoshida A. Identification of genotypes of blood group A and B. Blood 1980; 55:119-123.

12. Race C and Watkins WM. The enzymic products of the human A and B blood group genes in the serum of "Bombay" O_h donors. FEBS Lett 1972;27:125-130.

13. Mulet C, Cartron JP, Badet J, Salmon C. Activity of α-2-L-fucosyl-transferase in human sera and red cell membranes. A study of common ABH blood donors, rare "Bombay" and "Parabombay" individuals. FEBS Lett 1977;84:74-78.

14. Mourant AE, Kopec AC, Domaniewska-Sobczak K. The distribution of the human blood groups and other polymorphisms. 2nd ed. London: Oxford University Press, 1976.

15. Beck ML. The polyagglutinable red cell. In: The investigation of typing and compatibility problems caused by red blood cells. Washington, DC: American Association of Blood Banks, 1975:1-3.

16. Gerbal A, Maslet C, Salmon C. Immunological aspects of the acquired B antigen. Vox Sang 1975;28:398-403.

17. Mallory DM. Problems in the hemagglutination reaction. Part 1: false positive reactions due to drugs, dyes, and interfering substances. In: A seminar on polymorphisms in human blood. Washington, DC: American Association of Blood Banks, 1975:129-141.

9

The Rh System

The Rh system is so complex, and certain aspects of its genetics, nomenclature and antigenic interactions are so unsettled, that any attempt at full coverage in this manual would be unrealistic. The aim in this chapter will be to concentrate on commonly encountered observations, problems and solutions, without exhaustive theoretical considerations. More information is in the literature listed at the end of this chapter.

Rh-Positive and Rh-Negative

The unmodified descriptive terms *Rh-positive* and *Rh-negative* refer to the presence or absence of the red cell antigen now almost universally called D. An earlier name for D, Rh_0, has fallen largely into disuse, but remains of historical interest. To minimize confusion, the CDE nomenclature of Fisher and Race is used almost exclusively in this chapter, but sometimes it is necessary to use a combination of CDE and Rh-Hr terminology to facilitate understanding. Table 9-1 gives the equivalent names and may be used when needed for reference.

Discovery of D

The first human example of the antibody directed at the D antigen was reported in 1939 by Levine and Stetson,[1] who found it in the serum of a woman whose fetus had fatal hemolytic disease of the new-

born. In 1940, by immunizing guinea pigs and rabbits with the red cells of rhesus monkeys, Landsteiner and Wiener[2] raised an antibody that agglutinated the red cells of approximately 85% of humans tested. They called the determinant, apparently common to all rhesus monkeys and 85% of humans, the *Rh factor*. The connection between the two antigens and the clinical importance of the Rh factor were recognized the same year, when Levine and Katzin[3] found several postpartum women whose sera contained similar antibodies, at least one of which gave reactions that were parallel to those of the animal anti-rhesus sera. Also in 1940, Wiener and Peters[4] observed examples of human anti-Rh in Rh-negative patients who had received ABO-compatible transfusions of Rh-positive blood. Later evidence established that the antigens detected by animal anti-rhesus and human anti-D are not identical, but by that time the Rh blood group system had already received its name.

Clinical Significance

The D antigen is, after A and B, the most important red cell antigen in transfusion practice. Unlike the situation with A and B, persons whose red cells lack the D antigen do not regularly have anti-D in their serum. Formation of the antibody almost always results from exposure, through

Table 9-1. Equivalent Notations in the Rh Blood Group System

Numerical Designation	CDE	Rh-Hr	Other	Numerical Designation	CDE	Rh-Hr	Other
Rh1	D	Rh_0		Rh22	CE	rh*	Jarvis
Rhw1	D^u	$\mathfrak{R}h_0$		Rh23	D^w		Wiel
Rh2	C	rh'		Rh24	E^T		
Rh3	E	rh"		Rh25			LW
Rh4	c	hr'		Rh26	"c-like"		Deal
Rh5	e	hr"		Rh27	cE	rh_{ii}*	
Rh6	ce	hr		Rh28		hr^H	Hernandez
Rh7	Ce	rh_i		Rh29			total Rh
Rh8	C^w	rh^{w1}		Rh30	DCor		Go^a
Rh9	C^x	rh^x		Rh31		hr^B	
Rh10	ce	hr^v	V	Rh32		$\bar{\bar{R}}^N$‡	Troll
Rh11	E^w	rh^{w2}		Rh33		R_0^{Har}	Hill
Rh12	G	rh^G		Rh34		Hr^B	Bastiaan
Rh13	†	Rh^A		Rh35			1114
Rh14	†	Rh^B		Rh36			Be^a
Rh15	†	Rh^C		Rh37			Evans§
Rh16	†	Rh^D		Rh38			Duclos
Rh17		Hr_0		Rh39	"C-like"		
Rh18		Hr		Rh40			Targett
Rh19		hr^S		Rh41	"Ce-like"		
Rh20	e^s		VS	Rh42	Ce^s	rh_i^s	Thornton
Rh21	C^G			Rh43			Crawford

The table is compiled from the findings of the ISBT Working Party on Terminology for Red Cell Surface Antigens at a meeting held in August 1982.

*The Rh-Hr designations for Rh22 and Rh27 were the subject of a personal communication from Dr A.S. Wiener (1972).

†Categories I through VI of Tippett and Sanger[28,29] include these subdivisions of the D antigen, but the notations are not directly comparable.

‡Rh32 is a low frequency antigen that is a product of the predominantly black gene $\bar{\bar{R}}^N$, the other products of which include a reduced expression of C and e. The antibody that defines Rh32 has come to be called, perhaps rather misleadingly, "anti-$\bar{\bar{R}}^N$."

§Rh37 is the low-frequency antigen Evans, which occurs in association with the ·D· haplotype. This is similar to −D−, except for the presence of the Evans antigen and a lesser exaltation of D activity.

either transfusion or pregnancy, to immunizing red cells possessing the D antigen. A high proportion of D− subjects so exposed will produce anti-D. The immunogenicity of D, that is to say the likelihood of its provoking an antibody if introduced into a D− recipient, is greater than that of virtually all other red cell antigens studied. Of D− persons who receive a single unit of D+ blood, 50-75% can be expected to develop anti-D.[5,6] Accordingly, the blood of all recipients and donors is routinely tested for D, so that D− recipients can be identified and given D− blood.

Soon after anti-D was discovered, family studies showed that the D antigen is genetically determined, and that the gene controlling its production behaves like an autosomal dominant. The *Rh* genes have been shown to reside on chromosome 1.[7,8] With only a few interesting exceptions, persons who have the gene for D will have the antigen directly detectable on their red cells.

Other Important Antigens

More frequent and sophisticated pretransfusion testing, as well as investigations of transfusion reactions, soon revealed antibodies that identified antigens showing a recognizable association with D. By the mid-1940's, four additional antigens had been recognized as belonging to what is now called the Rh system[9-12]; subsequent new discoveries have brought the total of Rh-related antigens to over 40 (Table 9-1). The reader should be aware that these exist, but the five principal antigens and their specific antibodies are likely to account for more than 99% of the clinical work in the Rh field.

After D, the next four antigens to be recognized were C, E, c and e. The association of these antigenic factors suggests that immunologic activity of Rh arises from surface material with several determinant areas. Some antigenic associations include D and some do not. Combinations that do not include D nevertheless possess activity at other sites. The composition of these antigenic configurations is genetically determined. In terms of the five main antigens under discussion, a single gene (or gene complex) will determine the production or nonproduction of D, together with the production of either C or c and E or e. Many variations or combinations have been recognized and investigated, but these five antigens and the comparatively common antibodies that characterize them are the backbone of the Rh blood group system.

Inheritance and Nomenclature

Genes and Dosage

The genetic material that determines all constituents of an Rh haplotype is transmitted inseparably. It is best to think of a single gene as determining the composition of each combination of antigens, although it is convenient, if not strictly correct, to think of subloci as responsible for individual antigens. A person inherits one Rh gene from each parent. If these are identical the individual is homozygous for that gene and all the products of the gene will be expressed in double dose on that person's red cells. When the genes inherited from each parent are not identical, the person is heterozygous for two different genes and, since the *Rh* genes are codominant, the products of both will be expressed on that person's red cells. Antigens that are products of both genes will be present in double dose, while those produced by only one of the pair of genes will be present in single dose. In this context, the terms *homozygous* and *heterozygous* may be used in reference to an imagined sublocus. Thus, to be "homozygous for *D*" means that the person's two *Rh* genes both code for the production of D, not necessarily that both *Rh* genes are the same.

Serologic Reactivity

Testing red cells with specific Rh antisera gives reaction patterns that do not consistently parallel antigen dose. This is because the expression of these gene products is sometimes influenced by interaction between the two genes, or interaction between subloci of the same gene. This subject is treated in greater detail on page 132.

Attempts to isolate the Rh antigens for chemical study have met with limited success, so it is not clear how genetic information is translated into serologically demonstrable characteristics. An ambitious conceptual model of the Rh system has been advanced by Rosenfield and coworkers.[13] The interested reader should consult this paper for details.

Terminology

Three systems of nomenclature have been used to express genetic and serologic information about the Rh system.

Systems Notations

The Rh-Hr terminology derives from the work of Wiener,[14] who believed that the immediate gene product is a single entity he called an *agglutinogen*. According to Wiener's concept, each agglutinogen is characterized by numerous individual serologic specificities called *factors*, each of which is recognized by its own specific antibody. What Wiener called agglutinogens are now called *haplotypes*, and what Wiener called *factors* are now called *antigens*.

The CDE terminology was introduced by British workers Fisher and Race,[15] who postulated three closely linked loci. The same letter designation is used for both gene and gene product, except that, by convention, the symbols for genes are always printed in italics.

Rosenfield and coworkers[13,17] proposed a system of nomenclature based simply on serologic observations. The symbols were not intended to convey genetic information, but merely to facilitate the recording of phenotypic data. Antigens are numbered, generally in order of their discovery or of their admission to the Rh system, and their presence on the red cells is designated by the use of the appropriate numbers following the prefix Rh and a colon. A negative symbol preceding a number indicates the absence of that antigen.

It is useful to be familiar with both the CDE and Rh nomenclatures, and it may be helpful to have some knowledge of the numerical system (below). Table 9-2 shows the most common combinations of anti-gens determined by allelic gene complexes. Table 9-3 shows the reaction patterns of various cells tested with the five principal antisera, together with the descriptive terms used for phenotype in the three systems of nomenclature.

Phenotypic Notations

For informal designation of phenotype, particularly in conversation, many workers use a shorthand system based on Wiener's Rh-Hr notations and used by the English in the 1940's. These do not fit into any nomenclatural system, but they convey information in a convenient and efficient fashion. In Wiener's terminology, genes were designated by single italic letters: R for genes that include $Rh_o(D)$ among their products and r for genes that do not determine Rh_o, with various superscript symbols (R^1, R^2, R^o, R^z, r', r'', r and r^y) to denote the different alleles. The gene products or, by extension, the haplotypes, were designated by roman type Rh and rh with subscripts to indicate the different haplotypes. Again, a capital letter R was used when the gene product included $Rh_o(D)$. The symbols for individual factors were roman characters in boldface type, with **Rh$_o$** representing D and **rh'**, **rh''**, **hr'** and **hr''** representing C, E, c and e, respectively.

Table 9-2. Frequencies of the Principal Rh Genes (or Gene Complexes)

Wiener Terminology		Fisher-Race Terminology		Frequency in US Population, in %			
Allele	Major Antigenic Specificities	Gene Combination	Antigenic Specificities	Whites	Blacks	Native Americans	Orientals
R^1	Rh$_o$,rh',hr''	CDe	C,D,e	0.42	0.17	0.44	0.70
r	hr',hr''	cde	c,e	0.37	0.26	0.11	0.03
R^2	Rh$_o$,hr',rh''	cDE	c,D,E	0.14	0.11	0.34	0.21
R^o	Rh$_o$,hr',hr''	cDe	c,D,e	0.04	0.44	0.02	0.03
r'	rh',hr''	Cde	C,e	0.02	0.02	0.02	0.02
r''	hr',rh''	cdE	c,E	0.01	0.00	0.06	0.00
R^z	Rh$_o$,rh',rh''	CDE	C,D,E	0.00	0.00	0.06	0.01
r^y	rh',rh''	CdE	C,E	0.00	0.00	0.00	0.00

All figures were calculated from Mourant et al[16] and represent averages of several series in each case. Those for Native Americans are averaged from a total of 15 series and, in view of large regional variations, may be misleading.

Table 9-3. Determination of Some Rh Phenotypes from the Results of Tests with the Five Principal Rh Antisera

Antisera					Phenotypes in three nomenclatures		
Anti-D	Anti-C	Anti-E	Anti-c	Anti-e	Rh-hr	CDE	Numerical
+	+	0	+	+	Rh_1rh	CcDe	Rh:1,2, −3,4,5
+	+	0	0	+	Rh_1	CDe	Rh:1,2, −3, −4,5
+	+	+	+	+	Rh_1Rh_2	CcDEe	Rh:1,2,3,4,5
+	0	0	+	+	Rh_0	cDe	Rh:1, −2, −3,4,5
+	0	+	+	+	Rh_2rh	cDEe	Rh:1, −2,3,4,5
+	0	+	+	0	Rh_2	cDE	Rh:1, −2,3,4, −5
+	+	+	0	+	Rh_zRh_1	CDEe	Rh:1,2,3, −4,5
+	+	+	+	0	Rh_zRh_2	CcDE	Rh:1,2,3,4, −5
+	+	+	0	0	Rh_z	CDE	Rh:1,2,3, −4, −5
0	0	0	+	+	rh	ce	Rh: −1, −2, −3,4,5
0	+	0	+	+	rh′rh	Cce	Rh: −1,2, −3,4,5
0	0	+	+	+	rh″rh	cEe	Rh: −1, −2,3,4,5
0	+	+	+	+	rh′rh″	CcEe	Rh: −1,2,3,4,5

The shorthand phenotype notations employ single letters R and r in roman type, with subscripts, or occasionally superscripts, to indicate antigenic combinations. These subscripts are based approximately on the notations shown in the first column of Table 9-2. Thus R_1 indicates C, D and e together; R_2 indicates c, D and E; r indicates c and e; R_0 indicates c, D and e; and so on. In Table 9-3, the shorthand notations for the first five phenotypes would be R_1r, R_1R_1, R_1R_2, R_0, and R_2r.

Phenotype and Genotype

In clinical practice, only five reagent antisera are readily available. Routine pretransfusion studies include only tests for D; other antisera are used principally in the resolution of antibody problems or in family studies. The assortment of antigens detected on a person's red cells constitutes that person's phenotype. Since any one antigen may derive from any of several different genes, identifying antigens does not always allow the genotype to be deduced with certainty. Presumptions regarding the most probable genotype rest on knowledge of the frequency with which particular antigenic combinations derive from a single gene complex. Inferences about

genotype are useful in population studies and in the investigation of disputed parentage. Such analyses are also used to predict whether the sexual partner of a woman with Rh antibodies is likely to transmit the genes that will result in offspring negative for the particular antigen.

Unique Problem of D

Determining whether a person has one gene or two that code for C and c, and for E and e, is relatively easy in most cases; the required antisera are available and the red cells may be tested readily for both C and c and both E and e. In the case of the D antigen, however, only its presence or absence can be determined. If D is absent, it is normally correct to assume that the person tested possesses two genes that code for haplotypes lacking D. If D is present there is no simple serologic technique to establish whether two genes are present that code for D, or whether the antigenic material is the product of only one such gene. No antibody has been found that reacts specifically with a product common to all gene complexes that code for haplotypes lacking D, and dosage studies utilizing titrations of anti-D reagents do not give reliable information.

Position Effect

Position effect reflects interaction between genes. If the interaction is between genes on the same chromosome, or between their products, it is called a "*cis* effect." If a gene or its product interacts with the *Rh* gene on the opposite chromosome, it is called a "*trans* effect." Examples of both effects were first reported in 1950 by Lawler and Race,[18] who noted as a *cis* effect that the E antigen produced by the *cDE* (R^2) gene is quantitatively weaker than E produced by *cdE* (*r″*). They noted as *trans* effects that both C and E are weaker when they result from the genotype *CDe/cDE* (R^1R^2) than when the genotypes are *CDe/cde* (R^1r) or *cDE/cde* (R^2r), respectively.

Homozygous and Heterozygous Expression of D

Most D − persons are homozygous for the gene *r*, which produces c and e but no D. Less often, a gene that does not produce D may produce C or E (*r′* and *r″*, respectively). The gene that produces both C and E but not D (*r^y*) is quite rare. In any event, the determination of genotype is relatively simple when the red cells are D −. In the case of D + bloods, however, the determination of genotype is considerably more difficult. Since there is no consistently reliable serologic method to distinguish between red cells with D antigen resulting from one gene and those with D as a product of two genes, a person whose red cells are D + can be assigned a genotype only by inference from the frequencies with which the individual Rh gene complexes occur in the population (see Table 9-2).

Effect of Race

As an example, a person whose red cells are of the phenotype D + C + E − c − e + is most likely to have the genotype R^1R^1 (*CDe/CDe*), in which case a gene coding for D will be passed to all offspring. A somewhat less likely alternative, since the gene *r′* is infrequent in most populations, is that the genotype is $R^1r′$ (*CDe/Cde*). The racial origin of the person concerned should influence deductions about genotype, because the frequencies of the Rh genes differ with ethnic origin. For example, a white person with the phenotype D + C − E − c + e + would probably be R^0r (*cDe/cde*) because *r* is much more common than R^0 among whites; but a black person of the same phenotype would be almost equally likely to be R^0R^0 (*cDe/cDe*) as R^0r (*cDe/cde*).

Effect of Gene Frequency

An individual of the phenotype D + C + E + c + e + (line 3 of Table 9-3) could have any one of several genotypes. The genotype most likely to produce this phenotype in any population is R^1R^2 (*CDe/cDE*), as R^1 and R^2 are the most common *Rh* genes. Since both genes code for D, the inference usually made in this situation is that the person is homozygous for D, although actually heterozygous for both R^1 and R^2. Some less likely alternatives could mean that the person is heterozygous for D. For example, the true genotype could be $R^1r″$ (*CDe/cDE*), *r′*R^2 (*Cde/cDE*) or R^zr (*CDE/cde*), but *r′*, *r″* and R^z are uncommon in all populations. An even less likely possibility is R^0r^y (*cDe/CdE*).

Table 9-4 gives the frequencies of the more common genotypes in D + persons, together with the likelihood that cells of each phenotype have homozygous or heterozygous expression of D. The figures given are for whites and blacks. In other racial groups the likelihood of being heterozygous for D is reduced because, as shown in Table 9-2, genes that code for the absence of D are even less frequent than among blacks.

Weak Expression of D (D^u)

Not all D + red cell samples react equally well with every anti-D blood grouping serum. Most D + cells show clearcut macroscopic agglutination after centrifugation of cells with serum, and can readily be classified as D +. Cells that are not

Table 9-4. Frequencies of the More Common Genotypes in D-Positive Individuals

| Phenotype | | Genotype | | Genotype Frequency %* | | Likelihood of Zygosity for D % | | | |
| | | | | | | Whites | | Blacks | |
CDE	Rh-hr	CDE	Rh-hr	Whites	Blacks	Homo-	Hetero-	Homo-	Hetero-
CcDe	Rh₁rh	CDe/cde	R¹r	31.1	8.8				
		CDe/cDe	R¹R⁰	3.4	15.0	10	90	59	41
		Cde/cDe	rR⁰	0.2	1.8				
CDe	Rh₁	CDe/CDe	R¹R¹	17.6	2.9	91	9	81	19
		CDe/Cde	R¹r'	1.7	0.7				
cDEe	Rh₂rh	cDE/cde	R²r	10.4	5.7	10	90	63	37
		cDE/cDe	R²R⁰	1.1	9.7				
cDE	Rh₂	cDE/cDE	R²R²	2.0	1.2	87	13	99	1
		cDE/cdE	R²r"	0.3	<0.1				
CcDEe	Rh₁Rh₂	CDe/cDE	R¹R²	11.8	3.7				
		CDe/cdE	R¹r"	0.8	<0.1	89	11	90	10
		Cde/cDE	r'R²	0.6	0.4				
cDe	Rh₀	cDe/cde	R⁰r	3.0	22.9	6	94	46	54
		cDe/cDe	R⁰R⁰	0.2	19.4				

*Calculated from the gene frequencies given in Table 9-2. For the rare phenotypes and genotypes not shown in this table consult the reference books listed at the end of this chapter.

immediately agglutinated cannot as easily be classified as D−, however, because some D+ cells that react with anti-D may not be directly agglutinated. The cells are D+ because the D antigen is present, but additional testing may be required to demonstrate the presence of a weakly expressed D antigen. Variable reactivity with anti-D sera is usually designated by the collective term Dᵘ.

Genetically Transmissible Dᵘ

Dᵘ phenotypes can arise from several different genetic circumstances. Some *Rh* genes appear to code for a weakly reactive D antigen. This characteristic, which appears to be essentially quantitative, follows the regular pattern of Mendelian dominant inheritance and is fairly common in blacks, often appearing as the product of a deviant *R⁰* (*cDe*) gene. Transmission of a gene for weakened D is considerably less common in whites. When it occurs it is more often the product of a deviant *R¹* (*CDe*) or *R²* (*cDE*) gene, either

of which is considerably more common among whites than *R⁰*.

Most of these genetically determined weak D antigens, which are sometimes referred to as *low-grade Dᵘ*, give either negative or very weak reactions in direct agglutination tests with the majority of anti-D sera, but are usually readily detected when the same reagents are used in an antiglobulin procedure.

Dᵘ as Position Effect

Perhaps the best-known example of position effect (discussed above) is weakening of the D antigen by "C in *trans*." The observation that red cells representing the genotype *CDe/Cde* (*R¹r'*) appear to show weakened expression of D was explained in 1955 by Ceppellini and his associates[19] as being due to the effect of *C* on the expression of *Rh* genes on the opposite chromosome. Similar depression of D is seen when other *Rh* genes are accompanied by *Cde*. For example, red cells resulting from *CDe/cde* have the same antigens as those resulting from *Cde/cDe*, but the D antigen is perceptibly weaker in the latter case.

This kind of weakened D antigen is often referred to as *gene interaction D^u*, or *high-grade D^u*, and it seems likely that this was the kind of D^u observed by Stratton when he coined the term on observing variable reactivity with anti-D sera in 1946.[20] Stratton's study was carried out exclusively with saline-reactive anti-D sera, which sometimes give negative reactions with cells belonging to this class of D^u. Potent high-protein reagents now used for most D grouping tests may not give weaker than normal reactions with red cells of this kind, which thus go unrecognized. A similar minor depression of D antigen reactivity is associated with the presence of a low-frequency antigen called Targett (Rh40).[21]

Significance of D^u in Donors

D^u is not to be considered an antigen separate from D itself, but merely a weaker form of D. The widely held belief that D^u blood should not be administered to D− recipients rests on the possibility that, since D^u cells are D+, albeit weakly so, they may elicit an immune response to D. The possibility of such a response may be more apparent than real, as the D^u form of the D antigen seems to be substantially less immunogenic than "normal" D. Experimental transfusion of 68 units of D^u blood into 45 D− recipients (15 of whom were admittedly receiving immunosuppressant therapy) failed to produce a single example of anti-D, although one person in the series made anti-E and a second made anti-K.[22] It now seems probable that an earlier report[23] of "anti-CD" produced in response to CD^ue red cells may in reality have described anti-G (see below).

A more important consideration than the potential immunogenicity of D^u could be the fact that D^u cells may suffer accelerated destruction if introduced into the circulation of a recipient whose serum already contains anti-D. A severe hemolytic transfusion reaction has been reported in these circumstances,[24] and a case of

hemolytic disease of the newborn occurred in a D^u infant whose D− mother had been immunized by the cells of a D+ fetus during an earlier pregnancy.[25]

Subdivisions of D

The concept that the D antigen is a mosaic comprising a number of genetically determined components was devised to explain the fact that some people with D+ red cells produced anti-D that was nonreactive with their own cells. Wiener and Unger[26,27] proposed that the D antigen on normal D+ red cells includes all the components of the mosaic, to which they gave the designation "Rh_o-associated cognate specificities: Rh^A, Rh^B, Rh^C and Rh^D." In rare cases, one or more of these components may be missing from D+ red cells. Some such bloods show unremarkable positive reactions when tested with anti-D sera, whereas others may react weakly with anti-D and therefore invite classification as D^u.

Though phenotypically similar to the low-grade D^u mentioned above and perhaps indistinguishable from it except with special anti-D sera, the important distinction is that these examples of the D antigen are *qualitatively* different from normal, whereas in the low-grade D^u referred to earlier the distinction is *quantitative*. These true *variants* of D are sometimes collectively referred to as D^mosaic, to distinguish them from D^u. Individuals of the D^mosaic phenotypes, since their red cells lack portions of D, sometimes respond to a transfusion of Rh-positive blood or to a fetal-maternal hemorrhage from a D+ fetus by producing antibodies directed at the portions of the antigen not present on their own cells. When this occurs the antibody is indistinguishable from anti-D, except that it is nonreactive with the patient's own D+ cells and with others that lack the same components.

Tippett and Sanger[28] classified persons of these uncommon D+ phenotypes into six numbered categories, and the same authors[29] have subsequently subdivided these primary classifications in the light of further serologic evidence. Although arrived at by different criteria, the classifications of Tippett and Sanger, and those of Wiener and Unger,[27] are not fundamentally irreconcilable.

Significance of D^u in Recipients

The status of a transfusion recipient whose cells are D^u is sometimes a topic of debate. Theoretically such a patient, being $D+$, can receive Rh-positive blood without the risk of being immunized. Yet if the D^u status of the cells should mean that they are D^{mosaic}, the possibility exists that transfusion of Rh-positive blood could elicit a form of anti-D. This possibility exists equally for persons whose red cells react strongly with anti-D sera yet represent a form of D^{mosaic}.

Standards[30] requires that donor bloods be tested for D^u and labeled as $D+$ if the test is positive. Since recipients need not be so tested, most D^u patients will be recorded as $D-$ and will be given Rh-negative blood. Many transfusionists believe that the safest and most efficient routine is to give Rh-negative blood to patients whose cells are not directly agglutinated by anti-D serum. On the other hand, others consider this practice wasteful of Rh-negative blood, and regularly issue Rh-positive blood for D^u recipients. If D^u patients are to receive Rh-postive blood, it is important to safeguard against careless or incorrect interpretation of the D^u test. Rh-negative recipients erroneously classified as D^u and given Rh-positive blood sustain the risk of immunization to D. Precautions to be taken might include testing with two anti-D sera and requiring that both give unequivocal macroscopic reactions at the indirect antiglobulin phase before the patient is classified as D^u. These tests must not be examined microscopically, as it is safer in case of any doubt to assume that the patient is D-negative. (See Chapter 16 for discussion of microscopic examination of D^u tests in prenatal and postpartum blood specimens.)

Other Rh Antigens

The number of identified Rh antigens now exceeds 40, but most of these are of little more than academic importance. Table 9-1 lists most of the antigens sufficiently well-characterized to have been allocated names and/or numbers. The advantages of a numerical system of nomenclature are obvious at these esoteric levels. A few of the antigens and some of the phenotypes deserve additional comments. The interested reader should refer to books listed at the end of this chapter, or to the papers of Rosenfield and his colleagues[13,17,31] for references other than those given.

Compound Antigens

The material on the red cell surface that displays Rh activity has numerous possible antigenic subdivisions. Each gene or gene complex determines a single surface structure, of which some portions are more likely than others to generate an immune response. The product of the gene R^1 (*CDe*) possesses antigenic activity defined as D, C and e. It also includes Ce (rh$_i$) a compound product that always accompanies C and e when they are determined by the same gene. Cells having C and e determined by separate genes, as for example in a person of the genotype R^zr (*CDE/cde*), do not have the Ce antigen. Similar compound antigens exist for c and e determined by the same gene (the antigen called ce, or f), for c and E (cE), and for C and E (CE).

Although antibodies directed at these compound antigens are encountered less commonly as single specificities than those against the five basic antigens, it would not be correct to consider them rare. Such antibodies may be concealed within sera containing antibodies of the more obvious specificities; only absorption with selected cells would demonstrate their presence. Anti-ce may be present, for example, as a component of some anti-c and anti-e sera but the matter has little practical significance; the additional antibody would not confuse the reaction patterns given by anti-c and anti-e because it is exceedingly rare for a cell to be c − (or e −) and at the same time be ce +. An example of this rare event results from the very uncommon gene cD −, which is known to produce c and a weak ce antigen but no e.[32]

Serologic Significance

Many examples of anti-C used as reagent antisera contain as their predominant component anti-Ce (more often called anti-rh$_i$). If the cells being tested possess C as a product of R^z (CDE) or r^y (CdE), reagent "anti-C" consisting largely of anti-Ce would give weaker than normal reactions that might lead to negative interpretation. Since the cells most likely to be used for the positive control for anti-C are Ce + as well as C + (ie, CDe/cde, CDe/cDE or Cde/cde), a reassuringly strong reaction would be observed in the control test. The reaction with C + Ce − cells, by contrast, would be significantly weaker, take longer to develop or, in the worst case, not develop at all. This situation could lead to a false-negative test result, and to the possibility of a serious misinterpretation in investigating disputed parentage. The remedy is to confirm negative anti-C results with particular care when the test cells are E + and, if possible, to use C + Ce − cells as a control. Weak expression of C is also a feature of some phenotypes that occur predominantly in blacks, often accompanied by atypical expression of e (see below).

When correctly identified as such, antibodies specific for compound antigens can sometimes be very useful in determining genotype. For example, if tests are limited to the five basic antisera, the cells of a CDE/cde person are phenotypically identical to those of a CDe/cDE person. The use of anti-ce would draw the required distinction, however, as the former cells would be ce + and the latter ce −. A pure example of anti-Ce would be equally informative in this situation, as it would give reactions opposite to those of anti-ce.

Inferences about Structure

The existence of compound antigens provides a clue to the structure of Rh-active material on the cells. Whatever the overall configuration of the surface structure, it appears that C/c and E/e activities are in close spatial association. No compound antigens have been recognized that suggest a similar association between D/not D and E/e. Some workers find it more logical to write the gene product of, for instance, R^1 as DCe rather than as CDe, of R^2 as DcE rather than as cDE, and so on, to reflect this apparent spatial contiguity.

Deletions

Rare genes exist that code for Rh material lacking activity at the E/e site, or at the sites of both C/c and E/e. Some portions of the surface configuration are not detectable, leaving D (or C/c and D) as the only remaining site(s). The haplotypes C^{W}D −, cD −, − D − and ·D· have all been reported but are exceedingly uncommon.

Cells that lack any Rh antigens other than D may show exceptionally strong D activity, an observation that may allow such cells to be recognized during routine testing. More often, however, the − D − phenotype is identified in the course of studies to investigate an unexpected antibody in the person's serum. The specificity of the antibody may be complex, since the subject's red cells lack all Rh antigens except D. A single antibody with anti-Hr$_0$ (anti-Rh17) specificity is often made by persons of this rare phenotype, although some such sera have been reported to contain apparently separable specificities, such as anti-e.

The ·D· haplotype is similar in most respects to − D −, except that the D antigen is not exalted to the same degree, and ·D· cells may be agglutinated weakly by some examples of anti-Rh17. A distinguishing characteristic of ·D· cells is that they possess a low-frequency antigen known as Evans.[33,34]

The Antigen G and Crossreactions

The G antigen cannot be fitted neatly into the concept of three antigenic regions. G is almost invariably present on red cells possessing either C or D, so that antibodies against G appear superficially to be anti-C + D. The anti-G activity cannot, however, be separated into anti-C and anti-D. The fact that G appears to exist as an entity common to C and D explains the fact that D − persons immunized by C − D + red cells sometimes appear to make anti-C + D. It may also explain why D − persons who are exposed to C + D − red cells may develop antibodies appearing to contain an anti-D component.

Rare cells have been described that possess G but lack D altogether and show greatly diminished or altered expression of C.[35] The D − G + phenotype also occurs in blacks, but is evidently not quite the same as when it occurs in whites.[36] Cells also exist that express at least a part of D but lack G entirely.[37,38,39]

Variant Antigens

There must be innumerable subtle differences in composition among various Rh gene products. Although red cells from most people give straightforward reactions with common antibodies, those from some give atypical reactions, and others stimulate the production of antibodies that do not react with red cells of common Rh phenotypes. It has been convenient to consider C and c, and E and e, as antithetical activities at specific surface sites. This scheme can be expanded to include alternative antigenic activities that seem to reside at the same site, but are determined by genes coding for activity distinct from the common Rh determinants.

Atypical activity at the e site is fairly common in blacks. Several distinct patterns have been identified, such as hr^S − and hr^B −. Diminished C and markedly diminished e activity are among the features of products of the $\overline{\overline{R}}{}^N$ gene, which also determines a low-frequency antigen,

Rh32. Among whites, a weakened e antigen is among the products of genes that determine the Rh33 ($R_o{}^{Har}$) and the Be^a (Berrens) antigens.

Antigens that behave on most occasions as if they had an antithetical relationship to C/c or E/e have been found, mainly in whites. The most common is C^w, which occurs in 2% or more of some white populations. Table 9-1 lists many of the separate antigens that have been found to belong to the Rh system and have contributed to the advancing complexity of the system and its nomenclature.

The LW Antigen

As work progressed on the Rh system, evidence accumulated that the antigen identified by some of the animal antisera of Landsteiner and Wiener[2] was not, after all, identical to that defined by the human antibody reported by Levine and Stetson.[1] Specificity appeared at first to be similar because D + red cells gave significantly stronger reactions with the animal antisera than D − cells, which were accordingly interpreted as negative by the original investigators. It is now recognized that the antigen identified on rhesus monkey cells is present on nearly all human cells, although D − cells from adults have comparatively weak reactivity.[40] Red cells from umbilical cord blood, both D + and D −, are strongly reactive. Since the term Rh was so firmly established for the antigenic system first defined by human anti-D, Levine and his associates[41,42] suggested the name LW, in honor of Landsteiner and Wiener, for the antigen characterized by the original animal anti-rhesus sera.

LW Phenotypes

Rare persons exist whose cells lack the LW antigen, yet have normal Rh antigens, with or without D. These people can form alloanti-LW,[42] and this antibody shows the same graded reactivity with D + and D − red cells as the animal antisera. The notations LW_1 and LW_2 were adopted to describe, respectively, the strong LW reactivity of D+ cells and the comparatively weaker LW reactivity of adult D− cells. The notation LW_3 was used to describe the phenotype of people who made anti-LW and whose cells did not react with the antibody, and LW_4 was applied to describe the phenotype of the one LW-negative proposita (Mrs. Big.) whose serum contained a potent form of anti-LW that agglutinated LW_3 cells,[43] as well as LW_1 and LW_2 cells. Mrs Big.'s LW− status was originally recognized when her blood was investigated after her newborn infant was found to have a weakly positive direct antiglobulin test and her serum was found to contain potent anti-LW with a titer of 32,000 against D+ and 400 against D− red cells.[44]

Anti-LW has sometimes been identified in sera from LW+ people,[45,46] whose red cells, at the time of antibody formation, were either transiently LW− or showed feeble reactivity with anti-LW sera. In these cases the normal LW+ status of the cells has been observed to return as the antibody disappears.

Antithetical Antigens

In 1981, a new blood group antigen called Ne^a was reported, with a frequency of approximately 5% in the Finnish population.[47] Anti-Ne^a showed variation in strength of reactivity similar to that of anti-LW,[48] suggesting a relationship between Ne^a and LW. With adult Ne(a+) red cells, agglutination was consistently stronger if the D antigen was present than if it was absent; and Ne(a+) cord red cells showed strong agglutination irrespective of D status. Tests on blood from 11 unrelated LW_3 persons showed that all were Ne(a+), and family studies confirmed that LW and Ne^a are products of allelic genes. Accordingly, Sistonen and Tippett[49] proposed that the names of the antigens should be changed to reflect the proven relationship. Thus, the antigen formerly called LW becomes LW^a and that formerly called Ne^a becomes LW^b.

The red cells of Mrs Big, the LW− proposita mentioned earlier whose red cells had been classified as LW_4, were found to give negative reactions with anti-Ne^a as well as anti-LW; therefore her cells are to be considered LW(a−b−), and her antibody may be thought of as anti-LW^{ab}. Cells from persons with the transiently acquired form of LW− are also LW(a−b−), as are those of Rh_{null} people, whose LW− state was formerly designated by the term LW_0. Sera from transiently LW− subjects may contain either anti-LW^a or anti-LW^{ab} for the duration of their LW(a−b−) status. The new terminology for LW phenotypes is shown in Table 9-5.

Genetic Independence

The genes determining LW^a and LW^b activity are not part of the Rh system. Genetic independence was established by studying families in which the gene responsible for the inherited LW− condition was shown to segregate independently of the Rh genes.[42,50] This independence has been confirmed in several of the Finnish families studied with anti-LW^a and anti-LW^b.[49] Phenotypically, however, the gene products are obviously related. Not only are both LW^a and LW^b activity always weaker in adult D− cells than in adult D+ cells, but cells lacking demonstrable Rh antigens also lack LW^a and LW^b. The basis for the interaction is not clear. The LW^a gene appears to require for its expression some product of Rh gene activity.

Rh_{null} Syndrome and Rh_{mod}

Genetic Constitution

The literature reports at least 22 persons in 14 families whose red cells appear to have no Rh antigens at all.[51] A number of others are also known but have not been reported. The term used to describe this phenotype is Rh_{null}. Numerous studies have revealed that it may be produced by two different genetic mechanisms. In the more

Table 9-5. LW Phenotypes and Genotypes Expressed in the New and Old Nomenclatures

Old Phenotype		New Phenotype	Old Genotype	New Genotype
LW+ in D+	LW_1	LW(a+b−) or LW(a+b+)	*LWLW* or *LWlw*	*LW^aLW^a*, *LW^aLW^b* or *LW^aLW*
LW+ in D−	LW_2	LW(a+b−) or LW(a+b+)	*LWLW* or *LWlw*	*LW^aLW^a*, *LW^aLW^b* or *LW^aLW*
Most LW−	LW_3	LW(a−b+)	*lwlw*	*LW^bLW^b* or *LW^bLW*
LW− (Big.)	LW_4	LW(a−b−)	*lwlw*	*LWLW*

common *regulator type* of Rh_{null}, the absence of a very common regulator gene, X^1r, prevents expression of the person's perfectly normal genes at the Rh locus on chromosome 1. Such persons appear to transmit normal *Rh* genes to their offspring, in a manner roughly analogous to that in which the *A* or *B* genes are transmitted by people of the Bombay phenotype. These Rh_{null} subjects are thought to be homozygous for X^Qr, a rare allele of X^1r that segregates independently of genes of the Rh system. In some cases, parents or offspring of people with the regulator type of Rh_{null} show overall depression of their Rh antigens; this finding is consistent with being heterozygous for a regulator gene.

The other form of Rh_{null} occurs in persons homozygous for an amorphic gene ($\bar{r}$) at the Rh locus itself. The gene appears to have no product detectable with Rh antisera. In these cases, which are considerably rarer than the regulator type, parents and offspring are obligate heterozygotes for the amorph, and their phenotypes invariably reflect the presence of a single Rh haplotype, namely that inherited from the parent whose Rh antigens are normal. Thus, the red cells of obligate $\bar{r}$ heterozygotes will never be both C+ and c+, nor E+ and e+.

Red Cell Abnormalities

Whatever the genetic origin, red cells lacking Rh antigens have membrane abnormalities that shorten their survival. Severity of hemolysis and anemia varies among affected persons, but stomatocytosis, shortened red cell survival and variably altered activity of other blood group anti-

gens, especially S, s and U, have been consistent features.

Serologic Observations

A few Rh_{null} probands were recognized because their sera contained Rh antibodies, but some came to light when routine Rh phenotyping of their cells revealed the absence of Rh antigen activity. In three reported cases, the discovery resulted from deliberate testing for Rh antigens in patients who presented with hemolytic anemia. The antibodies produced by immunized Rh_{null} people have varied in specificity from apparently identifiable anti-e or anti-C to several examples that reacted with all cells tested except those of other Rh_{null} people. The specificity of this antibody is considered to be "anti-total Rh," which in the numerical nomenclature is identified as anti-Rh29.

Rh_{mod}

The Rh_{mod} phenotype represents a less complete type of suppressed *Rh* gene expression. The genetic basis appears to be similar to that of the regulator Rh_{null}, and the name X^Qr has been given to the unlinked recessive modifier gene thought to be responsible.[52] Unlike Rh_{null} cells, those classified as Rh_{mod} do not completely lack Rh and LW antigens. These show much reduced and sometimes varied activity, depending on the Rh system genes the proband possesses and on the potency and specificity of the antisera used in testing. Sometimes the Rh antigens are so weak as to require fixation-elution techniques to demonstrate their presence. As in Rh_{null}, hemolytic anemia is a feature of the Rh_{mod}

condition. It may be appropriate to think of the two abnormalities as being essentially similar and as differing only in degree.

Rh Antibodies

Except for some examples of anti-E and anti-C^w that occur without known stimulus, most Rh antibodies result from immunization by pregnancy or transfusion. D is considered to be the most potent immunogen, followed by c and E.[53] Although a few examples of Rh antibodies give strong reactions as saline agglutinins, most react best in high protein, antiglobulin or enzyme test systems. Even sera containing strong saline-reactive anti-D usually react to higher dilutions by the antiglobulin test. Some workers find enzyme techniques especially useful for detecting weak or developing Rh antibodies.

Immunization usually persists for many years. Even if levels of circulating antibody fall below detectable thresholds, subsequent exposure to the antigen often results in a rapid secondary immune response. With exceedingly rare exceptions, of which the anti-CD serum Ri is the example most often quoted, Rh antibodies do not bind complement when they combine with their antigens, at least to the extent recognizable by techniques currently used. The Ri antibody is additionally atypical of most Rh antibodies in that it shows a strong prozone when titrated by the bovine albumin test procedure.[54]

Dosage Effect

Anti-D seldom shows any difference in reactivity between cells with homozygous or heterozygous expression of the D antigen, although variably strong reactions may be observed with cells representing certain genotypes. For example, R_2R_2 cells have more D antigen sites than R_1R_1 cells and may therefore show higher titration scores with anti-D sera. Dosage effect can sometimes be demonstrated with some antibodies directed at the E, c or e antigens and, occasionally, at the C antigen. Determin-

ing the number of antigen sites requires specialized techniques, such as radioisotope labeling, immunoferritin localization or automated procedures.[55,56]

Unsuspected Concomitant Antibodies

Some Rh antibodies occur commonly together, and the components are not invariably of equal strength. For example, an R_1R_1 person who has made immune anti-E has almost certainly been exposed to c as well as E; anti-c is almost invariably present in addition to anti-E, although the anti-c component may be substantially weaker and may not be detectable at the time the anti-E is found. This antibody combination may cause a hemolytic transfusion reaction following transfusion of seemingly compatible E−, c+ blood. It is not a sound principle to select, as a routine practice, donor blood negative for antigens against which the recipient *might* produce antibodies, but the R_1R_1 recipient with detectable anti-E is a case that merits special consideration. Since anti-c occurs so commonly with anti-E in immunized people whose cells are E− and c−, it is prudent to select blood of the patient's own R_1R_1 phenotype for transfusion, even when the presence of anti-c cannot be demonstrated by the test procedures routinely used.

Serum that contains clearly detectable anti-c does not as consistently contain anti-E, as the patient can easily have been exposed to c without being exposed to E. Perhaps as many as one fifth of sera containing anti-c contain anti-E as well, but the presence of the second antibody is difficult to demonstrate unless an E+c− panel cell is available to be tested. Some commercial reagent red cell panels include an R_1R_z (*CDe/CDE*) cell suspension for this purpose, but these cells are quite rare and it is difficult for manufacturers to procure them consistently. The issue is not important, however, as unsuspected anti-E in a serum known to contain anti-c is extremely unlikely to cause adverse serologic or clinical effects when c— donor units are selected for transfusion, precisely because the R_1R_z phenotype is so rare. To place matters in sensible perspective, there is less clinical importance in definitively demonstrating anti-E in a serum known to contain anti-c than in identifying anti-Kp^a or anti-C^w, for example, as an unsuspected contaminant.

Rh Grouping Tests

Routine red cell grouping for donors and patients involves only the D antigen, with techniques to demonstrate D^u being required for donor bloods. Tests for the other Rh antigens are performed when there are specific reasons for additional testing, such as in identification of unexpected antibodies, obtaining compatible blood for a patient with an antibody, investigations of disputed parentage or other family studies, selecting a panel of donors known to lack certain antigens or in attempting to determine whether a person is probably homozygous or heterozygous for *D*. In selecting blood for a recipient whose serum contains a comparatively weak Rh antibody, testing with reagent antisera may allow more reliable detection of antigen-negative cells than relying merely on a negative crossmatch. Testing the antibody-maker's own cells may help to provide confirmation of specificity, and will suggest which other Rh antibodies might develop.

Prudent Use of Resources

Routine testing for Rh antigens other than D is not recommended, except when there are clearly defined indications. Besides the expenditure of time and money involved in unnecessary testing, excessive testing wastes scarce resources. Reagent anti-e sera, in particular, should be used sparingly, as there is sometimes a shortage of suitable raw material for their manufacture. In most cases, it may be assumed without actual testing that cells negative for the E

antigen are e+. This practice preserves precious supplies of anti-e for cases in which testing for the e antigen is specifically indicated, as it may be for E+ blood samples, or where there is good reason to suspect a deletion at the *E/e* sublocus.

Anti-D Sera for Slide or Rapid Tube Test (High-Protein Antisera)

Reagents designated for slide or rapid tube test contain macromolecular additives and give rapid, reliable results when used in accordance with manufacturers' directions. Because the high molecular weight medium may cause spontaneous agglutination of red cells coated with immunoglobulin, as in autoimmune conditions and hemolytic disease of the newborn, antisera with these additives may produce false-positive reactions. A D— patient whose cells were thus agglutinated spontaneously might receive transfusions of Rh-positive blood and be stimulated to produce anti-D. To detect false-positive agglutination due to high protein additives in the reagent formula, it is essential when testing patients to test the cells simultaneously against an immunologically inert reagent identical in formulation to the anti-D serum being used except for lacking the antibody component. If aggregation of the red cells occurs in the control test, the result of the anti-D test may not be valid. It will be possible in most cases to determine the D antigen status of the cells by further testing with other reagents, as detailed under "False Positives" on pages 143-4.

The Control

Several circumstances may cause false-positive results in tests using reagents designed for slide or rapid tube tests. Besides the above-mentioned spontaneous agglutination of immunoglobulin-coated red cells, factors in the patient's own serum may affect the test, since cells are frequently tested unwashed or suspended in their own serum or plasma. Strong autoagglutinins, abnormal serum proteins that promote rouleaux formation, or antibodies directed at an additive in the reagent may all cause cellular aggregation that could be mistaken for specific agglutination mediated by anti-D. The best way to detect possibly invalid reactions in anti-D testing is to use as the immunologically inert control reagent the actual diluent used for manufacturing the particular anti-D reagent. This material contains the same additives present in the anti-D serum except for the antibody component, and can therefore be expected to potentiate spurious agglutination to the same degree as the anti-D reagent itself.

Manufacturers offer their own high-protein diluents as control reagents; anti-D tests performed on patients' cells with slide or rapid tube test sera must be controlled with this material. If the diluent control for a particular manufacturer's anti-D serum is not available, it is better to use the control reagent of another manufacturer than to use reagent bovine albumin for the control test. The nature and concentration of the additives differ significantly among different manufacturers' reagents, however, so using the control reagent from one manufacturer may not invariably detect all possible false-positive reactions due to elements in another manufacturer's anti-D serum. Using 22% or 30% bovine albumin detects even fewer false positives, however,[57,58] since reagent bovine albumin solutions do not contain high molecular weight potentiators and immunoglobulin-coated red cells may not undergo spontaneous agglutination to the same degree as in the antiserum diluent.

Tube Testing

Most slide or modified tube test anti-D reagents can be used in tube tests with red cells suspended in saline, in serum or in plasma, but this should be confirmed by reading the manufacturer's directions before use. The recommended test procedure may vary somewhat among manufacturers, but the following is representative of methods in current use.

1. Place one drop of anti-D serum in a clean, labeled test tube.
2. Place one drop of the appropriate control reagent in a second labeled tube.
3. Add to each tube one drop of a 2-5% suspension (in saline, serum or plasma) of the red cells to be tested; alternatively, use separate applicator sticks to transfer the equivalent amount of red cells to each tube.
4. Mix gently and centrifuge for 30 seconds at approximately 900 to 1000 × g.
5. Gently resuspend the cell button and examine for agglutination. If a stick was used to transfer the cells, adding one drop of saline to each tube before resuspending the cell button will provide more fluid to aid resuspension.
6. Record test and control results.

Interpretation Agglutination in the anti-D tube and a smooth suspension in the control tube constitutes a positive test result. If there is agglutination in the control tube, the anti-D test result must not be interpreted as positive without further testing (see below).

A smooth suspension of cells in both the anti-D and control tubes is a negative test result. Although blood from patients may be designated as D− at this point, donor bloods must be further tested for D^u. The original test mixture may be used for the indirect antiglobulin phase of D^u testing, providing the manufacturer's directions state that the antiserum is suitable for the D^u test (see page 144 for details of D^u testing).

Slide Testing

The slide test requires a high concentration of cells and protein, and an optimum temperature of 37 C. The viewing surface should be kept lighted at all times to maintain a temperature of 45 to 50 C, which allows optimally rapid warming of the test mixture to 37 C. Because the slide test must be read within 2 minutes, the cells and serum on the glass slide must reach 37 C quickly. The slide test has the serious disadvantage that drying of the reaction mixture can cause aggregation of the cells that may be misinterpreted as agglutination. The tube test is preferred for this reason. As with the tube test, the procedures recommended by different manufacturers may not be precisely the same. The particular manufacturer's directions should always be consulted before performing the test, but the following method is representative of those in current use.

1. Place one drop of anti-D serum on a clean, labeled slide.
2. Place one drop of the appropriate control reagent on a second labeled slide.
3. To each slide add two drops of a well-mixed 40-50% suspension (in their own or group-compatible serum or plasma) of the red cells to be tested.
4. Thoroughly mix the cell suspension and reagent, using a clean applicator stick for each slide, and spreading the reaction mixture over most of the surface area of the slide.
5. Place both slides on the viewing box simultaneously and tilt gently and continuously to observe for agglutination. Most manufacturers stipulate that the test must be read within 2 minutes because drying of the reaction mixture may cause formation of rouleaux, which may be mistaken for agglutination.
6. After no longer than 2 minutes, interpret and record the results of the reactions on both slides.

Note: Do not allow the cell/serum mixture to come into contact with the hands, because of the hepatitis risk.

Interpretation Agglutination with anti-D serum and a smooth suspension on the control slide constitutes a positive test result. Drying around the edges of the reaction mixture must not be confused with agglu-

tination. If there is agglutination on the control slide, the anti-D test must not be interpreted as positive without further testing (see below).

A smooth suspension of cells with both anti-D and the control reagent is a negative test result. If testing for D^u is indicated, a tube test must be performed (see page 144).

Considerations with D^u

A reliable D^u test cannot be performed on a slide, although weak D^u cells sometimes give a direct agglutination reaction in slide testing and may be mistaken for normal D+ cells when tested by this method. When D^u cells are agglutinated in a slide test, the agglutination is invariably weaker than that seen with normal D+ cells. This distinction may not be recognized, however, unless the test on the D^u cells is compared against simultaneously performed tests on normal D+ cells. Cells demonstrating the stronger (gene interaction) form of D^u commonly give the same strength of reaction as normal D+ cells when tested with high-protein anti-D reagents, whether the test is performed on a slide or in a tube. As a result, this form of diminished D antigen most often passes for normal D. Accordingly, references to D^u from this point will be confined to low-grade D^u, the form requiring an indirect antiglobulin test for its reliable detection in tube tests.

Misleading Results

Causes of false reactions in Rh grouping are dealt with comprehensively in the "Additional Considerations" section on page 149. Certain problems are unique to high-protein reagents, however, and it may be helpful to discuss these separately.

False Positives

1. Either immunoglobulin coating the patient's cells or factors in the patient's serum causing cellular aggregation can cause agglutination in the control tube containing immunologically inert reagent. Serum factors can be excluded

by washing the cells thoroughly, using warm saline if cold agglutinins are known or suspected to be present, and then retesting the washed cells in a tube test. It is not necessary at this point to use a saline-reactive antiserum. Retesting may be performed with the original high-protein serum, providing the manufacturer's directions state that the product is suitable for use with saline-suspended cells. The control test must again be performed concurrently. If the control test now gives a negative result and agglutination still occurs in the anti-D test, the cells are D+. If agglutination still occurs in the control test it is most likely that the cells are coated with immunoglobulin. In such cases, the cells may be tested with a saline-reactive antiserum (see below).

2. If cells and antiserum are incubated together for too long before the test is read, the high-protein reagent may cause rouleaux to form. This may occur rapidly, particularly on a warm slide, as evaporation causes drying which in turn increases the concentration of protein in the reaction mixture. Rouleaux may be mistaken for agglutination, so it is important not to exceed the manufacturer's recommendation to interpret the test within a fixed time period, usually 2 minutes.

3. Small fibrin clots from the blood specimen, or clots that develop if the specimen is incompletely coagulated when tested, may give the appearance of agglutination.

False Negatives

1. Too heavy a suspension in the tube test, or too weak a cell suspension in the slide test, may result in poor agglutination. To achieve the required 40-50% cell suspension for the slide test, whole blood from a severely anemic patient may need to be concentrated by centrifuging and removing some of the plasma before testing.

2. Cells in a saline suspension may react poorly with some antisera. Saline suspensions must not be used for the slide test.

3. Cells possessing comparatively weak expression of the D antigen may not react well within the 2-minute limit of the slide test or upon immediate centrifugation in the tube test.

Testing for D^u

Cells classified as low-grade D^u possess the D antigen but expressed so weakly that they are not directly agglutinated by most anti-D sera. D^u can be recognized most reliably by the indirect antiglobulin test after incubating the test cells with anti-D serum. Not every anti-D serum is suitable for the D^u test, either because testing by the manufacturer has not shown reliable reactions with D^u cells, or because the antiserum contains other antibodies reactive by the antiglobulin test. The manufacturer's package insert will state whether the reagent may be used for D^u testing.

Note: If the original anti-D test was performed by the tube test technique, the same tube may be used directly for the D^u test, providing the manufacturer's directions so state. In this case, proceed directly to step 4 of the following procedure, after recording the original anti-D tube test as negative.

1. Place one drop of anti-D serum in a clean, labeled test tube.

2. Place one drop of the appropriate control reagent in a second labeled test tube.

3. To both tubes add one drop of a 2-5% suspension in saline of the red cells to be tested. A direct antiglobulin test may be performed on the cells being tested instead of the control test, if desired, but it is better to perform an indirect antiglobulin test with the control reagent, as this ensures that all the components of the antiserum that might cause a false-positive result are represented.

4. Mix and incubate both tubes for 15-30 minutes at 37 C, according to manufacturer's directions.
5. Centrifuge for 30 seconds at 900 to 1000 × *g*.
6. Gently resuspend the cell button and examine for agglutination. If strong agglutination of the test cells is observed at this point, record the test sample as D+. There is no need to proceed with the antiglobulin phase of the test.
7. If the test cells are not agglutinated, or show doubtful agglutination, wash the cells 3-4 times with large volumes of saline.
8. After the final wash, decant the saline completely and blot the rims of the tubes dry.
9. Add 1-2 drops of anti-human globulin serum, according to manufacturer's directions. Either a polyspecific or anti-IgG reagent may be used.
10. Mix gently and centrifuge for 15 seconds at 900 to 1000 × *g*.
11. Gently resuspend the cell button, examine for agglutination and record the test result.
12. If the test result is negative, the reaction may be confirmed by adding known IgG-sensitized red cells, recentrifuging and reexamining for agglutination. The development of agglutination at this point confirms the presence of active anti-human globulin in the test mixture.

Interpretation Either a diluent control test or a direct antiglobulin test must accompany the D^u test procedure. Agglutination in the anti-D tube and none in the control tube constitutes a positive test result. The blood must be classified as D+. It is incorrect to report D^u cells as being "D-negative, D^u-positive." A negative result is absence of agglutination in the test with anti-D. This means that the cells do not have D activity and are to be classified as D−. If the control test is positive, no valid interpretation of the D^u test can be made. In this situation, Rh-negative blood should be given if the test cells are from a patient; if the cells are from a donor the cells should not be used for transfusion.

Causes of false-positive and negative antiglobulin tests are discussed in Chapter 6.

Anti-D Sera for the Saline Tube Test

Saline-agglutinating Rh antiserum should be used when the control system for high-protein anti-D gives a positive test that persists even when washed red cells are tested. The usual cause is immunoglobulin attached to the cells (see Chapter 6 for causes of a positive direct antiglobulin test). Cells with a positive direct antiglobulin test can usually be tested successfully with antisera that contain saline-agglutinating antibodies and no additives that promote spontaneous agglutination of immunoglobulin-coated cells.

The test must be performed on a saline suspension of well-washed cells; a wise precaution is a concurrent control test, using a solution of bovine albumin at a protein concentration approximately that of the saline-reactive anti-D. Manufacturers usually recommend a suitable concentration of bovine albumin for the control test. Potentiators likely to enhance spontaneous agglutination are not normally used in saline-reactive antisera, but if such additives are present the fact should be stated in the "Reagent Description" section of the package insert.

Two kinds of saline-reactive Rh antisera are now available, and important differences exist between them. Traditional saline reagents are made from raw material containing predominantly IgM antibodies, which naturally agglutinate antigen-positive cells suspended in saline. A comparatively recent introduction has been antisera made from IgG antibodies that have been chemically modified to convert them into direct saline agglutinins.

IgM Antisera

Saline-reactive antisera prepared from IgM antibodies have always been relatively scarce because suitable raw material is scarce. Such reagents are usually reserved for testing red cell samples that cannot be tested reliably with antisera containing a high concentration of protein. These saline-reactive antisera invariably require the test to be incubated at 37 C, usually for 15 minutes or longer, and they are unsuitable for slide tests. Antisera of this kind cannot be used for the D^u test, even when the cells being tested do not have a positive direct antiglobulin test, because IgM antibodies generally perform poorly in the indirect antiglobulin test.

Chemically Modified IgG Antisera

Saline-reactive antisera prepared from IgG antibodies became commercially available toward the end of 1979. The IgG antibodies in the raw material are converted to direct saline agglutinins by chemical reduction of their interchain disulfide bonds, as described by Romans and colleagues.[59] This is usually achieved by treating the serum with a sulfhydryl compound, such as dithiothreitol or dithioerythritol. Pirofsky and Cordova[60] reported 2-mercaptoethanol to have the same effect on nonagglutinating antibodies as early as 1963, although this was later dismissed as being a nonspecific, nonimmunologic phenomenon.[61]

Chemical Considerations

Substances that convert IgG antibodies into direct saline agglutinins are the same agents that abolish that ability by IgM antibodies. Cleaving disulfide bonds depolymerizes the larger IgM molecules and nullifies the advantage of their greater size. In the case of IgG, mild reduction of the disulfide bonds that link the heavy chains (see Fig. 9-1) gives greater flexibility to the hinge region of the molecule. This greater flexibility allows the antigen combining sites situated at the terminal end of each Fab portion to span a greater distance and thus to agglutinate in a saline test medium red cells possessing the corresponding antigen. Oxidation reverses the chemical reaction, so an alkylating agent is added to give permanence to the chemical modification. The reactants are removed by dialysis before final formulation of the antiserum, usually in a medium that includes bovine albumin at a protein concentration approximately equivalent to that of human serum, but sometimes at a higher concentration (see below).

Serologic Considerations

Saline-reactive antisera made from reduced and alkylated IgG antibodies show stronger reactivity than those prepared from IgM antibodies, and are usually suitable for tests performed on a slide. They are more abundantly available than the IgM kind, and may be confidently used when immunoglobulin coating precludes the use of high-protein anti-D on a red cell sample. These chemically modified anti-D sera are just as suitable as high-protein reagents for the detection of D^u by the indirect antiglobulin test although, naturally, a D^u test is not possible if the cells have a positive direct antiglobulin test. In such circumstances, a negative result in testing with either sort of saline-reactive anti-D merely indicates that the cells are *probably* D − . If from a recipient, Rh-negative blood should be selected for transfusion. This would not be an issue if the cells were from a donor, as blood with a positive direct antiglobulin test is unsuitable for transfusion.

Control for Low-Protein Reagents

When antisera manufactured from chemically modified IgG first became available, they were marketed at a total protein concentration approximating that of human serum. False-positive reactions due to spontaneous agglutination of immunoglobulin-coated red cells occur no more often with this kind of reagent than with other saline-reactive antisera. False-posi-

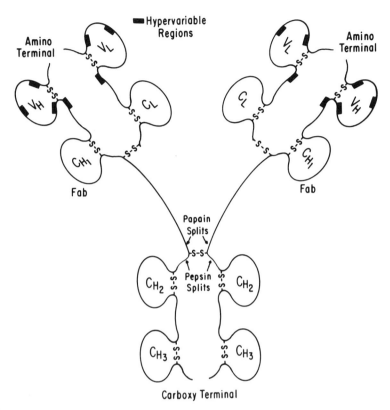

Figure 9-1. In chemically modified IgG molecules, the disulfide bonds shown holding the two heavy chains in close proximity undergo changes that allow greater separation of the chains, hence of the Fab portions of the molecule.

tive reactions still occur, in any saline reactive test system, if the red cells are tested unwashed and the sample contains cold autoagglutinins or a protein imbalance causing rouleaux. A suitable concurrent control to identify such false reactions could be observation of ABO grouping results. Absence of agglutination in either the anti-A or anti-B tube demonstrates absence of spontaneous agglutination, and no separate control test need routinely be performed. For cell samples that show agglutination in all tubes (ie, give the reactions of group AB, Rh-positive), a concurrent control must be performed if the test cells are from a patient. A suitable control is to centrifuge the cell suspension with its own serum, or with 6-8% bovine albumin at the same time the anti-D test is centrifuged. If the test is one of several requiring incubation before centrifugation, any test performed concurrently that gives a negative result serves as an adequate control. A separate control test is only required in the case of a red cell sample that gives positive reactions with all the Rh antisera (ie, $D + C + E + c + e +$).

Control for Medium-Protein Reagents

Some manufacturers now prepare antisera containing chemically modified IgG in a diluent having a level of protein between that of human serum and that of high-protein reagents. It is important not to confuse this type of antiserum with the kind formulated in a low-protein diluent, as the higher protein concentration may cause spontaneous agglutination of at least some immunoglobulin-coated cells. The incidence of false reactions from this cause may be less than when a high-protein reagent is used, but a parallel control test with a suitably formulated control reagent is nevertheless required when testing patients. The need for a control will be stated in the manufacturer's instructions. This kind of antiserum is more closely akin to those designed for the slide or rapid tube test than to those made from IgM.

D Grouping in Hemolytic Disease of the Newborn

Since the red cells of an infant suffering from hemolytic disease of the newborn will be coated with immunoglobulin, a saline-reactive antiserum is usually necessary for Rh testing. Occasionally, the cells may be so heavily coated with antibody that all antigen sites are occupied, leaving none to react with a saline-reactive antiserum of appropriate specificity. This "blocking" phenomenon should be suspected if the infant's red cells have a strongly positive direct antiglobulin test, yet give a negative result when tested with a saline-reactive antiserum of the same specificity as the maternal antibody. Blocking occurs most commonly when the mother's antibody is anti-D, and it is usually possible to obtain the correct result with a saline anti-D serum after first eluting some of the maternal antibody from the cord cells at 45 C. (Refer to Special Methods section, page 417, for details and the precautions needed.) Elution liberates enough antigen sites to permit grouping, but heat treatment of red cells must be carried out cautiously because overexposure to heat may destroy Rh receptors.

Tests for Antigens Other than D

Reagent antisera are available to test for the other principal Rh antigens: C, E, c and e. These may be obtained either as saline agglutinins or as high-protein sera for the slide or rapid tube test. High-protein antisera of any specificity are prone to the same causes of false results as high-protein anti-D sera and therefore require a comparable control test. A negative reaction in the control for anti-D serum cannot uncritically be applied to tests for other Rh antigens, because results with anti-D are usually obtained after immediate centrifugation, while tests for the other Rh antigens are usually incubated for a period at 37 C before being centrifuged and read. A valid control procedure must be performed concurrently with the test being controlled, using the same duration and conditions of incubation, and be interpreted together with the actual test.

Rh grouping sera may show weak or negative reactions with red cells possessing variant antigens. This is especially true of testing for the e antigen in blacks, among whom variants of e are relatively common. It is impossible to obtain anti-e sera that react strongly and consistently with the various qualitative and quantitative variants of e that occur in persons of African descent. Variant reactivity with anti-C sera may also be seen when testing the red cells of blacks, and those of any race when the genes *CDE* or *CdE* are involved. Variant E and c antigens have been reported, but are considerably less common.

Precautions for Using Sera

Whatever antisera are used, the manufacturer's directions must be carefully followed. The indirect antiglobulin technique must not be used unless the serum is described explicitly by the manufacturer as suitable for this use. Antisera for the other Rh antigens are more likely to contain antiglobulin-reactive contaminating specificities than is anti-D serum. For laboratories using these reagents only rarely, positive and negative controls should be tested in parallel with the test cells. The positive control cells should be known to have heterozygous expression of the antigen concerned, or be known to show weak reactivity with the antiserum. If these reagents are used regularly, they should be included in the routine quality assurance program.

Additional Considerations in Rh Testing

The problems with high-protein anti-D antisera already listed apply equally to reagents of other specificities, and also to reagents made from chemically modified IgG if the formulation includes macromolecular additives or a total protein concentration much exceeding that of normal human serum. The following limitations are common to all blood grouping procedures, including those performed with high-protein reagents.

False-Positive Reactions

The following circumstances can produce false-positive cell grouping results.

1. The wrong antiserum was inadvertently used. The *Code of Federal Regulations* (21CFR 660.28a1) permits a system of color-coding for the labels of certain blood grouping sera. In the Rh system, color-coded labels may be used for high-protein and chemically modified antisera. For anti-D the approved color is grey; for anti-C, pink; for anti-E, brown; for anti-c, lavender; for anti-e, green; and for anti-CDE, orange. It is important, however, to read the label each time the serum is used; label color or the location of the vial in a rack must not be relied upon to ensure selection of the correct reagent.
2. An unsuspected antibody of another specificity is present in the reagent. FDA regulations require that antisera be tested by the manufacturer to confirm

the absence of antibodies for antigens having a frequency of 1% or more in the general US population, but only by the test procedures recommended for use with the particular reagent. Use by an unauthorized test method may give rise to false results.

Antibodies for antigens having a frequency of less than 1% in the population may occasionally cause false-positive reactions, even when the manufacturer's directions are scrupulously followed. Though these antigens occur infrequently, antibodies to them are remarkably common, even in subjects who have no history of pregnancy or transfusions. Mixtures of several such antibodies are not rare, and it must be assumed that these arise through some stimulus other than exposure to human red cells. There is evidence that this phenomenon occurs with greater frequency in sera from people who have produced an immune blood group antibody, and it is precisely these sera that are used to manufacture most blood grouping reagents. It would not be reasonable to expect manufacturers to exclude from their products all antibodies directed at low-frequency antigens. Fortunately, cells possessing these antigens are rarely encountered; for this reason, however, routine quality assurance programs offer no protection.

In performing crucial antigen groupings, workers routinely perform tests in duplicate, using antisera from different sources. This reduces the likelihood of a false classification, as discrepant reactions between two antisera of a given specificity would alert the serologist to the need for further testing. A major limitation of duplicate testing as a safeguard, however, is that reagents from different manufacturers are not necessarily prepared from antibody provided by different donors. The scarcity of donors with acceptable titers of such relatively uncommon specificities as anti-C and anti-e, in particular, may lead to the same raw material being used by several manufacturers. Ostensibly different reagents may thus contain the same contaminating antibody.

3. Polyagglutinable red cells may demonstrate agglutination with any reagent containing human serum. Although antibodies that agglutinate these surface-altered cells are present in most adult human sera, these only rarely cause problems with reagent antisera, as ageing, dilution and various steps in the manufacturing process tend to eliminate these predominantly IgM antibodies. Polyagglutinability is more likely to become apparent in tests with ABO reagents than with Rh antisera, because ABO sera are seldom diluted significantly in manufacture and a room temperature test is optimal for the reactivity of antibodies to polyagglutinable cells. The situation will usually be obvious when the results of cell and serum grouping tests are observed to disagree.

4. Autoagglutinins and abnormal proteins in the test serum may cause false-positive reactions when the cells are tested unwashed. This cause of false reactions will usually be recognized through a discrepancy between cell and serum grouping results in the ABO test. Should such a discrepancy be observed, retesting the cells after thorough washing in isotonic saline will in most cases give correct test results.

5. Reagent vials may become contaminated with bacteria, with foreign substances, or with antiserum from another vial. This can be prevented by using careful technique. Droppers should never be removed from more than one reagent at a time, and periodic inspection of the contents of vials for visual evidence of deterioration should become second nature. A point to remember with high-protein antisera is that bacterial contamination may not cause recognizable turbidity, as the refractive index of bacteria is similar to that of the material itself.

False-Negative Reactions

The following circumstances can produce false-negative cell grouping results.

1. The wrong antiserum or some other similarly colored reagent was used, being mistaken for the required antiserum. Vial labels should be checked carefully at each use. The reagents most likely to be mistaken for each other are anti-human globulin, bovine albumin, anti-D and its diluent control.

2. Antiserum was not added to the tube, for instance to one of a long row of tubes. A good habit to cultivate is always to place serum in tubes first, checking each tube for the presence of serum before adding the cell suspension.

3. A specific antiserum fails to react with a variant form of the antigen. For example, anti-e sera may not react consistently with variant e antigens that are relatively common in blacks. Less commonly, an anti-E serum may react weakly or not at all with the E^w antigen.

4. An antiserum containing antibody that is predominantly directed at a compound Rh antigen may fail to give a reliably detectable reaction with cells carrying the individual antigens as separate gene products. This occurs most often with anti-C sera, which almost invariably give stronger reactions with C inherited as a product of R^1 or r' than when C is a product of R^z or r^y.

5. The manufacturer's directions were not followed, and the antiserum was used incorrectly. For example, the wrong proportions of serum to cells were used, or incubation was at the incorrect temperature or for the wrong duration.

6. Unduly hard shaking in resuspending the cell button after centrifugation may disperse weak agglutination.

7. Immunoglobulin in an antiserum may have deteriorated due to contamina-

tion or improper storage. Chemically modified IgG antibody appears to be particularly susceptible to destruction by certain proteolytic enzymes, as might be produced by bacteria.

References

1. Levine P, Stetson RE. An unusual case of intragroup agglutination. JAMA 1939;113:126-127.

2. Landsteiner K, Wiener AS. An agglutinable factor in human blood recognized by immune sera for rhesus blood. Proc Soc Exp Biol NY 1940;43:223.

3. Levine P, Katzin EM. Isoimmunization in pregnancy and the variety of isoagglutinins observed. Proc Soc Exp Biol NY 1940;43:343-346.

4. Wiener AS, Peters HR. Hemolytic reactions following transfusions of blood of the homologous group, with three cases in which the same agglutinogen was responsible. Ann Int Med 1940;13:2306-2322.

5. Diamond LK. Erythroblastosis fetalis or hemolytic disease of the newborn. Proc Roy Soc Med 1947;40:546-550.

6. Pollack W, Ascari WQ, Crispen JK, O'Connor RR, Ho TY. Studies on Rh prophylaxis: II. Rh immune prophylaxis after transfusion with Rh-positive blood. Transfusion 1971;11:340-344.

7. Ruddle F, Ricciuti F, McMorris FA, et al. Somatic cell genetic assignment of peptidase C and the Rh linkage group to chromosome A-1 in man. Science 1972;176:1429-1431.

8. Marsh WL, Chaganti RSK, Gardner FH, Mayer K, German J. Mapping human autosomes: evidence supporting assignment of rhesus to the short arm of chromosome No. 1. Science 1974;183:966-968.

9. Race RR, Taylor GL. A serum that discloses the genotype of some *Rh*-positive people (letter). Nature 1943;152:300.

10. Race RR, Taylor GL, Cappell DF, McFarlane MN. Recognition of a further common *Rh* genotype in man. Nature 1944;153:52-53.

11. Levine P. On Hr factor and Rh genetic theory. Science 1945;102:1-4.

12. Mourant AE. A new rhesus antibody (letter). Nature 1945;155:542.

13. Rosenfield RE, Allen FH Jr, Rubinstein P. Genetic model for the Rh blood group system. Proc Nat Acad Sci USA 1973;70:1303-1307.

14. Wiener AS. Genetic theory of the Rh blood types. Proc Soc Exp Biol NY 1943;54:316-319.

15. Race RR. The Rh genotypes and Fisher's theory. Blood 1948;3(suppl 2):27-42.

16. Mourant AE, Kopec AC, Domaniewska-Sobczak K. The distribution of human blood groups and other polymorphisms. 2nd ed. London: Oxford University Press; 1976:351-505.

17. Rosenfield RE, Allen FH Jr, Swisher SN, Kochwa S. A review of Rh serology and presentation of a new terminology. Transfusion 1962;2:287-312.

18. Lawler SD, Race RR. Quantitative aspects of Rh antigens. Proceedings of the International Society of Hematology 1950:168-170.

19. Ceppellini R, Dunn LC, Turri M. An interaction between alleles at the Rh locus in man which weakens the reactivity of the Rh$_o$ factor (D^u). Proc Nat Acad Sci USA 1955;41:283-288.

20. Stratton F. A new Rh allelomorph. Nature 1946;158:25.

21. Lewis M, Kaita H, Allerdice RW, Bartle A, Squires WG, Huntsman RG. Assignment of the red cell antigen Targett (Rh40) to the Rh blood group system. Am J Hum Genet 1979;31:630-633.

22. Schmidt PJ, Morrison EG, Shohl J. The antigenicity of the $\Re$h$_o$ (D^u) blood factor. Blood 1962;20:196-202.

23. Van Loghem JJ. Production of Rh agglutinins anti-C and anti-E by artificial immunization of volunteer donors. Br Med J 1947;ii:958-959.

24. Diamond LK, Allen FH Jr. Rh and other blood groups. N Engl J Med 1949;241:867-873.

25. Mollison PL, Cutbush M. La maladie hémolytique chez un enfant D^u. Rév Hématol 1949;4:608-612.

26. Wiener AS, Unger LJ. Rh factors related to the Rh$_o$ factor as a source of clinical problems. JAMA 1959;169:696-699.

27. Wiener AS, Unger LJ. Further observations on the blood factors Rh^A, Rh^B, Rh^C, and Rh^D. Transfusion 1962;2:230-233.

28. Tippett P, Sanger R. Observations on subdivisions of the Rh antigen D. Vox Sang 1962;7:9-13.

29. Tippett P, Sanger R. Further observations on subdivisions of the Rh antigen D. Ärztl Lab 1975;23:476-480.

30. Schmidt PJ, ed. Standards for blood banks and transfusion services. 11th ed. Arlington, VA: American Association of Blood Banks 1984.

31. Allen FH Jr, Rosenfield RE. Review of Rh serology. Eight new antigens in nine years. Hematologia 1972;6:113-120.

32. Tate H, Cunningham C, McDade MG, Tippett PA, Sanger R. An Rh gene complex cD −. Vox Sang 1960;5:398-402.

33. Contreras M, Armitage S, Daniels GL, Tippett P. Homozygous ·D·. Vox Sang 1979;36:81-84.

34. Contreras M, Stebbing B, Blessing M, Gavin J. The Rh antigen Evans. Vox Sang 1978;34:208-211.

35. Allen FH Jr., Tippett PA. A new Rh blood type which reveals the Rh antigen G. Vox Sang 1958;3:321-330.

36. Kevy SV, Schmidt PJ, Leyshon WC. A second example of the blood type rh^G. Vox Sang 1959;4:257-266.

37. Stout TD, Moore BPL, Allen FH Jr, Corcoran P. A new phenotype D + G − (Rh:1, − 12). Vox Sang 1963;8:262-268.

38. Shapiro M. Serology and genetics of a "new" blood factor: hr^H. J Forens Med 1964;11:52-66.

39. Zaino EC. A new Rh phenotype, Rh_o rh, G-negative. Transfusion 1965;5:320-321.

40. Beck ML. The LW system: a review and current concepts. In: Walker RH, ed. A seminar on recent advances in immunohematology. Washington, DC: American Association of Blood Banks; 1973:83-100.

41. Levine P, Celano MJ, Vos GH, Morrison J. The first human blood, ---/---, which lacks the D-like antigen. Nature 1962;194:304.

42. Levine P, Celano MJ, Wallace J, Sanger R. A human "D-like" antibody. Nature 1963;198:596-597.

43. Swanson JL, Azar M, Miller J, McCullough JJ. Evidence for heterogeneity of LW antigen revealed in a family study. Transfusion 1974;14:470-474.

44. deVeber LL, Clark G, Hunking M, Stroup M. Maternal anti-LW. Transfusion 1971;11:33-35.

45. Chown B, Kaita H, Lowen B, Lewis M. Transient production of anti-LW by LW-positive people. Transfusion 1971;11:220-222.

46. Giles CM, Lundsgaard A. A complex serological investigation involving LW. Vox Sang 1967;13:406-416.

47. Sistonen P, Nevanlinna HR, Virtaranta-Knowles K, et al. Ne^a, a new blood group antigen in Finland. Vox Sang 1981;40:352-357.

48. Sistonen P. A phenotypic association between the blood group antigen Ne^a and the Rh antigen D. Med Biol 1981;59:230-233.

49. Sistonen P, Tippett P. A "new" allele giving further insight into the LW blood group system. Vox Sang 1982;42:252-255.

50. Swanson J, Matson GA. Third human "D-like" antibody or anti-LW. Transfusion 1964;4:257-261.

51. Moulds JJ. Rh_nulls: amorphs and regulators. In: Walker RH, ed. A seminar on recent advances in immunohematology. Washington, DC: American Association of Blood Banks 1973:63-82.

52. Chown B, Lewis M, Kaita H., Lowen B. An unlinked modifier of Rh blood groups: effects when heterozygous and when homozygous. Am J Hum Genet 1972;24:623-637.

53. Giblett E. Blood group antibodies causing hemolytic disease of the newborn. Clin Obstet Gynecol 1964;7:1044-55.

54. Waller M, Lawler SD. A study of the properties of the rhesus antibody (Ri) diagnostic for the rheumatoid factor and its application to Gm grouping. Vox Sang 1962;4:591-606.

55. Masouredis SP. Quantitative and ultra-structural aspects of red cell membrane Rh antigens. In: Walker RH, ed. A seminar on recent advances in immunohematology. Washington, DC: American Association of Blood Banks 1973:41-62.

56. Berkman EM, Nusbacher J, Kochwa S, Rosenfield RE. Quantitative blood typing profiles of human erythrocytes. Transfusion 1971;11:317-332.

57. White WD, Issitt CH, McGuire D. Evaluation of the use of albumin controls in Rh typing. Transfusion 1974;14:67-71.

58. Reid ME, Ellisor SS, Frank BA. Another potential source of error in Rh-hr typing. Transfusion 1975;15:485-488.

59. Romans DG, Tilley CA, Crookston MC, Falk RE, Dorrington JK. Conversion of incomplete antibodies to direct agglutinins by mild reduction: evidence for segmental flexibility within the Fc fragment of immunoglobulin G. Proc Nat Acad Sci USA 1977;74:2531-2535.

60. Pirofsky B, Cordova MR. Bivalent nature of incomplete anti-D (Rh_o). Nature 1963;197:392-393.

61. Mandy WJ, Fudenberg HH, Lewis FB. On "incomplete" anti-Rh antibodies: mechanism of direct agglutination induced by mercaptoethanol. J Clin Invest 1965;44:1352-1361.

Suggested Additional Reading

- Issitt PD. Serology and genetics of the rhesus blood group system. Cincinnati: Montgomery Scientific Publications; 1979.

- Mollison PL. Blood transfusion in clinical medicine. 7th ed. Oxford: Blackwell Scientific Publications; 1983:330-401,675-687.

- Race RR, Sanger R. Blood groups in man. 6th ed. Oxford: Blackwell Scientific Publications; 1975: Chapter 5.

10

Other Blood Groups

In addition to antigens of the ABO and Rh blood group systems, over 300 others can be detected on human red cells. Some, due to a readily perceived relationship with each other, have been organized into additional blood group systems, whereas others have yet to be allocated to an established system. A few antigens occur on the red cells of almost all persons and are known as high-incidence or *public* antigens. Others, of low incidence, are sometimes called *private* antigens.

Each of the known blood group antigens was initially identified through the detection of its specific antibody in a serum. Some of these antibodies are exceedingly rare, while others are comparatively common. This chapter is devoted primarily to those antibodies most likely to be seen in routine blood banking. The blood group systems to which they belong are discussed in chronologic order of their discovery. Other antigens are mentioned briefly at the end of the chapter, and the interested reader is referred to the cited sources for detailed information, including original references. Tables listing phenotype frequencies among blacks and whites in the US population are given in or adjacent to the sections dealing with the appropriate blood group systems. Frequencies among

other racial groups in the population are not given, as data are scanty and such wide differences exist among groups of diverse Asian or native American origin that generalization about the incidence of phenotypes is unwarranted. A summary of the serologic behavior and characteristics of the major antibodies is shown in Table 10-11 later in this chapter (see page 172).

The MNSs Blood Group System

Anti-M and Anti-N

The M and N antigens were discovered in 1927, when Landsteiner and Levine obtained the antibodies defining them by immunizing rabbits with human red cells. Anti-M is detected quite frequently in human sera, usually occurring as a saline agglutinin in antibody tests performed at room temperature. Most examples of this antibody occur without a red cell-induced stimulus, although anti-M is often wholly or partly IgG. The ability to agglutinate M+ cells in a saline test is not necessarily an indication that a given example of anti-M is wholly IgM. As with the A and B antigens of the ABO system, the M anti-

155

gen occurs in sufficient density on the cells that agglutination in a saline test may occur even when the antibody is wholly IgG. With some examples of anti-M, agglutination is strongest if the pH of the test system is reduced to around 6.5.

Anti-M is rarely significant clinically, although examples recognized in tests incubated at 37 C or in antiglobulin testing should be considered potentially significant. In a few exceptional cases, anti-M detectable by the indirect antiglobulin test has caused hemolytic disease of the newborn.[1]

By contrast, anti-N is comparatively rare, and is frequently IgM. Anti-N typically behaves like a cold agglutinin, although more powerful and potentially significant examples have been observed uncommonly in individuals of the rare phenotypes $M + N - S - s - U -$ and $M + N - S - s - U + w$. The presence of an anti-N-like agglutinating antibody in some hemodialysis patients, first reported in 1972,[2] was associated with the reuse of formaldehyde-sterilized dialyzer membranes.[3] The stimulus to antibody formation appears to be formaldehyde-induced alteration of the 'N' antigen,[4] a determinant present on both N+ and N− red cells (see page 158).

Antibodies Showing Dosage

The M and N antigens behave like products of paired allelic genes, in that they bear an obvious allelic relationship. With rare exceptions, red cells type as $M + N -$, $M - N +$ or as $M + N +$. These phenotypes represent, respectively, homozygosity for M and N, and heterozygosity for both genes. Some individual examples of anti-M and anti-N demonstrate dosage, showing significantly greater reaction strength and higher titration scores against red cells from homozygotes than against cells from heterozygotes. Licensed antisera rarely demonstrate dosage, having been selected and standardized to give good reactions with all cells possessing the rel-

evant antigen, although with dilution, dosage may become apparent. It is not uncommon, however, to encounter a patient serum containing anti-M or, much less frequently, anti-N that reacts only with cells possessing homozygous expression of the specific antigen. In such cases, the specificity of the antibody may not be immediately apparent from the reaction pattern obtained with a cell panel.

Reagent Antisera

Blood grouping sera are available commercially for the detection of M and N antigens. Most are produced by immunizing rabbits and absorbing the resulting immune antibodies to yield antisera giving the expected reactions. Human antisera and lectin reagents are also available, of which the most widely used is the anti-N-like extract of Vicia graminea seeds. Research with murine hybridoma cell lines is yielding monoclonal antibodies apparently having anti-M and anti-N specificity. In most cases, reagents from these different sources will give concordant reactions, but occasional discrepancies may result from relatively subtle differences in specificity. Since almost all human red cells contain some N antigen, for a reason that is explained later, anti-N reagents may react weakly with cells from persons homozygous for the M gene. Interpretation of reactions with anti-M and anti-N reagents always requires special care, and it is particularly important that the manufacturer's instructions be carefully followed.

Variant Antigens

Discrepant phenotyping results may occur when variants of the M and N antigens are present. For example, the M^g antigen, product of a very rare allele at the M/N locus, reacts neither with anti-M nor with anti-N reagents. The cells of a person with the genotype M^gN will give the reactions $M - N +$, leading to the false conclusion that the genotype is actually NN. Parentage could be falsely excluded if M^g were inherited from a person of the genotype M^{g}M but thought to be MM because the cellular reactions were M + N −. Anti-M^g occurs in 1-2% of human sera, usually as a saline agglutinin in sera from persons who have had no red cell-induced stimuli; however, the rarity of the M^g antigen makes the frequency of anti-M^g largely a matter of academic curiosity.

S, s and U Antigens

The antigens S and s are produced by a pair of allelic genes at a locus apparently closely linked to that of M/N. An example of linkage disequilibrium is seen in the fact that the gene complex that produces N with s is five times more common than that producing N with S. A small proportion of blacks type as S − s −. In most cases S − s − cells are also negative for a high-frequency antigen called U, and persons of this phenotype may make anti-U. Some S − s − cells are U +, however, but the U antigen on these cells may be so weakly expressed that adsorption and elution techniques are needed to demonstrate its presence.

Table 10-1 shows the frequencies of the different phenotypes in the MNSs system.

Antibodies to S, s and U

Unlike anti-M and anti-N, antibodies to S, s and U usually occur following red cell stimulation. All are capable of causing hemolytic transfusion reactions and hemolytic disease of the newborn. Although a few saline-reactive examples have been reported, antibodies to S, s and U are usually detected by the indirect antiglobulin test. Anti-S occurs about as infrequently as anti-N. Anti-s is seen less often, perhaps partly because the s − phenotype is less frequent than S −, but perhaps also because the s antigen is less immunogenic than S. Anti-U is found comparatively rarely, but should be considered when serum from a previously transfused or pregnant black person contains antibody to a high-frequency antigen. It may not be possible to type the patient's red cells for U, but the probability that they are U − can be established by proving they are S − s −.

Biochemistry of MNSs System

Glycophorin A

Antigens of the MNSs system are associated with red cell membrane sialoglycoproteins (SGP) called *glycophorin A* and *glycophorin B*, molecules susceptible to cleavage at varying positions by certain proteases. M and N antigen activity resides on glycophorin A, also called MN SGP, of which approximately 500,000 copies are present on each cell. This has a molecular weight of 31,000 and consists of 131 amino acids, with approximately 60% of its total mass

Table 10-1. Phenotypes and Frequencies in the MNSs System

| | | Reactions with Anti- | | | | Phenotype Frequency % | |
M	N	S	s	U	Phenotype	Whites	Blacks
+	0				M + N −	28	26
+	+				M + N +	50	44
0	+				M − N +	22	30
		+	0	+	S + s − U +	11	3
		+	+	+	S + s + U +	44	28
		0	+	+	S − s + U +	45	69
		0	0	0	S − s − U −	0	Less than 1
		0	0	(+)	S − s − U + w	0	Rare

composed of carbohydrate. The structure penetrates the membrane, with the carboxy terminal extending into the cytoplasm, and a hydrophobic segment consisting of 23 amino acids embedded within the lipid bilayer.

Blood group antigen activity resides on the external segment, a sequence of approximately 70 amino acids with carbohydrate side chains attached within the first 50 residues. When glycophorin A carries M antigen activity (glycophorin A^M) the first amino acid residue is serine and the fifth is glycine. When it carries N antigen activity (glycophorin A^N), leucine and glutamic acid replace serine and glycine at positions one and five, respectively.

Glycophorin B

Glycophorin B (Ss SGP) is smaller, and there are fewer copies per cell than glycophorin A, approximately 100,000. Glycophorin B is thought to carry U activity as well as S and s antigen activity and possesses, at the amino terminal, a segment consisting of 26 amino acids that duplicate the sequence of glycophorin A^N. This accounts for the presence of an N-like antigen ('N') on almost all red cells regardless of MN type. U− red cells, which are considered by some investigators to lack glycophorin B altogether, lack not only S and s activity, but also lack 'N.' Glycophorin B derived from S+s− red cells has been found to differ from that derived from S−s+ red cells in the substitution of methionine for threonine at position 29.

Variant Glycophorins

Studies on sialoglycoproteins isolated from red cells positive for certain low frequency antigens of the MNSs system suggest that these characteristics reflect subtle changes in amino acid sequences, either of glycophorin A or glycophorin B, accompanied by differences in the carbohydrate side chains. More pronounced sialoglycopro-

tein modifications occur in hybrid molecules considered to arise from crossing-over between genes coding for glycophorin A and glycophorin B. Such hybrids have occasionally been noted to carry a low frequency antigen.

Three low frequency antigens known to reside on hybrid sialoglycoproteins are Hil, Stones (St^a) and Dantu. The Dantu antigen,[5] which occurs predominantly in blacks, is of particular interest because the glycophorin B portion of the hybrid carries an antigen reactive with a proportion of anti-s sera, but U antigen activity is not present. The result, in appropriate circumstances, may be a phenotype hitherto considered not to exist, namely S−s+U−, of which at least four examples have been recognized to date, two in people who made anti-U. (John Moulds, personal communication).

Proteolytic Enzymes

Since certain proteolytic enzymes cleave red cell membrane sialoglycoproteins, reactivity with anti-M and anti-N is abolished by enzyme techniques commonly used in blood group antibody tests. This feature sometimes helps to identify these antibodies. The effect of enzymes on tests for the S and s antigens is less firmly established. Some investigators have found that enzyme treatment destroys the reactivity of S+ cells with anti-S, but reactivity of anti-s with s+ cells seems to be little affected by enzyme treatment of the cells.[6] On the other hand, some examples of anti-S appear to agglutinate enzyme-treated cells irrespective of their S antigen status, except that, if the enzyme treated cells are U− as well as S−, no agglutination occurs. As a consequence, these examples of anti-S could be mistaken for anti-U in an enzyme test system.[7] The U antigen itself is unaffected by enzyme treatment (see Table 10-11).

The effect of different enzymes on the reactivity of MNSs system antigens reflects the point at which the particular enzyme cleaves the SGP and the position of the antigen relative to the cleavage site. Figure 10-1 is a diagrammatic representation of glycophorin A and glycophorin B, showing antigen locations and enzyme cleavage points. The diagram is from Ellisor,[8] who cites the original references.

Satellite Antigens

The MNSs system includes a series of so-called satellite antigens. Though mainly of very low frequency, these may assume clinical significance on rare occasions. Like anti-M[g], many of the corresponding antibodies occur relatively often as non-red-cell-stimulated agglutinins, but antiglob-

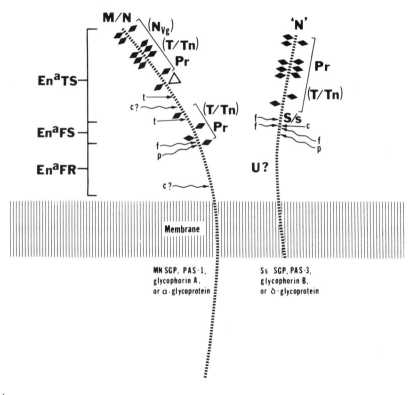

Legend:

◆	alkali-labile tetrasaccharides	← enzyme cleavage site on intact red cells	c = chymotrypsin
△	alkali-stable oligosaccharide	← enzyme cleavage site on SGP extracts and approximate site on intact red cells	f = ficin
()	cryptantigens		p = papain
			t = trypsin

Figure 10-1. Diagrammatic representation of M/N and S/s sialoglycoproteins in the red cell membrane including antigen locations and enzyme cleavage sites.

ulin-reactive examples have very uncommonly been implicated as the cause of hemolytic disease of the newborn. Reaction patterns with certain antisera suggest that several low-frequency antigens of the MNSs system are interrelated, forming the Miltenberger subsystem; some of these antigens appear to occur more commonly among populations of Oriental origin than in other population groups. Other low-frequency antigens have been assigned to the MNSs system by linkage data acquired through family studies. For some, recent biochemical data indicate that one or more amino acid substitutions, variation in the extent or type of glycosylation, or the existence of a hybrid sialoglycoprotein influence reactivity of the particular low-frequency determinant.

The P Blood Group System

The P_1 antigen, originally called P, was discovered by Landsteiner and Levine in 1927, in the series of animal experiments that also led to the discovery of M and N. The designation P was later reassigned to an antigen present on almost all human red cells. Cells lacking P_1 but shown to possess P may be designated P_2. P_1 is present on the red cells of approximately 80% of whites and 94% of blacks.

Anti-P_1

The serum of P_2 persons commonly contains anti-P_1. In fact, if sufficiently sensitive techniques are applied, it is likely that anti-P_1 would be detected in the serum of virtually every P_2 person. The antibody reacts optimally at 4 C but may occasionally be detected at 25 C. Anti-P_1 is rarely seen in tests performed strictly at 37 C. As anti-P_1 is almost invariably IgM, it does not cross the placenta; therefore, it has not been reported as the cause of hemolytic disease of the newborn. Anti-P_1 has very rarely been reported as causing hemolysis in vivo.

The strength of P_1 reactivity varies among different cell samples, and reactivity tends to diminish when red cells are stored. These characteristics sometimes create difficulties, both in testing cells for the antigen and in the identification of the antibody. Anti-P_1 blood grouping sera are usually sufficiently potent to detect weak forms of the antigen, but occasional blood samples may be falsely classified as P_1-, particularly after prolonged storage. An antibody weakly reactive on room temperature testing can often be shown to have anti-P_1 specificity by lowering incubation temperature or by using enzyme-treated cells. Hydatid cyst fluid or commercially available P_1 substance derived from pigeon eggs inhibit in vitro reactivity of anti-P_1. Inhibition may be a useful aid to the identification of anti-P_1, especially if the antibody is present in a serum with antibodies of other specificities.

Biochemistry of P and ABO Systems

Antigens of the P system share with glycolipid ABH antigens a common precursor, lactosylceramide. Sequential addition of several sugars leads to globoside, which is the P antigen present on almost all P_1+ and P_1- red cells. A different sequence of sugars results in the production of paragloboside, which is the P_1 antigen. A proposed scheme of biosynthetic pathways, compiled by Beattie,[9] is shown in Fig 10-2.

Rare Phenotypes

Several very rare phenotypes exist in the P system. The P^k antigen results from absence of the terminal sugar that leads to P reactivity. Persons whose red cells have P^k instead of P consistently have a strong IgM alloanti-P, which reacts with P_1+P+ and P_1-P+ cells. The biphasic autohemolysin of paroxysmal cold hemoglobinuria (PCH) is often but not invariably of this specificity. Unlike the anti-P of P^k people and the anti-P that is part of anti-PP_1P^k (see below), the autoanti-P of PCH is IgG.

Also very rare are persons whose red cells are P_1-P-P^k-. This phenotype, also

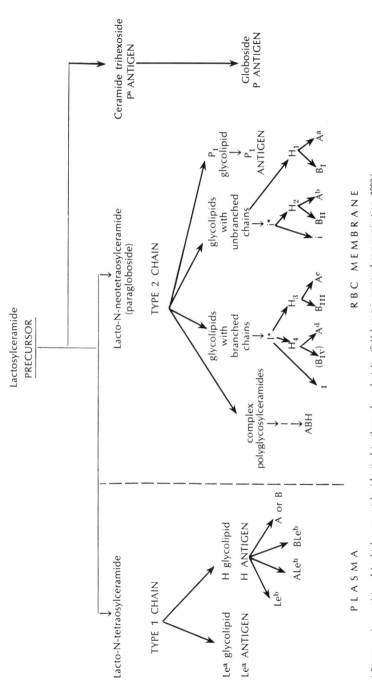

* Precursor forms of i and I which may not be identical to the end product Ii. (S Hakomori, personal communication, 1980.)

Figure 10-2. Proposed biosynthetic pathways of glycolipid antigens of human red blood cell membranes and plasma.

called p, is characterized by the presence of a strong hemolytic IgM antibody with anti-PP$_1$P^k activity. This antibody, which was formerly called anti-Tj^a, has caused hemolytic transfusion reactions and, occasionally, hemolytic disease of the newborn.[10,11] There is a curious association between anti-PP$_1$P^k and abortion occurring early in pregnancy in p women. Race and Sanger[1] cite an accumulation of data to support the association, although it is not clear that the maternal antibody causes early fetal death.

The different phenotypes of the P blood group system are shown in Table 10-2.

Lutheran Blood Group System

The first example of anti-Lu^a was found in 1945, in a serum that contained several other antibodies. The phenotypes of the Lutheran system, as defined by anti-Lu^a and anti-Lu^b, are shown in Table 10-3. The Lu(a−b−) phenotype is very rare and may arise from two distinct genetic circumstances. In one, a presumably amorphic Lutheran gene *Lu* is inherited from both parents. In the other, the negative phenotype is inherited as a dominant characteristic attributed to the independently segregating inhibitor gene *In(Lu)*, which prevents the normal expression of Lutheran and certain other blood group genes.

Lutheran system antibodies are not often encountered. Both anti-Lu^a and anti-Lu^b occur in subjects with no known red cell stimulation. Lutheran antigens are poorly developed at birth, so it is not surprising

that anti-Lu^a has not been reported as the cause of hemolytic disease of the newborn. Neither has this antibody been associated with hemolytic transfusion reactions. Anti-Lu^b, on the other hand, has been reported to cause diminished survival of transfused red cells and mild hemolytic disease of the newborn. Most examples of anti-Lu^a and some of anti-Lu^b will agglutinate saline-suspended red cells possessing the relevant antigen, producing small to moderately sized, loosely agglutinated clumps of cells superimposed on a background of unagglutinated cells. This mixed-field appearance is characteristic of reactions with Lutheran antibodies.

Associated Antigens

A series of high-frequency antigens (Lu4, 5, 6, 7, 8, 11, 12 and 13) have been assigned to the Lutheran system because the corresponding antibodies do not react with cells of the Lu(a−b−) phenotype. However, as the *In(Lu)* gene also appears to modify the expression of antigens belonging to other blood group systems (notably Au^a, P$_1$, and i), it is not certain that all these antigens belong to the Lutheran system. Two low-frequency antigens (Lu9 and Lu14) have gained admission to the Lutheran system because each has shown an apparently antithetical relationship with one of the previously mentioned high-frequency antigens, Lu9 with Lu6 and Lu14 with Lu8.

Kell Blood Group System

The K (Kell) antigen was first demonstrated in 1946, through an antibody that

Table 10-2. Phenotypes and Frequencies in the P System

	Reactions with Anti-				Phenotype Frequency %	
P$_1$	P	P^k	PP$_1$P^k	Phenotype	Whites	Blacks
+	+	0	+	P$_1$	79	94
0	+	0	+	P$_2$	21	6
0	0*	0	0	p		
+	0	+	+	P$_1$^{k}	All extremely rare	
0	0	+	+	P$_2$^{k}		

*Usually negative, occasionally weakly positive

Table 10-3. Phenotypes and Frequencies in the Lutheran System in Whites

| Reactions with Anti- | | Phenotype | Phenotype |
Lu^a	Lu^b	Phenotype	Frequency %
+	0	Lu(a + b −)	0.15
+	+	Lu(a + b +)	7.5
0	+	Lu(a − b +)	92.35
0	0	Lu(a − b −)	very rare

Insufficient data exist for the reliable calculation of frequencies in blacks.

caused hemolytic disease of the newborn. The gene responsible (*K*) is present in 9% of whites and a somewhat lesser number of blacks. The existence of the expected allele (*k*) was confirmed when an antithetical relationship was established between K and the antigen detected by anti-Cellano (anti-k), which reacted with the red cells of over 99% of the random population.

Anti-K and Anti-k

The K antigen is strongly immunogenic, and it is therefore not surprising that anti-K is frequently found in sera from transfused patients. In a few cases, anti-K has appeared as a saline agglutinin in sera from subjects never exposed to a red cell stimulus, but most examples detected are of immune origin and are reactive by the indirect antiglobulin test; some bind complement. Anti-K has caused hemolytic transfusion reactions on numerous occasions, both immediate and delayed. Since 90% of donors are K −, it is not difficult to find compatible blood for patients with anti-K, or to select K − blood in those special circumstances in which it is desirable to avoid transfusing cells that might be immunogenic. Anti-K has been observed as a saline-reactive antibody, but most examples are detected by the indirect antiglobulin test and follow known immunizing stimuli. Anti-k has clinical and serologic characteristics similar to anti-K, but occurs much less frequently because only about one person in 500 is negative for the k antigen.

Other Antigens

Other antithetical antigens of the Kell system include Kp^a and Kp^b, and Js^a and Js^b. These antigens, along with K and k, are inherited as if controlled by linked alleles, somewhat analogous to the antigens of the Rh system. A third allele at the *Kp^a/Kp^b* locus is considered[12] to produce the antigen Kp^c, which was first recognized in 1946 and originally called Levay. Unlike findings in the Rh system, not all the theoretically possible phenotype combinations have been recognized in the Kell system. For example, Kp^a and Js^a have never been found together. Kp^a is predominantly an antigen found in whites, and Js^a is predominantly found in blacks. The phenotype K + Kp(a + b −) has also not been found. Table 10-4 shows the phenotypes of the Kell system, defined separately by the three pairs of reciprocally related antibodies. The table also includes K$_o$, of which the distinguishing feature is that the cells lack the principal antigens of the system and may be thought of as Kell$_{null}$ (analogous to Rh$_{null}$). For simplicity, the various other high-frequency and low-frequency Kell system antigens are not included in the table.

Other Antibodies

Anti-Kp^a, anti-Kp^b, anti-Js^a, and anti-Js^b are all much less common than anti-K, but show similar serologic characteristics and are considered clinically significant. Any of them may occur following transfusion or fetomaternal immunization. Their frequency is influenced by the immunogenicity of the particular antigen and by differences in the distribution of the relevant

Table 10-4. Phenotypes and Frequencies in the Kell System

K	k	Reactions with Anti- Kpᵃ	Kpᵇ	Jsᵃ	Jsᵇ	Phenotype	Frequency % Whites	Blacks
+	0					K+k−	0.2	rare
+	+					K+k+	8.8	2
0	+					K−k+	91	98
		+	0			Kp(a+b−)	rare	0
		+	+			Kp(a+b+)	2.3	rare
		0	+			Kp(a−b+)	97.7	100
				+	0	Js(a+b−)	0	1
				+	+	Js(a+b+)	rare	19
				0	+	Js(a−b+)	100	80
0	0	0	0	0	0	K₀	exceedingly rare	

negative phenotypes among transfusion recipients and of the positive phenotypes among donors. The Js^a antigen is present on red cells from 20% of blacks; Kp^a occurs in 2% of whites but is rare in blacks. Thus, 80% of blacks and 100% of whites could form anti-Js^a if transfused with Js(a+) cells. Anti-Kp^a could theoretically be formed by 98% of white and 100% of black recipients of the cells from the 2% of whites who have the antigen. These antibodies are rarely seen, due probably to low immunogenicity and infrequency of the antigens on antibody screening cells.The occurrence of anti-Js^b and anti-Kp^b is similarly influenced by the incidence of the reciprocal negative phenotypes and the immunizing potential of the respective antigens. Patients immunized to the high-frequency antigens k, Kp^b and Js^b, or to any high-frequency antigen, present a problem that may require assistance from a rare donor file should transfusion be required.

Numerical Nomenclature

As in the Rh system, a numerical nomenclature has been proposed[13] to denote the antigens of the Kell system. K1, K2, K3, K4, K6 and K7 refer, respectively, to K, k, Kp^a, Kp^b, Js^a and Js^b. K5 was allocated to Ku, the antigen thought to be defined by the antibody that K_0 persons may form when immunized. Anti-Ku (anti-K5) is probably not directed at a single deter-

minant, as most examples appear to be mixtures of Kell system antibodies, reacting with red cells of all Kell phenotypes. In this respect, anti-Ku is similar to anti-Rh29 of the Rh system. K_0 is not strictly comparable with Rh_{null}, however, because K_0 cells do possess an antigen of the Kell system called Kx, whereas Rh_{null} cells appear to have no identifiable Rh system antigens.

As in the Lutheran system, several high-frequency antigens have been assigned to the Kell system because the identifying antibodies were found to give negative reactions with K_0 cells. The high-frequency antigen K11 and the low-frequency antigen K17 (Wkᵃ) bear an antithetical relationship, establishing the presence of a fourth pair of linked allelic genes at the Kell locus.

The Kx Antigen

Kx seems to be a precursor in the biosynthetic pathways of the Kell system.[14] Determined by a gene on the X chromosome designated X^1k, it is normally present on granulocytes and fibroblasts. Except in the K_0 phenotype, Kx is found only in trace amounts on red cells, since products of the autosomal Kell system genes convert it to antigens of the Kell system. A curious association exists between presence of Kx and cellular function, but the nature of this association remains unclear. In the absence of X^1k, the granulocytes lack Kx and, additionally, have defective intracellular bactericidal activity, such that they can phagocytize microorganisms but are unable to mobilize the enzyme pathways necessary to kill them. This defect of granulocyte function produces the condition called chronic granulomatous disease (CGD).

The McLeod Phenotype

Red cells that lack Kx completely have shortened survival, decreased permeability to water and acanthocytic morphology, as well as markedly depressed expression of Kell system antigens. This constellation of red cell abnormalities is called the McLeod phenotype, perhaps a rather misleading term, since the depressed antigens present depend on the Kell genes present in the particular subject. Persons with McLeod red cells also have a poorly defined abnormality of the neuromuscular system, characterized by persistently elevated serum levels of the enzyme creatine phosphokinase (CPK) and, in older people, disordered muscular function.

Other Variant Alleles

Not all sufferers from CGD have depressed Kell system antigens on their red cells, nor do all persons of the McLeod phenotype have clinical manifestations of CGD. There are several variant alleles of the Kx-determining gene on the X chromosome. Because females who possess one of the abnormal genes always have a normal gene on the other X chromosome, the clinical syndromes described above occur only in males, but cell studies on carrier females have revealed the presence of a population of abnormally functioning blood cells. The variant genes and the effects they are considered to produce are shown in Table 10-5.

Another phenotype characterized by weak expression of Kell system antigens has recently been described[15] in an elderly woman whose red cells were morphologically normal and whose serum contained an antibody directed at a high-freqency antigen evidently related to the Kell sys-

tem. Unlike McLeod cells, those of the Day phenotype, as it was called, exhibit Kx antigen activity elevated even beyond that on K_O cells. The possibility of homozygosity for a new allele was raised by the fact that her parents were first cousins.

Biochemical Manipulation

Kell system antigens are inactivated by treating red blood cells with 2-amino-ethylisothiouronium bromide (AET). This provides a useful method of artificially preparing red cells lacking Kell system antigens as an aid to the identification of Kell-related antibodies. AET treatment may impair the reactivity of certain other antigens, however, so the association of an antibody with the Kell system because of reduced reactivity with AET-treated cells is only tentative. ZZAP, a mixture of cysteine-activated papain and dithiothreitol,[16] also destroys Kell system antigens.

Lewis Blood Group System

Closely related to the ABH antigens, the Lewis antigens arise when fucose is attached to N-acetylglucosamine of the type 1 oligosaccharide chain (page 118). The fucosyl transferase determined by the Le gene produces Le^a in individuals who lack the Se gene. Simultaneous presence of the H, Se and Le genes produces Le^b, which has fucose moieties attached both to the terminal galactose and the N-acetylglucosamine. Because red cell membranes possess no type 1 chains, Lewis antigens are not intrinsic to the cell membrane. As glycosphingolipids carried in plasma, they are adsorbed to the red cell surface.

Lewis Antibodies

Lewis antibodies occur sporadically, almost exclusively in Le(a−b−) persons, and usually without a known red cell stimulus. People whose red cell phenotype is Le(a−b+) do not make anti-Le^a because Le^a is part of their antigenic constitution and is present in their saliva. It is extremely unusual to find anti-Le^b in the serum of a

Table 10-5. Sex-Linked Genes that Influence the Expression of Kx

Gene	Kx on Granulocytes	Kx on Red Cells	Kell Antigens on Red Cells	Elevated Serum CPK	Chronic Granulomatous Disease
X^1k	yes	trace	normal	no	no
X^2k	no	no	severely depressed	yes	yes (Type II)
X^3k	no	trace	normal	no	yes (Type I)
X^4k	yes	no	severely depressed	yes	no

Le(a + b −) person. Anti-Le^a and anti-Le^b may occur in serum either individually or in combination. The Lewis antibodies are almost always IgM and do not cross the placenta. Because of this, and because the Lewis antigens are poorly developed at birth, this system is not implicated in hemolytic disease of the newborn. Lewis antibodies may bind complement; some fresh sera that contain anti-Le^a, or, very occasionally, anti-Le^b may cause in vitro hemolysis of incompatible red cells. In vitro hemolysis is more often seen with enzyme-treated cells than with untreated cells.

Most Lewis antibodies agglutinate saline-suspended red cells of the appropriate phenotype; agglutinates are often fragile and easily dispersed if the red cell button is not resuspended very gently after centrifugation. Agglutination is sometimes seen after incubation at 37 C, but rarely of the strength seen in tests incubated at room temperature. Some examples of anti-Le^a, and less commonly anti-Le^b, produce a positive indirect antiglobulin reaction, providing complement is present in the reaction mixture and polyspecific antiglobulin serum is used.

Table 10-6. Phenotypes and Frequencies in the Lewis System

Reactions with Anti-			Adult Phenotype Frequency %	
Le^a	Le^b	Phenotype	Whites	Blacks
+	0	Le(a + b −)	22	23
0	+	Le(a − b +)	72	55
0	0	Le(a − b −)	6	22

Anti-Le^b

Sera with anti-Le^b can be divided into two categories. The more common examples react best with cells of group O and A$_2$; these have been designated anti-Le^{bH}. Those that react equally well with the Le^b antigen on cells of all ABO phenotypes are called anti-Le^{bL}. Anti-Le^{bH} but not anti-Le^{bL} is neutralized by saliva from group O Le(a − b −) persons who are secretors of H substance.

Anti-Le^c and Anti-Le^d

Two additional antibodies have been given names in the Lewis system, although the products with which they react are not determined by Lewis genes. Anti-Le^c has been reported once in a human subject as a cold agglutinin.[17] This antibody agglutinates the red cells of Le(a − b −) people who lack the Se gene and are therefore nonsecretors of H substance. The antibody called anti-Le^d agglutinates the red cells of Le(a − b −) secretors. The product with which "anti-Le^d" reacts has been identified as the type 1 oligosaccharide chain with a fucose at the H-active site but none at the Lewis-active site; hence the antibody should more correctly be viewed as a form of anti-H (see page 119). The material reactive with anti-Le^d seems to be the type 2 chain, with no added fucose moieties. No example of "anti-Le^d" has been reported in humans, but both anti-Le^c and "anti-Le^d" have been successfully produced by goats injected with saliva from, respectively, nonsecretors and secretors of H with the Le(a − b −) phenotype.[18]

In Vivo Neutralization

Lewis antigens are reversibly adsorbed to the red cell surface from the surrounding plasma. Transfused red cells assume the Lewis phenotype of the recipient within a few days of entering the circulation. Lewis antibodies in a recipient's serum are readily neutralized by Lewis blood group substance in donor plasma, and largely for this reason, it is exceedingly uncommon for Lewis antibodies to cause hemolysis of transfused Le(a+) or Le(b+) cells. Antibodies that cause hemolysis in vitro or give strong reactions in the indirect antiglobulin phase of the crossmatch, however, have been associated with post-transfusion hemolysis.

Transfusion Practice

It is not considered necessary to prescreen donor blood for the absence of Lewis antigens. For a patient with anti-Le^a or anti-Le^b, the reactions seen in a standard crossmatch provide a good index of transfusion safety.[19,20] Some workers have reported successful neutralization of Lewis antibodies by transfusing plasma containing Lewis substance before performing the crossmatch and transfusing Lewis-positive blood.[21] Many transfusionists, however, regularly give Le(a−b+) blood, compatible by routine crossmatch, without this precaution.

Lewis Reactivity in Children

Red cells from newborn infants usually give weak or negative reactions with both anti-Le^a and anti-Le^b, but react more strongly with sera that agglutinate both Le(a+b−) and Le(a−b+) adult cells. These sera are considered to contain not separable anti-Le^a and anti-Le^b, but activity against a determinant called Le^x,[22] which is present on cord cells and also on adult cells that are either Le(a+) or Le(b+). Reliable Lewis grouping of young children may not be possible, as the reactions often do not reflect the correct adult phenotype before the age of about 6 years.

Among small children the incidence of Le^a is high and that of Le^b is low. The phenotype Le(a+b+) may be observed as a transient phase in children whose adult phenotype will be Le(a−b+).

Duffy Blood Group System

The antigens Fy^a and Fy^b are determined by a pair of codominant alleles located on chromosome 1. *Fy*, a third allele at this locus, with a high frequency among blacks, produces no Fy^a or Fy^b antigen (Table 10-7). Black individuals who are Fy(a−b−) are thought to be homozygous *FyFy*.

Antibodies to Fy Antigens

Both anti-Fy^a and anti-Fy^b cause both hemolytic disease of the newborn and hemolytic transfusion reactions. Anti-Fy^a is quite commonly encountered, anti-Fy^b considerably less so. These antibodies react best by the indirect antiglobulin test. The antigen sites are destroyed by most enzymes used in serologic tests, so Duffy antibodies usually give negative reactions in enzyme test procedures.

Effect of Zygosity

Weak examples of anti-Fy^a or anti-Fy^b may give convincing reactions only with cells that have a double dose of the antigen. In white populations, red cells that have only one of the two antigens can safely be assumed to come from persons homozygous for the gene and to have a double dose of the antigen. In blacks, however, the *Fy* gene is so common that red cells

Table 10-7. Phenotypes and Frequencies in the Duffy System

Reactions with Anti-			Adult Phenotype Frequency %	
Fy^a	Fy^b	Phenotype	Whites	Blacks
+	0	Fy(a+b−)	17	9
+	+	Fy(a+b+)	49	1
0	+	Fy(a−b+)	34	22
0	0	Fy(a−b−)	v.rare	68

having only one of the two antigens are usually from persons heterozygous for *Fy*, and the active antigen is present only in single dose. In identifying Duffy antibodies, it can be important to know the racial origin of the cells on antibody identification panels. Clues that a panel cell donor may be black are the R$_o$, S−s− or Fy(a−b−) phenotypes, or the presence of the V, VS or Js^a antigens.

Rarely Encountered Antibodies

Black subjects who are Fy(a−b−) do not often make Duffy system antibodies. It was a rare white person of the Fy(a−b−) phenotype who first made anti-Fy3, an exceedingly uncommon antibody that acts like a combination of anti-Fy^a and anti-Fy^b, although the specificities cannot be separated by absorption and elution. Unlike anti-Fy^a and anti-Fy^b, however, anti-Fy3 reacts well with enzyme-treated Fy(a+) or Fy(b+) cells. Fy3 is considered to be an enzyme-resistant antigen present on all Fy(a+) and Fy(b+) cells but absent from Fy(a−b−) cells.

Two further rare antibodies have been described, both of which were reactive against papain-treated cells. One, anti-Fy4, reacts strongly with cells of the Fy(a−b−) phenotype, as well as with some Fy(a+b−) and some Fy(a−b+) cells from blacks, but never with Fy(a+b+) cells. On this evidence, Fy4 is considered to be the product of an allele that, in the homozygous state, is responsible for the Fy(a−b−) phenotype in blacks. The other antibody, anti-Fy5, is similar to anti-Fy3, except that it gives negative reactions with Rh$_{null}$ cells, as well as those of Fy(a−b−) blacks. This antibody was observed to react with the cells of a white Fy(a−b−) person, which provided a hitherto unrecognized distinction between the Fy(a−b−) phenotype so common in blacks and the one so rare in whites. It has been postulated that Fy5 is formed by interaction of Rh and Duffy gene products.[23]

Biologic Effects of Fy Antigens

The Fy^a and Fy^b antigens seem to be important in the process whereby malarial parasites gain entry to red cells. The Fy(a−b−) phenotype appears to provide resistance to certain forms of malarial infection. It was observed in 1975[24] that Fy(a−b−) cells resisted infection by the monkey malarial parasite, *Plasmodium knowlesi*, and that parasitism of Fy(a+) cells was markedly reduced when cells were coated with anti-Fy^a. *Plasmodium knowlesi* does not infect humans; the same resistance evidently applies to infection with *P. vivax* but not with *P. falciparum*.[25] There are areas of Africa where 100% of the native population is Fy(a−b−); *P. vivax* has not been found in these areas, although other species of *Plasmodium* are present and infective. In one investigation, 11 blacks were exposed to the bites of mosquitoes infected with *P. vivax*. All six who had Duffy antigens on their red cells developed *Plasmodium vivax* infection, but the five whose red cells were Fy(a−b−) did not.[26]

Kidd Blood Group System

Anti-Jk^a and Anti-Jk^b

Anti-Jk^a was first recognized in 1951, in the serum of a woman who had given birth to a child with hemolytic disease of the newborn. Two years later, the antithetical anti-Jk^b was found in the serum of a patient who had suffered a transfusion reaction. Both antibodies react best by the indirect antiglobulin test, but saline reactivity is sometimes observed in freshly drawn specimens. These antibodies are often weak when first detected and, perhaps because of complement-dependence, may become undetectable on storage. Even freshly drawn sera containing weak anti-Jk^a or anti-Jk^b may manifest a dosage effect, reacting only with cells expressing a double dose of the antigen.

Effects of Complement

Antiglobulin serum containing an anti-complement component is sometimes needed for the reliable detection of these inconsistently reactive antibodies. Anti-Jk[a] and anti-Jk[b] sera that have lost their reactivity during storage can sometimes be revived by adding fresh human serum as a source of complement, or by the use of an enzyme antiglobulin technique. Adding fresh serum, however, dilutes what may already be a weakly reactive antibody, and may not be successful if the serum has become anticomplementary during storage.

A method that has proved satisfactory with some complement-dependent antibodies is the two-stage antiglobulin test of Polley and Mollison.[27] The principle of this method, which may be helpful when antibody presence is suspected but elusive, is that the cells are first incubated with the test serum in the presence of EDTA, which allows antibody uptake but prevents complement from being bound. The cells are then washed and reincubated with immunologically inert fresh human serum as a source of complement. After rewashing, a suitable antiglobulin serum is added in the usual way.

Clinical Significance

The Kidd antibodies occasionally cause hemolytic disease of the newborn, but this is usually mild. These antibodies are notorious, however, for involvement in severe hemolytic transfusion reactions, especially in delayed reactions. These occur when antibody developing rapidly in an anamnestic response to antigens on transfused cells destroys the still-circulating cells. In some reported cases, retesting the patient's pretransfusion serum has confirmed that the antibody was indeed undetectable in the original compatibility tests. Events of this kind highlight the importance of consulting previous records before selecting blood for transfusion; in some cases of delayed hemolytic reactions the

Table 10-8. Phenotypes and Frequencies in the Kidd System

Reactions with Anti-			Adult Phenotype Frequency %	
Jk[a]	Jk[b]	Phenotype	Whites	Blacks
+	0	Jk(a+b−)	28	57
+	+	Jk(a+b+)	49	34
0	+	Jk(a−b+)	23	9
0	0	Jk(a−b−)	exceedingly rare	

antibody had previously been detected and identified.

Genes and Phenotypes

The four phenotypes defined by the reactions of anti-Jk[a] and anti-Jk[b] are shown in Table 10-8. The Jk(a−b−) phenotype, extremely rare except in some populations of Pacific Island origin, is apparently the result of homozygosity for the silent *Jk* allele, although the possibility of an inhibitor gene effect has not been excluded with certainty. Sera from some of these rare Jk(a−b−) people have been found to contain an antibody that reacts with all Jk(a+) and Jk(b+) cells, but not with Jk(a−b−) cells. Although a minor anti-Jk[a] or anti-Jk[b] component is sometimes separable, most of the reactivity has been directed at an antigen called Jk3, which is considered to be present on both Jk(a+) and Jk(b+) cell, in a manner analogous to that of Fy3 on Fy(a+) and Fy(b+) cells. Anti-Jk3 is most often immune in origin, but in one case an IgM example of the antibody was detected in a male Jk(a−b−) patient who had no history of transfusion.[28] Curiously, the man had a Jk(a−b−) sister who had been pregnant seven times but had produced no antibody.

Additional Pairs of Antithetical Antigens

So far this chapter has been devoted to blood group systems of which the principal antibodies may be seen fairly frequently in the routine blood grouping laboratory. Other systems of genetically determined antigens also exist and the

Table 10-9. Phenotype Frequencies in Other Blood Group Systems in which Antithetical Antibodies are Known

System	Reactions with Anti-		Phenotype	Phenotype Frequency in Whites*
Diego	Di^a	Di^b		
	+	0	Di(a + b −)	0†
	+	+	Di(a + b +)	very rare†
	0	+	Di(a − b +)	100
Cartwright	Yt^a	Yt^b		
	+	0	Yt(a + b −)	91.9
	+	+	Yt(a + b +)	7.9
	0	+	Yt(a − b +)	0.2
Dombrock	Do^a	Do^b		
	+	0	Do(a + b −)	17.2
	+	+	Do(a + b +)	49.5
	0	+	Do(a − b +)	33.3
Colton	Co^a	Co^b		
	+	0	Co(a + b −)	89.3
	+	+	Co(a + b +)	10.4
	0	+	Co(a − b +)	0.3
	0	0	Co(a − b −)	very rare
Scianna	Sc1	Sc2		
	+	0	Sc:1, − 2	99.7
	+	+	Sc:1,2	0.3
	0	+	Sc: − 1,2	very rare
	0	0	Sc: − 1, − 2	very rare

*There are insufficient data for reliable calculation of frequencies in blacks.
†The Di^a antigen has a much higher frequency in orientals and native Americans.

reader should be aware of them. Antibodies directed at these determinants may occur on rare occasions, perhaps especially in sera containing multiple specificities. The antigens themselves may be important in genetic investigations and population or family studies.

The phenotype frequencies in the Dombrock system are similar to those of Duffy, while those in the Cartwright and Colton systems parallel the frequencies of K and k. The Diego system is useful as a racial marker, with the Di^a antigen being almost entirely confined to populations of Mongolian origin, including native Americans. All these antigens, and those of the Scianna system, appear to be less immunogenic than those of the other major blood group systems, and their antibodies are of special interest because of their rarity. When present, these antibodies are often found in sera containing one or more other antibodies, perhaps because an immune response to multiple antigens implies unusual susceptibility to producing blood group antibodies. Table 10-9 lists the phenotype frequencies for these systems among whites.

The Sex-Linked Blood Group Antigen Xg^a

In 1962, an antibody was discovered that identified an antigen more common among women than among men. This would be expected of an X-borne characteristic,

Table 10-10. Frequencies of the Xg(a +) and Xg(a −) Phenotypes in White Males and Females

| Phenotype | Phenotype Frequency % | |
	Males	Females
Xg(a +)	65.6	88.7
Xg(a −)	34.4	11.3

Frequencies are based on combined results of testing nearly 7,000 random bloods from populations of Northern European origin. Insufficient data exist for reliable calculation of frequencies in blacks.

because females inherit an X chromosome from each parent, whereas males inherit X only from the mother. The antigen is called Xg^a, in recognition of its X-borne manner of inheritance. Table 10-10 gives the phenotype frequencies among white males and females in the American population.

Anti-Xg^a is an uncommon antibody that usually reacts only by the indirect antiglobulin technique, although at least three examples are known that agglutinated saline-suspended cells. Enzymes most often used in serologic tests appear to alter the antigen, so negative reactions are to be expected in enzyme test systems. This antibody has not been implicated in hemolytic disease of the newborn or hemolytic transfusion reactions, but it is evidently capable of binding complement and one example has been reported as an autoantibody.[29] Anti-Xg^a may be useful for tracing the transmission of genetic traits associated with the X chromosome, although linkage with the Xg locus has been demonstrated for few traits, so far.

The I/i Antigens

Oligosaccharide Structures

Antibodies directed at the I/i antigens are probably the unexpected antibodies most frequently encountered when serologic tests are performed at room temperature. The type 2 oligosaccharide chains carrying the terminal sugars that determine ABH specificity include multiple β-glcNAc(1-3) β-gal(1-4) units. The antigenic activity called i resides in a straight-chain oligosaccharide with only two such units. On adult red cells, many of these linear chains are modified and have a branched structure consisting of β-gal(1-4) β-glcNAc (1-6) linked to an internal galactose. I specificity derives from the branched structure, and heterogeneity observed among different anti-I sera may reflect the fact that different ones recognize different portions of the branched oligosaccharide chain.

Antigens and Antibodies

Anti-I is usually identified by its failure to react with red cells from cord blood. Fetal red cells are rich in i but lack branched oligosaccharide chains and therefore have a poorly developed I antigen. During the first two years of life, the I antigen gradually develops, and there is concomitant loss of i. Thus, the red cells of most adults are strongly reactive with anti-I and only weakly reactive with anti-i. Rare adults have cells that are not I +. These i$_{adult}$ people usually have anti-I as an alloantibody in their serum, but this may be so weak in some cases as to require an enzyme technique for its detection. If tests are performed at 4 C, most I + people can be shown to have autoanti-I in their serum.

Autoanti-i less often causes cold autoimmune hemolytic anemia than does anti-I. On rare occasions it may be seen as a relatively weak cold autoagglutinin reacting only at 4-10 C. Patients with infectious mononucleosis often have transient anti-i in their sera.

Complex Reactivity

Such specificities as anti-IH and anti-IP$_1$ probably recognize branched structures that have been further modified by transferases for H and P$_1$, respectively. Anti-IH occurs quite commonly in sera from A$_1$ people and, as would be expected, reacts most strongly with red cells that are strongly H + as well as I +.

Table 10-11. Serological Behavior of the Principal Antibodies of the Different Blood Group Systems

Antibody	In vitro Hemolysis	Saline 4 C	Saline 22 C	Albumin 37 C	Albumin AGT	Enzyme 37 C	Enzyme AGT	Associated with HDN*	Associated with HTR†
Anti-M	0	Most	Some	Few	Few	0	0	Few	Few
Anti-N	0	Most	Few	Occ.	Occ.	0	0	Rare	?
Anti-S	0	Few	Some	Some	Most	see text		Yes	Yes
Anti-s	0	0	Few	Few	Most	see text		Yes	Yes
Anti-U	0	0	Occ.	Some	Most	Most	Most	Yes	Yes
Anti-P$_1$	Occ.	Most	Some	Occ.	Rare	Some	Few	No	Rare
Anti-P	Some	Most	Some	Some	Some	Some	Some	No	?
Anti-PP$_1$P^k	Some	Most	Some	Some	Some	Some	Some	Rare	?
Anti-Lu^a	0	Some	Most	Few	Few	Few	Few	No	?
Anti-Lu^b	0	Few	Few	Few	Most	Few	Few	Mild	Yes
Anti-K	0		Few	Some	Most	Some	Most	Yes	Yes
Anti-k	0		Few	Few	Most	Some	Most	Yes	Yes
Anti-Kp^a	0		Some	Some	Most	Some	Some	Yes	?
Anti-Kp^b	0		Few	Few	Most	Some	Some	Yes	Yes
Anti-Js^a	0		Few	Few	Most	Few	Few	Yes	?
Anti-Js^b	0		0	0	Most	Few	Few	Yes	?
Anti-Le^a	Some	Most	Most	Some	Many	Most	Most	No	Few
Anti-Le^b	Occ.	Most	Most	Few	Some	Some	Some	No	No
Anti-Fy^a	0		Rare	Rare	Most	0	0	Yes	Yes
Anti-Fy^b	0		Rare	Rare	Most	0	0	Yes	Yes
Anti-Jk^a	Some		Few	Few	Most	Some	Yes	Yes	Yes
Anti-Jk^b	Some		Few	Few	Most	Some	Most	Yes	Yes
Anti-Xg^a	0		Few	Few	Most	0	0	No report	
Anti-Di^a	0		Some	Some	Most	Some	Some	Yes	Yes
Anti-Di^b	0				Most	Some	Some	Yes	Yes
Anti-Yt^a	0		0	0	Most	0	Some	No	?
Anti-Yt^b	0				All			No report	
Anti-Do^a	0		0	0	Some	Some	Most	?	Yes
Anti-Do^b	0				All		All	No report	
Anti-Co^a	0		0	0	Some	Some	Most	Yes	?
Anti-Co^b	0		0	0	Some	Some	Most	No report	
Anti-Sc1	0				All			No report	
Anti-Sc2	0		Some	Some	Most	Most	Most	No report	

*Hemolytic disease of the newborn
†Hemolytic transfusion reactions
The reactivity shown in the Table is based on the tube methods in common use. If tests are carried out by more sensitive test procedures (such as in capillary tubes, in microtiter plates or by the albumin layering method), direct agglutination (prior to the antiglobulin phase) may be observed more often with some antibodies. Blank spaces indicate a lack of sufficient data for generalization about antibody behavior.

Serologic Behavior

In some cases, the antiglobulin phase of testing is positive but this rarely indicates true reactivity at 37 C. Most often, these antiglobulin reactions occur because complement remains attached to the cell surface although the reactive antibody dissociates when the cells are incubated at 37 C. This problem can usually be avoided by warming the serum and cells to 37 C before mixing them, and performing all phases of the antiglobulin test, including centrifugation and washing, strictly at 37 C.

Table 10-12. Amounts of I/i Antigens on Different Human Red Cells

Phenotype	Antigen	
	I	i
I$_{adult}$	Much	Trace
i$_{cord}$	Little	Much
i$_{adult}$	Trace	Much

A clue to the identity of anti-IH may be the observation that antibody screening tests performed on group O cells, show aggtutination, but crossmatches with A$_1$ cells are uniformly negative or only weakly reactive. Cells of group A$_1$, although I +, react poorly with anti-IH because their H antigen is weak. Anti-IH does not react with group O cells from cord blood or from i$_{adult}$ persons because, although the H antigen is present, I is either absent or shows substantially diminished expression.

Anti-I is a common antibody, but usually occurs as a cold agglutinin having a narrow thermal range and a low titer, less than 64 at 4 C. Anti-I assumes pathologic significance in many cases of cold autoimmune hemolytic anemia, in which it behaves as a complement-binding antibody with a high titer and a wide thermal range.

Summary of Reactions

As an aid to the identification of these antibodies, Table 10-12 shows the relative amounts of I and i antigen on different

Table 10-13. Some Examples Illustrating the Serologic Behavior of the I System Antibodies with Saline Red Cell Suspensions

		Anti-I	Anti-i
4 C	I$_{adult}$	4 +	0–1 +
	i$_{cord}$	0–2 +	3 +
	i$_{adult}$	0–1 +	4 +
22 C	I$_{adult}$	2 +	0
	i$_{cord}$	0	2–3 +
	i$_{adult}$	0	3 +

human red cells. Table 10-13 provides examples that are meant to illustrate the serologic behavior of anti-I and anti-i at 4 C and at 22 C. The strengths of reactivity are purely relative. Strong examples of the antibodies may not show these clearcut differences without titration studies at different temperatures.

High-Frequency Antigens

Genetic Considerations

Persons who make alloantibody to a specific blood group antigen necessarily have red cells lacking that antigen. For this reason, antibodies directed at high-frequency antigens are rarely encountered. When they do occur, however, it may be exceedingly difficult to find compatible blood. The patient's family, especially siblings, is usually the most promising source of potential donors. Absence of a high-frequency antigen usually implies homozygosity for the rare gene that determines absence of that antigen. Both parents of the patient are usually heterozygous for this gene, so there is one chance in four that each sibling will, like the patient, be homozygous for the rare gene and negative for the antigen. In the extremely unlikely event that one of the parents is homozygous for the rare gene, the chance for a sibling to be homozygous increases to one in two. Table 10-14 lists some of the antigens of high frequency, defined as occurring in 99.9% or more of the general population.

Serologic Considerations

The antibodies corresponding to these antigens usually react best by the indirect antiglobulin technique, although a few examples of anti-Ge (Gerbich) and most anti-Ve (Vel) may agglutinate saline-suspended cells. Despite its occurrence after known immunizing stimuli, anti-Ve is most commonly of the IgM type and has not been reported to cause hemolytic disease of the newborn. The antibody has, how-

Table 10-14. Antigens of High Frequency Apparently Unrelated to the Principal Blood Group Systems

Augustine (At^a)*	Jacobs (Jr^a)
Cromer (Cr^a)*	Joseph (Jo^a)*
En^a#	Langereis (Lan)
Gerbich (Ge)	Ok^a
Gregory (Gy^a) and Holley (Hy)†	Vel (Ve)

Cells negative for the antigens listed occur with a frequency of less than 1 in 2,000 in the general population.

*The At(a −), Cr(a −) and Jo(a −) phenotypes are found predominantly in blacks.

†Gy^a and Hy are bracketed because Gy(a −) cells occurring in whites are also Hy −, although the Hy − phenotype is otherwise a predominantly black characteristic. The cells of Hy − blacks are only weakly Gy(a +). The Ok(a −) phenotype has so far been reported in only one family, of Japanese origin.[30]

#The En(a −) phenotype is associated with abnormal or absent glycophorin A, the MN sialoglycoprotein, and comes about through several genetic causes. Common to all En(a −) cells is a reduced charge at the cell surface, resulting from lowered sialic acid. Thus, the cells may behave with some antibodies as if enzyme treated.

ever, been implicated in hemolytic transfusion reactions. Anti-Ve binds complement, and in vitro hemolysis of incompatible cells is often seen when testing freshly drawn serum containing this antibody. Reactivity of anti-Ve is usually enhanced by enzymes.

Of the antigens listed in Table 10-14, Gerbich (Ge) and Vel (Ve) merit additional explanation. The Ge − phenotype is clearly heterogeneous, because some antibodies identified as anti-Ge react with some cells described as Ge −. A somewhat similar situation has been reported in the Ve − phenotype, but here the evidence for heterogeneity is less clearcut. It seems likely that distinctions inferred from reactions by different anti-Ve sera could result from quantitative variability in expression of the Ve antigen. Further details are to be found in the reference books listed at the end of this chapter.

Antigens of Comparatively High Frequency Defined by "High-Titer-Low-Avidity" Antibodies

Serologic Behavior

Among the most frustrating problems encountered in testing sera for unexpected antibodies are those created by the so-called *high-titer-low-avidity* (HTLA) antibodies. These reactions are invariably observed in the antiglobulin phase of testing, but they are commonly feeble, variable and sometimes irreproducible. The HTLA antibodies are not always of high titer, but the name derives from observations that feeble reactions seen with undiluted serum often persist in serum subjected to considerable dilution. This suggests that the relatively unconvincing initial reactions reflect either low affinity of the antibodies or weak cellular expression of the antigen, rather than limited antibody concentration. These antibodies, though of debatable clinical significance, react with antigens having a fairly high frequency in the population. When the antibody has been identified, blood can normally be issued without further delay, but tests to determine antibody specificity may cause delay in issuing blood for transfusion. The antigens generally included as defined by high-titer-low-avidity antibodies are listed in Table 10-15, together with their approximate frequencies in the population.

Ch^a and Rg^a

The Chido and Rodgers antigens are part of the C4 molecule of human complement,[31] and are not intrinsic to the red cell membrane. Ch^a and Rg^a seem to reside on the C4d fragment,[32] and many examples of the corresponding antibodies agglutinate saline suspensions of red cells coated heavily with C4. Because C4 is present in human serum, anti-Ch^a (anti-Chido) and anti-Rg^a (anti-Rodgers) are neutralized by serum or plasma from persons positive for

Table 10-15. Blood Group Antigens of Fairly High Frequency that are Defined by High-Titer-Low-Avidity Antibodies

Antigens	Phenotypes	Approximate Frequency %	
		Whites	Blacks
Chido (Ch^a)	Ch(a+)Rg(a+)	95	
and	Ch(a−)Rg(a+)	2	
Rodgers (Rg^a)	Ch(a+)Rg(a−)	3	
	Ch(a−)Rg(a−)	very rare	
Cost-Stirling (Cs^a)	Cs(a+)Yk(a+)	82.5	95.6
and	Cs(a+)Yk(a−)	13.5	3.2
York (Yk^a)	Cs(a−)Yk(a+)	2.1	0.6
	Cs(a−)Yk(a−)	1.9	0.6
Knops-Helgeson (Kn^a)	Kn(a+)McC(a+)	97	95
and	Kn(a+)McC(a−)	2	4
McCoy (McC^a)	Kn(a−)McC(a+)	1	1
	Kn(a−)McC(a−)	rare	rare
John Milton Hagen (JMH)	JMH+	99.9	
	JMH−	0.1	

the relevant antigen, who comprise the majority of the population. Aids in the identification of these antibodies are that they agglutinate C4d-coated red cells in a saline test system and that most randomly selected sera neutralize their reactivity (see Special Methods section, page 456).

The Sd^a Antigen

Sd^a (Sid) is another antigen of fairly high frequency that is widely distributed in mammalian tissues and body fluids.[33] The antigen is variably expressed on the red cells of Sd(a+) individuals and may disappear transiently during pregnancy. The strongest expression of Sd^a has been observed on red cells of the Cad phenotype, which are agglutinated by the *Dolichos biflorus* lectin and by a high proportion of human sera.[34]

Antibody Behavior

Anti-Sd^a is most often detected when antiglobulin tests are examined microscopically, but most examples would be equally demonstrable if the cell button in a saline agglutination test were examined microscopically after resuspension. Mixed-field agglutination is the characteristic reaction, with relatively small, tightly agglutinated clumps of cells present against a background of free cells. These agglutinates are refractile, and often present a shining appearance when viewed microscopically. A single example of anti-Sd^a tested against different red cells often gives agglutination reactions of different strength.

Red Cell and Urine Reactivity

The frequency of Sd(a−) bloods is generally considered to be around 9%, but weak positives are often difficult to distinguish from negatives. Among pregnant women, the incidence of the Sd(a−) phenotype is variously reported to be from 30 to 75%. Urine from guinea pigs and from Sd(a+) humans inhibits the reactivity of anti-Sd^a, but urine from Sd(a−) people is noninhibitory. When populations are screened by urine testing, the true incidence of Sd(a−) appears closer to 4% than to 9%.

The inhibitory substance in guinea pig and in human Sd(a+) urine has been identified as a configuration of the Tamm and Horsfall urinary glycoprotein; the immunodominant sugar is N-acetylgalactosamine.[35] Urine can inhibit agglutination by antibodies other than anti-Sd[a], however, for nonimmunologic reasons such as salt concentration or pH. Urinary inhibition studies may not yield reliable results unless the urine sample is first adjusted for pH and then dialysed against phosphate-buffered saline.[36]

Clinical Significance

Though reported once as causing a hemolytic transfusion reaction,[37] anti-Sd[a] is widely believed to have no clinical significance. However, cells of the rare Sd(a + +) phenotype, or the even rarer Cad cells, may have decreased survival in the circulation of a patient whose serum contains potent anti-Sd[a].

Low-Frequency Antigens

Many low-frequency antigens have been recognized in addition to a growing number that have been assigned to the MNSs system. Table 10-16 lists those that have been studied and shown to be inherited in a straightforward dominant manner. Antibodies specific for these low-frequency characteristics react with so few random bloods that they virtually never cause difficulties in selecting blood for transfusion. These antibodies are of interest to the blood banker, however, because of the relatively high frequency with which they occur, often without an identifiable antigenic stimulus.

Significance of Antibodies

Antibodies to low-frequency antigens are encountered by chance in antibody screening or compatibility testing, when a screening cell or a donor cell selected for crossmatching happens to be positive for the corresponding antigen. Since routine antibody screening tests rarely detect such antibodies, the crossmatch affords the only opportunity to detect an incompatibility,

Table 10-16. Antigens of Very Low Incidence that Appear to be Unrelated to the Principal Blood Group Systems

Ahonen (An[a])	Lewis II (Ls[a])
Batty (By)*	Livesay (Li[a])
Biles (Bi[a])*	Moen (Mo[a])
Bishop (Bp[a])	Orriss (Or[a])
Box (Bx)	Peters (Pt[a])
Chr[a]	Radin (Rd)*
Duch (Dh[a])	Redelberger (Rb[a])
Froese (Fr[a])*	Reid (Re[a])*
Good*	Rosenlund (Rl[a])
Griffiths (Gf)	Swann (Sw[a])
Heibel*	Torkildsen (To[a])
Hey	Traversu (Tr[a])
Hov*	van Vugt (Vg[a])
Hughes (Hg[a])	Waldner (Wd[a])
Hunt (Ht[a])*	Webb (Wb)
Jensen (Je[a])	Wright (Wr[a])*
Jn[a]	Wulfsberg (Wu)

The antigens listed occur with a frequency of 1 in 500 or less in the population.
*Antibodies to these antigens have been noted to arise in response to fetomaternal immunization, and in some cases to have caused hemolytic disease of the newborn.

should a donor blood positive for the appropriate antigen be selected for transfusion. The chance of choosing donor blood positive for that antigen, however, is quite remote.

Antibodies to low-frequency antigens may also be present as unsuspected contaminants in blood grouping sera, and may cause false-positive reactions if the cells tested contain the antigen. Replicate testing with antisera from different manufacturers may not invariably detect this source of error, since the same donor may be the source of antibody-containing serum used by several manufacturers.

Occurrence and Behavior

In some cases, antibodies to low-frequency antigens are seen as saline agglutinins, but they can also occur as IgG antibodies reactive only at the antiglobulin phase of testing, even in persons lacking a history of exposure to red cells. It is not uncommon for many of these antibodies to be present together in a single serum; multiple specificity is especially likely in sera from patients with autoimmune hemolytic anemia. Indeed, whether or not there is clinical evidence of disease, autoantibodies in a serum are frequently accompanied by a mixture of alloantibodies directed at low-frequency antigens. These are usually separable from the autoantibody, and from each other, by absorption using appropriate red cells.

The Bg Antigens

Antibodies directed at certain leukocyte antigens sometimes cause confusing reactions in serological tests with red cells. The so-called *Bg antigens* are expressed to variable degrees on red cells, with the result that reactions of differing strength are observed when a single serum containing "anti-Bg" is tested with different red cells positive for that Bg antigen. Reactivity is most commonly observed in the indirect antiglobulin test, but sufficiently potent anti-Bg sera may cause direct agglutination of red cells with unusually enhanced expression of the Bg antigens.

At least three separate antigens have been recognized, called Bg^a, Bg^b and Bg^c, but confident and precise classification is made difficult by the weak expression of these antigens on some red cells, and by multiple specificity amongst different examples of the "Bg" antibodies. These antibodies may also occur as unsuspected contaminants in blood grouping sera, where they may cause false-positive reactions with cells having unusually strong expression of the corresponding Bg antigen. The red cell antigen Bg^a appears to correspond with the leukocyte antigen HLA-B7; Bg^b with HLA-B17; and Bg^c with HLA-A28. A fourth antibody in some anti-leukocyte sera has been shown to react with the red cells of persons with the leukocyte antigen HLA-A10.

Determinants on Other Cellular Elements of Human Blood

Some red cell antigens are shared with other tissues, while those of the HLA system (see Chapter 11) are present on most human cells other than mature erythrocytes. Certain additional determinants recognized on other cellular elements of human blood deserve at least brief treatment in this chapter, since they may assume clinical significance in recipients who produce antibodies to them.

Granulocyte Antigens

The procedures used to demonstrate antigens on granulocytes are somewhat less straightforward and perhaps less reproducible than those used in red cell testing. Agglutination tests in tube, capillary or microplate tests use heat-inactivated serum in the presence of EDTA. For nonagglutinating antibodies, useful procedures are surface-binding tests utilizing either fluorescein-labeled antiglobulin serum or an enzyme-linked immunoassay (ELISA) procedure as label. Successful in some cases has been a granulocytotoxicity test comparable to lymphocytotoxicity procedures developed for the detection of HLA antigens on lymphocytes. Certain functional assay procedures have also been developed, but these are technically difficult to perform and are beyond the scope of most blood transfusion service laboratories. Details, test procedures and references are given by Thompson and Severson.[38]

Antigens Shared with Erythrocytes

Red cell determinants that have been demonstrated on granulocytes include I/i, U, Jk3, Kx and Ge. With the exception of I and i, which have been detected by leukoagglutination and cytotoxicity methods, all have been demonstrated only by absorption/elution techniques.

Antigens Shared with Lymphocytes and Other Tissues

The HLA antigens exist on most tissue cells. Some may be demonstrated on granulocytes by leukoagglutination with suitable antisera. Sera containing strong and specific lymphocytotoxic antibodies may, however, give negative reactions with granulocytes, even by granulocytotoxicity tests.

Antigens of Mature Granulocytes

In immune neutropenia, leukoagglutination or immunofluorescence techniques have sometimes demonstrated antibodies specific for several determinants present only on mature granulocytes. These include NA_1 and NA_2, which are thought to be reciprocally related; NB_1, product of a second locus; ND_1 and NE_1; 9a; and a series of related antigens called *Human Granulocyte Antigen (HGA)*: HGA-1 and five "allelic" antigens, HGA-3a, -3b, -3c, -3d and -3e, which are sometimes associated with febrile transfusion reactions as well as immune neutropenia. Antibodies directed at the HGA-3 series of antigens are not reactive as agglutinins. Original references to the antigens listed are cited by Thompson and Severson[38]; an additional discussion of neutrophil antigens and their significance is presented by Clay and McCullough.[39]

The antigens 5a and 5b appear to be independent of other systems. They are considered to be products of allelic genes, and antibodies directed at them are usually detected by agglutination methods. Such antibodies occasionally occur in women after pregnancy and may be associated with febrile transfusion reactions.

Platelet Antigens

Platelet antibody testing may be carried out by a variety of test procedures, as summarized by Schiffer,[40] who cites original references for the antigens listed. Testing for platelet antibodies has little benefit for the majority of patients, but may be a useful adjunct to HLA matching in selecting compatible platelets for recipients with alloantibodies directed at platelet antigens.

Besides antigens shared by platelets with other tissue cells, four platelet-specific antigen systems have so far been described.

The Pl^A System comprises two antigens: Pl^{A1} and Pl^{A2}, which have frequencies in the population of 97% and 27%, respectively.

The DUZO System includes only one antigen that has been recognized to date, with a frequency of approximately 22% in the population.

The Ko System includes two antigens, Ko^a and Ko^b, which occur in, respectively, 17% and 99% of the population, and may be detected by an agglutination test with suitable antibodies.

The PlE System includes the antigens Pl^{E1} (99%) and Pl^{E2} (5%), which are usually demonstrated most reliably by a complement fixation test.

References

1. Race RR, Sanger R. Blood groups in man. 6th ed. Oxford: Blackwell Scientific Publications; 1975.

2. Howell ED, Perkins HA. Anti-N-like antibodies in the sera of patients undergoing chronic hemodialysis. Vox Sang 1972;23:291-299.

3. Harrison PB, Jansson K, Kronenberg H, Mahoney JF, Tiller D. Cold agglutinin formation in patients undergoing haemodialysis. A possible relationship to dialyzer reuse. Aust NZ J Med 1975;5:195-197.

4. Dahr W, Lynen R, Gallasch E, Moulds JJ, Uhlenbruck G. Autoantibodies in dialysis patients. In: Roelcke D, Engelfriet CP, Hollander L, eds. Erythrozyten-Autoantikörper induzierte Mechanismen des Erythrozytenabbaus. Molter Heidelberg Symposium 1978:41-48.

5. Contreras M, Green C, Humphreys J, et al. Serology and genetics of an MNSs-associated antigen, Dantu. Vox Sang 1984;46:377-386.

6. Issitt PD, Jerez G. Absorption of unwanted antibodies from sera containing MNS or Duffy group antibodies without the need for selecting "appropriately negative" cells. Transfusion 1955;6:155-159.

7. Case J. The behavior of anti-S antibodies with ficin-treated human red cells. In: Abstracts of volunteer papers. 30th Annual Meeting of the American Association of Blood Banks, Atlanta, 1978 (abstract No. S-17).

8. Ellisor S. Action and application of enzymes in immunohematology. In: Bell CA, ed. A seminar on antigen-antibody reactions revisited. Arlington, VA: American Association of Blood Banks; 1982:133-174.

9. Beattie KM. Perspectives on some usual and unusual ABO phenotypes. In: Bell CA, ed. A seminar on antigens in blood cells and body fluids. Washington, DC: American Association of Blood Banks; 1980:97-149.

10. Levene C, Sela R, Rudolphson Y, Nathan I, Karplus M, Dvilansky A. Hemolytic disease of the newborn due to anti-PP₁Pk (Anti-Tjᵃ). Transfusion 1977;17:569-572.

11. Levine P. Comments on hemolytic disease of the newborn due to anti-PP₁Pk (Anti-Tjᵃ). Transfusion 1977;17:573-578.

12. Gavin J, Daniels GJ, Yamaguchi H, Okubo Y, Seno T. The red cell antigen once called Levay is the antigen Kpᶜ of the Kell blood group system. Vox Sang 1979;36:31-33.

13. Allen FH, Rosenfield RE. Notation for the Kell blood group system. Transfusion 1961;1:305-307.

14. Marsh WL, Oyen R, Nichols ME, Allen FH. Chronic granulomatous disease and the Kell blood groups. Br J Haematol 1975;29:247-262.

15. Brown A, Berger R, Lasko D, et al. The Day phenotype: A "new" variant in the Kell blood group system. Bl Transf Immunohaematol 1982;25:619-627.

16. Branch DR, Petz LD. A new reagent (ZZAP) having multiple applications in immunohematology. Am J Clin Path 1982;78:161-167.

17. Gunson HH, Latham V. An agglutinin in human serum reacting with cells from Le(a-b-) non-secretor individuals. Vox Sang 1972;22:344-353.

18. Potapov MI. Production of immune anti-Lewis sera in goats. Vox Sang 1972;30:211-213.

19. Waheed A, Kennedy MS, Gerhan S. Transfusion significance of Lewis system antibodies: report on a nationwide survey. Transfusion 1981;21:542-545.

20. Issitt PD. Antibodies reactive at 30 C, room temperature and below. In: Clinically significant and insignificant antibodies. Washington, DC: American Association of Blood Banks; 1979:13-28.

21. Mollison PL. Blood transfusion in clinical medicine. 7th ed. Oxford: Blackwell Scientific Publications; 1983:611-613.

22. Archilla MC, Sturgeon P. Leˣ, the spurned antigen of the Lewis blood group system. Vox Sang 1974;26:425-438.

23. Colledge KI, Pezzulich M, Marsh WL. Anti-Fy5, an antibody disclosing a probable association between the Rhesus and Duffy blood groups. Vox Sang 1973;24:193-199.

24. Miller LH, Mason SJ, Dvorak JA, McGinniss MH, Rothman IK. Erythrocyte receptors for *Plasmodium knowlesi* malaria: Duffy blood group determinants. Science 1975;189:561-563.

25. Spencer HC, Miller LH, Collins WE, et al. The Duffy blood group and resistance to *Plasmodium vivax* in Honduras. Am J Trop Med Hyg 1978;27:664-670.

26. Miller LH, Mason J, Clyde DF, McGinniss MH. The resistance factor to *Plasmodium vivax* in blacks: the Duffy blood group FyFy. New Engl J Med 1976;295:302-304.

27. Polley MT, Mollison PL. The role of complement in the detection of blood group antibodies. Special reference to the antiglobulin test. Transfusion 1961;1:9-11.

28. Arcara PC, O'Connor MA, Dimmette RM. A family with three Jk(a-b-) members. (abstract) Transfusion 1969;9:282.

29. Yokoyama M, Eith DT, Bowman M. The first example of auto anti-Xgᵃ. Vox Sang 1967;12:138-139.

30. Morel PA, Hamilton HB. Okᵃ: an erythrocyte antigen of high frequency. Vox Sang 1979;36:182-185.

31. O'Neill GJ, Yang SY, Tegoli J, Berger R, Dupont B. Chido and Rodgers blood groups are antigenically distinct components of human complement C4. Nature 1978;273:668-670.

32. Tilley CA, Romans DG, Crookston MC. Localization of Chido and Rodgers determinants of the C4d fragment of human C4. Nature 1978;276:713-715.

33. Morton JA, Pickles MM, Terry AM. The Sdᵃ blood group antigen in tissues and body fluids. Vox Sang 1970;19:472-482.

34. Cazal P, Monis M, Caubel J, Brives J. Polyagglutinabilité héréditaire dominante: antigène privé (Cad) correspondant à un anticorps public et à une lectine de *Dolichos biflorus*. Rév Franç Transf 1968;11:209-221.

35. Soh CPC, Morgan WTJ, Watkins WM, Donald, ASR. The relationship between the N-acetylgalactosamine content and the blood group Sdᵃ activity of Tamm and Horsfall

urinary glycoprotein. Biochem Biophys Res Comm 1980;93:1132-1139.

36. Judd WJ. Urines for inhibition. Letter to the editor. Transfusion 1983;23:404-405.

37. Peetermans ME, Cole-Dergent J. Haemolytic transfusion reaction due to anti-Sd^a. Vox Sang 1970;18:67-70.

38. Thompson JS, Severson DC. Granulocyte antigens. In: Bell CA, ed. A seminar on antigens in blood cells and body fluids. Washington, DC: American Association of Blood Banks; 1980:151-187.

39. Clay ME, McCullough J. Isoimmune neonatal neutropenia. Immunohematology Check Sample. Chicago: American Society of Clinical Pathologists; 1982: Volume 25, Number 6.

40. Schiffer CA. Clinical importance of anti-platelet antibody testing for the blood bank. In: Bell CA, ed. A seminar in antigens in blood cells and body fluids. Washington, DC: American Association of Blood Banks; 1980:189-208.

11

The HLA System

Introductory Information

The HLA system comprises a group of glycoprotein antigens found on the surface membranes of all nucleated cells of the body, those of solid tissue and most of the circulating blood cells, namely lymphocytes, granulocytes, monocytes and platelets. Mature, nonnucleated red cells lack consistently demonstrable HLA antigens, but immature, nucleated red cells exhibit HLA reactivity. Antigens of the HLA system have been variously designated histocompatibility locus antigens, human leukocyte antigens, transplantation antigens and tissue antigens.

The antigens of the HLA system are second in importance only to the ABO antigens in influencing the survival of transplanted solid organs. Immunologic recognition of differences in HLA antigens is probably the first step in the rejection of transplanted tissue. The antigens of the HLA system are determined by genes present in the major histocompatibility complex (MHC) on the short arm of chromosome 6. Genes at the MHC contribute to recognition of nonself, to coordination of cellular and humoral immunity, to synthesis of several circulating proteins and, quite possibly, to genetic susceptibility to various diseases. HLA antigens are important in tissue and organ transplantation, platelet transfusion, disease associations and parentage testing.

Discovery

Delineation of the HLA system began in the 1950's when several investigators independently described leukoagglutinating antibodies in the sera of patients immunized by blood transfusion[1] or pregnancy.[2] Further studies revealed that these leukoagglutinins defined a series of polymorphic, genetically determined antigens.[3,4] By the early 1960's, an association between human leukoagglutinating antibodies and tissue transplantation was inferred from observations of accelerated skin graft rejection in recipients preimmunized with peripheral blood leukocytes.[5]

Technical Considerations

The agglutinating and complement fixation techniques originally employed led to difficulties in interpretation and reproducibility. In 1964, a microlymphocytotoxicity test was developed that uses lymphocytes and a microdroplet technique.[6] Lymphocytes, with their high surface density of HLA antigens, are well suited to this testing system, and a modified form of the original lymphocytotoxicity test is in common use today. The greater interlaboratory reproducibility achieved by microlymphocytotoxicity testing paved the way for an international WHO Terminology Committee, which was formed in 1967 to standardize the HLA nomenclature. As larger numbers of clearly defined antisera became available and as understanding of the genetics of the system improved, nomenclature has been expanded and systematized. The current classification of HLA antigens is outlined in Table 11-1.

Nomenclature

A number of genetic loci code for the HLA antigens, currently recognized in man as HLA-A, -B, -C, -D, -DR, DQ and DP. Clearly identified antigens are designated by a number following the letter that denotes the series, such as HLA-A1 and HLA-B8. Antigenic specificities not fully confirmed carry the additional letter "w" for "workshop," such as HLA-Bw22. When identification of the antigen becomes more definitive, the WHO Terminology Committee drops the "w" from the designation. The WHO Terminology Committee meets every few years to update the nomenclature by either dropping the "w" designations or by recognizing new specificities or loci. The numerical designations for the HLA-A and HLA-B specificities are not in sequence because numbers were assigned before the existence of two separate series was recognized.

Shared Determinants

Some of the antigens listed at the bottom of Table 11-1 represent broadly inclusive groups, called public specificities, in which more restricted specificities can be identified. For example, HLA-A9 includes HLA-A23 and HLA-A24. These subdivisions are known as "splits." The very broad specificities HLA-Bw4 and HLA-Bw6 include many splits, some of which have, themselves, been subdivided. These shared antigenic determinants on the public specificities contribute to extensive serological crossreactivity, as seen in Table 11-2.

Classification by Testing Technique

The HLA-A, B, C, DR and DQ (formerly called MB or DC) antigens are defined by

serum antibodies, usually in the microlymphocytotoxicity test, and are sometimes called serum-defined (SD) antigens. The HLA-D antigens are detected by a cellular response in which one individual's lymphocytes undergo the enlargement, proliferation, and DNA production described as blastogenesis when exposed to a foreign HLA-D antigen on another individual's lymphocytes in mixed lymphocyte culture (MLC). A test similar to the MLC, in which previously sensitized lymphocytes react to the test cells, is also used to detect the DP system antigens, formerly called SB antigens. These techniques will be discussed later in this chapter.

Recognition of DR

The D related (DR) locus was not defined until the late 1970's,[8] when certain sera, weakly reactive in the microlymphocytotoxicity test, were shown to react only with the B lymphocytes in preparations of peripheral blood lymphocytes. Testing these weakly reactive sera against a relatively pure suspension of B lymphocytes revealed a clear pattern of reactions that defined a set of antigens closely related to antigens of the D series, hence called D-related (DR) antigens. DR antigens are expressed primarily on B lymphocytes, monocytes and other tissue cells, but not on platelets, granulocytes or unstimulated T cells. The clinical significance of the DR system lies mainly in organ transplantation. At its 1984 meeting, the WHO Terminology Committee[9] recognized as additional subsets of products related to D the antigenic system previously called DC or MB[10] and the antigens denoted as SB[11] or PL3. The three D-related subsets are now designated DR, DQ and DP. The antigenic supertypes designated MT2 and MT3[12] have been characterized as operationally supertypic specificities in the DR system, DRw52 and DRw53.

Biochemical Classes

The HLA antigens are sometimes divided into two classes according to biochemical

Table 11-1. Complete Listing of Recognized HLA Specificities as of July, 1984[8]

A	B		C	D	DR	DQ formerly DC or MB	DP formerly SB
A1	B5	Bw4	Cw1	Dw1	DR1	DQw1	DPw1
A2	B7	Bw6	Cw2	Dw2	DR2	DQw2	DPw2
A3	B8		Cw3	Dw3	DR3	DQw3	DPw3
A9	B12		Cw4	Dw4	DR4		DPw4
A10	B13		Cw5	Dw5	DR5		DPw5
A11	B14		Cw6	Dw6	DRw6		DPw6
Aw19	B15		Cw7	Dw7	DR7		
A23 (9)	B16		Cw8	Dw8	DRw8		
A24 (9)	B17			Dw9	DRw9		
A25(10)	B18			Dw10	DRw10		
A26(10)	B21			Dw11(w7)	DRw11(5)		
A28	Bw22			Dw12	DRw12(5)		
A29(w19)	B27			Dw13	DRw13(w6)		
A30(w19)	B35			Dw14	DRw14(w6)		
A31(w19)	B37			Dw15			
A32(w19)	B38(16)			Dw16	DRw52		
Aw33(w19)	B39(16)			Dw17(w7)	DRw53		
Aw34(10)	B40			Dw18(w6)			
Aw36	Bw41			Dw19(w6)			
Aw43	Bw42						
Aw66(10)	B44(12)						
Aw68(28)	B45(12)						
Aw69(28)	Bw46						
	Bw47						
	Bw48						
	B49(21)						
	Bw50(21)						
	B51 (5)						
	Bw52(5)						
	Bw53						
	Bw54(w22)						
	Bw55(w22)						
	Bw56(w22)						
	Bw57(17)						
	Bw58(17)						
	Bw59						
	Bw60(40)						
	Bw61(40)						
	Bw62(15)						
	Bw63(15)						
	Bw64(14)						
	Bw65(14)						
	Bw67						
	Bw70						
	Bw71(w70)						
	Bw72(w70)						
	Bw73						

The listing of broad specificities in parentheses after a narrow specificity, eg, HLA-A23 (9) is optional.

Table 11-1. Continued.

The following is a listing of these specificities which arose as clear-cut splits of other specificities.

Original Broad Specificities	Splits
A9	A23, A24
A10	A25, A26, Aw34, Aw66
Aw19	A29, A30, A31, A32, Aw33
A28	Aw68, Aw69
B5	B51, Bw52
B12	B44, B45
B14	Bw64, Bw65
B15	Bw62, Bw63
B16	B38, B39
B17	Bw57, Bw58
B21	B49, Bw50
Bw22	Bw54, Bw55, Bw56
B40	Bw60, Bw61
Bw70	Bw71, Bw72
DR5	DRw11, DRw12
DRw6	DRw13, DRw14
Dw6	Dw18, Dw19
Dw7	Dw11, Dw17

The following are the generally agreed inclusions of HLA-B specificities into Bw4 and Bw6.

Bw4: B5, B13, B17, B27, B37, B38(16), B44(12), Bw47, B49(21), B51(5), Bw52(5), Bw53, Bw57(17), Bw58(17), Bw59, Bw63(15).

Bw6: B7, B8, B14, B18, Bw22, B35, B39(16), B40, Bw41, Bw42, Bw45(12), Bw46, Bw48, Bw50(21), Bw54(w22), Bw55(w22), Bw56(w22), Bw60(40), Bw61(40), Bw62(15), Bw64(14), Bw65(14), Bw67, Bw70, Bw71(w70), Bw72(w70), Bw73.

The following specificities are generally agreed to be associated with DRw52 and DRw53:

DRw52: DR3, DR5, DRw6, DRw8, DRw11(5), DRw12(5), DRw13(w6), DRw14(w6)
DRw53: DR4, DR7, DRw9

Table 11-2. Known Cross-Reactive Associations of Specificities of HLA-A and -B Alleles

HLA-A Locus	HLA-B Locus
A1, A3, A10, A11, Aw36	B51, Bw52 (B5), Bw62, Bw63 (B15), B18, B35, Bw53
A2, A28	Bw62, Bw63 (B15), Bw67
A23, A24 (A9)	B7, B27, Bw55, Bw56 (Bw22), Bw60, Bw61 (B40), B13, Bw42, Bw47, Bw54
A25, A26, Aw34 (A10)	B8, B14, Bw59
A10, A32	B44, B45 (B12), B49, Bw50 (B21)
A30, A31, Aw33	B38, B39 (B16) B13, Bw60, Bw61 (B40), Bw41, Bw47, Bw48

Table 11-2 was adapted from Miller and Rodey.[7]

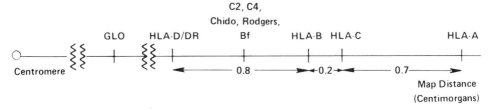

Figure 11-1. The location of the HLA and complement loci on the short arm of chromosome 6.

structure. Class I antigens, HLA-A, -B and -C, have a molecular weight around 56,000 and consist of two chains: a glycoprotein heavy chain and a beta microglobulin light chain.[13] They are found on all body tissue cells except the mature red cell, and are the major targets of rejection following tissue transplantation. Class II antigens, which include HLA-D antigens and those closely related to the HLA-D system (HLA-DR, DQ and DP), have a molecular weight of 63,000 and consist of two dissimilar glycoprotein chains designated α and β.[13] They are located on the cell membranes of B lymphocytes, activated T lymphocytes, monocytes, macrophages, dendritic cells, early hematopoietic cells and some tumor cells. They are apparently important in the initial part of the cellular immune response that recognizes nonself HLA antigens.

Genetics of the HLA Region

The HLA antigens are products of closely linked genes present on the short arm of chromosome 6 (see Fig 11-1) and transmitted en bloc. Each locus has multiple alleles and the traits they determine are codominant. The HLA system constitutes the most polymorphic blood group system

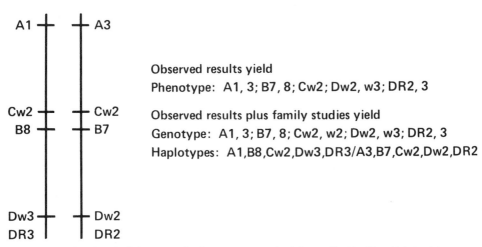

Figure 11-2. The linked alleles on each chromosome are haplotypes. To identify which haplotypes an individual possesses, one must know the antigens present and also the inheritance pattern in the specific kindred.

known in humans. Each individual has two examples of chromosome 6, one from each parent. The genes of the MHC of each chromosome are inherited as a unit, called the *haplotype,* meaning half of the genotype. In the illustration, Fig 11-2, one chromosome contains the haplotype HLA-A1, B8, Cw2, Dw3, DR3; the other haplotype includes HLA-A3, B7, Cw2, Dw2, DR2.

Haplotyes and Genotypes

Each person has two chromosomes containing HLA genes, hence two HLA haplotypes. These determine the observable traits, which can be identified to yield the individual's *phenotype.* The phenotype reflects observation of test results and does not always allow direct inference of the genotype. Some genes determine traits that cannot be detected by the antigen testing system employed. It may not be possible to tell whether an individual is homozygous for a given allele, or whether an unidentified gene is present. Family studies are necessary to determine an individual's complete genetic makeup and, often, to determine which combinations of observed antigens constitute the haplotype units.

Inheritance of Haplotypes

Figure 11-3 illustrates inheritance of haplotypes. Each child receives one chromosome, hence one haplotype, from each parent. Each parent has only two examples of chromosome 6, so in a single mat-

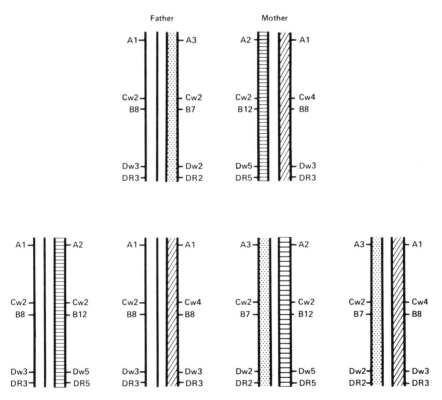

Figure 11-3. Offspring of a single mating pair must have one of only four possible combinations of haplotypes, assuming there has been no crossing over.

Crossing-over, the Exchange of Linked Genes

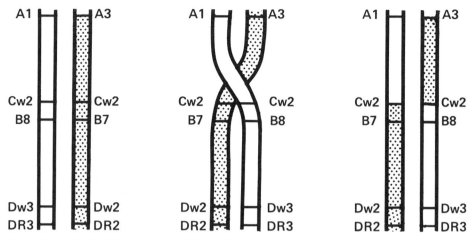

Figure 11-4. New haplotypes are formed if crossing over occurs during meiosis.

ing, only four combinations of haplotypes are possible in the offspring; each child will have one of those four. Two parents having five offspring will have at least two children with an identical HLA type, an important factor in selecting compatible donors for transplantation.

Crossing Over

Figure 11-4 shows an example of chromosome *crossover*, in which segments containing linked genetic material are exchanged between the two chromosomes during germ cell division. These recombinations are then transmitted as new haplotypes to the offspring. Crossover frequency is directly related to the distance between genes. The HLA-A and HLA-B loci, for example, are close together and the crossover rate is only 0.8%. The possibility of recombination must be considered in any family studies.

Linkage Disequilibrium

Alleles of the HLA system exhibit *linkage disequilibrium*, in which certain alleles occur together more often than would be expected by chance. Expected HLA haplotype frequencies may be calculated by multiplying the frequencies for each gene within a population. Certain allele combinations occur with increased frequency in certain racial groups, and constitute common haplotyes in those populations. For example, in Caucasians, the overall frequency of HLA-A1 is 0.15 and that of HLA-B8 is 0.10; therefore, 1.5% (0.15 × 0.10) of all Caucasian HLA haplotypes should contain both HLA-A1 and HLA-B8. The actual frequency of the A1 and B8 combination, however, is 7-8% in the Caucasian population, much higher than the expected 1.5%. This is an example of linkage disequilibrium, with alleles exhibiting nonrandom association. Linkage disequilibrium in the HLA system is important in studies of parentage, because haplotype frequencies in the relevant population make transmission of certain gene combinations more plausible than others.

Techniques for Detection of HLA Antigens

Lymphocytotoxicity

The standard technique used to detect HLA-A, B, C, DR and DQ antigens is the microlymphocytotoxicity test. Lymphocytes are used because a relatively pure suspension can be readily isolated from anticoagulated peripheral blood by the Ficoll-Hypaque centrifugation separation technique.[7] For HLA-DR and DQ typing, the peripheral blood lymphocytes are further manipulated to yield an enriched B cell preparation for testing with suitable reagents. A concentrated suspension of peripheral blood lymphocytes is placed in wells on a microtiter plate. HLA antiserum of known specificity is added to each well. If the lymphocyte possesses the antigen corresponding to the antibody present in the antiserum, the antibody will bind to the cell. Rabbit complement is then added to the wells and, if sufficient antibody is bound to the lymphocyte membrane, complement binds to the system and injures the cell membrane. Cell injury is detected by the dye exclusion test, which exploits the fact that intact cells exclude the macromolecules of vital dyes. Injured cells, however, are penetrated by vital dyes such as eosin-y or trypan blue, and appear as opaque cells of the appropriate color. Uninjured cells exposed to the dye appear colorless and refractile.

Enhancement by Antiglobulin Serum

Many technologists also add an antiglobulin test to the microlymphocytotoxicity test to make the test system more sensitive. Anti-kappa or anti-lambda antibodies will bind to HLA antibodies and may convert some noncytotoxic antibodies to cytotoxic antibodies.[14] Antiglobulin serum, however, produces an increase in cell injury unrelated to antibody specificity. The antiglobulin test is not used in routine antigen typing, but is useful in detecting sub-threshold levels of antibody during crossmatching.

Sources of Serum

HLA grouping sera are obtained from multiparous women exposed to antigen-bearing cells during pregnancy and from multi-transfused patients repeatedly exposed to HLA-containing blood elements. Monoclonal HLA antibodies are currently being developed and may be in wide use in the near future.

Mixed Lymphocyte Culture (MLC) Tests

The HLA-D system is determined by cellular events in mixed lymphocyte culture (MLC) tests, rather than by antibody-mediated lymphocytotoxicity. In the MLC, lymphocytes from two individuals are cultured together, allowing mutual exposure to cell surface antigens that, if not identical, provoke lymphocyte enlargement and proliferation within 5 days. This blast transformation and DNA synthesis is measured by adding tritiated thymidine to the maximally stimulated mixed lymphocyte culture after 5 to 7 days; uptake of the radiolabeled material is proportional to DNA synthesis in the dividing cells. The lymphocyte reaction occurs without preimmunization and mimics a primary immune response. Presumably, the T lymphocytes proliferate in response to foreign D and DR antigens carried on B lymphocytes. In tests for D antigens, cells homozygous for a single D antigen are employed to discriminate the presence or absence of that antigen on the cells under consideration.

Donor-Recipient Testing

In tests to determine compatibility between a recipient and prospective organ donor, the donor cell line is pretreated with mitomycin C or with x-irradiation to prevent proliferation in response to the recipient's antigens. A unilateral reaction thus occurs in which the treated donor cells act only as stimulator and the noninhibited lymphocytes of the recipient respond to foreign antigens present on the stimulating cells.

A test in which one set of cells is inhibited is called a *one-way MLC*, because only one of the cells can respond to a D or DR antigen difference. When DNA synthesis is not inhibited, the test is called a *two-way MLC*, since each set of cells will react to the presence of different D and DR antigens. Kidney transplants from recipient/donor pairs with low reactivity in the two-way MLC have better survival than those showing high reactivity.[15]

Because the MLC takes several days to perform, it is used to select living, related prospective donors, and is not practical for selecting cadaver transplants.

Primed Lymphocyte Typing

Primed lymphocyte typing (PLT) is a faster method for D antigen testing,[12] but it is more expensive and more complex than the routine MLC test. If cells in an MLC are continued in culture for 9 to 14 days, the stimulator cells die and the responder cells, although still viable, cease to proliferate actively. These "primed" responder cells undergo very rapid proliferation if again exposed to the D antigen present on the original stimulating cell. This technique gives results within 24 hours rather than 5-7 days, but the results, although closely associated with HLA-D results, are not identical. The PLT system defines the system of antigens designated DP (formerly SB).

Cell-Mediated Lympholysis in the Cellular Immune Response

The cell-mediated lympholysis (CML) test[16] illuminates another facet of cellular immune function. The CML is used to define cytotoxic T cell ("killer cell") function, in which responding T cells directly kill the target cells. The responder lymphocyte is sensitized by 5 days of culture with a mitomycin-treated stimulator cell having a different D antigen. At the end of this time are added ^{51}Cr-labeled cells from the original stimulator cell line, which have been treated with phytohemagglutinin, an agent that induces blast transfor-

Table 11-3. Differential Effects of Class I and Class II Antigens on MLC and CML

	Cell		Test Results	
	Responder	Stimulator	MLC	CML
1.	$A_1B_1D_1$	+ $A_1B_1D_1$m	−	−
2.	$A_1B_1D_1$	+ $A_2B_2D_2$m	+	+
3.	$A_1B_1D_1$	+ $A_1B_1D_2$m	+	−
4.	$A_1B_1D_1$	+ $A_2B_2D_1$m	−	−

MLC: mixed lymphocyte culture
CML: cell-mediated lympholysis
Class I antigens: HLA-A, -B
Class II antigens: HLA-D
m: cell treated with mitomycin C
+: positive response, −: no response

mation and enhances HLA-D surface expression. Upon contact with these ^{51}Cr-labeled antigenically enhanced cells, the sensitized responder cells attack and kill them by cell-mediated lympholysis, an endpoint detected by release of ^{51}Cr.

CML studies[16] have yielded important information about HLA antigens, mixed lymphocyte culture results, and cytotoxic T cell response, as shown in Table 11-3. Line 1 shows that when cells with identical Class I (HLA-A and HLA-B) and Class II (HLA-D) antigens are mixed, neither MLC nor CML is reactive. Line 2 demonstrates that when both Class I and Class II antigens are different, both MLC and CML testing show a positive response. Line 3 shows that a positive MLC response occurs with a Class II antigenic disparity, but if the cells have the same Class I antigens there is no CML response. Line 4 demonstrates that difference in Class I antigens does not, in and of itself, provoke CML. The cells must also differ in Class II antigens before CML occurs between cells with dissimilar Class I antigens. It appears that the Class II antigen difference produces a positive MLC result before CML takes place, but the target of CML seems to be the Class I and not the Class II antigens. The association of CML reactivity with graft survival is ambiguous, and remains under investigation.

HLA Testing and Transplantation

Transplantation of foreign tissue induces in the recipient both humoral and cellular immune responses which lead to graft rejection. The severity of rejection may be reduced by: 1) close HLA-matching between the graft and the host; 2) giving steroids to decrease the humoral antibody response; and 3) inhibiting the cellular immune response with cyclosporin A, antithymocyte antilymphocyte globulin, or azothioprine.

Antigen Testing

Both host and transplanted tissue are ordinarily tested for ABO, HLA-DR, HLA-B and HLA-A, listed in decreasing order of probable importance. HLA-C testing is sometimes performed. The DQ and DP systems are under evaluation for their usefulness in predicting transplant survival, but there are problems in obtaining reproducible test results for these systems.[17] A positive crossmatch by microlymphocytotoxicity testing indicates preexisting antibodies and contraindicates performing the transplant. Incompatibility between donor and recipient in the ABO, HLA-DR, or HLA-A, -B, -C systems poses the possibility of hyperacute rejection.[13]

Blood Transfusion in Kidney Transplantation

In the early 1970's, many potential kidney recipients were transfused preferentially with frozen red cells to minimize HLA immunization from exposure to white cells and platelets. Interestingly, however, kidney graft survival was poorer in these patients than in patients multiply transfused with whole blood or packed cells.[18] As a result, some investigators[19] deliberately transfused potential kidney trans-

plant patients with nonfrozen transfusion components that contained abundant HLA-reactive material, and observed increased kidney graft survival.

Some current protocols to select living, related kidney donors include transfusing packed red cells from the potential donor in an attempt to induce HLA sensitization.[20] If the recipient produces HLA antibody, transplantation does not occur and both donor and recipient are spared major surgery before determining whether rejection will occur. If the recipient does not produce antibody, the likelihood of success in the subsequent transplantation is high. The mechanism by which blood transfusions enhance kidney graft survival remains an enigma. It is clear that patients differ in their tendency to produce antibodies after antigenic stimulation, and that response to antigens differs widely among individuals. Pretransfusing the patient with donor blood helps determine the antigenicity in the specific donor-recipient pair. Most protocols call for 3 aliquots of approximately 200 ml of blood to be transfused every 2 weeks,[20] with the patient screened for HLA antibodies after each transfusion. A positive crossmatch precludes the transplant because hyperacute rejection is likely to occur. HLA-A and -B typing is important in selecting donors for recipients with preexisting HLA antibodies, but its significance for nonimmunized donors is less apparent.

Red Blood Cell Antigens and Kidney Transplantation

ABO compatibility is probably the most important factor determining the immediate survival of organ and tissue transplants other than bone marrow. Since ABO antigens are expressed in varying amounts on all cells of the body, transplanted ABO-incompatible tissue comes into continuous contact with the recipient's ABO antibodies. For bone marrow transplants, unlike other organ transplants, HLA identity is more important than ABO. Successful

ABO-incompatible bone marrow transplants have been performed after serologic modification of the marrow and are being used more liberally.[21] Other red cell blood groups play no apparent role in transplant survival, except for Lewis (see below). This is probably due, at least in part, to the fact that few other red cell antigens are expressed on cells of solid organs.

Le(a−b−) recipients have had reduced survival of transplanted Le-positive kidneys; it has been suggested that such persons should receive kidneys only from Le(a−b−) donors.[22] Lewis antigens are soluble and present in body fluids as well as on cells. Renal epithelium appears to produce Lewis substance. Many kidney transplant centers now type for Lewis antigens and transplant only kidneys from Le(a−b−) donors to Le(a−b−) recipients.

There is no genetic or phenotypic relationship between the ABO, Rh or Lewis systems and the HLA complex. The red cell antigens in the Bg system are serologically related to certain HLA antigens, and probably represent a weak expression of remnant HLA substance on the red cell.[23,24] Bg^a correlates with HLA-B7; Bg^b correlates with HLA-B17; and Bg^c with HLA-A28.

HLA System and Response to Platelets

As many as 70% of patients receiving repeated transfusion of random-donor platelets become refractory to further random-donor platelet transfusions.[25] The refractory state exists when suitably preserved platelets no longer produce a reasonable platelet increment in the recipient. A lack of platelet increment after platelet transfusion may have an immune basis or be due to sepsis, high fever, disseminated intravascular coagulopathy, hypersplenism, complement-mediated destruction or a combination of these. Immune destruction sometimes correlates with immunization to the HLA system, but antibodies to platelet-specific antigens may also be involved. Single-donor HLA-matched platelets can be of benefit in many of these refractory patients. In one study,[26] which combined HLA typing and crossmatching with matching for platelet-specific antigens, there was a 90% success rate.

Donor Requirements

ABO antigens are, at most, weakly expressed on platelets and HLA-C, -D and -DR are not present on the platelet surface. HLA-A and -B antigens are important in selecting single-donor platelets. To ensure perfect HLA-A and -B matches for all recipients would require a donor pool larger than 10,000. Because some HLA antigens are weakly expressed on platelets, and many antigens exhibit crossreactivity (see Table 11-2), selective mismatching at the A and B locus may also provide a good platelet response. Therefore, a donor pool of about 1500 people[27] can provide sufficient donors for most transfusions. Even if all four HLA-A and HLA-B antigens are matched, 5-30% of patients still have a poor response.[28] This is apparently due to other immunological reactions, possibly involving platelet-specific antibodies.

Typing the Patient

Patients whose diagnosis or therapy makes subsequent thrombocytopenia likely should be HLA typed early, when enough lymphocytes are present in the peripheral blood to type. It is very difficult to get enough cells for HLA typing after intensive chemotherapy makes the patient pancytopenic. It is not usually necessary to begin therapy with HLA-matched platelets, but it is important to have typing data available if it later becomes necessary to select a compatible donor.

HLA and Disease

Many factors determine susceptibility to disease. For some conditions, an association exists between HLA phenotype and occurrence of clinical disease. Several possible mechanisms could link the HLA system with disease, especially those in which immune response to microorganisms is known or suspected to be involved: 1) genes that determine HLA antigens may be linked to genes controlling the immune response; 2) some HLA antigens may be antigenically similar to certain viruses, possibly causing altered response to these viruses; and 3) some HLA antigens may provide a receptor for certain viruses. Statistically significant associations have been noted between HLA antigens and a number of diseases,[29] most notably HLA-B27 with ankylosing spondylitis and Reiter's disease. The use of HLA profiles to identify individuals at risk is theoretical except for: 21-hydroxylase deficiency; idiopathic hemochromatosis; and C2 or C4 deficiency,[30] in which there is a very close association in individual families between transmission of these diseases and transmission of certain HLA haplotypes.

HLA typing is of only limited value in most diseases because the association is incomplete, often giving false negatives and false positives. The association in Caucasians of HLA-B27 and ankylosing spondylitis is instructive. The test is highly sensitive; more than 90% of Caucasian patients with ankylosing spondylitis possess the HLA-B27 antigen. On the other hand, specificity is low; only 20% of individuals with B-27 antigen will develop ankylosing spondylitis. Within affected families, transmission of B-27 antigen cannot be the only criterion for determining transmission of ankylosing spondylitis, since the association is not complete. HLA-B27 typing is most useful in differentiating ankylosing spondylitis from juvenile rheumatoid arthritis.

HLA phenotypes are used in assessing the relative risk of developing certain diseases, based on the cross-product ratio of a 2 × 2 contingency table, as shown in Table 11-4. The relative risk value indicates that a person who is HLA-B27 positive is 103.5 times more likely to develop ankylosing spondylitis than a person who is negative for the antigen.

Parentage Testing

HLA typing is very useful in parentage testing because: 1) the HLA system is highly polymorphic; 2) the antigens are well developed at birth; and 3) no single antigen occurs with a high frequency in any population. HLA typing alone can exclude about 90% of falsely accused males.[31] With the addition of red cell antigen typing, the exclusion rate is 95%, rising to over 98% when red cell enzymes and serum proteins are typed.[31] Statistics on HLA frequencies can be used to calculate the likelihood that a specific individual is, in fact, the parent of a specific child.[32] HLA haplotype frequencies are used in these calculations rather than gene frequencies, because linkage disequilibrium is so common in this genetic system, but gene recombination must be considered when haplotypes are scrutinized. HLA-A and -B are the only two loci usually studied in parentage

Table 11-4. Comparison of Associations of HLA-B27 and Ankylosing Spondylitis

| B27 | Ankylosing Spondylitis | | Totals |
	Yes (patients)	No (controls)	
positive	90 A	10 B	100 A + B
negative	8 C	92 D	100 C + D
Totals	98 A + C	102 B + D	200 N

$$\text{Relative risk (odds ratio)} = \frac{AD}{BC} = \frac{90 \times 92}{10 \times 8}$$

$$= \frac{8280}{80} = 103.5$$

Reproduced with permission from Rodey.[30]

testing because tests for other antigens are expensive and/or difficult to interpret. It is more practical to add tests for red cell antigens, red cell enzymes and serum proteins, than to do a complete HLA profile.

References

1. Dausset J, Nenna A. Presense d'une leucoagglutinine dans le serum d'un cas d'agranulocytose chronique. Compt Rend Soc Bio 1952;146:1539-1541.

2. Payne R, Rolfs MR. Fetomaternal leukocyte incompatibility. J Clin Invest 1958;37:1756-1763.

3. Dausset J. Iso-leuco-anticorps. Acta Haematol 1958;20:156-166.

4. Payne R, Hackel E. Inheritance of human leukocyte antigens. Amer J Hum Genet 1961;13:306-319.

5. Friedman EA, Retan JW, Marshall DC, Henry L, Merrill JP. Accelerated skin graft rejection in humans preimmunized with homologous peripheral leukocytes. J Clin Invest 1961;40:2162-2170.

6. Terasaki PI, Bernoco D, Park MS, Ozturk G, Iwaki Y. Microdroplet testing for HLA-A, -B, -C, and -D antigens, The Philip Levine Award Lecture. Am J Clin Pathol 1978;69:103-120.

7. Miller WV, Rodey G. HLA without tears. Chicago, IL: American Society of Clinical Pathologists; 1981.

8. Bodmer JG, Pickbourne P, Richards S. Ia serology. In: Bodmer WF, Batchelor JR, Bodmer JG, Festenstein H, Morris PH, eds. Histocompatibility testing 1977. Copenhagen: Munksgaard; 1977.

9. Bodmer WF, Albert E, Bodmer JG, et al. Nomenclature for factors of the HLA system, 1984. Hum Immunol 1984;11:117-125.

10. Duquesnoy RJ, Marrari M, Annen K. Identification of an HLA-DR-associated system of B-cell alloantigens. Transplant Proc 1979;11:1757-1760.

11. Shaw S, Pollack MS, Payne SM, Johnson AH. HLA-linked B cell alloantigens of a new segregant series: population and family studies of the SB antigens. Hum Immun 1980;1:177-185.

12. Park MS. Terasaki PI, Nakata S. Aoki D. Supertypic DR groups: MT1, MT2, and MT3. In: Terasaki PI, ed. Histocompatibility testing 1980. Los Angeles, CA: UCLA Tissue Typing Laboratory: 1980.

13. Fuller TC, Rodey GE. Specificity of alloantibodies against antigens of the HLA complex. In: Hackel E, Mallory D, eds. Theoretical aspects of HLA. Arlington, VA: American Association of Blood Banks; 1982.

14. Fuller TC, Phelan D, Gebel HM, Rodey GE. Antigenic specificity of antibody reactive in the antiglobulin-augmented lymphocytotoxicity test. Transplantation 1982;34:24-29.

15. Bach FH, van Rood JJ. The major histocompatibility complex genetics and biology. N Engl J Med 1976;295:806-813,872-878,927-936.

16. Kristensen T, Madsen M, Johnsen HE. Cell-mediated lympholysis. In: Dick HM, Kissmeyer-Nielsen F, eds. Histocompatibility techniques. Amsterdam: Elsevier/North-Holland Biomedical Press; 1979:87-110.

17. Singh G, Griffin M. B-lymphocyte typing (HLA-DR, MT, MB) interlaboratory reproducibility. Am J Clin Pathol 1983;79:569-573.

18. Opelz G, Terasaki PI. Poor kidney-transplant survival in recipients with frozen-blood transfusions or no transfusions. Lancet 1974;2:696-698.

19. van Rood JJ, Balner H, Morris PJ. Blood transfusion and transplantation. Transplantation 1978;26:275-277.

20. Salvatierra O Jr, Vincent F, Amend W, et al. Deliberate donor-specific blood transfusions prior to living related renal transplantation. Ann Surg 1980;192:543-552.

21. Lasky LC, Warkentin PI, Kersey JH, et al. Hemotherapy in patients undergoing blood group incompatible bone marrow transplantation. Transfusion 1983;23:277-285.

22. Oriol R, Opelz G, Chun C, Terasaki PI. The Lewis system and kidney transplantation. Transplantation 1980;29:397-400.

23. Morton JA, Pickles MM, Sutton L. The correlation of the Bg^a blood group with the HL-A7 leucocyte group: demonstration of antigenic sites on red cells and leucocytes. Vox Sang 1969;17:536-547.

24. Morton JA, Pickles MM, Sutton L, Skov F. Identification of further antigens on red cells and lymphocytes. Vox Sang 1971;21:141-153.

25. Silvergleid A. Clinical platelet transfusions. In: Silver H, ed. Blood, blood components and derivatives in transfusion therapy. Washington, DC: American Association of Blood Banks; 1980.

26. Brand A, van Leeuwen A, Eernisse JG, van Rood JJ. Platelet transfusion therapy. Optimal donor selection with a combination of lymphocytotoxicity and platelet fluorescence tests. Blood 1978;51:781-788.

27. Tomasulo PA. Management of the alloim-munized patient with HLA-matched plate-lets. In: Schiffer CA, ed. Platelet physiology and transfusion. Washington, DC: American Association of Blood Banks; 1978.

28. Schiffer CA, Dutcher JP, Hogge DE, Aisner J. Histocompatible platelet transfusion for patients with leukemia. Plasma Therapy and Transfusion Technology 1982;3:273-281.

29. Solheim BG, Ryder LP, Svejgaard A. HLA and disease associations. In: Ferrone S, Solheim BG, eds. HLA typing: methodology and clinical aspects, Volume II. Boca Raton, FL: CRC Press, Inc.; 1982.

30. Rodey G. Overview of HLA. Immunohema-tology Check Sample. Chicago, IL: American Society of Clinical Pathologists; 1983: Volume 26, Number 3.

31. Silver H, ed. Paternity testing. Washington, DC: American Association of Blood Banks; 1978.

32. Silver H, ed. Probability of inclusion in patern-ity testing. Arlington, VA: American Association of Blood Banks; 1982.

12

Pretransfusion Testing

The purpose of pretransfusion testing is to select for each recipient blood products that, when transfused, will have acceptable survival and will not cause clinically significant destruction of the recipient's own red cells. AABB *Standards*[1] states that the following procedures must be part of pretransfusion compatibility testing:

1. Positive identification of recipient and blood sample
2. Review of transfusion service records for results of previous testing on samples from the recipient
3. ABO and Rh grouping tests
4. Selection of blood products of appropriate ABO and Rh groups
5. Antibody detection tests using the recipient's serum or plasma
6. Tests with the recipient's serum or plasma and donor's red cells, ie, the major crossmatch
7. Labeling and issue of the blood products

Tests on donor blood are discussed in Chapter 1.

Transfusion is usually a beneficial and relatively safe procedure. Donor cells or, very rarely, the recipient's cells, do sometimes undergo accelerated destruction. Most hemolytic transfusion reactions result from identification errors,[2,3] but in some cases blood group antibodies exist that were not detected by standard serological techniques.[4] Despite advances in blood group serology, pretransfusion testing will not detect all unexpected red cell antibodies in the recipient's serum or guarantee normal survival of transfused red cells.[5] If performed properly, pretransfusion tests will:

1. Ensure that a patient is issued the designated blood products.
2. Verify in most cases that blood products are ABO-compatible.
3. Detect most of the commonly encountered antibodies in the recipient's serum.
4. Detect most antibodies in the recipient's serum, reactive by the crossmatch procedure used, directed against antigens on the donor's red cells.

Transfusion Request Forms

Blood request forms must contain sufficient information for positive identification of the patient. AABB *Standards* requires that at least the first and last names of the patient and the patient's unique hospital identification number be on the form.[1] Additional information such as sex and age of the patient, diagnosis, previous transfusion history, pregnancy history and the name of the requesting physician may be helpful in resolving problems should they occur. Blood request forms lacking the required information or containing illegible information must not be accepted by laboratory personnel.

195

Transmittals from a computer terminal are acceptable as long as the information is complete. Telephoned requests should be documented by a subsequently submitted completed blood request form. Personnel receiving the telephoned request should, as part of maintaining good records, note the caller's name and time the request is received in addition to the patient's name and identification number.

Blood Sample

Critical to safe transfusion is collecting a properly identified and labeled blood sample from the correct patient for pretransfusion testing. The person who draws the blood sample must positively identify the patient.
1. Compare the information on the request form with the information on the wristband. Do not collect a sample if there is a discrepancy between the two. Do not rely on a bed tag or on charts or records placed on the bed or nearby tables or equipment.

If the patient does not have a wristband:
2. Ask the patient to state his or her full name; never offer a name and ask the patient to confirm that it is correct.
3. Require confirmation of the patient's identity from someone who knows the patient and note on the request form who made the identification.

If the patient's identity is unknown:
4. Use the emergency identification attached to a patient. This emergency identification should be cross-referenced with the patient's name and identification number when they are known.

The phlebotomist should remind the staff that the patient should have a wristband to facilitate identification at the time of transfusion.

Labeling the Sample

The blood sample must be drawn into a stoppered tube. Before the phlebotomist leaves the bedside the tubes must be labeled with the patient's first and last names, identification number and the date.[1] Imprinted labels may be used if the information on the label is identical to that on the wristband and request form. There must be a way to identify the phlebotomist.[1] This can be done by initialing or signing either the tube label or the transfusion request form. Since the request form is a permanent record and the tube is discarded, signing the request form records the information in a more permanent fashion.

Nature of Specimen

It is permissible to collect a blood sample from an infusion line if the patient is receiving intravenous fluids. The tubing should be flushed with saline and the first few (5) ml of blood withdrawn should be discarded because the residual fluid in the line could interfere with serological testing.

Serum or plasma may be used for pretransfusion testing[1]; the same antibodies are present in both. Most blood bank technologists prefer serum because, with plasma, small fibrin clots sometimes form which are occasionally difficult to distinguish from agglutination. Fibrin can be a problem in samples that fail to clot, usually because the patient has been given heparin. In this situation thrombin or protamine sulfate can be added to the sample (see page 417 for procedures.)

Another reason technologists prefer serum is that antibodies demonstrable only through complement activation cannot be detected if plasma is used. Anticoagulants such as EDTA or citrate chelate calcium and prevent complement activation (see page 99 for a discussion of the role of complement in antibody detection).

Hemolyzed samples should not be used. Free hemoglobin in the serum may mask antibody-induced hemolysis. If there is no alternative to using serum that contains hemoglobin (eg, as in specimens from burn patients or those with acute hemolytic anemia) it is helpful to compare the size of the cell button in the tests (patient's serum) with a control (saline or antibody-free serum) to see whether red cells have been lysed.

Age of Specimen

For patients who have, within the preceding 3 months, been pregnant or received transfusions, the sample used for compatibility testing must be no more than 2 days old at the time the transfusion.[1] It is important that the sample used for serological tests reasonably represent the patient's current immunological status. Recent transfusion or pregnancy may stimulate appearance of unexpected antibodies. Since it is not possible to predict when such an antibody will be demonstrable, a 2-day limit has been somewhat arbitrarily selected. Many laboratory directors prefer to set a 2-day limit on all specimens used for pretransfusion testing to avoid problems that might occur because of recordkeeping errors or inaccurate history. If a fresh sample from a patient who has not been recently pregnant or transfused is unavailable, the director may approve the exception.

Specimens from Infants

The requirements for samples from neonatal recipients (less than 4 months old) are different and will be discussed in detail in Chapter 16. Briefly,
1. If there are no unexpected antibodies detected by initial tests and the infant receives no blood products containing clinically significant antibodies, antibody detection and crossmatching tests can be omitted throughout the 4-month neonatal period. The serum or plasma of either the mother or infant may be used for initial testing.
2. After the baby's ABO and Rh groups have been determined, ABO and Rh grouping tests may be omitted, provided the baby receives only red cells that are of the baby's ABO group or group O, and are either the baby's Rh group or Rh-negative.

Confirming Identification

When a sample is received in the laboratory, a qualified member of the staff must confirm that the information on the label and on the transfusion request form are identical. If there is any discrepancy or any doubt about the identity of the patient, a new sample must be obtained.[1] It is unacceptable for anyone to correct an incorrectly labeled sample.

Retaining and Storing Blood Samples

The recipient's blood specimen and a sample of the donor's red cells must be sealed or stoppered and kept at 1 to 6 C for at least 7 days after each transfusion.[1] The sample from the donor may be the remainder of the segment actually used in the crossmatch or a segment removed just before issuing the blood. If the original segment is saved, it must be placed in a sealed or stoppered tube; an intact segment removed before issuing is already sealed. Keeping the patient's and donor's samples makes it possible to do repeat or additional testing if the patient experiences an unfavorable response to the blood transfusion.

Previous Records

Compatibility testing must include checking previous transfusion service records for information on the recipient's past serological history.[1] If the patient has been previously tested, results of current testing must be compared with interpretation of previous testing. Concurrence between previous and current findings gives added assurance (but not proof) that there have been no identification errors and that tests have been correctly performed and interpreted. Discrepancies must be resolved before blood is issued.

Perhaps the most significant information to be gleaned from the records is the existence of clinically significant antibodies. The specificity of previously detected antibodies should be compared with presently detectable antibodies. Even if the current antibody detection test is negative, the antiglobulin phase of the crossmatch is required for such patients.[1] Blood lacking the particular antigen should be selected for transfusion even though red cells possessing the antigen may now be serologically compatible.

Serological Testing

The ABO and Rh groups of the intended recipient must be determined before blood is issued for transfusion. If the patient is to receive Whole Blood, Red Blood Cells or Platelet or Granulocyte Concentrates that contain 5 ml or more of red cells, the recipient's serum must, in addition, be tested for unexpected antibodies and for serological compatibility with the donor's red cells.[1]

Blood Grouping Tests

To determine the ABO group of the recipient, the red cells must be tested with anti-A and anti-B and the serum with A_1 and B red cells. The techniques and interpretation of the results are described on pages 114 and 121 in Chapter 8. Any discrepancy in test results should be resolved before blood is given. If the problem cannot be defined with certainty before transfusion, the patient should receive group O Red Blood Cells, which are safest in an emergency situation. See pages 122–126 for a discussion of ABO grouping problems.

The patient's red cells must be tested with anti-D but routine testing for other Rh antigens is not recommended. Tests with anti-D must be controlled to avoid incorrectly concluding that an Rh-negative individual is Rh-positive. See Chapter 10 for a discussion of Rh-grouping reagents and appropriate control techniques. If there is a problem in interpreting tests for D, the patient should be given Rh-negative blood until the problem is resolved.

It is not necessary to determine whether a recipient's red cells are of the D^u phenotype because no harm results from giving these individuals Rh-negative red cells. In some laboratories the test for the weaker expression of D, the D^u test, is done. Because patients of the D^u phenotype are Rh-positive, and they can receive Rh-positive blood and only rarely make anti-D.[6] Rh-negative blood can then be reserved for recipients whose cells lack the D antigen. Performing the D^u test routinely and then giving Rh-negative blood to patients of the D^u phenotype accomplishes no useful purpose. See page 132 for more discussion of the D^u phenotype.

Antibody Detection Tests
Clinically Significant Antibodies

AABB *Standards* requires that the serum or plasma of a recipient be tested against suspensions of group O red cells from individual donors. The cells are selected to possess the relevant blood group antigens for detection of clinically significant unexpected antibodies. Unexpected antibodies are those other than anti-A or anti-B. It is difficult to define "clinically significant" since the significance may depend on the specific clinical situation and on the condition of the patient. In general terms, an antibody is clinically significant if examples with that specificity are known to have caused a frank transfusion reaction or to have caused unacceptably short survival of transfused red cells. Again in general terms, antibodies that are reactive at 37 C and/or in the antiglobulin test are more likely to be significant than those reactive only at room temperature or below. The antiglobulin phase of testing is therefore required by AABB *Standards*. IgG-coated red cells must be used to detect false negative antiglobulin tests due to inactivation of anti-IgG in the antiglobulin reagent.

Practical Considerations

The antibody detection test, or antibody screen, may be done prior to or simultaneously with testing the patient's serum with donor's red cells. The advantage of doing an antibody screen is potential detection of antibodies that might not be detected in the crossmatch procedure. The reagent red cells used in the procedure (see below) are selected to possess antigens that may be absent from the donor's red cells, and they may possess stronger expression of a given antigen than is present on the donor's red cells. Antibody detection tests may also include additional techniques (eg, a two-stage enzyme technique) that would not be practical for testing a donor's red cells. Including antibody detection tests in the compatibility testing procedure may permit:

1. Detection of very weakly reactive antibodies that may not react with red cell samples from donors. If an antibody is detected and then identified, donor cells can be screened for the presence of antigen with reagent antibodies that usually give stronger reactions than antibodies in the patient's serum. Selecting antigen-negative blood prevents potentially harmful transfusion reactions.

2. Realization that a clinically significant antibody is present in ample time for identification of the antibody and location of compatible units. For example, if a patient has anti-E in his or her serum, 7 of 10 randomly selected donor units would lack E and be serologically compatible; the antibody might not be detected if the only test were crossmatching two units. If additional units were needed in an emergency, a unit of E-positive blood might be selected and given. Finding the antibody at the time of antibody detection tests allows the technologist the opportunity to test the units with reagent anti-E prior to release.

Reagent Red Blood Cells

Group O red cells suitable for antibody screening are available as commercially prepared products and are offered as a set of two or three vials, each containing cells from a single donor, or as a pool of equal volumes of cells from two donors. The pooled cells may be used only for testing serum samples from donors; in testing serum samples from recipients, separate screening cells are required because they provide greater sensitivity. The following antigens must be present on screening cells: D, C, E, c, e, M, N, S, s, P_1, Le^a, Le^b, K, k, Fy^a, Fy^b, Jk^a and Jk^b.[7] There is no requirement that certain other antigens be present (eg, Lu^a, V, C^w, Kp^a, Js^a) or that cells have homozygous expression of antigens of the Kidd, Rh or other systems.

Limitations of the Antibody Detection Test

The antibody screening test cannot detect all antibodies of potential clinical significance. Antibodies reactive with low-incidence antigens are likely to be missed. If the screening cells have heterozygous expression of an antigen, the test will miss antibodies that react only with cells with homozygous expression of a particular antigen. Some clinically significant antibodies, notably in the Rh, Kell, Duffy and Kidd systems, react better, or only, with cells having a double dose of the corresponding antigen; it is therefore desirable that donors of screening cells be apparently homozygous for the genes controlling expression of these antigens. Donors of the appropriate genotypes are in short supply, and it is difficult for manufacturers to provide cells of ideal phenotype if the set includes cells from only two donors. In order to provide cells with a double dose of the significant antigens, it may be necessary to use cells from three donors.

The decision to use cells from three donors rather than two in an antibody screening procedure should be based on circumstances in an individual laboratory. If the antiglobulin phase of the crossmatch is not done routinely, the laboratory director may wish to select screening cells that possess selected low-incidence antigens and stronger expression of some antigens.

Practical Considerations

Commercially prepared reagent red cells are suspended in a preservative solution. When not in use, they should be refrigerated. Aliquots may be washed and resuspended in saline or low ionic strength salt solution (LISS). They should not be stored in these wash solutions beyond the time recommended by the manufacturer because they may be bacterially contaminated when prepared, and in LISS some antigens, Fy^a in particular, deteriorate more rapidly. Reagent red cells may be as many as 7 weeks old at the expiration date. They should not be used for routine tests beyond this date because the strength of some antigens decreases on storage. The loss may be more pronounced on the red cells of some donors than on others.

Crossmatching Tests

Unless the situation is urgent, the recipient's serum or plasma must be tested with the donor's red cells before Whole Blood and Red Blood Cell components are given; ie, a major crossmatch must be done. The sample from the recipient must be as described on page 196, and the donor's red cells must be from an originally attached donor segment. The methods used must include those that will demonstrate ABO incompatibility and detect clinically significant unexpected antibodies and include an antiglobulin test *unless both* of the following conditions are met.

1. No clinically significant antibodies are detected in antibody screening tests.
2. There is no record that a clinically significant antibody has at any time been detected.

When these two requirements are met, the antiglobulin phase of the crossmatch is not required. Rarely is a clinically significant unexpected antibody detected by the antiglobulin phase of the crossmatch when the antibody detection test is negative.[9] The decision to omit the antiglobulin phase of the crossmatch for patients who meet these criteria must be made by the medical director. Some of the points worth considering before making this decision are:

1. The incidence of incompatible crossmatches when antibody detection tests are negative and the reasons for these results in the individual laboratory.
2. The sensitivity of the antibody detection procedure used in the laboratory.
3. The potential benefits of omitting a routine antiglobulin crossmatch in the laboratory, eg, saving technologist time and reagents, and utilizing blood more effectively.

If clinically significant antibodies are detected in the screening procedure, the antiglobulin phase of the crossmatch is required. The tests to demonstrate ABO incompatibility are required at all times. The most important reason to do a crossmatch is to do a final check on ABO blood group compatibility.

It is not necessary to test the recipient's red cells with the donor's serum or plasma, ie, perform a minor crossmatch. Antibody detection tests have already been done on samples from donors whose history indicates the likelihood of having clinically important antibodies. When antibodies are detected in a unit of blood, components are prepared that contain minimal amounts of plasma and the label indicates that the antibody screening test was positive.[1]

The methods used for crossmatching tests may be the same as those used for antibody detection or they may differ. Recommended procedures for both are given on pages 208–210.

Autologous Control

In some laboratories the patient's red cells and serum are tested, as an autologous control, by the same methods used for the crossmatch and antibody detection tests. This procedure is often used to detect antibody coating red cells in the patient's circulation, either his own cells or transfused donor cells. Autoantibody, or alloantibody in the case of a recently transfused patient, may not be free in the serum because it is present in very low concentration and is all bound to the red cells. See page 243 for further discussion. A direct antiglobulin test (DAT) accomplishes the same purpose as the autologous control.

AABB *Standards* does not require that an autologous control or DAT be done. Judd and his coworkers[10] have suggested that including the autologous control or DAT as part of routine pretransfusion testing is of limited value, and that it may be more appropriate to include this procedure only when the patient has been recently transfused.

Selection of Units
ABO Group

Whenever possible, patients should receive blood components of their own ABO group. When this is not possible, blood of alternative ABO groups may be selected. If the component to be transfused contains a large number of red cells, the donor's red cells must be ABO-compatible with the recipient's plasma. For plasma-containing products, there is a possibility of damage to the recipient's red cells. Therefore the recipient's red cells should be compatible with ABO antibodies in the donor's plasma. ABO blood group requirements for components and acceptable alternative ABO groups are summarized in Table 12-1.

Rh Group

Rh-positive blood should be selected for an Rh-positive recipient. Rh-negative blood is acceptable but, except in special circumstances, better reserved for Rh-negative recipients. Rh-negative blood should be selected for Rh-negative recipients to avoid immunizing the recipient to the D antigen. Ocassionally, ABO-compatible Rh-negative blood may not be available. In this situation there should be consultation with the patient's physician, who may prefer postponing transfusion over transfusing Rh-positive blood. However, if transfusion is urgently required, there may be no alternative. The risk of immunization, up to 70–80% in some circumstances,[11] may be less critical than the risk of not transfusing. Depending on the dose of red cells given, it may be appropriate to administer Rh Immune Globulin to a D-negative patient who has received D-positive blood products.[1] See page 291 for further discussion.

Blood Administered After Non-Group-Specific Transfusion

It is often desirable to return to transfusion of group-specific blood after administering blood of an ABO group other than the patient's own. Whether or not ABO group-specific blood can safely be given depends on the presence or absence of anti-A and/or anti-B in current samples of the recipient's blood.[12] When serum from a freshly drawn sample is compatible in the antiglobulin phase with red cells of the patient's original ABO group, group-specific blood may be issued for transfusion. If the crossmatch is incompatible because of ABO antibodies, transfusion should be continued with red cells of the alternative compatible ABO group.

If the change in blood group involved only the Rh system, the change back to Rh group-specific blood is simple since antibodies are not expected to be present in the plasma of either recipient or donor. This situation may, however, be complicated if a patient has received blood of an Rh group other than his own before testing is done. This may make it difficult to determine his correct Rh group. An Rh-negative recipient may, in fact, have been transfused with Rh-positive blood. The recipient's true Rh group can be established only by testing autologous cells from a sample collected prior to transfusion or autologous cells harvested from a recently collected sample.[13] (See pages 419–421 for the procedure.) If there is a question about the recipient's Rh group, it is safer to transfuse Rh-negative blood.

Table 12-1. Selection of Components When ABO-Identical Donors Are Not Available

Component	ABO Group of Recipient	Acceptable Alternative Blood Group of Donors	Rationale[1]
Whole Blood	O, A, B, AB	None	Must be identical to recipient
Red Blood Cells	O	None	Must be compatible with the recipient's plasma
	A	O	
	B	O	
	AB	A, B or O*	
Granulocyte† Concentrate	O	None	‡Contaminating red cells must be compatible with the recipient's plasma
	A	O	
	B	O	
	AB	A, B or O	
Single Donor Plasma, Single Donor Fresh Frozen Plasma	O	A, B or AB	Should be compatible with the recipient's red cells
	A	AB	
	B	AB	
	AB	None	
Platelet Concentrate†	O	A, B or AB	All ABO groups acceptable; components compatible with recipient's red cells preferred
	A	B or AB	
	B	A or AB	
	AB	A, B or AB	
Single Donor Cryoprecipitate	O	O, A, B or AB	All ABO groups acceptable
	A		
	B		
	AB		

*Components of any group are acceptable, but only one of the three should be used for a given recipient if possible. Group A is more abundant than B. Group O components should be reserved for group O recipients.
†Since a large volume of plasma is administered, components compatible with recipient's red cells are preferred.
‡Compatibility of donor's red cells becomes an issue only if component contains 5 ml or more of red cells.

Other Blood Groups

It is not necessary routinely to select units of blood on the basis of other blood groups. However, if the recipient has an unexpected antibody considered to be clinically significant, antigen-negative blood must be selected for transfusion. If the antibody is weakly reactive or no longer demonstrable, it is necessary to use reagent antisera to screen donor units for the required phenotype. If, on the other hand, the antibody reacts well with antigen-positive red cells, a more economical approach is to screen units with the patient's serum, and then use reagent antiserum to confirm that the compatible units lack the antigen in question.

Techniques for Antibody Detection Tests and Crossmatching

There are numerous serological techniques suitable for detection of blood group antibodies. To select blood for a recipient, it is best to use the method(s) that 1) will detect as many clinically significant antibodies as possible; 2) will not detect "nuisance" antibodies; and 3) will allow prompt delivery of blood to the recipient. Greater sensitivity is required in testing recipients' specimens than in testing samples from blood donors and prenatal samples from obstetrical patients. Very low levels of antibody in the plasma of a donor will not harm a recipient and would be most unlikely to cause intrauterine red cell destruction. Detection of very low levels of antibody in a recipient's serum, however, is important because transfusion of antigen-positive red cells may result in rapid production of antibody with subsequent red cell destruction. The same procedure may be used for all categories of specimens, provided it is appropriately sensitive.

The methods selected for antibody detection and crossmatching tests may be the same or they may differ. It may be practical, for example, to use an enzyme technique for antibody detection tests but not for crossmatching tests. Room temperature tests may be preferred to detect ABO incompatibility and thus be appropriate for crossmatching but unnecessary for antibody detection tests. Regardless of the procedures chosen, the antibody detection method must demonstrate clinically significant unexpected antibodies and must include an antiglobulin test. In addition, the crossmatch must demonstrate ABO incompatibility.[1] Several commonly used methods are described below.

General Considerations
Labeling Tubes

Each tube used for serological tests should be labeled, before use, with recipient's initials (or other identifying information) and the donor unit number or reagent red cell identification number. The position of a tube in a rack or centrifuge head should not be used to identify the contents of a tube.

Volume of Serum

Instructions for most serological procedures call for 2 drops of serum. Taswell

and his coworkers[4] have presented data that the volume dispensed in 2 drops is insufficient to provide an optimum ratio of antibody to antigen in some cases; they found some alloantibodies detectable only when the volume of serum was increased to 3 or 4 drops. If antibody is present in low concentration, increasing the serum-to-cell ratio will increase the amount of antibody uptake per cell. See page 231 for further discussion.

Beattie[14] has demonstrated tremendous variability in serum-to-cell ratios resulting from differences in drop size. Drops of serum dispensed from some disposable Pasteur pipettes tend to be small and highly variable, while drops delivered from droppers in reagent vials tend to be large. It is important to standardize the volume of serum and cells used in routine test systems.

Cell Suspension

The red cells used for crossmatching should be obtained from a sealed segment of tubing originally attached to the blood container. The cells should be washed at least once and resuspended to 2–4% in saline or low ionic strength salt solution. Washing the donor's red cells removes plasma and can prevent formation of small fibrin clots.

Since the ratio of serum to cells markedly affects the sensitivity of agglutination tests, it is best to use the weakest cell suspension that can easily be observed for agglutination. Agglutination is dependent on a minimum number of antibody molecules per cell. If too many cells are present in the serum-cell mixture, weak antibodies may be missed because too few antibody molecules are bound to each cell. Although suspensions of 2 to 4% are acceptable, many workers find that the 2% concentration gives the best results.

Reading and Interpretation of Reactions

In serological testing, the hemolysis or agglutination that constitutes the visible endpoint must be described accurately and consistently. Using a light source and optical aid enhances sensitivity and consistency. If both hemolysis and agglutination are possible, the supernatant should be observed for free hemoglobin immediately after centrifugation and then the cells should be gently dispersed to observe for agglutination. The manner in which cells are dislodged from the bottom of the tube affects detection of agglutination. The tube should be held at a sharp angle so that the fluid cuts across the cell button as the tube is gently tilted. When cells no longer adhere to the tube, gentle tilting or shaking should be continued until there is an even suspension of cells or agglutinates. Overshaking may break up large agglutinates or disperse weakly cohesive agglutinates.

The strength of agglutination or degree of hemolysis observed with each cell sample must be recorded as the test is read. All personnel in a laboratory should use the same interpretations and notations and be consistent in grading reactions. Consistency in grading is especially important in antibody identification. A code in common use is given on page 462.

Some laboratories prefer to use a scoring system to indicate reaction strength. An example of one such system is given on page 240. Microscopic observation may be useful in distinguishing rouleaux from true agglutination and detecting specific patterns of agglutination characteristic of some antibodies, eg, mixed-field pattern with anti-Sd[a].

Saline Testing

The simplest serological method is the saline technique. The recipient's serum is mixed with saline-suspended cells. The tube may be centrifuged immediately or incubated at room temperature prior to centrifugation. ABO incompatibilities and antibodies reactive at room temperature (eg, anti-M, anti-P_1, anti-Le[a], etc) are most often detected at this phase. Some workers use saline testing at room temperature for crossmatching to detect ABO incompati-

bility but have deleted it from antibody detection tests to avoid finding antibodies, active only at room temperature, that have no clinical significance.

The serum-cell mixture is usually incubated only at 37 C. Some antibodies directly agglutinate (eg, anti-K, anti-D) or lyse (eg, anti-Le[a], anti-PP_1P^k) antigen-positive cells after incubation at this temperature. Most often, however, antibodies bind to the red cells during incubation but are not demonstrable until the antiglobulin phase of testing. If tests are incubated at both room temperature and 37 C, two sets of tubes are usually prepared. One set is incubated at room temperature; the other set at 37 C to avoid positive antiglobulin reactions due to complement binding by cold agglutinins.

Method

1. Add 2-3 drops of serum to properly labeled tubes.
2. Add 1 drop of 2–4% suspension of red cells (reagent or donor) and mix.
3. Centrifuge for the time and at the speed determined by quality control testing. Observe for hemolysis and agglutination. Grade and record results.
4. Incubate at 37 C for 30 minutes (or 15 minutes at room temperature).
5. Centrifuge; observe for hemolysis and agglutination; record results.

Interpretation

Agglutination or hemolysis is a positive test. Absence of agglutination or hemolysis does not mean, however, that antibody has not bound to the cells. It may be necessary after incubation at 37 C to perform the antiglobulin test to detect these antibodies.

Albumin-Enhanced Agglutination

Since 1945, bovine serum albumin solutions have been used to enhance direct agglutination of red cells by antibodies of the IgG class.[15,16] Albumin can be used as an additive to the serum-cell mixture or can be layered on the cell button.[17] The addition technique given below is more frequently used in the United States, but the layering method is probably the more sensitive method for detecting direct agglutination by Rh antibodies and by occasional examples of anti-Fy[a] and anti-K.[18] (See page 451 for a description of the layering method). Polymerized albumin solutions enhance direct agglutination more effectively than unmodified albumin.[19,20]

In the 1960s, Stroup and MacIlroy[21] and Griffitts and coworkers[22] reported enhanced reactivity of many antibodies when albumin was included in the test system. Some of these antibodies were reactive in the antiglobulin phase after a shorter incubation time than when no albumin was included. These results suggested increased antibody uptake in the presence of albumin. Later it was shown that the effect of albumin itself on the first stage of the reaction is minimal.[23] The increased antibody uptake reported earlier[21,22] may have been a function of the ionic strength of the albumin diluent.[20] The effect of ionic strength on antibody uptake is discussed below. There is still controversy concerning the action of albumin in hemagglutination. For a discussion of the mechanisms involved the reader should see reviews by Steane[24] and Case.[18]

Method

1. Add 2–3 drops of serum to properly labeled tubes.
2. Add 1 drop of 2–4% cell suspension to each tube.
3. Add 22%, 30% or polymerized albumin according to the manufacturer's instructions.
4. Mix and incubate at 37 C for 15–20 minutes.
5. Centrifuge; observe for presence of hemolysis and agglutination; grade and record results.

Interpretation

Agglutination or hemolysis is a positive result.

Low Ionic Strength Salt (LISS) Solutions

Allowing the antigen-antibody reaction to occur in low ionic strength conditions shortens the incubation time required for the detection of most antibodies.[25–28] Enhancement of hemagglutination and of antibody uptake have also been reported.[29] See pages 83–85 for a discussion of physicochemical factors affecting the antigen-antibody reaction. Low ionic strength salt (LISS) solutions can be prepared in the laboratory (see page 424) or can be purchased for use as wash solutions or additives. Procedures for using wash solutions and additives are given below.

Several important factors must be considered when using LISS in serological tests. Adding additional serum to the LISS system increases the ionic strength of the mixture. The shortened incubation period and enhanced sensitivity depend upon strict maintenance of the desired ionic conditions. It is therefore important to adhere to the procedure recommended by the manufacturer or established in the individual laboratory. It may be convenient to prepare LISS-suspended screening cells sufficient for one working day, but these may be used only on the day of preparation. Some antigens may deteriorate after prolonged incubation in LISS.

LISS-Suspended-RBCs Technique

1. Wash red cells once with a LISS solution. Decant supernatant completely.
2. Resuspend red cells to 2–4% in LISS solution.
3. Add 2 drops of serum to a labeled tube.
4. Add 2 drops of LISS-suspended cells. Mix completely.
5. Centrifuge immediately. Examine the supernatant for hemolysis; resuspend the cells and observe for agglutination. Grade and record observed results.
6. Incubate tube 5–15 minutes at 37 C according to manufacturer's directions.
7. Centrifuge and examine the supernatant for hemolysis; resuspend the cells

and observe for agglutination. Grade and record observed results.

LISS Additive Technique

1. Wash red cells at least once with normal saline and resuspend to 2–4% in saline.
2. Add 2 drops of serum to a labeled tube.
3. Add 1 drop of saline-suspended cells.
4. Add 2–4 drops of low ionic medium, depending on manufacturer's directions. Mix completely.

The remainder of the procedure is the same as steps 5–7 given above.

Interpretation

Hemolysis or agglutination is a positive test.

Antiglobulin Test

The antiglobulin technique is required when testing samples from recipients for the presence of unexpected antibodies and for serological compatibility with red cells from donors in some cases (see above). See Chapter 6 for a complete discussion of the antiglobulin test.

Method

1. Incubate serum and cells (using saline, albumin or LISS procedures described above) at 37 C. The optimum incubation time recommended varies according to the reaction medium. A 10-minute incubation is adequate for LISS-suspended cells[29]; 15 minutes is commonly used if albumin is added[21]; 30 minutes may be required to achieve the same level of sensitivity if the saline procedure is used.[22]
2. After centrifugation and examining the reaction mixture for hemolysis and agglutination, resuspend the cells as completely as possible.
3. Fill the tube with saline, centrifuge, decant saline and resuspend the cells. Repeat 2–3 times.
4. Following the final wash, decant all saline. Blot the rim of the tube.

5. To the dry cell button, add the amount of antiglobulin reagent recommended by the manufacturer. Mix thoroughly.
6. Centrifuge, gently resuspend cells and observe for agglutination. Record results.
7. Add 1 drop of IgG-coated cells to all negative tests.[1] Centrifuge and read for agglutination. If the IgG-coated cells are not agglutinated, the test is not valid and must be repeated from the beginning. It is not necessary to add antibody-coated cells to tubes in which the test is positive. See page 96 for discussion of the use of IgG-coated cells.

Interpretation

Agglutination by antiglobulin serum of cells incubated with serum is a positive test.

Antiglobulin Reagent

Either anti-IgG or a polyspecific antiglobulin reagent that contains anti-IgG and anti-C3d may be used for the antiglobulin phase of antibody detection and crossmatching tests. The polyspecific reagent, since it contains anti-C3 activity, will detect those rare antibodies demonstrable only because they activate complement. Many of the antibodies detected by polyspecific but not by anti-IgG reagents have Kidd blood group specificity.[30] Although some antibodies are detected by both polyspecific and anti-IgG reagents, stronger reactions are occasionally obtained with polyspecific antisera.[30,31] Consequently some laboratory workers prefer using polyspecific antiglobulin antisera. See Chapter 6 for more information on the antiglobulin test.

The disadvantage of using antiglobulin reagents that contain anti-complement reactivity is that clinically insignificant "nuisance" antibodies, eg, cold reactive auto-anti-I, are detected. The director of the transfusion service may consider that the benefits of polyspecific reagents in detecting the rare complement-dependent antibodies are outweighed by the amount of time expended resolving problems caused by nuisance antibodies. The decision on which antiglobulin reagent to use is usually based on the incidence of detecting clinically insignificant antibodies and on which other procedures are used. For example, some antibodies reacting best with polyspecific reagent might be expected to react as well or better in an enzyme technique. (See below.)

Enzyme Techniques

Techniques employing proteolytic enzymes to enhance hemagglutination were first described in 1947.[32] Enzyme techniques strengthen the reactions seen with many antibodies, and there are a few blood group antibodies demonstrable only when enzyme techniques are used, notably in the Rh and Kidd systems. The exact mechanism by which enzymes enhance antibody reactivity is not clearly understood. The proposed mechanisms have been recently reviewed by Ellisor.[33]

An enzyme method should never be the only technique used for antibody detection because antigenic determinants such as M, N, S, Fy^a, and Fy^b are usually destroyed, and antibodies recognizing these antigens would not be detected. Enzyme techniques may be used routinely in addition to other methods, and they are helpful additional techniques for use when increased sensitivity is desired, eg, in investigating delayed transfusion reactions when antibody reactivity is not detected by other methods.

Several proteolytic enzymes (papain, bromelain, trypsin, ficin) are suitable for blood bank use. Papain and bromelain are usually added directly to a serum-cell mixture (one-stage technique); papain, ficin and trypsin are used in a two-stage technique to treat the red cells before serum is added. The one-stage technique is less sensitive than the two-stage method because serum proteins serve as substrate in addition to RBC membrane proteins, and there is less modification of the membrane. It is, however, a more convenient procedure. The two-stage method, in addition to being more sensitive, has the additional advantage that the enzyme-modified cells can be tested prior to use to ensure that optimal modification has been achieved (see page 426).

Enzyme solutions and reagent red cells pretreated with enzymes are commercially available. Instructions for the preparation and use of papain and ficin are on pages 425–427. It is important to follow the designated methods for use, either those of the manufacturer or those adopted in the laboratory in which solutions are prepared.

Two-Stage Technique

1. Add 2 drops of serum to a labeled tube.
2. Add 1 drop of a 2–4% suspension of enzyme-pretreated red cells.
3. Mix and incubate at 37 C for 15–30 minutes.
4. Centrifuge. Examine the supernatant for hemolysis; resuspend the cells and observe for agglutination.
5. Perform the antiglobulin test.

Note: Hemolysis or agglutination at any stage of testing constitutes a positive test. Some antibodies directly agglutinate enzyme-treated cells but do not give a positive result in the antiglobulin phase, either because they are of the IgM class or because they elute during washing. These results are particularly common with Rh antibodies. Other antibodies are demonstrable only in the antiglobulin phase of an enzyme-modified procedure.

Low Ionic Polycation Tests

The manual Polybrene® test[34] (MPT) and the low ionic polycation[35] (LIP) test are rapid but sensitive methods to detect most blood group antibodies. The procedures vary (see pages 452–453 for methods) but are based on the same principles. Reagents for the MPT are commercially available.

Method

1. Sensitization. The serum-cell mixture is incubated with a large volume of a low ionic medium for 1 or 5 minutes

at room temperature or 37 C, depending on the specific procedure.

2. Aggregation. Red cells are aggregated (*not* agglutinated) by the addition of polycation, Polybrene® or protamine sulfate. The mixture is centrifuged and the supernatant decanted.

3. Disaggregation. Either citrate or phosphate buffer is added to the button of aggregated cells. Cells free of antibody are easily disaggregated and resuspended when the tubes are gently shaken. Antibody-coated cells, however, remain agglutinated.

4. Antiglobulin test. Tubes can be discarded at this point in testing, or the antiglobulin test can be performed on the cells. Cells are washed 3-4 times with the appropriate solution, and anti-IgG added to the dry cell button. Reagents containing anti-complement activity should not be used because complement may be nonspecifically fixed to the cells during incubation in the low ionic medium.

Interpretation

Hemolysis or agglutination at any stage of testing is a positive test.

Most blood group antibodies are detected after the first stage of testing (disaggregation). Agglutination is frequently stronger at this phase than after the antiglobulin test. With some antibodies the antiglobulin test may even be negative after positive results in the disaggregation phase. Some antibodies are, however, optimally reactive by the antiglobulin technique.

The low ionic polycation tests are very sensitive techniques for detection of most blood group antibodies. Some antibodies, particularly those with Rh specificity, may be demonstrable only by these methods, but antibodies reacting with Kell blood group antigens react less well by these methods than by standard procedures. In general, examples of anti-K, anti-k, etc. react very weakly or not at all at the first stage of testing and are slightly less reactive in the antiglobulin phase than they

are by a saline, albumin or LISS antiglobulin technique.

Suggested Procedure for Routine Antibody Detection Tests

Each of the techniques described above (saline, albumin, LISS, antiglobulin, enzyme, low ionic polycation) is advantageous for demonstrating antibodies with particular serological characteristics. The characteristics of the ABO and Rh antibodies are described in Chapters 9 and

Table 12-2. Acceptable Procedures for Routine Antibody Detection Tests

Method 1

1. Label 2 or 3 tubes (one for each reagent red cell)
2. Add 2 drops of serum to each tube
3. Add 2 drops of 2–4% LISS-suspended reagent red cells to each tube
4. Incubate for 10–15 minutes at 37 C
5. Centrifuge and read
6. Perform the antiglobulin test
7. Add IgG-coated red cells to negative antiglobulin tests

Method 2

1. Label 2 or 3 tubes (one for each reagent red cell)
2. Add 2 drops of serum to each tube
3. Add 1 drop of 2–4% saline-suspended reagent red cells to each tube
4. Incubate for 30 minutes at 37 C
5. Centrifuge and read
6. Perform the antiglobulin test
7. Add IgG-coated red cells to negative antiglobulin tests

Method 3

1. Label 2 or 3 tubes (one for each reagent red cell)
2. Add 2 drops of serum to each tube
3. Add 1 drop of 2–4% saline-suspended reagent red cells to each tube
4. Add 2 or 3 drops of 22% or 30% bovine serum albumin
5. Incubate for 15 minutes at 37 C
6. Centrifuge and read
7. Perform the antiglobulin test
8. Add IgG-coated red cells to negative antiglobulin tests

Table 12-3. One Acceptable Crossmatching Method to Demonstrate ABO Incompatibility and Clinically Significant Antibodies, Including an Antiglobulin Test

1. Label 1 tube for each donor sample to be tested
2. Add 2 drops of serum to each tube
3. Add 2 drops of 2–4 % LISS-suspended donor red cells to each tube
4. Centrifuge immediately and read*
5. Incubate for 10–15 minutes at 37 C
6. Centrifuge and read
7. Perform the antiglobulin test

*Optional step in testing. Trudeau et al[36] have demonstrated that a room temperature crossmatch is unnecessary for detection of ABO errors when LISS-suspended red cells are used.

Table 12-4. Crossmatching Method to Demonstrate ABO Incompatibility*

1. Label 1 tube for each donor sample to be tested
2. Add 2 drops of serum to each tube
3. Add 1 drop of 2–4% saline-suspended red cells to each tube
4. Incubate 5 minutes at room temperature†
5. Centrifuge and read

*Acceptable method if antibody detection tests are negative and if patient has no history of clinically significant antibodies.
†An immediate spin test is acceptable, but the incubation improves sensitivity of the test if the recipient has a weakly reactive anti-A or -B or if the donor's red cells have a weak expression of an antigen, eg, the A antigen on A_2B red cells.

10. Table 10-11 on page 172 summarizes the serological behavior of antibodies of the other major blood groups.

Before deciding upon routine procedures for antibody detection, the blood bank director must decide which antibodies are significant and should be sought in routine testing. It will be necessary to give this decision particularly careful consideration if the antiglobulin phase of the crossmatch is not done routinely for patients whose antibody detection test is negative. Once a procedure has been adopted, the method must be described in the procedure manual and each member of the staff must know and follow the directions as written. Examples of three acceptable antibody detection procedures are given in Table 12-2.

Suggested Procedures for Routine Crossmatching Tests

The methods used to test the recipient's serum with the donor's red cells must demonstrate ABO incompatibility; the crossmatch procedure must demonstrate clinically significant antibodies and must include the antiglobulin test *unless* the prospective recipient has no clinically sig-

nificant antibodies in the antibody detection tests and has no history of having had such antibodies.[1] The methods adopted for use in a laboratory will depend on whether the medical director has chosen to omit the antiglobulin phase of the crossmatch under permissible conditions, and whether or not each patient currently has or in the past had clinically significant antibodies. Both situations are discussed and suggested procedures are given below.

Method of Demonstrating ABO Incompatibility and Clinically Significant Antibodies, Including an Antiglobulin Test

The procedure outlined in Table 12-3 meets the requirements stated in AABB *Standards* in all routine situations. Depending on workload and staffing it may be as convenient and cost-effective to include an antiglobulin test routinely as part of the crossmatch as to omit this phase of testing. The antiglobulin phase of the crossmatch does sometimes uncover clinically significant antibodies in a patient whose antibody screening test is negative, albeit very rarely,[9] and the medical director may prefer to continue this phase of testing. Some of the reasons for incompatible crossmatches and negative antibody detection tests are discussed below in the section on interpretation of results.

Method of Demonstrating ABO Incompatibility

When the crossmatch is performed only to detect an ABO incompatibility between the recipient's serum and donor's red cells, the procedure given in Table 12-4 is acceptable. Since the testing is done at room temperature, alloantibodies other than anti-A, anti-B or anti-A,B may be detected that were not detected in the antibody detection tests. See the section on interpretation for a discussion.

Interpretation of Antibody Screening and Crossmatch Results

Negative Antibody Screen, Compatible Crossmatches

The vast majority of samples tested have a negative antibody screen and the crossmatches with donor's red cells are compatible. These tests are of great value, but, as discussed above, they do not guarantee absence of antibody or normal red cell survival. A negative antibody screen, for example, does not necessarily mean that the serum contains no red cell antibodies, only that there are no antibodies that react with the screening cells by the techniques employed. A compatible crossmatch should be interpreted in a similar fashion.

Additional Testing

If clinical circumstances are suspicious (eg, the patient fails to have the expected rise in hemoglobin) or other laboratory findings warrant additional investigation, the routine testing protocol should be expanded. For example, for patients in whom destruction of transfused cells is suspected, more sensitive techniques such as enzyme, manual Polybrene[34] or low ionic polycation (LIP)[35] methods, may be appropriate for investigating the suspected transfusion reaction; if these tech-

niques are revealing, they should be used to crossmatch additional units, if needed. In some cases, all the antibody may be bound to the transfused cells and an eluate will have to be tested to demonstrate the antibody causing destruction. The DAT may or may not be positive, depending on the concentration of antibody. In other cases in vivo cell survival studies would be required to select compatible units.[5] (See pages 487–488.)

Positive Antibody Screen, Incompatible Crossmatches

Alloantibodies, autoantibodies, problems with reagents (red cells or additives) and rouleaux formation may cause the antibody screen, the crossmatch or both to be positive. If the antibody detection tests are positive, a crossmatch including an antiglobulin test must be done.[1] The procedure given in Table 12-3 is acceptable. Whatever the cause, the problem should be identified prior to issuing blood for transfusion, unless the need for transfusion is urgent. If there is not time to identify the problem and locate serologically compatible blood, a transfusion service physician should advise the patient's physician of the potential risks involved in transfusion in such a case. Often the risk of death due to transfusing incompatible blood may be less than the risk of death due to depriving the patient of oxygen-carrying capacity.[37]

Alloantibodies

When unexpected alloantibodies are present, the antibody screen will usually be positive; crossmatches may or may not be incompatible depending on the frequency(ies) of the particular antigen(s) involved. The autologous control will be negative unless the patient has been recently transfused. When the screen is positive, it is necessary to:
1. Identify the specificity of the antibody(ies), if possible. (See Chapter 13.)
2. Use appropriate reagent antisera to test red cells from units found to be serologically compatible. Alternatively, units

can be screened with reagent antisera first and then crossmatched with the recipient's serum. The decision to screen with recipient's serum or reagent antisera should be based on the strength with which the patient's serum reacts, the volume of serum available from the recipient (eg, is the recipient an adult with bad veins or a neonate) and the availability and cost of the antisera. Testing with reagent antiserum is desirable because the reagent serum frequently reacts more strongly than the patient's serum with donor red cells having weak expression of the antigen. It is not necessary to confirm crossmatch compatibility of units with reagent antisera if the antibodies are not clinically significant, eg, most examples of anti-P_1,[38] anti-Le[a] or -Le[b].[39]

3. Estimate the likelihood of finding compatible blood in available inventory and, if necessary because of the frequency distribution of the antigens, request assistance from the blood supplier or Rare Donor File.

If multiple antibodies are present, if an antibody reacting with a high-incidence antigen is present or if the antibody is present in very low concentration, it may not be possible to identify the antibody(ies) with available resources. If time permits, a sample can be sent to a reference laboratory for additional work. If the only antibody present reacts with a high-incidence antigen, siblings are the most promising source of compatible blood.

Alloantibody, Positive Autologous Control

An alloantibody may cause a positive reaction with autologous control cells in patients who have received blood or components within the preceding 2 to 3 months.

1. Alloantibody in the patient's serum may be reacting with transfused donor cells. Mixed-field agglutination is usually noted because only those cells positive for the antigen react with the antibody.

These results are often found in patients experiencing delayed hemolytic transfusion reactions. The antibody directed against the donor cells may be present in such low concentration in the serum that it can be demonstrated only in an eluate prepared from the antigen-positive cells. See pages 429–433 for discussion of elution techniques. It is often necessary to use sensitive enhancement techniques to demonstrate antibody in the eluate or serum.

Alloantibody reacting with circulating donor cells can be easily misinterpreted as autoantibody. It is important to differentiate the two because selection of blood for transfusion differs in the two situations. In most circumstances it is not necessary to attempt to find donor blood compatible with an autoantibody; with alloantibodies it is important to identify the specificity, and if clinically significant, transfuse blood that lacks the corresponding antigen. The patient's diagnosis and transfusion history may help in making the distinction, as well as the specificity of the antibody. If anti-Fy[a] is eluted from the red cells, for example, it would be most unlikely to be autoantibody. An antibody of apparent anti-e specificity, however, might be either alloantibody or autoantibody.

2. There may have been alloantibody present in transfused plasma products, which may be reacting with the recipient's cells. Depending on the concentration of the antibody and its clinical significance, one might choose to give antigen-negative red cells. If antibody is present in the serum, the antibody screen and crossmatches will probably be positive, and antigen-negative blood would be selected until the antibody is no longer demonstrable.

Cold-Reactive Autoantibodies

Potent cold-reactive autoantibodies may cause problems with ABO and Rh grouping, antibody detection, antibody identification and/or crossmatching. The most common specificity for autoantibody is anti-I, but transfusion of i blood is unnecessary. The most important considerations are accurate determination of the patient's ABO and Rh groups and detection of any alloantibodies are present. A detailed discussion of this problem is found in Chapter 14. Briefly:

1. Obtain red cells free of autoantibody by collecting and maintaining the sample at 37 C until the serum and cells are separated. Wash the cells several times with warm saline. The saline-suspended cells should not agglutinate after centrifugation. If agglutination persists, washing with warm saline may not have adequately removed the cold-reactive antibody from the cells. Treatment with dithiothreitol[40] (DTT) will disperse the cells when the warm wash technique is ineffective. See page 463 for discussion. Use either washed or DTT-treated red cells with controls for blood grouping tests.

2. Obtain serum from a sample that has been allowed to clot at room temperature or in the refrigerator. Some of the autoantibody will be autoabsorbed from the serum.

3. Perform antibody detection and crossmatching tests strictly at 37 C using a prewarmed technique (See Table 12-5). Using an anti-IgG reagent for the antiglobulin test avoids detecting complement activated by cold-reactive antibody.

4. Perform autoabsorption techniques, if needed. This is unnecessary in most cases because using prewarmed testing and/or anti-IgG reagents eliminates most testing problems.

Warm-Reactive Autoantibodies

Warm-reactive autoantibodies rarely cause discrepancies in ABO grouping tests, but commonly cause problems in Rh grouping tests if the reagent anti-D contains a lot of potentiator. Using an anti-D reagent

that contains a minimal amount of potentiator (eg, chemically-modified anti-D) will give valid results in most cases. If autoantibody is present in the serum, antibody screening tests will be positive and crossmatches incompatible. See Chapter 14 for a complete discussion. To select blood for a patient with warm-reactive autoantibodies:

Table 12-5. Prewarmed Technique for Antibody Detection and Crossmatching Tests

1. Label one tube for each reagent and donor red cell sample to be tested.
2. Add 1 drop of 2–4% saline-suspended red cells to each tube. Note: LISS is not recommended because reactivity of cold autoagglutinins may be enhanced.
3. Place the tubes containing the cell suspensions and a separate tube containing a small volume of the recipient's serum in a 37 C incubator; incubate 5–10 minutes.
4. Transfer 2 drops of the prewarmed serum to each tube containing prewarmed red cell suspension. Mix without removing the tubes from the incubator.
5. Incubate at 37 C for 30 minutes.
6. Without removing the tubes from the incubator, fill each tube with prewarmed (37 C) saline. Centrifuge, wash 2 or 3 additional times with 37 C saline.
7. After decanting all saline from the last wash, add the antiglobulin reagent; centrifuge and read.
8. Add IgG-coated red cells to negative antiglobulin tests.

Note: If agglutination occurred after 37 C incubation in the initial tests, it may have been caused either by the cold-reactive autoantibody or a 37 C-reactive agglutinating alloantibody. The prewarmed procedure described above does not allow for the detection of these alloantibodies. To demonstrate these antibodies, testing, including centrifugation, has to be done at 37 C. Alternatively, if time permits, a tube containing prewarmed mixture of serum and cells can incubate at 37 C for 60–120 minutes to allow the cells to settle. The cells can be examined for agglutination by resuspending the cell button without centrifugation.

1. Test serum, autoabsorbed if necessary, for the presence of alloantibodies with screening cells and donor red cells.
2. Prepare an eluate and examine for blood group specificity.

The blood selected for transfusion should, most importantly, be compatible with any alloantibodies present; selecting blood "most compatible" with the autoantibody is a matter of preference. See Chapter 14.

Rouleaux

Rouleaux formation is a property of serum that causes all cells tested to appear agglutinated at room temperature and at 37 C. Because serum is removed by washing, rouleaux formation does not affect the antiglobulin test. Classically, the flat surfaces of the cells adhere to each other, giving "coin-like" stacks that are easily recognized. Rouleaux activity is harder to identify when the cells adhere in irregular clumps that resemble agglutination. To disperse rouleaux, two techniques are useful:

1. Add 1–3 drops of saline to the tube. Rouleaux tend to disperse, but antibody-mediated agglutination remains.
2. Use the saline replacement technique as described on page 452, if rouleaux persist despite addition of saline.

Reagent-Related Problems

Antibodies to a variety of drugs and additives can cause positive results in antibody screening and/or compatibility tests. When all the reagent red cells are positive and all the donor red cells are compatible, an antibody reactive with a substance in the red cell preservative solution should be suspected. In some cases the reagent red cells will not react if they are washed with normal saline before testing and testing can be completed with this minor modification. Since preservative solutions vary from manufacturer to manufacturer, it may be helpful to use cells from another manufacturer if washing does not solve the problem.

With some reagent-related problems, all tests that employ the reagent will be positive. For example, agglutination in all tubes that contain serum, cells and reagent albumin suggests an antibody against sodium caprylate. Some patients have antibody against this compound, which is used as a stabilizer in reagent albumin. To resolve crossmatch problems associated with antibody to sodium caprylate use one of the following approaches:

1. Omit albumin from screening test and crossmatch and prolong incubation at 37 C to at least 30 minutes.
2. Use an albumin reagent that does not contain sodium caprylate.
3. Use a LISS technique for antibody screening and crossmatch.

An antibody to a constituent of some LISS solutions, eg, thimerosal, has also been described. Again, all crossmatches and tests with reagent red cells and autologous cells will be positive. Using a procedure that does not include LISS will circumvent the problem. See the review by Pierce[41] for more information.

Negative Antibody Screen, Incompatible Crossmatch(es)

Some positive reactions occurring in the crossmatch but not the antibody screen may be due to clinically significant antibodies.[9,42] Therefore the cause should be investigated. Depending on the phase of testing in which the incompatibility was detected, it may be necessary to do one or more of the following tests:

1. Repeat ABO grouping tests on the donor's sample.
2. Perform a direct antiglobulin test on the donor's red cells.
3. Test the patient's serum with a panel of reagent red cells or other selected red cells.

Crossmatch(es) Incompatible at Room Temperature

In the following situations the antibody screen may be negative but one (or more) of the crossmatches is (are) incompatible at room temperature.

1. Donor red cells are ABO incompatible: In this situation the first thing to do is confirm the donor's ABO group. Labeling errors are more likely to cause this problem than technical errors. Most ABO antibodies present in a recipient's serum react strongly at room temperature and also at 37 C or in the antiglobulin test with most mislabeled A, B or AB red cells. Rarely, a unit of blood from a donor whose red cells have a weak expression of A or B antigens (eg, A_x) are incorrectly labeled as group O. In this case, the crossmatch with group O serum may be weakly incompatible only at the antiglobulin phase.

2. Anti-A_1 in the serum of A_2 or A_2B individuals: If room temperature testing is done, anti-A_1 will be commonly encountered. Some, but not all, group A donor units may be incompatible. If the antibody reacts only at room temperature, it is not considered clinically significant, but if it is reactive at 37 C, blood lacking the A_1 antigen should be given.[43]

3. Other alloantibodies reactive at room temperature: If the antibody detection test does not include a room temperature phase, antibodies such as anti-M may first be detected by a room temperature crossmatch. Performing antibody detection and identification tests at room temperature and then testing the donor red cells for the corresponding antigen usually resolves the problem.

4. Polyagglutinable red cells: All normal adult sera contain varying levels of antibodies (eg, anti-T, anti-Tn, anti-Tk, anti-Cad) that recognize and agglutinate red cells with altered surface reactivity that renders them polyagglutinable. These antibodies are rarely a problem because most red cells do not manifest the corresponding antigens. Polyagglutinable cells, however, react with these antibodies either because they

have acquired antigenic reactivity (T, Tn, T^k) or, more rarely, because the donor has inherited such an antigen.

Polyagglutinable donor red cells may first be detected in the crossmatch. The problem might appear to result from an antibody to a low-frequency antigen because the recipient's serum is nonreactive with antibody screening cells, panel cells and all other donors' red cells. The antibodies that recognize polyagglutinable red cells are direct agglutinins that react best at room temperature so it is most common to see reactivity in the immediate spin or room temperature phase of the crossmatch. Rabbit sera contain anti-T, anti-Tn and others,[44] so these altered cells may react with antiglobulin reagents and the crossmatch may be incompatible at the antiglobulin phase.

Polyagglutinability often results from the action of bacterial enzymes. Cells from a healthy donor virtually never have this form of activation in vivo. In vitro activation is now very rare, because using sealed segments for compatibility testing eliminates the kind of contamination that sometimes affected stored pilot tubes. The other forms of polyagglutinability (eg, Tn, Cad) occur as often among donors as among patients, but all these forms of polyagglutination are also very rare.

See page 428 for a description of a procedure to recognize polyagglutinable red cells. For more information the reader should see the AABB workshop manual edited by Beck and Judd.[45]

Crossmatch(es) Incompatible at the Antiglobulin Phase

If an antiglobulin test is part of the crossmatch procedure, some of the following situations may be encountered.

1. Donor red cells have a positive DAT: Acceptable donors occasionally have red cells that are coated with IgG and/or complement and cause incompatibility

in the antiglobulin phase of the cross-match. These units are not identified during processing since a direct anti-globulin test (DAT) is not performed routinely. The problem can be quickly and easily identified by performing a DAT on the cells. Since the unit will be incompatible with the serum of all recipients, it is usually discarded.

2. Antibody reactive only with cells having strong expression of a particular antigen: A random donor's red cells may have stronger expression of a particular antigen than do the screening cells, either because of dosage, (eg, Rh, Kidd, Duffy antigens) or because of intrinsic variation in strength (eg, P_1). If the patient's serum contains an antibody that reacts only with cells having strong expression of the antigen, the crossmatch may be positive and the antibody screen may be negative. The antibody can usually be identified by testing a full panel of red cells since some of the panel cells are likely to have a double dose or strong expression of the antigen in question. It may be necessary, however, to use a more sensitive technique for identification.

3. Antibody reactive with low-frequency antigen: Antibodies to some of the low-incidence antigens are relatively common as non-red-cell-stimulated antibodies. Anti-Wr^a, for example, may be present in as many as 1% of sera.[46] Low-incidence antigens may be present, unsuspected and unidentified, on either antibody detection cells or donor cells, causing unexpected positive reactions with sera containing these antibodies.

Positive Antibody Screen, Compatible Crossmatches

If all reagent red cells are positive but many or all of the crossmatches are compatible, antibodies of one of the following specificities may be responsible:

Anti-H

Group O cells have large amounts of H antigen; A_1 and A_1B cells have very little H. Serum containing anti-H will agglutinate all group O reagent red cells, but will not agglutinate A_1 and A_1B donor cells. Since A_2 cells have substantial amounts of H, a crossmatch with A_2 cells may be incompatible. Anti-H does occur in the serum of group B people, but less often than in A_1 and A_1B. Anti-H found in A_1, A_1B and B sera is usually reactive only at room temperature and is not clinically significant. The anti-H in the serum of an O_h person is significant; the prospective recipient would appear to be group O, but antibody screening cells and all group O donor cells would be strongly agglutinated.

Anti-Le^{bH}

This antibody reacts with Le(b+) cells that are group O, but not with A_1 or A_1B cells that are Le(b+). It is most often made by group A_1 or A_1B individuals. Anti-Le^{bH} is often reactive at room temperature but may be detected in the antiglobulin phase if the anti-human serum contains anti-complement reactivity. It is not necessary to screen compatible A_1 or A_1B donor units for Le^b.

Antibodies to Constituents of Reagents

Antibodies to drugs and additives can cause positive results with prepared reagent cells but be nonreactive with donor cells suspended in a different medium.

Autologous Control

An autologous control, consisting of the recipient's red cells and recipient's serum tested in parallel with the antibody screening test and crossmatches, often gives useful information. As discussed in preceding sections, it will be positive if:

1. The patient's red cells have a positive direct antiglobulin test caused by autoantibody or, in the case of a delayed

hemolytic transfusion reaction, alloantibody.

2. The patient's serum causes all cells to rouleaux.
3. The patient's serum has an antibody to an additive in the potentiating medium or saline.

There is no requirement that an autologous control be routinely performed, but as discussed in Chapter 13, the procedure should be part of antibody identification tests.[2]

Massive Transfusion

Massive transfusion is defined as infusion, within a 24-hour interval, of a volume of blood approaching or exceeding replacement of the recipient's total blood volume.[1] This may occur unexpectedly in surgical and medical emergencies and/or in planned circumstances such as cardiac and vascular surgery. Exchange transfusion of an infant is also a massive transfusion.

Following massive transfusion, there is so little of the patient's blood left that complete crossmatching has little benefit. The pretransfusion sample no longer represents currently circulating transfused blood, and sensitive antiglobulin testing on the current specimen accomplishes virtually nothing.[47] It is only important to confirm ABO compatibility of subsequently transfused blood. This may be accomplished by either:

1. Performing the room temperature crossmatch
2. Confirming the donor's ABO group by testing the cells with reagent anti-A and anti-B blood grouping sera

With the recent change in *Standards*,[1] performing only an immediate spin crossmatch is acceptable in many situations in addition to massive transfusions.

If unexpected alloantibody was present in the patient's pretransfusion sample, abbreviating the crossmatch is acceptable following massive transfusion. Donor blood shown by testing with reagent serum to lack the corresponding antigens may be transfused after testing only for ABO compatibility.

The procedures to use in these situations should be selected by the blood bank physician, should be in writing, and should be followed consistently by all laboratory personnel.

Labeling and Release of Blood

A blood transfusion form indicating the recipient's name, identification number and ABO and Rh groups must be completed for each unit of donor blood or component.[1] The form must also include: 1) donor identification number, 2) donor ABO and Rh groups, 3) interpretation of crossmatching testing and 4) identification of the person performing the crossmatch tests. When blood must be issued before compatibility problems are resolved, the status of the serologic findings must be indicated on the blood transfusion form.[1]

Prior to issuing a unit of blood, blood bank personnel must:

1. Securely attach to the unit of blood a label or tag that contains:
   a. the recipient's first and last names and identification number
   b. the donor blood number assigned by the transfusing or collecting facility
   c. interpretation of the crossmatch tests and identification of the person performing the crossmatch tests
2. Check the blood expiration date to avoid issuing an outdated unit.
3. Inspect the unit to make certain it does not have abnormal color or appearance.
4. Indicate on an appropriate form:
   a. name of the individual issuing blood
   b. date and time blood was issued
   c. the person to whom blood was issued

Final identification of the recipient and the blood container rests with the transfusionist, who must identify the patient and donor unit and certify that identifying forms, tags and labels are in agreement. See pages 285–287 for procedures to be followed.

Release of Blood in Urgent Situations

When there is a desperate requirement for blood, the patient's physician must weigh the hazard of transfusing uncrossmatched or partially crossmatched blood against the risk of waiting while testing is completed. When blood is released before the crossmatch is completed, the records must contain a statement of the requesting physician indicating that the clinical situation was sufficiently urgent to require release of blood.[1] Such a statement does not absolve the blood bank from its responsibility to issue properly labeled donor blood of an ABO group compatible with the patient. When urgent release is requested:

1. Issue uncrossmatched blood, if necessary, and immediately begin compatibility testing procedures. Blood released should be:
   a. ABO- and Rh-group compatible, if there has been time to perform ABO and Rh testing on the patient's current blood specimen. Previous records must not be used to determine which blood group to issue, nor may the patient's blood group be taken from other records such as cards, dog tags or driver's license.
   b. Group O Red Blood Cells, if the patient's ABO group is unknown. It is preferable to give D-negative blood if the patient's Rh group is unknown, especially if the patient is a young woman.
   c. Group A or B Red Blood Cells for group AB recipients if group AB donor blood is unavailable.
2. Indicate in a conspicuous fashion on the attached tag or label that compatibility testing had not been completed at the time of issue.

3. Complete compatibility tests promptly. If incompatibility is detected at any stage of testing, immediately notify the patient's physician and blood bank physician.

If the patient dies from a medical problem unrelated to the blood transfusion, it is not necessary to complete pending compatibility tests. This decision rests with the physician responsible for the transfusion service. If there is any reason to suspect that transfusion aggravated the original problem or contributed to death, all testing should be completed.

Effective Blood Utilization

Increasing blood demands and limited blood resources have made blood bankers increasingly conscious of the need to use blood efficiently. In many operating rooms it has been standard practice to have blood crossmatched and reserved for every individual patient as a "standby" precaution. Since most of these units were not used, the crossmatches and the expanded inventory needed to meet these demands were wasted resources. Keeping blood reserved for a patient unlikely to use it makes the blood unavailable for a patient whose need is immediate and makes it more likely that the blood will outdate without being transfused. Reducing the number of unnecessary crossmatches reduces outdating and also leads to efficient use of technologists' time, decreased requirements for reagents and disposable glassware and decreased costs of crossmatching.

Elective operations are those for which most unnecessary crossmatches are done.[48,49] Transfusion service directors, in conjunction with the appropriate clinicians, should analyze their records of crossmatches and transfusions to see if improvement can be achieved. Two useful approaches are: 1) to establish realistic ordering levels for procedures that nearly always require blood, and 2) to provide a reliable emergency reserve system for procedures that rarely require blood.[48,49]

Standard Surgical Blood Orders

Blood ordering levels for common elective procedures can be developed from previous records of blood use. For each of the procedures designated, the transfusion service can crossmatch the agreed-upon standard number of blood units.[48]

Since surgical requirements vary among institutions, the standard blood orders should be based on local transfusion utilization patterns. The blood bank medical director, staff surgeons and anesthesiologists should agree on standard ordering levels, but there must be a way to modify the standard orders for patients with anemia, bleeding disorders or other conditions in which increased blood use is anticipated. As with other circumstances that require rapid provision of blood, the transfusion service staff must be prepared to provide additional blood if an unexpected problem requires blood use greater than the standard level. Standard blood order schedules are successful only when there is cooperation and confidence among the professionals involved in setting and using the guidelines.

Group and Screen

"Group and screen" (or "type and screen" or "type, screen and hold") is a shorthand notation for a policy in which crossmatched blood is not set aside for those patients undergoing surgical procedures that rarely require transfusion. Instead, the patient's blood sample is completely tested for ABO and Rh groups and unexpected antibodies and is kept in the blood bank for immediate crossmatching, should this prove necessary. For procedures like cholecystectomy, hysterectomy, thyroidectomy and others, blood is so seldom needed that specific preoperative crossmatching is inappropriate.[1] The blood bank must have appropriate donor blood available for all patients undergoing operations on a "group and screen" basis.

If transfusion becomes necessary, uncrossmatched ABO- and Rh-compatible blood can be released with 99.9% assurance of safety,[49] as long as the patient has no unexpected antibodies. A crossmatch to demonstrate ABO incompatibility can be completed prior to actual infusion of the product in most cases. If the patient does have blood group alloantibodies, donor blood known to lack the corresponding antigens must be available. In some institutions blood is crossmatched prior to surgery if alloantibodies are present.

References

1. Schmidt PJ, ed. Standards for blood banks and transfusion services. 11th ed. Arlington, VA: American Association of Blood Banks, 1984.

2. Honig CL, Bove JR. Transfusion-associated fatalities: review of Bureau of Biologics reports 1976–8. Transfusion 1980;20:653–661.

3. Schmidt PJ. The mortality from incompatible transfusion. In: Sandler SG, Nusbacher J, Schanfield MS, eds. Immunobiology of the erythrocyte. New York: Alan R Liss, 1980:251–261.

4. Taswell HF, Pineda AA, Moore SB. Hemolytic transfusion reactions: frequency and clinical and laboratory aspects. In: Bell CA, ed. A seminar on immune-mediated cell destruction. Washington, DC: American Association of Blood Banks, 1981:71–92.

5. Baldwin ML, Barrasso C, Ness PM, Garratty G. A clinically significant erythrocyte antibody detectable only by ^{51}Cr survival studies. Transfusion 1983;23:40–44.

6. Issitt PD. Serology and genetics of the Rhesus blood group system. Cincinnati: Montgomery Scientific Publications, 1979:34.

7. Code of federal regulations. Title 21, vol 6, parts 660.6-660.36. Washington, DC: US Govt Printing Office, 1981.

8. Ellisor SS. The selection of reagent red cells and antibody potentiating reagents. In: Considerations in the selection of reagents. Washington DC: American Association of Blood Banks, 1979:83–91.

9. Oberman HA, Barnes BA, Steiner EA. Role of the crossmatch in testing for serologic compatibility. Transfusion 1982;22:12–16.

10. Judd WJ, Butch SH, Oberman HA, Steiner EA, Bauer RC. The evaluation of a positive

direct antiglobulin test in pretransfusion testing. Transfusion 1980;20:17–23.

11. Pollack W, Ascari WQ, Crispen JF, O'Connor RR, Ho TY. Studies on Rh prophylaxis. II: Rh immune prophylaxis after transfusion with Rh positive blood. Transfusion 1971;11:340–344.

12. Barnes A Jr, Allen TE. Transfusions subsequent to administration of universal donor blood in Viet Nam. JAMA 1968;204:695–697.

13. Wallas CH, Tanley PC, Gorrell LP. Recovery of autologous erythrocytes in transfused patients. Transfusion 1980;20:332–336.

14. Beattie K. Control of the antigen-antibody ratio in antibody detection/compatibility tests. Transfusion 1980;20:277–284.

15. Diamond LK, Denton RL. Rh agglutination in various media with particular reference to the value of albumin. J Lab Clin Med 1945;30:821–830.

16. Cameron JW, Diamond LK. Chemical, clinical and immunological studies of the products of human plasma fractionation. XXIX: Serum albumin as a diluent for Rh typing reagents. J Clin Invest 1945;24:793–801.

17. Case J. The albumin layering method for D typing. Vox Sang 1959;4:403–405.

18. Case J. Potentiators of agglutination. In: Bell CA, ed. Seminar on antigen-antibody reactions revisited. Arlington, VA: American Association of Blood Banks 1982:99–132.

19. Jones JM, Kekwick RA, Goldsmith KLG. Influence of polymers on the efficacy of serum albumin as a potentiator of "incomplete" Rh agglutinins. Nature (London) 1969;224:510–511.

20. Reckel RP, Harris J. The unique characteristics of covalently polymerized bovine serum albumin solutions when used as antibody detection media. Transfusion 1978;18:397–406.

21. Stroup M, MacIlroy M. Evaluation of the albumin antiglobulin technic in antibody detection. Transfusion 1965;5:184–191.

22. Griffitts JJ, Frank S, Schmidt, P. The influence of albumin in the antiglobulin crossmatch. Transfusion 1964;4:461–468.

23. Leikola J, Perkins HA. Red cell antibodies and low ionic strength: a study with enzyme-linked antiglobulin test. Transfusion 1980;20:224–228.

24. Steane EA. Red blood cell hemagglutination: a current perspective. In: Bell CA, ed. Seminar on antigen-antibody reactions revisited. Arlington, VA: American Association of Blood Banks 1982:67–98.

25. Elliot M, Bossom E, Dupuy ME, Masouredis SP. Effect of ionic strength on the serologic behavior of red cell isoantibodies. Vox Sang 1964;9:396–414.

26. Hughes-Jones NC, Polley MJ, Telford R, Gardner B, Klein-Schmidt G. Optimal conditions for detecting blood group antibodies by the antiglobulin test. Vox Sang 1964;9:385–395.

27. Löw B, Messeter L. Antiglobulin tests in low-ionic strength salt solutions for rapid antibody screening and crossmatching. Vox Sang 1974;26:53–61.

28. Moore HC, Mollison PL. Use of a low-ionic strength medium in manual tests for antibody detection. Transfusion 1976;16:291–296.

29. Fitzsimmons JM, Morel PA. The effects of red blood cell suspending media on hemagglutination and the antiglobulin reaction. Transfusion 1979;19:81–85.

30. Howard JE, Winn LC, Gottlieb CE, Grumet FC, Garratty G, Petz LD. Clinical significance of the anti-complement component of antiglobulin antisera. Transfusion 1982;22:269-272.

31. Wright MS, Issitt PD. Anticomplement and the antiglobulin test. Transfusion 1979;19:688–694.

32. Morton JA, Pickles MM. Use of trypsin in detection of anti-Rh antibodies. Nature 1947;159:779–780.

33. Ellisor SS. Action and applications of enzymes in immunohematology. In: Bell CA, ed. Seminar on antigen-antibody reactions revisited. Arlington, VA: American Association of Blood Banks, 1982:133–174.

34. Lalezari P, Jiang AF. The manual Polybrene test: a simple and rapid procedure for detection of red cell antibodies. Transfusion 1980;20:206–211.

35. Rosenfield RE, Shaikh SH, Innella F, Kaczera Z, Kochwa S. Augmentation of hemagglutination by low ionic conditions. Transfusion 1979;19:499–510.

36. Trudeau LR, Judd WJ, Oberman HA. Is a room temperature crossmatch necessary for the detection of ABO errors? Transfusion 1983;23:237–239.

37. Grindon AJ. The decision to transfuse: role of the immunohematology laboratory. Lab Med 1982;13:270–271.

38. Cronin CA, Pohl BA, Miller WV. Crossmatch compatible blood for patients with anti-P_1. Transfusion 1978;18:728–730.

39. Waheed A, Kennedy MS, Gerhan S, Senhauser DA. Transfusion significance of Lewis system antibodies. Success in transfusion with

crossmatch-compatible blood. Am J Clin Pathol 1981;76:294–298.

40. Reid M. Autoagglutination dispersal utilizing sulphydryl compounds. Transfusion 1978;18:353–355.

41. Pierce SR. Anomalous blood bank results. In: Dawson RB, ed. Trouble-shooting the crossmatch. Washington, DC: American Association of Blood Banks, 1976:85–114.

42. Mintz PD, Haines AL, Sullivan MF. Incompatible crossmatch following nonreactive antibody detection test: frequency and cause. Transfusion 1982;22:107–110.

43. Mollison PL. Blood transfusion in clinical medicine. 7th ed. Oxford: Blackwell Scientific Publications, 1983:291–292.

44. Beck ML, Hicklin BL, Pierce SR. Unexpected limitations in the use of commercial anti-globulin reagents. Transfusion 1976;16:71–75.

45. Beck ML, Judd WJ, eds. Polyagglutination. Washington, DC: American Association of Blood Banks, 1980.

46. Dunsford I. The Wright blood group system. Vox Sang 1954;4:160–163. (OS)

47. Oberman HA, Barnes BA, Friedman BA. The risk of abbreviating the crossmatch in urgent or massive transfusion. Transfusion 1978;18:137–141.

48. Friedman BA, Oberman HA, Chadwick AR, Kingdom KI. The maximum blood order schedule and surgical blood use in the United States. Transfusion 1976;16:380–387.

49. Boral LI, Henry JB. The type and screen: a safe alternative and supplement in selected surgical procedures. Transfusion 1977;17:163–168.

13

Identification of Unexpected Alloantibodies

Unexpected alloantibodies are antibodies, other than naturally occurring anti-A or -B, that react with antigens not present on red cells of the antibody producer. Such antibodies are found in approximately 0.3% to 2% of the population, depending upon the incidence of previous transfusions and pregnancies in the population studied and the sensitivity of the test methods.[1,2] Immunization to red cell antigens occurs through pregnancy or transfusion or following deliberate injection with immunogenic material. In some instances the immunizing event is unknown.

Screening tests to detect unexpected antibodies are required in pretransfusion testing and desirable in prenatal care. Although not required, antibody screening tests are performed on most donor bloods. Determining the specificity of antibody is particularly important in pretransfusion and prenatal testing. Some specificities have little clinical significance. Identifying the specificity of significant antibodies makes it possible to test donor blood more accurately for absence of the corresponding antigen(s). Weakly reactive antibodies may fail to react when donor cells are tested with the prospective recipient's serum, whereas tests with potent reagent antisera may demonstrate the antigen to be present. In prenatal testing, knowing the specificity and immunoglobulin class of an antibody helps predict the likelihood of hemolytic disease of the newborn. It is not crucial to identify unexpected antibodies in donor bloods, but this often allows procurement of reagent antisera or teaching samples.

General Procedures

Blood Samples

Ten ml of clotted blood usually supplies sufficient serum for identifying simple antibody specificities, but complex problems may require additional serum. Blood anticoagulated with EDTA is preferred for studies on the autologous red cells, to avoid the possibility of complement attaching to the red cells (see Chapters 6 and 14). Antibody studies can be performed on serum or plasma. Most workers prefer using serum (see Chapter 12), and the term "serum" will be used throughout this chapter.

Medical History

It is useful to know a patient's clinical diagnosis, transfusion history, obstetrical history and drug therapy. Recent transfusion complicates obtaining autologous cells, and it may be necessary to use red cell separation techniques (see page 419). The presence of autoantibodies, often associated with diseases of the lymphoreticular system or induced by drugs such as α-methyldopa, will dictate the use of other procedures discussed in Chapter 14.

Methods

Serum should be tested at all test phases at which antibody activity was initially detected. Using different test phases and such additional procedures as extended incubation periods, cold temperatures or enhancement methods may uncover additional antibodies or enhance the reactivity of the antibody initially detected.

Enzyme techniques offer substantial advantages in antibody identification studies. The reactivity of some antibodies, such as Rh antibodies and complement-binding examples of anti-Le^a and anti-Jk^a, is enhanced in enzyme tests. In contrast, enzyme treatment denatures some blood group antigens, especially M, N, S, Fy^a and Fy^b.[3] Comparing results of tests with and without enzymes can provide clues to identification, and may clarify ambiguous results.

Reagent Red Cells

The serum under investigation is ordinarily tested by the desired techniques against a panel of eight or more group O red cell samples of known antigen composition. Such panels may be obtained from commercial sources or may be assembled from samples obtained locally. A list is provided with each commercially prepared panel that shows, in moderate detail, the phenotype of each red cell sample.

To be useful, a reagent red cell panel must permit confident identification of those clinically significant alloantibodies that are most frequently encountered, such as anti-D, -E, -K and -Fy^a. The red cell phenotypes should be such that for a serum containing a single antibody, the presence of most other alloantibodies can be at least tentatively excluded. A distinct pattern of reactivity should be apparent for each of the commonly encountered alloantibod-

ies; for example, the K+ samples should not be the only ones that are also E+. There must be sufficient numbers of informative red cells that chance alone can be excluded (see page 227) as the cause for seemingly definitive patterns associated with most of the antigens listed in Table 13-1.

Autologous Control

It is important to know how the serum under investigation reacts with the autologous red cells. This helps determine whether alloantibody, autoantibody, or both, are present (see Table 13-2). Serum that reacts only with reagent red cells usually contains only alloantibody; reactivity with both reagent and autologous red cells suggests the presence of autoantibody, or auto- plus alloantibody. A patient with alloantibodies directed against recently transfused red cells may have a positive autologous control because circulating donor red cells are coated with alloantibodies. This may be misinterpreted as being due to autoantibody. A detailed transfusion history is especially important in patients whose red cells are coated with antibody in vivo (see Chapter 14).

The autologous control should be included in antibody identification studies, even if it was already performed during antibody detection tests, because useful information can arise from comparing concurrent reactions of the autologous and reagent red cells.

The Positive Control

Additional testing may be needed if the autologous control is positive. Elution studies may be useful for recently transfused patients or to clarify inconclusive results of serum studies. For example, a weakly reactive alloantibody reacting with most but not all Fy(a+) red cells may be present in the serum of a recently transfused patient whose red cells manifest a positive autologous control. Since antibody reactivity tends to be significantly stronger in an eluate than in serum, it may

Table 13-1. A Reagent Red Cell Panel for Alloantibody Identification

Sample #	Rh Phenotype	Rhesus						Kell	Duffy		Kidd		P	Lewis		MN			
		C	Cw	c	D	E	e	K	Fya	Fyb	Jka	Jkb	P1	Lea	Leb	M	N	S	s
1	r′r	+	0	+	0	0	+	0	+	0	+	+	+	0	+	+	+	0	+
2	R1wR1	+	+	0	+	0	+	+	+	+	0	+	+	+	0	+	+	+	+
3	R1R1	+	0	0	+	0	+	0	+	+	+	+	0	0	+	+	0	+	0
4	R2R2	0	0	+	+	+	0	0	0	+	0	+	+	+	0	0	+	0	+
5	r″r	0	0	+	0	+	+	0	+	+	0	+	0	0	+	+	+	+	0
6	rr	0	0	+	0	0	+	0	0	+	+	0	+	0	0	+	+	0	+
7	rr	0	0	+	0	0	+	+	0	+	+	0	+	0	+	+	0	+	0
8	rr	0	0	+	0	0	+	0	+	0	0	+	+	+	0	0	+	0	+
9	rr	0	0	+	0	0	+	0	0	+	+	0	0	0	+	0	+	+	0
10	R0r	0	0	+	+	0	+	0	0	0	+	+	+	0	0	+	+	+	+

be possible to confirm anti-Fy^a specificity in the eluate. In other instances, free autoantibody may cause weak serum reactivity and a potent autoantibody can be revealed by elution.

Absorption studies may be necessary to establish that autoantibodies are not masking coexisting alloantibodies. The need for such studies on transfusion candidates cannot be overemphasized (see Chapter 14). Procedures for the detection of alloantibodies in the presence of cold-reactive autoantibodies include: 1) cold autoabsorption, 2) prewarmed techniques, 3) heterologous absorption with rabbit red cells, and 4) the use of anti-IgG rather than polyspecific antiglobulin serum. The latter two are especially suitable for recently transfused patients since the circulating red cells used for absorp-

tion contain transfused cells that might adsorb clinically significant alloantibodies. Procedures to detect concomitant alloantibodies in the presence of warm-reactive autoantibodies are discussed in detail on pages 253–255.

Interpreting Serologic Results

Alloantibodies of certain blood group specificities often display consistent serologic characteristics (Table 10-11). In interpreting the results of serum studies, it is important to look for these characteristics and to examine the phenotypes of both reactive and nonreactive red cell samples. The following should be considered:

1. What is the effect of temperature, suspending medium or proteolytic enzymes on the reactions of individual red cell samples?
2. Does the strength of agglutination vary among reactive red cell samples?
3. Is hemolysis present?
4. Are the autologous red cells reactive or nonreactive?

The general serologic characteristics of blood group antibodies are given in Chapters 8, 9, and 10. With these data, and the results of tests against a reagent red cell panel, it usually is possible to identify an antibody, or to select additional reagent red cells or procedures that can be used for conclusive identification. Table 13-3 includes an approach to interpreting the

Table 13-2. Patterns of Serum Reactivity

Reagent Red Cells	Autologous Red Cells	Interpretation
+	0	Alloantibody
0	+	Autoantibody*
+	+	Autoantibody* or Autoantibody* and Alloantibody

*may be interpreted as alloantibody in recently transfused patients due to circulating donor red cells

Table 13-3. A Sequential Approach to Resolving Alloantibody Problems

Reagent Red Cells:	Eliminate from initial consideration antibodies to antigens present on nonreactive samples.
Autologous Red Cells:	Eliminate from consideration antibodies to antigens present on autologous red cells.
Enzyme-Treated Red Cells:	Examine phenotypes (eg, S, Fy^a) of samples that react when untreated, but are nonreactive (or weaker) in enzyme tests. Eliminate from consideration antibodies (eg, anti-Rh) that, if present, should have reacted with antigens present on nonreactive enzyme-treated samples.
Reaction Patterns:	Examine reaction patterns at each test phase; keep in mind possible specificities involved; consider possible specificities relative to test phase and manner of reactivity (eg, direct agglutination with anti-P$_1$, hemolysis at 37°C with anti-Le^a, nonreactivity of anti-Fy^a in enzyme tests).
Additional Tests:	Test sufficient red cell samples of appropriate phenotypes to obtain a p (probability) value less than 1/20 for each suspected antibody. Test serum against red cells carrying a double dose of antigens to which the serum may contain antibodies, if such red cells were not among previously nonreactive samples. Test autologous red cells with additional antisera (if necessary) to show absence of all antigens to which the serum contains antibodies.

results of alloantibody identification tests and selecting additional tests for confirmation. These, and other considerations, are discussed more fully below.

Single Alloantibodies

The specificity of a single alloantibody is usually apparent from the pattern of reactive and nonreactive test results. For example, serum reacts at the antiglobulin phase only with cells 4 and 5 of Table 13-1. The two reactive samples are both E+ and all nonreactive samples are E−. The test phase at which the reactions are observed is consistent with an antibody with Rh blood group specificity. Antibodies that should react with antigens present on the E− samples can be excluded from consideration. For example, anti-K, if present, would react with samples 2 and 7. The presence of anti-E does not appear to mask the presence of other antibodies. Providing the autologous red cells are E−, the identification of alloanti-E in this instance can be established using a single panel of reagent red cells.

Identification of single antibodies may not always be this straightforward. Some important considerations in studies involving single antibodies are discussed below.

Reactions at an Unexpected Test Phase

An antibody may react in an unexpected manner. For example, since anti-P$_1$ antibodies are optimally reactive at or below 22 C, anti-P$_1$ specificity might not be suspected initially if a serum reacts only in the antiglobulin phase. Similarly, most examples of anti-S antibodies react only by the indirect antiglobulin technique, but occasional saline-agglutinating examples occur. The test phase at which a serum reacts can suggest specificity, but the possibility of exceptional behavior must be considered.

Variations in Antigen Expression

With some antibodies, cells carrying the corresponding antigen may not react, or the strength of observed reactions varies with red cells of the same phenotype. This may be due to the phenomenon known as dosage, in which some antibodies react preferentially with red cells from individuals homozygous for the allele determining presence of the antigen. The antibody may not react with red cells from individuals heterozygous for the same gene, presumably carrying a single dose of the antigen.

Some antibodies, including those to I, Le^a, Le^b, Sd^a, Lu^a, Lu^b, Vel, Yt^a, Hy^a, McC^a, Cs^a, Ch^a and Rg^a antigens, react more weakly with cord blood red cells than with red cells from adults. The I, P$_1$, Le^a and Sd^a antigens may be expressed to varying degrees on red cells from different adult donors; such expression is unrelated to zygosity. Some antigens deteriorate more rapidly than others during storage, and the rate of antigen deterioration varies among red cells from different donors. The use of enhancement techniques often helps resolve problems associated with variations in antigen expression (see pages 231–232).

No Discernible Specificity

Other factors besides variations in antigen expression may contribute to the difficulty in interpreting antibody identification test results. If reagent cells are incorrectly phenotyped, clear-cut reactive and nonreactive tests are obtained in a pattern that cannot be interpreted. Nebulous reaction patterns that do not fit any designated specificity may occur with antibodies such as anti-Bg that react with antigens on both leukocytes and red cells.

In other instances a serum may react with an antigen not listed on the antigen profile supplied by the reagent manufacturer; Yt^b is one example. Even though serum studies yield clear-cut reactive and nonreactive tests, anti-Yt^b may not be suspected. In such circumstances it is often useful to ascertain additional phenotype results from the manufacturer. An ambitious way to approach identification in this setting would be to test many ABO-com-patible cell samples to determine antigen frequency and provide information about specificities that the unknown antibody plausibly could have. If the appropriate antiserum is available, reactive and nonreactive red cell samples can be phenotyped, as can the autologous red cells. Such problems will often have to be referred to an Immunohematology Reference Laboratory.

ABO Group of Tested Red Cells

Serum may react with all or most group O reagent cell samples, but not with red cells of the same ABO phenotype as the autologous red cells. This occurs most frequently with anti-H, -IH or -Le^{bH} antibodies. Groups O and A$_2$ red cells have large amounts of H antigen; A$_1$ and A$_1$B red cells carry very little H (see Chapter 8). Serum that contains anti-H or -IH will, therefore, react strongly with group O reagent red cell samples, but weakly or not at all with autologous and donor cells of group A$_1$ or A$_1$B. Similarly, anti-Le^{bH} reacts strongly with group O, Le(b+) red cells, but is usually nonreactive with Le(b+) red cells from A$_1$ or A$_1$B individuals. In pretransfusion testing, such antibodies should be suspected when antibody detection studies using group O red cells are strongly reactive, but serologically compatible group A$_1$ or A$_1$B donor bloods can be obtained without difficulty.

Excluding Additional Antibodies

Other antibodies may be present in a serum that displays a reaction pattern indicating a single antibody. This consideration is obvious when the serum contains antibody to a high-incidence antigen and reacts uniformly with all red cell samples. In more routine situations it is easy to overlook additional antibodies, particularly if they are weakly reactive. Knowing the phenotype of the autologous red cells may help predict the specificities of additional antibodies that might be present. It may be necessary to test the serum against additional reagent red cell samples. Such red cells should be selected to ensure the differentiation and detection of antibodies to those antigens listed in Table 13-1. Red cells carrying a double dose of the relevant antigens are especially helpful. For example, if the serum of an $M + N + S - s +$, $Fy(a-b+)$, $Jk(a-b+)$, $K-$ individual appears to contain anti-Jk^a, testing the serum against $Jk(a-)$ red cells from individuals homozygous for S, and Fy^a would help exclude the presence of anti-S and anti-Fy^a. $K+$, $k-$ red cells may, however, be difficult to obtain to exclude anti-k.

In routine patient-care situations, excluding antibodies to antigens of relatively low incidence, such as anti-C^w, -Kp^a and -V, has little clinical importance. These antibodies are uncommon, and the corresponding antigens are present on the red cells of less than 2% of the random population. If present, these antibodies would be detected if donor red cells carrying the antigen are subjected to compatibility testing.

Special Considerations with Rh Antibodies

Some special considerations apply to Rh antibodies of certain specificities. If the serum of a transfusion candidate contains anti-E, it is important to consider the additional presence of anti-c. The Rh phenotype of the patient's red cells should be determined; if they are of the R_1R_1 phenotype, lacking c and E antigens, the anti-E will most likely be accompanied by anti-c.[4] The anti-c may be less reactive than the anti-E, and more sensitive methods such as enzyme techniques may be required to demonstrate its presence. Even when anti-c is not detectable, it is advisable to select $c-$, $E-$ blood for transfusion to R_1R_1 patients with anti-E, since anti-c is a common cause of delayed hemolytic transfusion reactions.

The reverse situation causes less of a problem. If anti-c is identified, the additional presence of anti-E may not be ascertained unless rare R_zR_1 red cells are used.

Note that Table 13-1 does not include such a sample, nor is it necessary to test all anti-c sera from transfusion candidates against R_zR_1 red cells. Failure to detect anti-E in the serum of an R_1R_1 patient with anti-c does not pose a major transfusion hazard; almost all $c-$ donor units also will be $E-$. Further, anti-E, if present, would be detected on the rare occasion that an R_zR_1 donor unit might be selected by chance for compatibility testing.

Phenotype of Autologous Red Cells

Once an alloantibody has been identified, the autologous red cells should be tested for the corresponding antigen. This is an important confirmatory test. With rare exceptions, when alloantibody is present in the serum, the corresponding antigen should be absent from the autologous red cells. For example, if the serum from a nontransfused individual appears to contain anti-Fy^a but the autologous red cells have a negative direct antiglobulin test and type as $Fy(a+)$, the data are clearly in conflict and further testing with additional reagent red cells is necessary.

In recently transfused individuals, the patient's pretransfusion sample should be tested, if available. If necessary, the patient's red cells can be separated from the transfused red cells. Procedures for this are discussed on pages 419–421.

Probability

Conclusive antibody identification requires testing the serum against sufficient reagent red cell samples that lack, and sufficient that carry, the relevant antigens to ensure that an observed pattern of reactivity does not result from chance alone. Table 13-4 shows the probabilities of various combinations of reactive and nonreactive tests, as calculated by Fisher's exact method for estimating probabilities. The method is discussed more fully on pages 412–414.

The probability (p) values shown in Table 13-4 are the result of statistical tests that show the likelihood of a given set of results being due to chance alone. A p value of

Table 13-4. Probability of Identification for Combinations of Reactive and Nonreactive Tests

# Tested	# Reactive	# Nonreactive	p
6	4	2	1/15
6	3	3	1/20
7	5	2	1/21
7	4	3	1/35
8	7	1	1/8
8	6	2	1/28
8	5	3	1/56
8	4	4	1/70
9	8	1	1/9
9	7	2	1/36
9	6	3	1/84
10	9	1	1/10
10	8	2	1/45
10	7	3	1/120
10	6	4	1/210
10	5	5	1/252

1/20 (0.05) means that an identical set of results would be obtained by chance once in 20 similar studies; the odds are 19 to one that the interpretation of the data is correct. For example, if a serum agglutinates three reagent red cell samples that are D+ and fails to agglutinate three that are D−, then p is 1/20; therefore, there is a 19 to one probability that the antibody is anti-D.

A p of 1/20 (0.05) is the minimum value at which an interpretation is considered statistically valid. Most reagent red cell panels are limited in their ability to provide statistically conclusive identification of some blood group antibodies. For example, if a serum is tested against the panel of red cell samples shown in Table 13-1 and only sample 4 is nonreactive, there is a nine to one chance (p = 1/10) that the reactions are not due to anti-e. If, however, another e− sample was present in this panel and was also nonreactive, the p would change to 1/45.

It is important to remember these unavoidable limitations when only one panel of reagent red cells is available for testing. It is often necessary to test additional red cell samples that lack moder-ately high-incidence antigens such as e, before assigning conclusive specificity to an antibody.

Multiple Alloantibodies

When a serum contains two or more alloantibodies, serum studies on a single panel of reagent red cells may be difficult to interpret. Multiple alloantibodies usu-ally present in one or more of the follow-ing ways.
1. The observed pattern of reactive and nonreactive tests does not fit that of a single antibody.
2. Variations in reaction strength occur that cannot be explained on the basis of dosage.
3. Different red cell samples react at dif-ferent test phases.
4. Unexpected reactions are obtained when attempts are made to confirm the specificity of a suspected single anti-body. For example, if a serum sus-pected of containing anti-e reacts when tested against additional e− red cell samples, another antibody might be present; or alternatively, the suspected antibody might not be anti-e. Such a situation requires testing further e− red cell samples.

When multiple alloantibodies are pres-ent, an approach similar to that outlined in Table 13-3 can be used to determine the likely specificities involved, and to help decide what additional tests are necessary for conclusive identification. An example of such an approach is the following dis-cussion of findings shown in Table 13-5. The serum in this case contains anti-M, anti-Fy^a, and anti-Jk^a. The resolution of this case is as follows:
1. *Eliminate from initial consideration anti-bodies to antigens present on nonreactive reagent red cell samples.* Only sample 4 is nonreactive at all test phases. Thus, anti-c, -D, -E, -Fy^b, -Jk^b, -P$_1$, -Le^a, -N and -s can all be provisionally excluded from consideration at this time. These find-ings may be due to a mixture of anti-

Table 13-5. Example of Reactions Observed with Multiple Alloantibodies

Cell Number	Antigen																		LISS			Ficin	
	C	Cw	c	D	E	e	K	Fya	Fyb	Jka	Jkb	P1	Lea	Leb	M	N	S	s	RT	37	IAT	37	IAT
1	+	0	+	0	0	+	0	+	0	+	+	+	0	+	+	+	0	+	1+	0	3+	0	4+
2	+	+	0	+	0	+	+	+	+	0	+	+	+	0	+	+	+	0	1+	0	2+	0	0
3	+	0	0	+	0	+	0	+	+	+	+	0	0	+	+	0	+	0	3+	2+	3+	0	4+
4	0	0	+	+	+	0	0	0	+	0	+	+	+	0	0	+	0	+	0	0	0	0	0
5	0	0	+	0	+	+	0	+	+	0	+	0	0	+	+	+	+	0	1+	0	2+	0	0
6	0	0	+	0	0	+	0	0	+	+	0	+	0	0	+	+	0	+	1+	0	3+	*H	†
7	0	0	+	0	0	+	+	0	+	+	0	+	0	+	+	0	+	0	3+	2+	3+	*H	†
8	0	0	+	0	0	+	0	+	0	0	+	+	+	0	0	+	0	+	0	0	3+	0	0
9	0	0	+	0	0	+	0	0	+	+	0	0	0	+	0	+	+	0	0	0	3+	*H	†
10	0	0	+	+	0	+	0	0	0	+	+	+	0	0	+	+	+	+	1+	0	2+	0	4+
Auto	0	+	+	+	0	+	0	0		0		+	0	+	0	+	0	+	0	0	0	0	0

* denotes hemolysis RT = Room temperature IAT = Indirect antiglobulin testing
† = no cells left for testing 0 = no reaction 1–4 + = degree of agglutination

bodies to a number of different antigens, including C, Cw, e, K, Fya, Jka, Leb, M and S.

2. *Eliminate from consideration antibodies to antigens present on the autologous red cells.* Alloantibodies, by definition, cannot be made against antigens present on the autologous red cells. The phenotype of the autologous red cells indicates that antibodies to c, D, e, P1, N, Leb and s antigens should not be present in the serum.

3. *Examine the phenotypes of red cell samples that react when untreated but are nonreactive (or weaker) in enzyme tests.* Three samples (2, 5 and 8) fail to react at the antiglobulin phase with enzyme-treated cells, but these three samples are reactive in the untreated state. All three samples are Fy(a+), and samples 2 and 5 are also S+; anti-Fya is a likely specificity, but anti-S cannot be excluded on the basis of these reactions.

4. *Eliminate from consideration antibodies that, if present, should have reacted with antigens present on red cells nonreactive after enzyme treatment.* Anti-C, anti-Cw and anti-K can now be eliminated from consideration. Sample 2 carries all three antigens, and is nonreactive in enzyme tests. Enhanced reactions with enzyme-treated red cells

would have been expected if Rh antibodies were present, and Kell system antigens are not adversely affected by ficin. At this point in the investigation it is appropriate to consider antibodies to Fya, Jka, M or S as likely specificities. All of these antigens are absent from the autologous red cells. In order to ascertain which of these may be involved it is necessary to:

5. *Examine reaction patterns at each test phase; keep in mind possible specificities involved; consider possible specificities relative to test phase and manner of reactivity.* The results of LISS tests at room temperature suggest the presence of anti-M. Reagent red cell samples 4, 8 and 9 are nonreactive and are M − N + . Samples that are M + N + (1, 2, 5, 6 and 10) are weakly (1 +) reactive, and samples 3 and 7 are M + N − and are strongly (3 +) reactive. Further, only the two M + N − samples (3 and 7) are reactive in LISS tests at 37 C. This is a typical pattern of reactions of an anti-M showing dosage.

In the antiglobulin phase of testing with untreated red cells, only sample 4 is nonreactive. Although this sample is the only one that is e −, anti-e has already been eliminated from consideration, since the autologous red cells are e+. The reactions at the antiglobulin phase also fit for a mixture of anti-Fyᵃ and anti-Jkᵃ, and it can be noted that the three samples that give a 2+ reaction (2, 5, and 10) carry only a single dose of either Fyᵃ or Jkᵃ.

In enzyme tests, the three Jk(a+b−) red cell samples (6, 7 and 9) are hemolyzed after incubation at 37 C. A distinct anti-Jkᵃ reaction pattern is observed in ficin-antiglobulin tests (considering that both hemolysis and agglutination are manifestations of an antigen-antibody reaction). The serologic findings, therefore, suggest the presence of anti-M, anti-Fyᵃ and anti-Jkᵃ in this serum. For conclusive identification, it is necessary to:

6. *Test sufficient red cell samples of appropriate phenotypes to obtain a p value less than 1/20 for each suspected antibody.* A statistically valid interpretation of the data can be made for anti-M in room temperature tests and anti-Jkᵃ in ficin-antiglobulin tests. For anti-M, all three M− samples are nonreactive and all six M+ samples are reactive; p = 1/20. For anti-Jkᵃ, there are six reactive Jk(a+) samples and four nonreactive Jk(a−) samples; p = 1/20. However, in the antiglobulin phase with untreated red cells, three reactive Jk(a−) samples (2, 5 and 8) are Fy(a+) and the one nonreactive Jk(a−) sample (sample 4) is Fy(a−). The p value is only 1/4 for anti-Fyᵃ. Before anti-Fyᵃ specificity can be confirmed, at least two more Fy(a−), Jk(a−) samples must be tested and found to be nonreactive, to obtain a p of 1/20. M−N+ red cells may be required for these confirmatory studies, since it has yet to be established that the anti-M is solely reactive by direct agglutination tests.

7. *Test serum against red cells carrying a double dose of antigens to which the serum may contain antibodies, if such red cells have not already been tested.* The presence of anti-S has not been excluded, and further

tests with S+ red cells that lack M, Fyᵃ and Jkᵃ antigens should be undertaken. S+ s− red cells should be included in these studies, if available.

Although certain specificities are excluded from initial consideration because the corresponding antigens are present on nonreactive red cell samples, such exclusions should be confirmed with red cells carrying a double dose of the relevant antigens, if these are available. In this case, the phenotype of the autologous red cells does not preclude the presence of anti-E, but sample 4, carrying a double dose of E, is nonreactive at all test phases.

8. *Test autologous red cells with additional antisera (if necessary) to show absence of all antigens to which the serum contains antibodies.* It may be necessary to test the autologous red cells with additional antisera, to show that they lack all antigens corresponding to those antibodies present in the serum. If the approach shown in Table 13-3 has been followed, much of this testing will already have been performed; no further testing of the autologous red cells is required for the case study presented in Table 13-5.

This case illustrates the value of performing enzyme tests when alloantibody identification studies are undertaken, especially when multiple antibodies are present in a serum. Much valuable information can be obtained early in the investigation by performing at least limited phenotyping of the autologous red cells along with the serum studies. However, it must be stressed that not all problem cases can be resolved in this manner. Often, determining the specificity of some antibodies or excluding the presence of others requires use of some of the procedures described on pages 231–236.

Antibodies to High-Incidence Antigens

An alloantibody to a high-incidence antigen should be suspected when all reagent red cell samples are uniformly reactive, but the autologous control is nonreactive. These antibodies can often be identified with red cells of selected rare phenotypes, [eg, k − or Yt(a −)], and by demonstrating that the autologous red cells lack the appropriate high-incidence antigens.

Knowing the serologic characteristics of the antibody and the race of the antibody producer will help in planning additional tests. For example, reactivity in tests at room temperature suggests anti-H, -I, -Tj^a (-PP$_1$P^k); hemolysis at 37 C is observed with these antibodies and with anti-Jk3 and anti-Vel; reduced or absent reactivity in enzyme tests occurs with anti-Ch^a or -Rg^a, and some examples of anti-Yt^a; weak, nebulous reactions in the antiglobulin phase are often associated with so-called high-titer, low-avidity (HTLA) antibodies (eg, anti-Kn^a, -McC^a, -Yk^a, -Cs^a), but are also seen when polyspecific antiglobulin reagents are used on complement-binding autoantibodies, such as anti-I or anti-IH. In blacks, anti-U and -Js^b should be suspected; individuals lacking these antigens are almost always black.

Chapter 11 discusses the serologic characteristics of antibodies reacting with high-incidence red cell antigens. Methods for the evaluation of sera containing HTLA antibodies are given on pages 455–456. Such problems will often have to be referred to an Immunohematology Reference Laboratory.

The patient's siblings are often the best source of serologically compatible blood for patients with antibodies to high-incidence antigens. Rare phenotypes lacking high-incidence red cell antigens usually occur in individuals homozygous for a rare blood group gene, one inherited from each parent. Offspring of the same parents are far more likely to have inherited the same two rare genes than someone from the random donor population. In very rare circumstances blood from a parent may lack the same high-incidence antigen, as for example, in Lu(a − b −) phenotypes

resulting from inheritance of the dominant *InLu* gene (see page 162). Ordinarily, blood from each parent carries only a single dose of the relevant antigen, and may be preferable to random-donor blood if incompatible blood must be given in life-threatening situations. In addition, the AABB Immunohematology Reference Laboratory Program, in collaboration with the AABB and other rare donor files, can be extremely helpful in locating donors of the appropriate phenotypes when necessary (see pages 414–415).

Antibodies to Low-Incidence Antigens

When a serum sample reacts only with red cells from a single donor unit, possibilities to consider are that the donor red cells are ABO-incompatible, have a positive direct antiglobulin test, or are polyagglutinable. See page 214 for a discussion of polyagglutinable red cells.

Reactions between a serum and a single donor or reagent red cell sample are also associated with antibodies to low-incidence antigens. (See Chapter 11.) If red cells known to carry low-incidence antigens are available, the serum may be tested against them. Conversely, the one reactive red cell sample can be tested with known examples of antibodies to low-incidence antigens. Antibodies to several low-incidence antigens frequently occur together in a single serum, and the expertise and resources of an Immunohematology Reference Laboratory are usually required to confirm the suspected specificities. It is inappropriate to delay transfusion while such studies are undertaken.

Anomalous Serologic Reactions

Antibodies to a variety of drugs and additives can cause positive results in antibody detection and identification tests. Antibodies against substances used in the preparation of reagent red cells (eg, chloramphenicol, neomycin, tetracycline, hydrocortisone, lactose or EDTA) may cause agglutination of reagent red cells suspended in that manufacturer's preservative solution.[5,6] Reactions rarely occur if saline-washed red cells are used for testing, and the autologous control is nonreactive unless the autologous red cells are suspended in the manufacturer's red cell diluent or a similar preservative solution.

Antibodies to other reagent additives can cause agglutination of reagent, donor and autologous red cells. Several reports describe antibodies to sodium caprylate, a stabilizing agent added to some commercially prepared bovine albumin solutions; such antibodies cause direct agglutination and, rarely, reactivity in the antiglobulin phase when the test system contains added albumin. Agglutination is absent when other test procedures, such as saline or LISS tests, are employed. The autologous control reacts to the same degree as reagent or donor red cells, but a direct antiglobulin test performed on cells washed without contact with other reagents will be nonreactive.

In very rare situations, the age of the test red cells, or the fact that they have been washed in saline prior to use, may give rise to anomalous serologic reactions.[5] Antibodies to stored red cells can cause agglutination of reagent red cells by all techniques, and enhanced reactions will be observed in enzyme tests. Such reactivity is not affected by washing the red cells in saline, and the autologous control is usually nonreactive. No reactivity will be seen with tests on freshly collected red cells (eg, from freshly drawn donor or autologous blood samples). When antibodies to freshly washed red cells are encountered, antibody detection studies with unwashed reagent red cells will be nonreactive, but agglutination of freshly washed donor or autologous red cells will be seen.

For a detailed account of unusual serologic phenomena that are encountered in antibody detection and compatibility studies, the review by Pierce[6] is recommended.

Selected Serologic Procedures

Enhancement Techniques

When a pattern of weak reactions fails to indicate specificity, or when the presence of an antibody is suspected but cannot be demonstrated, the following procedures may be helpful.

Enzyme Techniques

Tests with proteolytic enzymes, if not used routinely, are a useful addition to antibody identification studies. Treating red cells with proteolytic enzymes enhances the reactivity of Rh antibodies and of complement-binding alloantibodies such as anti-Jk[a]. Procedures for the preparation and use of proteolytic enzyme solutions are given on pages 425–427.

Temperature Reduction

Many alloantibodies that react at room temperature react better at cold temperatures; specificity may only be apparent at 4 C. For tests at cold temperatures, an autologous control is especially important, because most sera contain cold-reactive autoantibodies. In some instances, the interference of autoantibodies can be avoided by incubating tests at 12 C rather than 4 C.

Increased Serum:Cell Ratio

Increasing the volume of serum incubated with a standard volume of red cells often enhances the reactivity of antibodies present in low concentration.[5] An acceptable procedure is to mix five to ten volumes of serum with one volume of a 2-5% saline suspension of red cells and incubate for 60 minutes at 37 C with periodic mixing to promote contact between red cells and antibody molecules. The serum should be removed before washing red cells for the antiglobulin test because the standard three to four wash phases may be insufficient when large quantities of serum are present. Additional wash phases are not recommended because bound antibody molecules may elute.

Increased Incubation Time

For some antibodies, particularly when saline or albumin tests are employed, a 15-minute incubation period is insufficient to achieve equilibrium, and the observed reactions may be weak. Extending the incubation time to 60 minutes may increase reactivity and help clarify the observed pattern of reactions.

Alteration of pH

The reactivity of certain antibodies, notably some examples of anti-M, is enhanced by decreasing the pH of the reaction medium to pH 6.5.[7] Thus, when anti-M specificity is suspected because only M + N − red cells are agglutinated, tests with acidified serum may reveal a definitive anti-M pattern of reactivity. Adding one volume of 0.2 N HCl to nine volumes of serum decreases the pH to 6.5. M − red cells should be tested against the acidified serum to check for nonspecific aggulutination.

Low Ionic Strength Salt (LISS) Procedures

Reactions of some blood group antibodies are stronger in a low ionic strength salt (LISS) medium. LISS reagents act by enhancing antibody uptake, the stage of the reaction that involves association of antibody molecules to red cells. A variety of LISS procedures have been described. Enhancement of the second, agglutinating phase of hemagglutination results from use of polycations such as protamine sulphate or Polybrene® to aggregate LISS-suspended antibody-coated red cells.[5] The nonspecific aggregation caused by polycations is easily dispersed by addition of phosphate buffer or sodium citrate-glucose solutions, allowing recognition of agglutination due solely to an antigen-antibody interaction. The red cells may subsequently be subjected to antiglobulin

testing. These methods are discussed in more detail in Chapter 12.

Use of Thiol Reagents

Thiol reagents, such as dithiothreitol (DTT) and 2-mercaptoethanol (2-ME), cleave intersubunit disulfide bonds of IgM molecules. Intact 19S IgM molecules are cleaved into 7S subunits, which have altered serologic reactivity.[5,8] The interchain bonds of 7S IgM subunits, and IgG and IgA molecules, are relatively resistant to such cleavage (see Chapter 5 for the structure of immunoglobulin molecules). The applications of DTT and 2-ME in immunohematology include:

1. Determining the immunoglobulin class of an antibody (see page 454 for method).
2. Dissociating red cell agglutinates caused by IgM antibodies, eg, the spontaneous agglutination of red cells by potent cold-reactive autoantibodies. See page 463.
3. Identifying specificities in a mixture of IgM and IgG antibodies, particularly when an agglutinating IgM antibody masks the presence of IgG antibodies.
4. Dissociating IgG antibodies from red cells with a mixture of DTT and a proteolytic enzyme (ZZAP reagent). See page 464.
5. Converting nonagglutinating IgG antibodies into direct agglutinins.[9] Commercially prepared typing reagents for use in rapid saline tube or slide tests have been manufactured in this manner. See page 146.

Soluble Blood Group Substances

Some blood group antigens exist in soluble form in such body fluids as saliva, urine or plasma. These substances are useful in antibody identification studies, either to confirm antibody specificity by inhibition or to neutralize antibodies that mask the presence of concomitant nonneutralizable antibodies. The following soluble blood group substances can be used in antibody identification tests:

1. Lewis substances. Le^a and Le^b substances are present in the saliva of persons of the appropriate Lewis phenotype. Le^a substance is present in the saliva of Le(a+b−) individuals, and both Le^a and Le^b substances are present in the saliva of Le(a−b+) individuals.[4,5] Saliva should be boiled immediately after collection to inactivate salivary enzymes, and should be rendered isotonic prior to use.[4] Commercially prepared Lewis substance is available.
2. P$_1$ substance. Soluble P$_1$ substance is present in hydatid cyst fluid. A reagent preparation derived from pigeons is commercially available.[5]
3. Sd^a (Sid) substance. Sd^a blood group substance is present in soluble form in various body fluids. The most abundant source is urine.[10] If anti-Sd^a is suspected, urine from a known Sd(a+) individual can be used to inhibit the antibody. Either saline or urine that does not contain Sd^a substance should be used as a negative control. Because urine may have an acidic pH and a high concentration of salts, it should be dialyzed for 48 hours against pH 7.3 phosphate buffered saline prior to use (see page 424 for preparation). Once dialyzed, Sd(a+) and Sd(a−) urines can be frozen in small aliquots for future use.
4. Chido and Rodgers substances. Among the antibodies most difficult to work with are those collectively known as the HTLA (high-titer, low-avidity) antibodies. Although undiluted serum gives weak (1+ to 2+) reactions by the indirect antiglobulin technique, weak reactions continue to be observed in tests with progressively diluted serum. Characteristically, these antibodies produce fragile agglutinates, and the reaction scores are low.[11] Anti-Ch^a and anti-Rg^a, unlike such HTLA antibodies as anti-Cs^a and anti-Kn^a, can be inhibited by plasma from Ch(a+), Rg(a+) individuals[12] (see page 456 for method).
   Chido and Rodgers antigens are epitopes on the plasma protein C4, the fourth component of human complement (C4).[13,14] Since trace amounts of C4 are present on normal red cells,[15] anti-Ch^a and anti-Rg^a react with normal red cells in the antiglobulin phase of testing. Red cells coated in vitro with excess C4 (see page 456) will be directly agglutinated by these antibodies. This is a useful test for rapid identification of anti-Ch^a and anti-Rg^a, and should be implemented at an early stage in the evaluation of sera suspected to contain HTLA antibodies.

Confirmation of Specificity

Antibody specificity can be confirmed if the appropriate soluble substance inhibits serologic reactivity. For example, if a serum is thought to contain anti-P$_1$ but there are insufficient P$_1$-negative red cell samples available for conclusive identification, inhibition of reactivity by soluble P$_1$ substance confirms the specificity. A volume of P$_1$ substance is added to the appropriate volume of serum (use volumes recommended by the manufacturer for commercially prepared substances), and the mixture is incubated at room temperature, as is a control test of serum plus saline. Following incubation, P$_1$ red cells are added to both mixtures. The tests are incubated at room temperature and subsequently examined for agglutination.

One of three reaction patterns will be observed:

	1	2	3
Serum + P$_1$ substance	0	+	0
Serum + saline (control):	+	+	0

The interpretation is as follows:

1. If agglutination is abolished by incubating P$_1$ substance with serum, and the control test remains reactive, the serum contains anti-P$_1$.
2. If both tests are reactive, possible interpretations are: a) the antibody is not anti-P$_1$; b) the serum contains a potent example of anti-P$_1$ and only partial

neutralization has occurred; c) the serum contains anti-P_1 plus additional antibody activity.

3. If both tests are nonreactive, the antibody may be present in such a low concentration that it cannot withstand dilution.

Neutralization of Antibodies

In a serum containing multiple antibodies, neutralizing one antibody with a soluble blood group substance facilitates recognition of other antibody specificities. For example, if a serum contains anti-P_1 and anti-S, the anti-S may not be apparent because there are no S + red cells that lack P_1 antigen among the available reagent red cell samples. If the anti-P_1 is neutralized with soluble P_1 substance, the presence or absence of anti-S can be confirmed with S + and S − reagent red cell samples, regardless of their P-system phenotype.

Inactivation of Kell-System Antigens

Antibodies to all antigens of the Kell system, except anti-Kx (K15), are nonreactive with red cells treated with 2-aminoethylisothiouronium bromide (AET).[16] Thus, if an antibody is suspected of having specificity directed toward an antigen in the Kell system (eg, anti-Kp^b), failure to react with reagent red cells treated with AET helps to confirm the suspicion of Kell-related specificity. However, AET may weaken the expression of other blood group antigens[17] so that loss of reactivity following AET treatment is not conclusive evidence for Kell-related specificity. A procedure for treating red cells with AET is described on page 453. Also, a panel of AET-treated red cells may be used to determine the presence of other, non-Kell-related antibodies in the presence of an antibody to a high-incidence Kell-system antigen.

AET treatment produces changes to red cells similar to those seen in paroxysmal nocturnal hemoglobinuria (PNH), such that red cells are sensitive to the presence of complement components activated by nonimmune mechanisms. An anti-IgG reagent should be used in tests with AET-treated red cells.[16]

Kell-system antigens are also denatured by treatment with ZZAP reagent, a mixture of proteolytic enzyme and sulfhydryl compound, as discussed on page 464. Red cells treated with ZZAP can be used to test for the presence of certain additional antibodies (eg, those to Rh and Kidd system antigens) in a serum containing antibody to a high-incidence Kell-system antigen. However, because of the proteolytic activity of ZZAP reagent, such red cells cannot be used to exclude the presence of antibodies to M, N, S, s, Fy^a and Fy^b antigens.

Absorption

Antibody can be removed from a serum by adsorption by red cells carrying the corresponding antigen. The antibody forms a complex with antigens of the red cell membrane; when red cells are separated from the serum, the antibody remains attached to the red cells. Subsequent elution of the bound antibody can often give additional useful information. Absorption techniques are useful in such situations as:

1. Removing autoantibody activity, to permit the detection of coexisting alloantibodies (see Chapter 14).
2. Removing unwanted antibody, especially anti-A or -B, from a serum that contains an antibody suitable for reagent use.
3. Confirming the presence of antigens on red cells through their ability to remove a specific serum antibody.
4. Confirming the specificity of an antibody, by showing that it can be adsorbed only by red cells of a particular blood group phenotype.
5. Separating multiple antibodies present in a single serum sample. Such studies require the use of combined absorption and elution tests, and are useful in the identification of complex mixtures of antibodies (see pages 237–238).

Technical Considerations

Absorption procedures are used for different purposes in different situations; no single procedure is satisfactory in all instances. The usual serum:red cell ratio is one volume of serum to an equal volume of washed, packed red cells. The incubation temperature should be that which is optimal for the reactivity of the antibody.

Pretreating the red cells with a proteolytic enzyme may enhance antibody uptake, and thereby reduce the number of absorptions required for complete removal of antibody. Since some antigens, such as M, N and Fy^a, are destroyed by proteases, antibodies directed against these antigens may not be removed by enzyme-treated red cells.

In separating mixtures of antibodies, selecting red cells of the appropriate phenotype is extremely important. At least one antibody specificity should be known or suspected in order to choose red cells that lack one antigen yet carry another. The red cells must be available in sufficient quantity; vials of reagent red cells will not suffice. Blood samples from staff members or donor units are the most convenient sources.

Absorption Procedure

1. Wash the selected red cells at least three times with saline. After the third wash, centrifuge the red cells for at least 5 minutes, and remove as much of the supernatant saline as is possible by suction. Residual saline may be removed by placing a narrow piece of filter paper into the red cells.

2. Mix appropriate volumes of the packed red cells and serum, and incubate at the desired temperature for 30 to 60 minutes. Absorption will be more effective if the area of contact between the red cells and serum is large; the use of a large bore test tube (ie, 13 mm or greater) is recommended. The tube of serum and cells should be mixed periodically throughout the incubation phase, preferably with a rotating device.

3. Centrifuge to pack the red cells tightly. To avoid antigen-antibody dissociation, centrifuge at the incubation temperature if possible.

4. Transfer the supernatant serum into a clean test tube, and label it as absorbed serum. If an eluate is to be prepared, save the red cells.

5. Test an aliquot of the absorbed serum to see if the procedure has removed all of the antibody, preferably against another aliquot of red cells from the sample used for absorption. Repeat the absorption process if necessary with a fresh aliquot of washed, packed red cells.

Elution

Elution techniques liberate antibody molecules from coated red cells; the intent of most elutions is to recover bound antibody in a usable form. Bound antibody may be released by changing the thermodynamics of antigen-antibody reactions, by neutralizing or reversing forces of attraction that hold antigen-antibody complexes together, or by disturbing the structural complementarity between an antigen and its corresponding binding site on an antibody molecule.[18]

A variety of methods have been described for eluting antibody from sensitized red cells, and some procedures are given on pages 429–433. Among those in popular use are the heat technique of Landsteiner and Miller,[19] the acid technique for stromal elution described by Jenkins and Moore,[20] and elution with organic solvents such as ether.[21] While no single method is best in all situations, heat elution appears most suited for the investigation of ABO hemolytic disease of the newborn, and elution with acid or an organic solvent is required for optimal elution of warm-reactive auto- and alloantibodies.[18]

Technical Considerations

Technical factors that impair the success of elution techniques include:

1. Incorrect technique. Depending upon the elution method used, such factors as incomplete removal of organic solvents and failure to render an eluate isotonic or to a neutral pH, may cause hemolysis or ambiguous ("sticky") results when the eluate is tested. Similarly, the presence of stromal debris may interfere with reading of tests. Careful technique and strict adherence to the protocol selected should eliminate such problems.

2. Incomplete washing. To ensure that an antibody present in an eluate originated from the surface of the cells and not from residual serum present around the cells, the sensitized red cells must be thoroughly washed prior to elution. Six washes with saline usually are adequate, but more may be needed if the red cells have been coated in vitro with a high-titer antibody. To monitor the efficacy of the washing process, the supernatant fluid from the final wash phase can be tested for antibody activity; it should be found nonreactive.

3. Binding of proteins to glass surfaces. If eluates are prepared from red cells coated in vitro with purified antibody and the same test tube used during the sensitization phase is also used for preparing the eluate, antibody bound nonspecifically to the test tube surface may dissociate during the elution and contaminate the eluate. To avoid such contamination, red cells should be transferred into a clean test tube for washing, before proceeding with preparation of the eluate.

4. Storage changes to organic solvents. Organic solvents, particularly ether, become acidic during storage, probably as a result of peroxide formation. This may result in apparent "nonspecificity" of eluates prepared with ether from an almost empty canister. Consequently, it is advisable to discard organic solvents from containers opened longer than 30 days.[18]

5. Dissociation of antibody prior to elution. This is not usually a problem with IgG antibodies, unless they have a low affinity for their respective antigens. It may, however, contribute to difficulties encountered when attempting to elute predominantly cold-reactive antibodies such as anti-A or anti-M. To minimize loss of antibody during the washing process, the use of cold (4 C) saline is recommended.

6. Instability of eluates. Dilute protein solutions, such as those obtained by elution into saline, are unstable. Eluates should be tested as soon after preparation as possible. Alternatively, eluates may be kept frozen following the addition of bovine albumin to a final concentration of 6% (wt/vol).

Applications

Elution techniques are useful for:

1. Investigation of a positive direct antiglobulin test (see Chapter 14).

2. Concentration and purification of antibodies, detection of weakly expressed antigens and identification of multiple antibody specificities. Such studies are used in conjunction with an appropriate absorption technique (see pages 237–238).

3. Preparation of antibody-free intact red cells for use in phenotyping or autologous absorption studies. Procedures used to remove cold- and warm-reactive autoantibodies from red cells are discussed on pages 463 and 417, and methods for autologous absorption of warm-reactive autoantibodies are given on page 463.

Combined Absorption-Elution Procedures

Combining absorption and elution can often be helpful in the detection of weakly expressed antigens on red cells or the identification of weakly reactive antibodies. An antibody that may not cause direct agglutination may be adsorbed by antigen-positive red cells. Reduced antibody reactivity in the absorbed serum and subsequent recovery of the antibody from the adsorbing red cells show that an antibody-antigen interaction has occurred. Combining absorption and elution may be invaluable in separating antibody mixtures in identification studies or reagent production.

Detection of Weak Antigens or Antibodies

A low serum:cell ratio (eg, 2:1 or less) is needed in absorption procedures to demonstrate the presence or absence of the corresponding antigen on red cells. Care should be taken not to dilute the serum, and hence the antibody, with residual saline from inadequately packed red cells. To check for such dilution the protein concentrations of the pre- and postabsorbed sera can be tested by refractometry. A postabsorption reduction in titration score of 10 or more, using the system described on page 240, is considered evidence that the adsorbing red cells possess the relevant antigen. In critical studies, control absorptions with red cells known to lack the antigen in question should be undertaken.

When antibody is to be recovered from the red cells by subsequent elution, a higher serum:cell ratio (eg, 5:1 or more) should be used to sensitize the red cells with antibody. The eluate so produced may be more potent than the original serum, since absorption followed by elution concentrates the antibody molecules.[18] Once prepared, the eluate should be tested against uncoated red cells from the same sample used for absorption, to establish recovery of the antibody.

Identification of Antibodies in Multispecific Sera

Absorption and elution may be used to identify individual specificities in sera containing multiple antibodies. Since these studies are tedious, they should be under-

taken when all other studies with multiple reagent red cell samples and enhancement procedures have failed to resolve the problem fully. In laboratories where this is frequently undertaken, phenotyping staff members is invaluable to obtain a source of adequately large volumes of red cells.

The choice of adsorbing red cells often has to be an inspired guess, influenced by the phenotype of the antibody producer; narrowing the range of possibly present antibodies helps in selecting additional red cell samples that can prove their presence or absence. As a general rule, red cells should be those that react weakly with the multispecific serum, on the assumption that these carry only one of the antigens with which the serum reacts.

The serum under investigation should be absorbed several times, until it no longer reacts with a fresh sample of the adsorbing red cells. Both the absorbed serum and an eluate prepared from the adsorbing red cells should be examined for antibody specificity. While it is to be hoped that one or both preparations will contain definable antibody specificity, this is not always the case. Some antibodies, particularly HTLA antibodies, are difficult to absorb and elute. Sometimes the absorbed serum is nonreactive, yet the eluate reacts with all reagent red cell samples. Such results may indicate the presence of antibody to a high-incidence antigen that is variably expressed on red cells, or may occur if the absorption process caused dilution of the serum antibody.

When the above studies are not informative, or when autoantibodies are present in the serum of a recently transfused individual so that autologous absorption is not appropriate (see Chapter 14), selective absorptions with R_1R_1, R_2R_2 and rr red cells may be helpful in identifying alloantibodies. Beattie[22] recommends using three K− red cell samples for this purpose, including among them one Jk(a−), one Jk(b−) and one Fy(a−) sample. The absorbed serum samples, and eluates prepared from red cells used in the first absorption, are then examined for antibody specificity.

Isolation of Specific Antibodies

Absorption and elution permit effective preparation of antisera for use with red cells of any ABO group. It is often difficult to obtain group A, B, or AB red cells that lack the relevant antigen needed for preparation by simple absorption of antisera to high-incidence antigens. An eluate prepared from group O red cells that react with the antibody in question should contain only the desired antibody, devoid of anti-A and anti-B. Antibodies purified in this manner can be preserved frozen if bovine albumin is added to bring the protein concentration to 6%. Frozen eluates of this sort are useful for phenotyping red cells from individuals whose serum appears to contain antibody to a high-incidence red cell antigen.

A similar approach can be applied to confirm the specificity of serologic reactions, particularly when a serum reacts with a number of reagent red cell samples that do not appear to share a common antigen. The serum may contain several antibodies to low-incidence antigens, or a single antibody to an unknown determinant for which the reagent red cells have not been tested. In the latter instance, but not the former, an eluate prepared after incubating the serum with one reactive red cell sample will react with all the other initially reactive cells.

Titration

The titer of an antibody is usually determined by testing serial two-fold dilutions of the serum against selected red cell samples. Results are expressed as the reciprocal of the highest serum dilution that causes macroscopically visible agglutination. Titration values can help quantify the relative antibody concentration in a serum, or the relative strength of antigen expression on red cells. Titration studies

are most frequently performed in the following situations:

1. Prenatal studies. The maternal serum containing alloantibodies is tested at intervals during pregnancy. The presence or absence of rising titers helps predict the likelihood of hemolytic disease of the newborn.

2. Antibody identification. Some antibodies agglutinate virtually all reagent red cell samples, but specificity is indicated by differences in reaction strength following dilution. For example, potent autoanti-I agglutinins may react in the undiluted state with both adult and cord blood red cells; in titration studies, the serum will be found to react at a higher dilution with adult $I+$ red cells than it does with i_{cord} red cells.

3. HTLA antibodies. The term "HTLA" is used to describe those antibodies that are weakly reactive in the undiluted state but, unlike most weakly reactive antibodies (eg, an anti-D with a titer of 4), react to a high titer (eg, 2000). Such antibodies include anti-Ch^a, -Rg^a, -Cs^a, -Yk^a, -Kn^a, -McC^a and -JMH. When weak reactions are observed in indirect antiglobulin tests, titration studies may establish whether the antibody displays HTLA characteristics.

At best, titration is a semiquantitative technique. Technical variables can greatly influence the results. For reliable results, these technical variables should be kept to a minimum.

1. Careful pipetting technique is essential. Recommended for use are automatic pipettes with disposable tips that can be changed after each dilution.

2. Incubation time, temperature and centrifugation times optimum for the antibody should be used consistently.

3. The age and concentration of the test red cells may affect the results. When the titers of several different examples of an antibody are to be compared, all sera should be tested against red cells (preferably freshly collected) from the same donor. If this is not practical, the

sera should be tested against a pool of reagent red cells from donors of the same apparent genotype. When a single serum is to be tested against different red cell samples, the samples should be collected and preserved in the same manner, and diluted to the same concentration, prior to use.

4. Completely reproducible results are virtually impossible to achieve. Comparisons are valid only when specimens are tested concurrently. When sequential prenatal serum samples are tested for changing antibody titer, samples should be frozen for comparison with subsequent specimens. Each new sample should be tested in parallel with the immediately preceding sample. In tests with a single serum against different reagent red cell samples, the same specimen of diluted serum must be used for all tests.

5. Measurements are more accurate with large volumes than with small volumes, and a master dilution technique gives more reliable results than individual dilutions for a single set of tests. If serum dilutions are to be tested against several reagent red cell samples, a sufficient volume of each dilution must be prepared so that the same dilution can be tested against each test red cell sample.

Technique for Master Dilution

The master dilution technique for titration is as follows:

1. Label test tubes according to the serum dilution (eg, 1 in 1, 1 in 2, etc.). A 1 in 1 dilution means one volume of serum undiluted; a 1 in 2 dilution means one volume of serum in a final volume of two, or a 50% concentration of serum in the diluent.

2. Deliver one volume of diluent (eg, 0.5% bovine albumin in saline) to all test tubes except the first tube (1 in 1).

3. Add an equal volume of serum to each of the first two tubes (1 in 1, 1 in 2).

4. Using a clean pipette, mix the contents of the 1 in 2 dilution several times, and

transfer one volume to the next tube (1 in 4 dilution).

5. Continue the same process for all dilutions, using a clean pipette for each transfer of diluted serum. Remove one volume of diluted serum from the final tube, and save for use if further dilutions are required.

6. Using separate pipettes for each dilution, transfer 0.1 ml of diluted serum into appropriately labeled test tubes. For each dilution to be tested, add 0.05 ml of the appropriate reagent red cell sample. The red cells should be prepared as a 2-5% suspension in the same diluent used to prepare the serum dilutions (eg, 0.5% bovine albumin in saline).

7. Mix well, and test by the appropriate technique.

8. Examine test results macroscopically, and grade and record the reactions. Since the prozone phenomenon (see page 82) may cause the reactions to be weaker with low serum dilutions than with the higher dilutions, it is preferable to commence reading with the tube containing the most dilute serum, and proceed to the most concentrated sample.

9. Report the results as the reciprocal of the highest dilution that produces agglutination. A titer is reported as 32, not 1 in 32 (see Table 13-6 for an example). If there is agglutination in the tube containing the most dilute serum, the end-point has not been reached, and additional dilutions must be prepared and tested.

In comparative studies, a difference in titer of at least two dilutions can be considered a significant difference. Variations in technical detail and inherent variability of the technique can cause duplicate results to differ by as much as one dilution.

Scoring

Titers alone can be misleading. Titration results can be expressed with more discrimination by assigning to each reaction a number based on the observed strength

Table 13-6. Examples of Antibody Titers and Scores

		Serum Dilutions								Titer	Score
		1/1	1/2	1/4	1/8	1/16	1/32	1/64	1/128		
Sample 1	Strength:	4+	3+	3+	2+	1+	1+	w	0	64	52
	Number:	12	10	10	8	5	5	2	0		
Sample 2	Strength:	4+	4+	4+	3+	3+	2+	1+	0	64	69
	Number:	12	12	12	10	10	8	5	0		
Sample 3	Strength:	1+	1+	1+	1+	w	w	w	0	64	30
	Number:	5	5	5	5	2	2	2	0		

of agglutination. The sum of these values represents the score, which is a semiquantitative measurement of antibody reactivity. A difference of 10 or more between different test samples has arbitrarily been deemed significant. In many laboratories, a scoring system similar to that described by Marsh[23] is used see page 462 for details).

Table 13-6 shows the results of titration studies on three sera, each with a titer of 64. The differences in score values, however, indicate substantial differences in reactivity. The results with sample 3 are characteristic of an HTLA antibody (eg, titer as high as 64, score only 30).

References

1. Giblett ER. Blood group alloantibodies: an assessment of some laboratory practices. Transfusion 1977;17:299-308.

2. Boral LI, Henry JB. The type and screen: A safe alternative and supplement in selected surgical procedures. Transfusion 1977;17: 163-168.

3. Ellisor SS. Action and applications of enzymes in immunohematology. In: Bell CA, ed. A seminar on antigen-antibody reactions revisited. Arlington, VA: American Association of Blood Banks, 1982:133-174

4. Issitt PD, Issitt CH. Applied blood group serology, 2nd ed. Oxnard, CA: Spectra Biologicals; 1975.

5. Mollison PL. Blood transfusion in clinical medicine, 7th ed. Oxford: Blackwell Scientific Publications; 1982.

6. Pierce SR. Anomalous blood bank results. In: Dawson RD, ed. Trouble shooting the crossmatch. Washington DC: American Association of Blood Banks; 1977:85-114.

7. Beattie KM, Zuelzer WW. The frequency and properties of pH-dependent anti-M. Transfusion 1965;5:322-326.

8. Freedman J, Masters CA, Newlands M, et al. Optimal conditions for use of sulphydryl compounds in dissociating red cell antibodies. Vox Sang 1976;30:231-239.

9. Romans DG, Tilley CA, Crookston MC, et al. Conversion of incomplete antibodies to direct agglutinins by mild reduction: evidence for segmental flexibility within the Fc fragment of immunoglobulin G. Proc Nat Acad Sci USA 1977;74:2531-2535.

10. Morton JA, Pickles MM, Terry AM. The Sd^a blood group antigen in tissues and body fluids. Vox Sang 1970;19:472-482.

11. Rolih SD, ed. High-titer low-avidity antibodies: recognition and resolution. Washington, DC: American Association of Blood Banks; 1979.

12. Crookston MC. Soluble antigens and leukocyte related antibodies. Part A. Blood group antigens in plasma: An aid in the identification of antibodies. In: Dawson RB, ed. Transfusion with "crossmatch incompatible" blood. Washington, DC: American Association of Blood Banks; 1975;20-25.

13. O'Neill GJ, Yang SY, Tegoli J, et al. Chido and Rodgers blood groups are distinct antigenic components of human complement C4. Nature 1978;273:668-670.

14. Tilley CA, Romans DG, Crookston MC. Localization of Chido and Rodgers to the C4d fragment of human C4 (abstract). Transfusion 1978;18:622.

15. Judd WJ, Kraemer K, Moulds JJ. The rapid identification of Chido and Rodgers anti-

bodies using C4d-coated red blood cells. Transfusion 1981;21:189-192.

16. Advani H, Zamor J, Judd WJ, Johnson CL, Marsh WL. Inactivation of Kell blood group antigens by 2-aminoethylisothiouronium bromide. Br J Haematol 1982;51:107-115.

17. Moulds J. Moulds M. Inactivation of Kell blood group antigens by 2-amino-ethylisothiou-ronium bromide (letter). Transfusion 1983;23:274-275.

18. Judd WJ. Elution of antibody from red cells. In: Bell CA, ed. A seminar on antigen-antibody reactions revisited. Arlington, VA: American Association of Blood Banks; 1982:175-221.

19. Landsteiner K, Miller CP Jr. Serological studies on the blood of primates. II. The blood

groups in anthropoid apes. J Exp Med 1925;42:853-862.

20. Rubin H. Antibody elution from red cells. J Clin Pathol 1963;1570-1573.

21. Jenkins DE Jr, Moore WH. A rapid method for the preparation of high potency auto- and alloantibody eluates. Transfusion 1977;17:110-114.

22. Beattie KM. Laboratory investigation and management of antibody specificities in warm autoimmune hemolytic anemia. In: Bell CA, ed. A seminar on laboratory management of hemolysis. Washington, DC: American Association of Blood Banks; 1979:105-150.

23. Marsh WL. Scoring of hemagglutination reactions. Transfusion 1972;12:352-353.

14

Investigation of a Positive Direct Antiglobulin Test and Immune Hemolysis

Significance of a Positive Direct Antiglobulin Test

A positive direct antiglobulin test (DAT) does not imply that an individual's red cells have a shortened survival. As many as 10% of hospital patients, and between 1 in 4000 to 1 in 9000 blood donors, may have a positive DAT without clinical manifestations of immune-mediated hemolysis.[1-4] A positive DAT, with or without associated shortened red cell survival, may be caused by the in vivo phenomena listed below, but in some cases no explanation is apparent.

1. Autoantibodies to intrinsic red cell antigens that coat red cells with immunoglobulins or complement, or both.[1,5,6]
2. Alloantibodies present in the recipient of a recent transfusion that react with antigens on donor red cells.
3. Antibodies transfused in donor plasma or plasma products that react with antigens on the recipient's red cells.
4. Maternal alloantibodies that cross the placenta and coat fetal red cells. These antibodies are often associated with hemolytic disease of the newborn.[7]
5. Antibodies directed against certain drugs, such as penicillin, that bind to red cell membranes.[8]

6. Red cell membrane modifications resulting from therapy with certain drugs, notably those of the cephalosporin group, leading to nonspecific adsorption onto red cells of proteins, including immunoglobulins.[8]
7. Drug-antidrug complexes that develop when a patient with suitable antibodies receives drugs such as quinidine and phenacetin.[8] These immune complexes cause complement components and sometimes IgG to be bound to red cells.
8. Antihuman species antibodies present in the equine antihuman-lymphocyte globulin sometimes given to recipients of organ and bone marrow transplants.[9]

The results of direct antiglobulin testing should reflect in vivo conditions; in vitro phenomena associated with the collection, storage or handling of blood samples can affect test results, and before further studies are undertaken on a patient with a positive DAT, causes of in vitro red cell coating should be excluded. False-positive DAT results are most often associated with the use of refrigerated, clotted blood samples, in which complement components coat red cells in vitro. Any positive DAT result obtained from a clotted blood sample should be confirmed using a freshly collected EDTA anticoagulated specimen. Causes of false-positive antiglobulin tests are discussed in Chapter 6.

Evaluation of a Positive DAT

Extent of Testing

Clinical considerations should dictate the extent to which a positive DAT is evaluated, and dialogue with the attending physician is important before any additional serologic tests are undertaken. Interpretation of serologic findings requires knowledge of the patient's diagnosis, drug therapy and recent transfusion history. The significance of serologic results should be evaluated in light of the patient's clinical condition, and laboratory data such as hematocrit, bilirubin, haptoglobin and reticulocyte count.

Answers to the following questions may help decide what investigations are appropriate when a positive DAT is encountered in patients other than newborns:

1. *Is there evidence of in vivo hemolysis?* Reticulocytosis, hemoglobinemia, hemoglobinuria, decreased serum haptoglobin, and elevated levels of serum unconjugated bilirubin or lactic dehydrogenase (LDH), especially LDH_1, may be associated with hemolysis.[1,10] If an anemic patient with a positive DAT manifests clinical signs and symptoms of hemolysis, it is appropriate to determine if the hemolysis has an immune basis. On the other hand, if there is no evidence of hemolysis, no further studies are necessary in most instances, except as detailed below.

2. *Does the patient's serum contain unexpected antibodies?* Serum antibodies may have coated circulating red cells, either the patient's own or transfused cells. Investigating a positive DAT may help identify the unexpected serum antibodies.

3. *Has the patient been recently transfused?* Many workers routinely attempt to determine the cause of a positive DAT or autologous control when the patient has been recently transfused. A positive test on a recipient of a recent transfusion may indicate an immune response to recently transfused red cells, with alloantibodies present that could jeopardize the safety of subsequent transfusions. Instances in which clinically significant alloantibodies would not also be detected during pretransfusion serum studies are, however, infrequent. Because of the costs involved in evaluating all positive tests, and the low yield of clinically significant results, some workers no longer advocate the routine performance of a pretransfusion DAT or autologous control.[11]

4. *Is the patient receiving any drugs, especially α-methyldopa (eg, Aldomet) or intravenous penicillin?* Approximately 3% of patients receiving intravenous penicillin and 15-20% of patients receiving α-methyldopa will develop a positive DAT,[1,8] but less than 1% of those patients who develop a positive DAT have hemolytic anemia. The attending physician should be alerted if a patient receiving α-methyldopa or intravenous penicillin develops a positive DAT, so that appropriate surveillance for hemolysis can be maintained.

5. *Is the patient receiving antilymphocyte globulin (ALG) or antithymocyte globulin (ATG)?* Patients receiving ALG or ATG produced in horses develop a positive DAT within a few days after such therapy is initiated.[9] ALT and ALG preparations have very high titers of antispecies antibodies, which coat the recipient's red cells. Many rabbit antihuman globulin reagents contain antihorse antibodies that react with the horse immunoglobulins.[12] Antihuman globulin reagents can be absorbed, before use, with red cells coated with ALG or ATG in vitro, or can be partially neutralized with horse serum.

Collection of Blood Samples

To ensure that a positive DAT represents in vivo conditions, not in vitro phenomena such as the uptake of complement components by clotted specimens, blood anticoagulated with EDTA should be obtained. This is used for direct antiglobulin testing, and provides a source of red cells for elution if required. A freshly collected clotted blood sample is needed for serum studies; if cold hemagglutinin disease or paroxysmal cold hemoglobinuria are suspected as causing the positive DAT, the clotted specimen should be maintained at 37 C until the serum has been separated.

Initial Serologic Studies

Once the decision has been made to evaluate a positive DAT, three areas of investigation are helpful in ascertaining the cause of in vivo red cell coating.
1. Tests with anti-IgG and anti-C3d antiglobulin reagents, to determine the types of protein coating the red cells (see Chapter 6).
2. Detection of unexpected serum antibodies. If they are found, antibodies should be studied at room temperature, 37 C and by an indirect antiglobulin technique with untreated group O reagent red cell samples; tests at 37 C and by the indirect antiglobulin technique with enzyme-treated red cells may also be useful.
3. Preparation and testing of an eluate prepared from the coated red cells. The eluate should be tested by an indirect antiglobulin test against a panel of untreated group O reagent red cell samples, and against enzyme-treated red cells, if available. Ideally, the latter should consist of R_1R_1, R_2R_2 and rr red cells, and include among them one K+, one Jk(a+b−) and one Jk(a−b+) sample. If warm-reactive autoantibodies are suspected, the designated Rh phenotypes afford maximal sensitivity for detecting autoantibodies with Rh-related activity (eg, autoanti-e). If

the patient has been recently transfused, the suggested phenotypes provide optimal sensitivity for detecting alloantibodies to Rh, Kell and Kidd system antigens. Such antibodies are frequently associated with an immune response to recently transfused red cells.

Further Studies

Depending on the initial results, further studies may be appropriate. For example, if alloantibody appears to be present in serum or eluate, or both, additional studies may be required to confirm specificity. Chapter 13 details the procedures involved in the identification of alloantibodies. If both serum and eluate are nonreactive at all test phases, and if the patient is known to have received intravenous penicillin, then tests with penicillin-coated red cells should be considered. If the patient received blood components of an ABO group other than his own, testing the eluate with group A and B red cells may indicate that passively acquired anti-A or anti-B is responsible for the positive DAT. *When no unexpected antibodies are present in the serum, when the patient has not been recently transfused, and when autoantibody is the only activity in the eluate, no further serologic testing is necessary.*

Some of the procedures used for differentiating between auto and alloantibody activity are discussed in Chapter 13. The remaining sections of this chapter describe procedures used to classify autoimmune and drug-induced hemolysis, and tests intended to ensure safe transfusion management of the patients concerned. Alloimmune hemolysis, resulting in hemolytic disease of the newborn or associated with an immune response to recently transfused red cells, is discussed in Chapters 16 and 17.

Immune Hemolysis

Immune hemolysis is shortened red cell survival resulting from an immune reaction. If bone marrow compensation is adequate, hemolysis may not result in anemia.

Hemolysis is but one cause of anemia, and there are many causes of hemolysis unrelated to immune reactions.[1,5,6,10] Serologic investigations do not determine whether or not a patient has hemolytic anemia. This diagnosis rests on clinical findings and such laboratory data as hemoglobin or hematocrit values; reticulocyte count; red cell morphology; bilirubin, haptoglobin and LDH levels; and, sometimes, red cell survival studies. The serologic findings help determine whether the hemolysis has an immune basis, and if so, what type of immune hemolytic anemia is present. This is important, since the treatment for each type is different.

Immune hemolytic anemia may be classified in various ways. One classification is shown in Table 14-1. In one series involving over 300 patients with immune hemolytic anemia, 70% had immune hemolysis associated with warm-reactive autoantibodies, 16% had cold hemagglutinin dis-

Table 14-1. Classification of Immune Hemolytic Anemia*

Autoimmune Hemolytic Anemia:
1. Associated with warm-reactive autoantibodies (WAIHA)
   a. primary (idiopathic)
   b. secondary (WAIHA present together with such conditions as lymphoma, SLE, carcinoma, etc.)
2. Associated with cold-reactive autoantibodies
   a. cold hemagglutinin disease (CHD)
      1) primary (idiopathic)
      2) secondary (CHD present together with such conditions as lymphoma, pneumonia, infectious mononucleosis)
   b. paroxysmal cold hemoglobinuria
      1) primary (idiopathic)
      2) secondary (PCH present together with such conditions as syphilis, viral infections)

Drug-Induced Hemolytic Anemia:
See table 14-4

Alloimmune Hemolytic Anemia:
1. Hemolytic disease of the newborn
2. Hemolytic transfusion reactions

*After Petz and Garratty.[1]

ease, 2% had paroxysmal cold hemoglobinuria, and 12% had drug-induced hemolysis.[1] Other reported series are similar.[13]

Warm Autoimmune Hemolytic Anemia

The most common type of immune hemolysis is warm autoimmune hemolytic anemia (WAIHA), associated with antibodies reactive at warm (37 C) temperatures. Typical serologic findings are given below.

Direct Antiglobulin Test

Three patterns of reactivity may be seen in WAIHA when monospecific anti-IgG and anti-C3d reagents are used. In 67% of cases red cells are coated with both IgG and complement; in approximately 20% of cases the red cells are coated with IgG alone, and in 13% only with complement.[1] Rarely, IgA or IgM coating can also be demonstrated and very rare cases have been described in which IgA or IgM was the only globulin present.[1,13,14]

Serum

Very little autoantibody may be free in the serum, as the autoantibody reacts optimally at 37 C and is being continuously adsorbed by red cells in vivo. Autoantibody tends to appear in serum when all the specific antigen sites on the red cells have been occupied, and no more can be found in vivo; hence, the DAT is strongly positive. Sera from approximately 50% of patients with WAIHA contain autoantibody that reacts with untreated red cells. The autoantibody is usually IgG, and is best demonstrated by indirect antiglobulin techniques. With more sensitive methods, notably testing enzyme-treated red cells, over 90% of sera can be shown to contain autoantibody. Antibodies that, in routine procedures, hemolyze or agglutinate untreated red cells are extremely rare, but approximately 15% of sera contain warm-reactive antibodies that hemolyze enzyme-treated red cells. Approximately one-third of patients with WAIHA also have cold-reactive autoagglutinins demonstrable in tests at 20 C, but this does not mean the patient has cold hemagglutinin disease (CHD) in addition to WAIHA. Cold agglutinin titers at 4 C are not elevated.[1] The serum may contain alloantibodies in addition to autoantibodies, or alloantibodies may be present alone.

Eluate

Autoantibody can be characterized only by making and examining an eluate. The presence of the IgG autoantibody on the red cells is best confirmed by elution with digitonin acid or an organic solvent such as ether (see pages 429–433). IgG may be present at such low levels that elution studies are nonreactive. If complement is the only protein coating the red cells, the eluate will have no serologic activity.

Specificity of Autoantibody

The specificity of autoantibodies associated with WAIHA is very complex.[1,15–17] Specificity is often directed against the Rh antigen complex, but this can only be determined if red cells of very rare phenotypes are available, such as -D-/-D- or Rh_{null}. Apart from Rh specificity, there have been other reports of warm-reactive autoantibodies with anti-U, -LW, -I^T, -K_p^b, -K13, -Jk^a, -Xg^a, -Ge, -En^a, -Wr^b, -A and -N specificites. Testing for such specificity is not routinely necessary.

Cold Hemagglutinin Disease

Cold hemagglutinin disease (CHD) is the most common type of hemolytic anemia associated with cold-reactive autoantibodies, and accounts for approximately 16% of all cases of immune hemolysis.[1,13] It occurs as an acute or chronic condition. The acute form is often secondary to lymphoproliferative disorders (eg, lymphoma), or *Mycoplasma pneumoniae* infection. The chronic form is often seen in elderly patients and results in a mild to moderate degree of hemolysis; Raynaud's phenomenon and hemoglobinuria may occur in cold weather. Typical serologic findings are discussed below.

Direct Antiglobulin Test

Complement is the only globulin detected on the red cells. The cold-reactive autoantibody is an IgM immunoglobulin that reacts with red cells in the peripheral circulation, where the temperature falls to 32 C, and binds complement components (C3 and C4, in particular) to the red cells at this temperature. As the red cells return to warmer parts of the circulation, the IgM immunoglobulin dissociates, leaving red cells coated only with complement. The components present on circulating red cells are C3d and C4d, resulting from the action of Factor I (see page 81). It is the anti-C3d component of polyspecific antiglobulin reagents that accounts for the positive DAT.

Serum

Cold-reactive IgM autoagglutinins associated with immune hemolysis are usually present at titers greater than 1000 when tested at 4 C. They rarely react in vitro with saline-suspended red cells at temperatures above 32 C, but if 30% bovine albumin is included in the reaction medium, 70% of clinically significant examples will react at 37 C.[18] Hemolytic activity against untreated red cells can sometimes be demonstrated at 20-25 C and, except in rare cases with anti-Pr specificity, enzyme-treated red cells are always hemolyzed in the presence of adequate complement. In chronic CHD the IgM autoagglutinin is usually a monoclonal protein of the kappa light chain type. Polyclonal IgM immunoglobulins (with normal kappa and lambda light chain distribution) are associated with the acute form of the disease. Rare examples of IgA and IgG cold-reactive autoagglutinins also have been described.

Eluate

If the red cells have been collected and washed at 37 C, no antibody reactivity will be found in the eluate, as only complement components are present on the red cells in vivo at 37 C.

Specificity of Autoantibody

The most common specificity associated with CHD is anti-I. Less commonly, anti-i specificity is found, usually associated with infectious mononucleosis. On rare occasions, cold-reactive autoagglutinins with anti-Pr (also called anti-Sp₁) specificity are seen (see pages 467-468).

Paroxysmal Cold Hemoglobinuria

The rarest form of autoimmune hemolytic anemia is paroxysmal cold hemoglobinuria (PCH). In the past, it was characteristically associated with syphilis, but this association is unusual nowadays. More commonly, PCH presents as an acute transient condition secondary to viral infections, particulary in young children. It can also occur as an idiopathic chronic disease in older people. Typical serologic findings are discussed below.

Direct Antiglobulin Test

The autoantibody in PCH is an IgG protein, but like IgM cold-reactive autoagglutinins, the IgG autoantibody in PCH reacts with red cells in colder parts of the body, causes complement components (C3 and C4) to be bound irreversibly to red cells, and then elutes at warmer temperatures. Consequently, only complement components are found coating red cells.

Serum

The IgG autoantibody in PCH is classically described as a biphasic hemolysin, since it binds to red cells at low temperatures and causes hemolysis only when red cells are warmed to 37 C. This is the basis of the diagnostic test for the disease, the Donath-Landsteiner test. Coating and complement binding are the usual properties of the autoantibody, but coating does not occur, in vitro, above 15 C. The autoantibody often agglutinates normal red cells at 4 C, but rarely at titers greater than 64.

Eluate

As in CHD, only complement components are present on red cells in vivo at 37 C. Consequently, eluates prepared from red cells of patients with PCH are invariably nonreactive.

Specificity of Autoantibody

The autoantibody of PCH has most frequently been shown to have anti-P specificity; it reacts with all red cells (including the patient's own red cells) except those of the very rare p or pᵏ phenotypes. Exceptional examples with anti-IH specificity have also been described.[7]

Classification of Autoimmune Hemolytic Anemias

Classifying autoimmune hemolytic anemias into one of the three major types described above, warm autoimmune hemolytic anemia (WAIHA), cold hemagglutinin disease (CHD), and paroxysmal cold hemoglobinuria (PCH), sometimes may be made easier by employing two additional tests, a "diagnostic" cold agglutinin titer, and the Donath-Landsteiner test for PCH. These procedures are described in detail on pages 457 and 458, and a summary of the Donath-Landsteiner test is given in Table 14-2. Table 14-3 summarizes serologic findings in each of these conditions.

Serologic Investigation of Blood Samples Containing Autoantibodies

Serologic techniques employed to investigate autoimmune hemolysis are directed at obtaining answers to the following questions:

Question #1: *Are the patient's red cells coated with antibody or complement, or both?*

Most commercially prepared polyspecific antiglobulin reagents detect IgG coating adequately, and the anticomplement activity of these products has improved in recent years. However, as discussed in Chapter 6, some polyspecific reagents may

Table 14-2. The Donath-Landsteiner Test for PCH

Tube #	Volumes of:			Incubation (minutes)	
	Patient's Serum	Fresh Normal Serum	P+ Red Cells	0 C[†]	37 C
*A1	10	none	1		
*A2	10	10	1	30	60
A3	none	10	1		
B1	10	none	1		
B2	10	10	1	90	none
B3	none	10	1		
C1	10	none	1		
C2	10	10	1	none	90
C3	none	10	1		

*The Donath-Landsteiner test is positive when there is hemolysis only in tubes A1 and/or A2.
†Tests incubated in melting ice.

detect complement coating only if the tests are incubated at room temperature for 5 to 10 minutes. This also applies to those rare cases of WAIHA in which IgA is present on red cells. A single nonreactive DAT obtained with a polyspecific antiglobulin reagent should not be considered definitive evidence against autoimmune hemolysis in a patient with clinical signs and symptoms. Rare cases of WAIHA exist in which the number of IgG molecules on the red cells is below the threshold of sensitivity for the DAT, and autoimmune hemolysis occurs in the absence of positive results in direct antiglobulin testing.[19]

Although the majority (87%) of WAIHA cases have both IgG and complement or IgG alone on the red cells, complement coating alone is seen in 13% of WAIHA cases, as well as in CHD and PCH.[1] Monospecific antiglobulin reagents (see Chapter 6) provide the best demonstration of these proteins. In some cases of WAIHA, IgA or IgM may be present in addition to IgG or complement, but this is quite uncommon.

The use of monospecific antiglobulin reagents requires some caution. Tests should be performed in parallel with a control, consisting either of saline or, preferably, the manufacturer's diluent for the antiglobulin serum. This control detects

autoagglutination, which may occur in CHD and, if not recognized, can lead to the incorrect conclusion that red cells are coated with both IgG and complement. Anti-IgG and anti-C3 reagents are the only currently available products licensed for use with human red cells. Other antiglobulin reagents (eg, anti-IgA, -IgM, -C4) are commercially available but, as they are prepared for use in precipitation tests such as immunodiffusion, their reactivity should be carefully standardized. They may contain antihuman species antibodies, which must be removed by absorption with uncoated human red cells or by diluting the reagent to a point at which the antihuman species activity is undetectable. Quality assurance must be precise. Agglutination is more sensitive than precipitation; a serum found to be monospecific by precipitation tests may react with several different proteins in antiglobulin tests using agglutination.[20]

Question #2: *Does the serum contain antibodies? If so, are these antibodies:*

agglutinating or nonagglutinating?

hemolytic in vitro?

optimally reactive at warm or cold (37 C or 4 C) temperatures?

autoantibodies?

alloantibodies?

Table 14-3. Serologic Findings in Autoimmune Hemolytic Anemia*

	WAIHA[†]	CHD[†]	PCH[†]
Direct Antiglobulin Test:	20% IgG alone; 67% IgG + C3; 13% C3 alone	C3 alone	C3 alone
Eluate:	IgG antibody	nonreactive	nonreactive
Immunoglobulin Type:	IgG (sometimes IgA or IgM, rarely alone)	IgM (rarely IgA)	IgG
Serum:	57% react by indirect antiglobulin techniques; 13% hemolyze enzyme-treated red cells at 37 C; 90% agglutinate enzyme-treated red cells at 37 C; 30% agglutinate untreated red cells at 20 C; rarely agglutinate untreated red cells at 37 C	cold-reactive antibody titer > 640 at 4 C; reacts up to 32 C; monoclonal protein (kappa light chain in chronic disease)	potent hemolysin but may agglutinate red cells at 4 C; classically referred to as biphasic hemolysin (ie, coats red cells at low temperatures, then hemolyzes them when warmed to 37 C); does not usually coat red cells above 15 C
Specificity:	usually within Rh system, but often combined with a "nonspecific" component; other specificities include anti-LW, -U, -En[a], "-Wr[b]", -I[T], -K, -Kp[b], Jk[a]	usually anti-I but can be anti-i; anti-Pr very rare	anti-P (ie, nonreactive with p and p[k] red cells)

*Data from Petz and Garratty.[1]
[†]WAIHA: Warm autoimmune hemolytic anemia; CHD: cold hemagglutinin disease; PCH: paroxysmal cold hemoglobinuria.

These questions can usually be answered from the results of serologic tests used for the detection and identification of unexpected antibodies (see Chapters 12 and 13).

Question #3: *Is antibody activity present in the eluate?*

If red cells are coated only with complement, as in CHD, PCH, and 13% of WAIHA cases, no antibody will be detected in the eluate. Autoantibody can sometimes be detected in eluates from these WAIHA cases if enzyme-treated red cells are used, particularly if the eluate is concentrated prior to testing. When antibody is found in an eluate from a recently transfused patient, its specificity should be examined to establish whether it is autoantibody or alloantibody made in response to the transfused red cells. If the DAT is strongly positive with anti-IgG, but the eluate is nonreactive with untreated and enzyme-treated red cells, the possibility of drug-associated hemolysis should be considered. See final sections of this chapter for appropriate tests.

Technical Considerations

The following technical variations may be useful additions to routine tests:

1. Prewarmed tests. Autoantibodies strongly reactive at room temperature may appear to react at 37 C unless temperature conditions are strictly controlled. This can confuse the classification of the autoimmune process and misrepresent the clinical significance of the autoantibody. The patient's serum and reagent red cells should be warmed to 37 C separately, prior to mixing. The tests should be centrifuged at 37 C, and red cells for indirect antiglobulin tests should be washed at 37 C with 4 C saline (see Chapter 12 for method).

2. Addition of complement. Patients with autoimmune hemolytic anemia sometimes have low serum complement levels. Antibody reactivity can sometimes be enhanced by adding fresh normal serum as a source of complement.

3. Acidification of serum. Some workers[1,5] prefer the pH of the test conditions to be between 6.5 and 6.8, as this seems optimal for detection of both cold- and warm-reactive hemolysins. This can be achieved by adding one-tenth volume of 0.2 N HCl to the serum.

4. Enzyme tests. Both warm- and cold-reactive autoantibodies may give enhanced reactions with enzyme-treated red cells. When serologic classification of the autoimmune process is difficult, tests with enzyme-treated cells may provide additional information. Autoantibodies are more likely to hemolyze enzyme-treated red cells than untreated red cells.

Determining Specificity of Warm-Reactive Autoantibodies

Determining the specificity of warm-reactive autoantibodies is usually of only academic interest, unless the patient is actively hemolyzing and requires blood transfusion. The undiluted serum or eluate usually reacts with all red cell samples of common Rh phenotypes, but strength of reactivity may vary. If red cells of such rare phenotypes as -D-/-D- or Rh_{null} are available, approximately 70% of warm-reactive autoantibodies can be shown to have an Rh-related specificity. Apparent clear-cut specificity such as anti-D, -C, -c, -E or -e, is present only rarely, with anti-e specificity being the most common. Occasional examples of autoantibodies with specificities for other blood group system antigens (U, LW, I^T, K, Kp^b, K13, Jk^a, En^a, "Wr^b," Xg^a, Ge, A, N) have also been reported. Rh-related specificity not apparent in tests with undiluted serum or eluate may become apparent after dilution or upon performing absorption and elution studies.

Dilution of Serum or Eluate

Titration studies may help to define relative Rh specificity when there is uniform reactivity with the undiluted serum or eluate. Serial two-fold dilutions of serum or eluate are tested by the indirect antiglobulin technique against group O reagent red cell samples of the phenotypes R_1R_1, R_2R_2 and rr (see page 465 for method). Rh-related specificity is inferred when the red cell samples react to different degrees. For example, the titer against R_1R_1 and rr (e-positive) red cells might be 64, compared with 8 obtained against R_2R_2 (e-negative) red cells. Testing a 1 in 16 dilution against a reagent red cell panel would demonstrate anti-e specificity. In this situation, the autoantibody is said to have relative anti-e specificity.

Absorption and Elution Studies

A better but more time-consuming way to determine specificity is to attempt isolation of different specificities by absorbing the serum or eluate with red cells of different phenotypes. Since Rh-related specificity is most common, selected Rh phenotypes (eg,

R_1R_1, R_2R_2, rr) are usually used, but cells expressing other antigens may be selected if indicated. Each absorbed specimen is then tested against a panel of reagent red cells to determine the specificity of those autoantibodies left unabsorbed. In addition, eluates prepared from the adsorbing red cells can be tested for specificity.

This method requires substantial quantities of red cells of selected phenotypes, and also requires a great deal of effort. However, the results can sometimes be rewarding in defining specificities within complex mixtures of warm-reactive autoantibodies.

Determining Specificity of Cold-Reactive Autoantibodies

The specificity of cold-reactive autoantibodies is not diagnostic for CHD. Autoanti-I antibodies may exist in healthy subjects. The nonpathogenic form of anti-I rarely reacts at 4 C at titers above 64 and is usually nonreactive with I-negative (i_{cord} and i_{adult}) red cells at room temperature. In contrast, the pathogenic form of anti-I that occurs in CHD may react quite strongly with I-negative red cells in tests at room temperature, while even stronger reactions are observed with I-positive red cells. Anti-i antibodies react in the opposite manner; they give much stronger reactions with I-negative red cells than they do with red cells that are I-positive.

I-positive and I-negative red cells differ from each other only in quantitative, not qualitative, expression of I and i antigens. Titration is required to determine the specificity of cold-reactive autoantibodies. A procedure for this is given on page 467.

Management of Patients with Autoantibodies

In pretransfusion tests on patients with autoantibodies, the following problems may arise:

1. Cold-reactive autoantibodies can cause discrepant ABO and Rh grouping results, either from autoagglutination of the patient's cells or agglutination of A and B red cells used in reverse grouping tests.
2. Red cells strongly coated with IgG may agglutinate spontaneously when exposed to the high protein content of some commercially prepared anti-Rh sera, resulting in discrepant Rh grouping results.
3. The presence of free autoantibody in the serum may make it virtually impossible to obtain serologically compatible blood for transfusion. Of particular concern in this situation is the possibility that autoantibody may mask the presence of a clinically significant alloantibody. Providing time permits, the presence or absence of alloantibody should be determined (see pages 463–466) before blood is transfused.

Although it is desirable to resolve these serologic problems in patients with autoantibodies, the delay imposed by efforts to find serologically compatible blood may in some cases cause greater danger to the patient than administration of serologically incompatible blood. Only clinical judgement can resolve this dilemma. Dialogue with the patient's physician is important.

Resolution of ABO Grouping Problems

ABO grouping problems associated with cold-reactive autoagglutinins may respond to several approaches. Often, it is only necessary to maintain the blood sample at 37 C immediately after collection and to wash the red cells with warm (37 C to 45 C) saline prior to testing. A negative control test, using 6% bovine albumin in saline to suspend the cells, will demonstrate residual autoagglutination. If the control test is nonreactive, the results obtained with anti-A and anti-B are valid. When autoagglutination still occurs, interpretation of the results can be difficult, but comparing the strength of the observed reactions may be informative.

Blood samples kept at room temperature or those containing potent cold-reactive autoagglutinins can be processed by incubating the red cells at 45 C for 5 to 10 minutes and then washing them several times in 45 C saline before testing. Alternatively, since these autoagglutinins are IgM proteins and thiol reagents dissociate IgM molecules, such reagents (eg, 2-mercaptoethanol or dithiothreitol) may be used to abolish autoagglutination, and permit accurate ABO grouping of the red cells (see page 463).

When the serum agglutinates group O reagent red cells, the results of reverse grouping tests may be unreliable. Repeat studies using prewarmed serum and group A and B red cells incubated at 37 C, or absorbed serum (either autoabsorbed or absorbed with homologous group O red cells), will often be informative.

Resolution of Rh Grouping Problems

Discrepant Rh grouping results may occur if cold-reactive autoantibodies spontaneously agglutinate the red cells. The procedures described for resolution of ABO grouping problems should be used. Red cells strongly coated with IgG (eg, in WAIHA) may spontaneously agglutinate when mixed with antisera containing high concentrations of proteins or other potentiators of agglutination. High-protein reagents designated for use by slide or rapid tube tests (sometimes referred to as modified-tube anti-Rh) are most likely to cause problems with IgG-coated red cells. The inclusion of appropriate controls or the use of chemically modified or saline-reactive reagents may be necessary to avoid erroneous results (see Chapter 9).

Detection of Alloantibodies in the Presence of Warm-Reactive Autoantibodies

If warm-reactive autoantibodies are present in the serum of a patient requiring transfusion, it is important to determine whether alloantibodies are also present. In initial studies, the presence of alloantibodies may be masked by autoantibody activity.

There are several ways to detect alloantibodies in the presence of warm-reactive autoantibodies. Some procedures involve the use of absorption techniques, the principles of which are discussed in Chapter 13. Several approaches are discussed below.

Testing the Patient's Cells

It can be helpful to know the blood group phenotype of the patient's own red cells. This permits prediction of those alloantibodies a patient is capable of producing. The possibility of antibody production exists for any blood group antigen absent from the patient's cells. When the red cells are coated with IgG, antiglobulin-reactive reagents such as anti-Fy^a or anti-Jk^a cannot be used unless the IgG is removed from the red cells prior to testing. A procedure for this, involving the use of chloroquine disphosphate, is given on page 418. It is possible to absorb the reagent antiserum with the patient's red cells, and test by titration for a decrease in reactivity, but this is time-consuming and requires large volumes of expensive antisera.

Autologous Absorption

The best way to detect alloantibodies in the presence of warm-reactive autoantibodies is to test serum after autologous absorption. Two procedures are given on pages 463–465. It is necessary to elute autoantibody from the red cells to make the sites available for in vitro autoantibody absorption, since maximal antibody attachment will have occurred at the 37 C in vivo conditions. In addition, treating the autologous red cells with proteolytic enzymes increases their capacity to adsorb autoantibody. The absorbed serum is examined for alloantibody activity after absorption has removed autoantibody.

Autologous absorption studies are most applicable when the patient has not been recently transfused; ie, there are no circulating transfused red cells that might adsorb an alloantibody. "Recent," in this context, usually means within the 3 to 4 month life span of normal red cells. Autologous absorption may be informative even a week or two after transfusion, although absence of alloantibody activity in autoabsorbed serum from a recently transfused patient cannot be considered conclusive evidence that alloantibody is absent.

It is also possible to separate the patient's own red cells from the transfused red cells and to use the harvested autologous red cells for autoadsorption. Small quantities (eg 0.2 ml) of autologous red cells can be harvested with either of the red cell separation techniques described on pages 419–421. Such red cells can be used for autologous adsorption of a small volume (eg, 6-8 drops) of serum using the procedure described on page 464. Simple antibody detection tests can then be done on the absorbed serum to determine the presence or absence of unexpected alloantibodies.

Homologous Absorption

Homologous absorption studies are appropriate when the patient has been recently transfused, or when insufficient red cells are available for autoabsorption. When the patient's Rh phenotype is not known, group O red cell samples of three different Rh phenotypes (R_1R_1, R_2R_2 and rr) should be selected. All should be K −, one should lack Jk^a, and another Jk^b, and one sample should be s −. These red cells, enzyme-treated to denature Fy^a, Fy^b and S antigens and to increase their absorptive capacity, are used to absorb separate aliquots of the patient's serum, one phenotype for each aliquot. Each aliquot may have to be absorbed two or three times. The absorbed aliquots are then tested against selected group O reagent red cells known either to lack or to carry common antigens of the Rh, MN, Kidd, Kell and Duffy blood group systems.

Absorbing the serum with different red cell samples provides a battery of absorbed specimens that can be used for antibody detection and identification purposes. For example, if the aliquot absorbed with K-negative red cells subsequently reacts only with K-positive red cells, the presence of alloanti-K can be inferred.

Untreated red cells may be used for homologous absorption, but are less efficient than enzyme-treated red cells in removing autoantibody. The phenotypes of these red cells should be selected to include samples lacking Fy^a, Fy^b and S antigens. When enzyme-treated red cells are used, they should be tested with reagent antisera to show that they lack Fy^a, Fy^b and S antigens; otherwise, alloantibodies to these antigens would be removed by the absorption process. Another modification of this homologous absorption technique is to treat the red cells with ZZAP reagent (a mixture of papain and dithiothreitol) prior to absorption (see pages 464–465). ZZAP-treated red cells lack M, N, S, Fy^a, Fy^b and all Kell system antigens except Kx.

The number of different red cell phenotypes required may be reduced if the patient's Rh phenotype is known. If the patient has been recently transfused, this can be determined after separating autologous from transfused red cells (see pages 419–421).

Dilution Technique

This is not the optimal way to detect alloantibodies in the presence of autoantibody (see page 465 for method); it is useful only when alloantibodies are present at a higher titer than autoantibodies.

Interpretation of Results

Autoantibody reactivity occasionally may be mistaken for alloantibody.[21] For example, the serum of an R_1R_1 patient may have apparent anti-c activity. Even though the patient's red cells lack the c antigen, the anti-c reactivity may in fact be due to warm-reactive autoantibody. That such reactivity is due to autoantibody can be determined by autologous and homologous absorption studies. In the situation mentioned, the apparent alloanti-c will be absorbed by both autologous and homologous R_1R_1 red cells, whereas true alloanti-c will be absorbed only by c-positive red cells.

Detection of Alloantibodies in the Presence of Cold-Reactive Autoantibodies

Potent cold-reactive autoagglutinins, like warm-reactive autoantibodies, may mask clinically significant alloantibodies. If the autoagglutinins are reactive at 32 C, or if they bind complement to red cells in the indirect antiglobulin test, it is advisable to absorb the serum at 4 C with the patient's own red cells (see page 466). This should uncover clinically significant alloantibodies. Complete absorption of high-titer cold-reactive autoagglutinins can be very time-consuming. Enzyme treatment of the patient's red cells often facilitates absorption of autoantibody.

If autologous absorption studies are inappropriate because of recent transfusion or if autoantibody cannot be completely removed, tests for alloantibody activity should be performed strictly at 37 C. The patient's serum and reagent red cells should be warmed to 37 C prior to mixing. Bovine albumin enhances the reactivity of cold-reactive autoantibodies,[18] and should not be used. If centrifugation at 37 C is impossible, tests can be incubated at 37 C for 1 to 2 hours and the settled red cells can be examined for agglutination without centrifugation. The red cells should be washed in saline at 37 C and then tested with antiglobulin serum. Some workers prefer to use anti-IgG at this stage, rather than a polyspecific antiglobulin serum, to avoid detecting any complement bound by the cold-reactive autoantibody. EDTA-anticoagulated plasma, or serum to which EDTA has been added (2 ml serum plus 0.25 ml 4.45% K_2EDTA),[22] can also be used to avoid interference by complement-binding autoantibodies.

Selection of Blood for Patients with WAIHA

It is best to avoid transfusing patients who have WAIHA. If transfusion is essential, the smallest volume of red cells necessary to maintain adequate oxygen transportation should be given. Serologically compatible blood may not be obtainable, and there is substantial risk that concomitant alloantibodies could cause a severe hemolytic transfusion reaction. The clinical need must justify the risk of transfusion, but needed transfusions should not be withheld because serologically compatible blood cannot be found. Clinical judgement must always be the deciding factor. The procedures described above to detect alloantibodies in the presence of autoantibody should be employed if time permits. If alloantibodies are present, blood lacking the corresponding antigen(s) should be selected for transfusion.

Autoantibody Reactivity

If the autoantibody has apparent specificity for a single antigen (eg, anti-e), blood lacking that antigen (R_2R_2) may be selected, since there is evidence that such red cells survive better than the patient's red cells.[1,7,15,23,24] However, Rh-negative patients with autoanti-e are usually given e-positive, D-negative blood, to avoid immunization to the D antigen. If titration techniques (see page 465) reveal only relative Rh specificity, the use of blood lacking the corresponding antigen is debatable. Limited data[1,5,24,25] suggest that such blood may survive longer than the patient's own red cells.

In many cases of WAIHA, no autoantibody specificity is apparent; the patient's serum reacts with all red cell samples tested to the same degree, or reacts with red cells from different donors to varying degrees for reasons seemingly unrelated to their respective Rh phenotype. In such cases, some workers test a large number of donor blood samples (eg, 12 to 20) and select those units that give the weakest reactions in vitro. There are no data to indicate better in vivo survival of these least-reactive red cells, but some workers feel more comfortable issuing the least incompatible units.

Other workers recommend ignoring any relative specificity of the autoantibody. After the presence of alloantibody has been excluded, they suggest selecting blood solely on the basis of matching the patient's Rh phenotype, to avoid possible subsequent development of Rh alloantibodies.[24,26] While data regarding the in vivo significance of warm-reactive autoantibody specificity are scanty, a significant minority of these autoantibodies react fairly specifically with one or another of the Rh antigens and there are no data to prove such specificity is insignificant.

Expected Results

In cases of severe and progressive anemia, it may be essential to transfuse blood reactive in vitro with the autoantibody. Warm-reactive autoantibodies are unlikely to cause an acute hemolytic transfusion reaction. Although red cell survival may not be normal, the temporary benefit may be of great value until some other therapy can effect a more lasting benefit.[1,5,6,24,26]

In summary, transfusion of patients with WAIHA should be undertaken only if absolutely essential, with the realization that the blood is not truly compatible and its effects are likely to be brief. The volume transfused should be the least amount required to maintain adequate oxygen transportation. An attempt should be made to differentiate autoantibody from alloantibody in the serum. If specificity is obvious, the appropriate donor blood should be selected. Blood should never be withheld from a patient with severe life-threatening anemia because autoantibodies cause in vitro incompatibility.

Selection of Blood for Patients with CHD

Patients suffering from CHD occasionally require transfusion. If the need arises, compatibility tests should be performed in ways that minimize the detection of the cold-reactive autoantibody, yet still permit the detection of clinically significant alloantibodies.

Autoabsorption and prewarmed techniques, as described above, are useful. Rabbit red cells may also be used to remove autoanti-I and -IH from sera[28]; a preparation of rabbit red cell stroma is commercially available.

Selection of Blood for Patients with PCH

Sera from patients with PCH will be compatible on routine crossmatching tests with random donor red cells. The causative antibody, demonstrated by the Donath-Landsteiner test described on page 457, rarely reacts as an agglutinin above 4 C. The antibody usually has anti-P specificity and does not react with p and p^k red cells. There is some evidence that transfused p red cells survive better than red cells of common P-system phenotypes.[27] These cells are extremely rare, however, and the transfusion of random donor blood should not be withheld from PCH patients requiring urgent transfusion.[1]

Red Cell Sensitization Induced by Drugs

Drugs sometimes induce the formation of antibodies, either against the drug itself or against intrinsic red cell antigens. Although most drugs have a molecular weight substantially below the 5000 dalton level usually considered the threshold for effective immunogenicity, they act as haptens (see Chapter 5), and elicit antibody after combination with a protein carrier. The antibody, once formed, can react with the small hapten independent of any protein attachment. Drugs may cause a positive DAT, which may or may not be accompanied by immune hemolysis, by one of four possible mechanisms (Table 14-4).

Mechanisms of Red Cell Sensitization
Drug Adsorption

Approximately 3% of patients receiving large doses of penicillin intravenously (eg, millions of units per day) develop a positive DAT, but less than 5% of these develop hemolysis, usually of the extravascular type.[1] The positive DAT results from adsorption of penicillin onto the red cells in vivo. If the patient has formed antibodies to the drug, the antipenicillin antibody reacts with the cell-bound penicillin and drug-coated red cells become coated with IgG (Fig 14-1). Complement is not usually involved. Hemolysis, if it occurs, is extravascular, probably by the mechanisms that damage red cells coated with IgG alloantibodies.

Drugs such as penicillin have several distinct haptenic groups. The major haptenic determinant is the benzyl-penicilloyl (BPO) group. With sufficiently sensitive techniques, most adult human sera can be shown to contain BPO antibodies. These are usually IgM and of low titer; however, some sera contain an IgG component. The

high incidence of penicillin antibodies probably reflects widespread environmental exposure to this drug.[8] Most clinically apparent allergic (ie, nonhemolytic) reactions to penicillin are due to IgE antibodies and occur unrelated to the presence of IgM or IgG antibodies.

The clinical and laboratory features of penicillin-induced immune hemolysis are:

1. The DAT is strongly positive due to IgG coating. Occasionally, complement coating also may be present, but this is usually very weak.[1]
2. Screening tests for unexpected antibodies are nonreactive unless alloantibodies are coincidentally present.
3. Antibody eluted from the red cells reacts with penicillin-coated red cells but not with untreated red cells.
4. A high-titer IgG anti-penicillin antibody is always present in the serum.
5. Hemolysis typically develops only in patients receiving very large doses of intravenous penicillin (millions of units daily for a week or more). When it occurs, the onset is subacute but it may be life-threatening if the etiology is unrecognized and penicillin administration is continued. Cessation of penicillin therapy is usually followed by cessation of hemolysis, but hemolysis

Table 14-4. Summary of Serologic Findings Associated with Drug-Induced Positive Direct Antiglobulin Tests

Mechanism	Example	DAT	Serum and Eluate
Drug adsorption	Penicillin, cephalosporins	IgG (C3 in addition, on some occasions[1])	Reacts with drug-coated red cells, but not with untreated red cells
Immune complex formation	Phenacetin, quinidine	C3 (IgG in addition, on some occasions[1])	Serum reacts with red cells only in the presence of the drug; eluate nonreactive
Nonimmunologic adsorption of proteins	Cephalosporins	IgG + C3 + albumin, etc.	Serum may contain a low-titer anti-drug antibody; eluate nonreactive
Induction of autoimmunity	α-methyldopa (eg, Aldomet)	IgG (C3 in addition, present only rarely[1])	Reacts with normal red cells in the absence of the drug

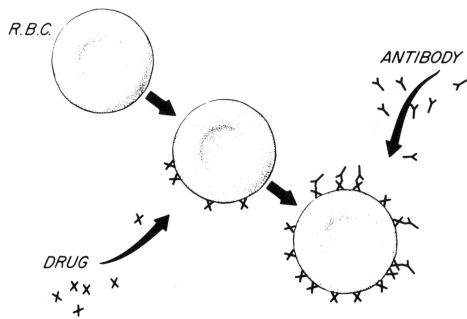

Figure 14-1. Drug adsorption mechanism. Anti-drug antibody binds with drug bound to the red cell surface. Anti-drug antibody does not bind to "drug-free" red cells.

of decreasing severity may persist for several weeks.

Immune Complex Adsorption

Some drugs do not bind to red cells, but have a high affinity for their specific antibodies and form antigen-antibody complexes that circulate in the plasma. These immune complexes attach nonspecifically to red cells and initiate complement activation on the red cell surface (Fig 14-2). This may lead to intravascular hemolysis. Red cells that are not hemolyzed have a positive DAT because of complement coating and, sometimes, immunoglobulin coating. Often complement is the only globulin demonstrable on the red cell surface because the immune complex binds loosely to the red cells. The immune complexes may dissociate after activating complement and go on to react with other red cells. This may explain why small amounts

of the drug can induce acute hemolytic episodes.

Many drugs have been described as causing a positive DAT, immune hemolysis or both, through this mechanism but most reports involve single cases. This mechanism is the one least often encountered in investigating drug-induced immune hemolysis. The characteristic observations are:

1. Acute intravascular hemolysis with hemoglobinemia and hemoglobinuria is the usual presentation. Renal failure occurs in approximately 50% of cases.
2. The patient may experience severe hemolytic episodes after taking only small quantities of the drug.
3. The antibody can be either IgM or IgG.
4. The red cells are often coated only with complement.
5. In vitro reactions such as agglutination, hemolysis and reactive indirect antiglobulin tests occur only when drug is

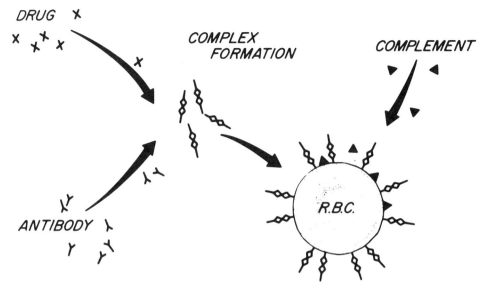

Figure 14-2. Immune complex mechanism. Complexes of the drug and anti-drug antibody attach to the red cell surface, where they initiate complement activation.

present in the incubation mixture with patient's serum and reagent red cells.

Nonimmune Adsorption of Proteins

Drugs of the cephalosporin type may alter red cell membranes in such a way that the red cells adsorb all proteins in a nonspecific manner (Fig 14-3). Red cells coated with cephalothin (Keflin) and incubated with normal plasma will adsorb albumin, IgA, IgG, IgM, α- and β-globulins (ie, complement).[8,29] When this occurs in vivo, a positive DAT can occur; antisera to any human serum protein, not just anti-IgG or anti-C3, will yield a positive test. This nonimmunologic adsorption of proteins does not seem to result in hemolysis.[1]

Cephalosporins can induce a positive DAT by the mechanism described for penicillin, in which antibody attaches to cell-bound drug. Antibodies induced by cephalosporin exposure crossreact with penicillin-treated red cells. Approximately 4% of patients receiving cephalosporins will develop a positive DAT.[29] There have been occasional reports of hemolysis resulting from cephalosporin

therapy but these have been associated with specific anti-cephalosporin antibodies, not with red cell membrane modification and nonimmunologic adsorption of proteins.

Induction of Autoimmunity

The first cases of WAIHA resulting from α-methyldopa (Aldomet) therapy were described in 1966. A closely related drug (L-dopa) has also been reported to cause a positive DAT and immune hemolysis, as has mefenamic acid (Ponstel), a drug unrelated to α-methyldopa.[1]

Following α-methyldopa therapy, autoantibodies are formed that react with intrinsic red cell antigens. They do not react with the drug in vitro, either directly or indirectly. The serologic findings are indistinguishable from those associated with WAIHA; often, the autoantibody can be found to have Rh-related specificity.[1] It has been suggested that the drug interferes with suppressor T-cell function allowing overproduction of autoantibody by B lymphocytes.[30]

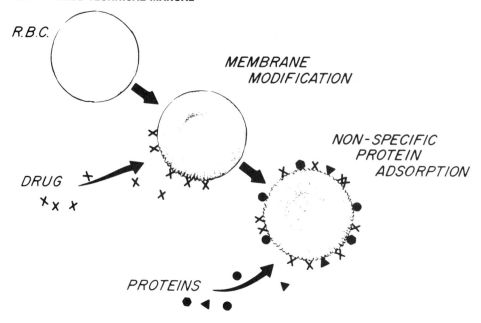

Figure 14-3. Nonimmunologic protein adsorption mechanism. Drug alters surface of red cells such that all proteins are adsorbed nonimmunologically.

Therapy with α-methyldopa accounts for more cases of drug-induced positive DAT and immune hemolysis than all the other drugs listed in Table 14-5 added together. In a series of 347 patients with immune hemolytic anemia,[1] 12% were drug-induced, and of these almost 70% were due to α-methyldopa; 23% were due to penicillin, and the remainder were associated with drugs that form immune complexes. The clinical and laboratory features associated with α-methyldopa-induced autoantibodies include:

1. Approximately 15% of patients receiving α-methyldopa develop a positive DAT, but only 0.5-1.0% of patients taking α-methyldopa develop hemolytic anema.

2. The red cells are usually coated only with IgG, but occasionally weak complement coating is also present.[1]

3. The DAT usually becomes positive only after 3 to 6 months of α-methyldopa therapy.

4. The development of a positive DAT is dose dependent; approximately 36% of patients taking 3 g of the drug daily develop a positive DAT, compared with 11% of patients receiving 1 g per day.

5. The antibodies in the serum and on the red cells are indistinguishable from those found in idiopathic WAIHA.

6. The strength of the positive DAT diminishes when α-methyldopa therapy is discontinued but disappearance may take from 1 month to 2 years. In patients with hemolysis, hematologic values usually improve within the first week or so after the drug is discontinued.

Laboratory Investigation of Drug-Induced Hemolysis

The most common drug-related problem encountered in the blood bank is a positive DAT, most often due to α-methyldopa, which induces autoantibodies reactive with

Table 14-5. Drugs that Have Been Reported to Cause a Positive Direct Antiglobulin Test and Hemolytic Anemia*

Fuadin (Stibophen)
Quinidine
p-aminosalicylic acid (PAS)
Quinine
Phenacetin
Penicillins
Chlorinated hydrocarbon insecticides (Dieldrin, Heptaclor, Toxaphene)
Antihistamines (Antazole, Antistin)
Sulfonamides
Isoniazid (INH, Rifamate, Nydrazid)
Chlorpromazine (Thorazine)
Pyramidon (Aminopyrin)
Dipyrone
Methyldopa (Aldomet, Aldoril, Aldoclor)
Melphalan (Alkeran)
Cephalosporins
Mefenamic acid (Ponstel)
Carbromal (Carbitral, Carbropent)†
Sulfonylurea derivatives (Diabenese, Tolbutamide)
Insulin
Levodopa (L-dopa, Sinemet)
Rifampin (Rifadin, Rifamate, Rimactane)
Methadone†
Tetracycline
Methysergide (Sansert)
Acetaminophen
Hydrochlorothiazide
Streptomycin
Procainamide (Pronestyl, Sub-Quin)
Ibuprofen
Hydralazine (Apresoline, Hydralazide, Unipres, Serpasil)
Probenecid (Benemid)
Fenfluramine (Pondimin)
Triamterene (Dyrenium)
Trimellitic anhydride
Nomifensine

After Petz and Swisher[24]
*Some brands are listed; however, it is impractical to list every drug by brand name. The American Drug Index (JB Lippincott, Philadelphia, 1979), for example, lists 235 products containing acetaminophen.
†Carbromal and methadone have been reported to cause a positive DAT but not hemolytic anemia.

intrinsic red cell antigens. Drugs of the α-methyldopa group can also cause reactive indirect antiglobulin tests in serum-cell mixtures without added drug. The serologic evaluation of drug-induced hemolysis is essentially the same as that used to investigate autoimmune hemolytic anemia:

1. Monospecific antiglobulin sera are useful for the DAT. Drugs that cause a positive DAT by the immune complex mechanism primarily bind complement to red cells, in contrast to positive DAT induced by penicillin or α-methyldopa, in which only IgG is usually bound. Red cells that have adsorbed proteins nonimmunologically react with some or all antiglobulin sera (eg, anti-IgG, -IgA, -IgM, -C3) and anti-albumin reagents.

2. The patient's serum should be tested for unexpected antibodies by the routine procedures used in pretransfusion studies (see Chapter 12). If the serum is nonreactive with untreated red cells, it should be tested against ABO-compatible red cells in the presence of any drug that the patient has been receiving. Techniques for testing may be those described in published cases, if the drug is one already reported as immunogenic. If such information is not available, an initial screening test can be performed with a solution of the drug at a concentration of approximately 1 mg/ml in phosphate-buffered saline.[31] A method is given on page 460. The physical properties of drugs, such as solubility and stability, may be found in the *Physicians' Desk Reference*,[32] the *Merck Index*,[33] or through consultation with the hospital pharmacist.

3. If these tests are not informative, an attempt should be made to coat normal red cells with the drug, and test the patient's serum and an eluate from the patient's red cells against the drug-coated red cells. This is the method of choice when penicillin or the cephalosporins are the suspected cause of the

positive DAT (see page 460). The definitive test for a penicillin-induced positive DAT is demonstration that the eluate reacts with penicillin-coated red cells but not with untreated red cells. Drugs that induce a positive DAT by the immune complex mechanism often bind only complement to red cells, so that the eluate is nonreactive, even when the drug is added to the test system.

Drugs that have been reported to cause a positive DAT and hemolytic anemia are shown in Table 14-5.

References

1. Petz LD, Garratty G. Acquired immune hemolytic anemias. New York: Churchill Livingstone; 1980.
2. Worlledge SM. The interpretation of a positive direct antiglobulin test. Br J Haematol 1978;29:157-162.
3. Judd WJ, Butch SH, Oberman HA, Steiner EA, Bauer RC. The evaluation of a positive direct antiglobulin test in pretransfusion testing. Transfusion 1980;20:17-23.
4. Freedman J. False-positive antiglobulin tests in healthy subjects and in hospital patients. J Clin Pathol 1979;32:1014-1018.
5. Dacie JV. The immune hemolytic anemias. II. The autoimmune hemolytic anemias. 2nd ed. New York: Grune and Stratton; 1962.
6. Pirofsky B. Autoimmunization and the autoimmune hemolytic anemias. Baltimore: Williams and Wilkins; 1969.
7. Mollison PL. Blood transfusion in clinical medicine. 7th ed. Oxford: Blackwell Scientific Publications; 1983.
8. Garratty G, Petz LD. Drug-induced immune hemolytic anemia. Am J Med 1975;58:398-407.
9. Swanson JL, Issitt CH, Mann EW, Condie RM, Simmons RL, McCullough J. Resolution of red cell compatibility testing problems in patients receiving anti-lymphoblast or anti-thymocyte globulin. Transfusion 1984;24:141-143.
10. Petz LD. The diagnosis of hemolytic anemia. In: Bell CA, ed. A seminar on laboratory management of hemolysis. Washington, DC: American Association of Blood Banks; 1975.
11. Judd WJ, Butch SH. Cost-containment in the blood bank: eliminating unnecessary serological testing. J Med Technol 1984;1:485-495.
12. Postoway N, Garratty G. Mechanisms causing positive antiglobulin tests subsequent to antilymphocyte globulin (ALG) administration. (abstract) Transfusion 1984;24:427.
13. Dacie JV. Autoimmune hemolytic anemia. Arch Intern Med 1975;135:1293-1300.
14. Sturgeon P, Smith LE, Chun HMT, Hurvitz CH, Garratty G, Goldfinger D. Autoimmune hemolytic anemia associated exclusively with IgA of Rh specificity. Transfusion 1976;19:324-328.
15. Issitt PD. Serology and genetics of the rhesus blood group system. Cincinnati: Montgomery Scientific Publications; 1979.
16. Issitt PD, Pavone BG, Goldfinger D, et al. Anti-Wr^b and other autoantibodies responsible for positive direct antiglobulin tests in 150 individuals. Br J Haematol 1976;34:5-18.
17. Vos GH, Petz LD, Garratty G, Fudenberg HH. Autoantibodies in acquired hemolytic anemia with special reference to the LW system. Blood 1973;42:445-453.
18. Garratty G, Petz LD, Hoops JK. The correlation of cold agglutinin titrations in saline and albumin with haemolytic anemia. Br J Haematol 1975;35:587-595.
19. Gilliland BC, Baxter E, Evans RS. Red cell antibodies in acquired hemolytic anemia with negative antiglobulin serum tests. N Engl J Med 1971;285:252-256.
20. Chaplin H. Clinical usefulness of specific antiglobulin reagents in autoimmune hemolytic anemias. Prog Hematol 1973;8:25-49.
21. Issitt PD, Zellner DC, Rolih SD, Duckett JB. Autoantibodies mimicking alloantibodies. Transfusion 1977;17:531-538.
22. Issitt PD, Smith TR. Evaluation of antiglobulin reagents. In: Myhre BA, ed. A seminar on performance evaluation. Washington, DC: American Association of Blood Banks; 1976.
23. von dem Borne AEG Kr, Engelfriet CP, Beckers D, van Loghem JJ. Autoimmune haemolytic anemias: biochemical studies of red cells from patients with autoimmune haemolytic anemia with incomplete warm autoantibodies. Clin Exp Immunol 1971;8:377-388.
24. Petz LD, Swisher SN. Blood transfusion in acquired hemolytic anemias. In: Petz LD, Swisher SN, eds. Clinical practice of blood transfusion. New York: Churchill Livingstone; 1981.
25. Salmon C. Autoimmune hemolytic anemia. In: Bach J.F, ed. Immunology. 2nd ed. New York: John Wiley & Sons; 1982.
26. Pirofsky B. Immune haemolytic disease: the autoimmune haemolytic anemias. Clin Haematol 1975;4:167-180.

27. Rausen AR, Levine R, Hsu TCS, Rosenfield RE. Compatible transfusion therapy for patients with PCH. Pediatrics 1975;55:275-278.

28. Marks MR, Reid ME, Ellisor SS. Adsorption of unwanted cold autoagglutinins by formaldehyde treated rabbit erythrocytes (abstract) Transfusion 1980;20:629.

29. Spath P, Garratty G, Petz LD. Studies on the immune response to penicillin and cephalothin in humans: 1. Optimal conditions for titration of hemagglutinating penicillin and cephalothin antibodies. J Immunol 1971;107:845-858.

30. Kirtland HH III, Mohler DN, Horwitz DA. Methyldopa inhibition of supressor lymphocyte function. A proposed cause of autoimmune hemolytic anemia. N Eng J Med 1980;302:825-832.

31. Garratty G. Laboratory investigation of drug-induced immune hemolytic anemias. Washington, DC: American Association of Blood Banks; 1979.

32. Physicians' Desk Reference. 38th ed. Oradell, NJ: Medical Economics; 1984.

33. Windholz M, ed. The Merck Index. 10th ed. Rahway, NJ: Merck & Co, 1983.

15

Blood Transfusion Practice

The general availability and safety of blood transfusion is a remarkable scientific achievement. Appropriate blood transfusion practice, however, requires the constant use of critical clinical judgement. The medical indications for every transfusion should be carefully evaluated, and each transfusion should be monitored for therapeutic effectiveness. Comparing posttransfusion laboratory studies with baseline pretransfusion values is the best way to assess efficacy of transfusion. Failure to achieve or maintain an expected hemoglobin value, platelet count or level of clotting factor activity should be investigated promptly and the cause determined.

While the basic indications for transfusion are to restore or maintain: 1) oxygen-carrying capacity, 2) blood volume, 3) hemostasis or 4) leukocyte function, the clinical variations on these few indications are endless. Numerous blood components are available (see Table 15-1), each with its own potential benefits and untoward effects. Providing astute consultation is one of the most important functions of the blood bank director and laboratory personnel.

Transfusion of Components Containing Red Cells

Effects of Transfusing Red Cells

Blood Volume
Transfusing a unit of whole blood (500 ml) rapidly, over 30 to 60 minutes, increases the blood volume by this amount. After approximately 24 hours, the blood volume returns to its pretransfusion level if hypovolemia was not initially present. Readjustment of the expanded blood volume may be delayed or abnormal in patients with chronic renal disease, congestive heart failure, chronic anemia or certain liver diseases. If acute volume expansion exceeds the compensatory capacity of the cardiovascular system, circulatory overload will develop, usually manifest as congestive heart failure, often with frank pulmonary edema.

Hemoglobin
The effects of red cell transfusion on the posttransfusion hemoglobin and hematocrit depend upon the recipient's clinical condition and pretransfusion blood volume, hemoglobin and hematocrit, and upon the hemoglobin and hematocrit of the donor unit. As shown in Table 15-2, whole blood produces greater expansion of blood volume, whereas infusion of red cells gives a larger immediate increase in hemoglobin. One unit of red cells should raise the nonbleeding adult patient's hemoglobin by about 1 gm/dl and the hematocrit by about 3%.

Survival of Transfused Red Cells
The normal red cell life span is approximately 120 days. Each unit of blood con-

Table 15-1. Blood and Blood Components

Proper Name*	Commonly Used Names
Whole Blood	Whole Blood
Red Blood Cells	Red Blood Cells, Packed Cells, Red Cell Concentrate
Red Blood Cells Frozen	Frozen Red Blood Cells
Red Blood Cells Deglycerolized	Deglycerolized Red Blood Cells, Thawed Red Blood Cells
Red Blood Cells Leukocytes Removed by Centrifugation	Leukocyte-Poor Red Blood Cells
Red Blood Cells Leukocytes Removed by Washing	Washed Red Blood Cells
Red Blood Cells Leukocytes Removed by Filtration	Leukocyte-Poor Red Blood Cells
Plasma	Single Donor Plasma
Liquid Plasma‡	Single Donor Plasma
Fresh Frozen Plasma§	Fresh Frozen Plasma
Cryoprecipitated AHF	Cryoprecipitate
Whole Blood Cryoprecipitate Removed	Modified Whole Blood
Platelet Rich Plasma	Platelet Rich Plasma
Platelets	Platelet Concentrate
Platelets Apheresis	Single-Donor Platelets, Apheresis Platelet Concentrates
Granulocytes† Apheresis	Granulocyte Concentrate
Granulocytes-Platelets† Apheresis	Granulocyte-Platelet Concentrate

*Designated by FDA
†These products are not recognized by the FDA. Names are as proposed for Uniform Labeling.
‡Stored at 1–6 C
§Stored at −18 C or lower

Table 15-2. Effects of Transfusion with Whole Blood or Red Blood Cells (Adult Recipient)

	Hemoglobin (g/dl)	Total Hemoglobin (g)	Blood Volume (ml)
Before Transfusion	8.0	400	5000
1 unit whole blood	8.4	460	5517
1 unit red blood cells	8.7	460	5300
After 24 hours (for both)	9.2	460	5000

tains red cells of all ages between 1 and 120 days. Red cells continue to age during storage. Following transfusion, senescent cells and nonviable red cells of any age are removed from the circulation within 24 hours. Surviving transfused cells are destroyed in a linear fashion with a mean half-life of 50 to 60 days.[1] Approximately 70-80% of red cells stored for 21 days in CPD or for 35 days in CPDA-1 survive normally in the recipient.[2,3] Cells stored in new additive solutions have 70-80% post-transfusion viability after as long as 49 days of storage. Transfused cells have shortened survival in patients with active bleeding and in those patients with hemolysis due to alloantibodies, autoantibodies or hypersplenism.

Indications for Transfusing Red Cells and Whole Blood

The patient's clinical condition, not a laboratory test result, is the most important factor determining transfusion needs. Many patients with asymptomatic anemia do not require transfusion. If the patient's major need is enhanced oxygen-carrying capacity, the component of choice is Red Blood Cells. If blood volume replacement is also necessary, whole blood transfusion may be optimal. Following acute blood loss, hemoglobin and hematocrit may remain normal or nearly normal for an hour or more, until there is equilibration between the intravascular space and the extravascular fluid. Patients with acute hemorrhage may require transfusion despite normal hemoglobin and hematocrit levels. It is unwise, however, to initiate blood transfusion too soon. In most patients loss of approximately 20% of blood volume can safely be corrected by crystalloid (electrolyte) solutions alone.[4,5]

When anemia develops slowly, compensatory mechanisms occur, such as increased cardiac output and a right shift of the oxyhemoglobin dissociation curve, which enhances oxygen delivery to the tissues. These mechanisms lessen somewhat the physiological impact of reduced hemoglobin levels. For patients with chronic anemia, it is important to diagnose and treat the cause of anemia, not merely restore hemoglobin by transfusion. Since transfusion may suppress erythropoiesis, it should be used only as the last resort.

There is no evidence that it is necessary to transfuse a patient to a "normal" hemoglobin prior to surgery. The time-honored threshold of 10 g/dl of hemoglobin seems to be based more on theory than on clinical or experimental evidence.[6] One study of 82 patients undergoing surgery with a mean hematocrit of 24.5% revealed no excess operative morbidity or postoperative mortality.[7] Preoperative transfusion for a patient with limited cardiac reserve may expand the intravascular volume to a degree that administering additional fluids during anesthesia when the patient is recumbent provokes congestive heart failure. It is similarly unnecessary to transfuse postoperatively just to achieve normal hematocrit values. Mortality rates, in one study, were lowest in that group of critically ill postoperative patients whose hematocrits were between 27 and 33%.[8]

Transfusion Order Schedule

Hospital transfusion committees often are responsible for establishing institutional transfusion policies, and the following strategies merit serious consideration: 1) establishment of a standard surgical blood order schedule (maximum surgical blood order schedule, MSBOS) that specifies the appropriate number of units to be cross-matched for commonly performed surgical procedures[9]; 2) use of "type and screen" for patients undergoing operations that rarely require transfusions[10]; and 3) use of predeposit autotransfusion and intraoperative salvage to decrease transfusion of stored bank blood.

Red Cell Components Available

Fresh Whole Blood

Use of freshly drawn whole blood less than 24 hours old is a vestige of past transfusion practice when appropriate components were not available. Processing donor blood, which includes typing for ABO and Rh antigens, antibody detection testing, hepatitis screening and syphilis testing, is rarely completed in less than 24 hours. Transfusing blood before necessary tests are complete carries a risk of hepatitis that outweighs any anticipated benefit.

There are no valid indications for specifically transfusing fresh whole blood. A request for fresh whole blood should be interpreted by the blood bank staff as a need for consultative help to establish a diagnosis and to plan specific component therapy. For thrombocytopenia, appropriate therapy is transfusion of platelet concentrates. For most such cases, one unit of fresh whole blood would not contain sufficient platelets to be effective. Similarly, fresh whole blood is impractical for replacement of deficient coagulation factors. If the deficit is greater than can be corrected with fresh frozen plasma, specific factor concentrates, if available, are preferred.

Whole blood less than 4-5 days old is the component of choice for exchange transfusion in newborns. Blood less than 7 days old ensures plasma electrolyte concentrations within limits that are tolerable for infants, and also ensures adequate red cell content of 2,3-diphosphoglycerate (2,3-DPG).

Stored Whole Blood

Whole blood, which provides both oxygen-carrying capacity and blood volume expansion, is indicated for actively bleeding patients who have lost over 25% of their blood volume. Depletion of intravascular volume, the pathogenesis of hypovolemic shock, is best treated by rapid restoration of blood volume. Acute massive blood loss is best treated with whole blood,[11] but if whole blood is not available, components must suffice. Red blood cells and crystalloid (electrolyte) solutions supplemented by colloid (protein) solutions, are usually less cost-effective than whole

blood,[12] and simultaneous use of fresh frozen plasma with red blood cells carries twice the risk of hepatitis transmission. Infusions to restore intravascular volume should be started immediately, beginning with readily available crystalloid solutions. If blood loss exceeds one-third of the patient's blood volume, crystalloid solutions alone will not sustain blood volume,[4] and colloid solutions will be necessary. Such circumstances are an indication for whole blood.

Whole Blood, Modified

Whole blood, modified, is prepared by returning the plasma to the red blood cells after removal of platelets and/or cryoprecipitate. This product has virtually the same hemostatic properties as stored whole blood.[13] Preparation of this product permits collection of platelets and cryoprecipitate, while ensuring a supply of whole blood for treating hemorrhage.

Red Blood Cells

Red Blood Cells is the component of choice to restore or maintain oxygen-carrying capacity. Patients who have chronic anemia, congestive heart failure, or are elderly or debilitated tolerate poorly rapid changes in blood volume. Transfusing red blood cells increases oxygen-carrying capacity with minimal expansion of blood volume. Nonhemolytic transfusion reactions occur less frequently after transfusion of red blood cells than after whole blood, probably because most platelets, granulocytes and plasma are removed.[14]

Exclusive use of red blood cells for transfusion during surgery is controversial. Patients with operative blood loss of only 1000 to 1200 ml seldom require red cell transfusion; electrolyte and/or colloid solutions provide adequate volume replacement.[4,5] A large national survey demonstrated that, of patients who did need transfusion, 65% used four units or less[15]; increasing oxygen-carrying capacity, not compensation for volume deficit, was the apparent indication. Most such patients should receive red blood cells and crystalloid solutions, but if significant volume expansion is required along with increased oxygen transport capacity, whole blood or whole blood, modified, should be transfused, if available, rather than red blood cells augmented by albumin solution or frozen plasma.

Additive and Rejuvenation Solutions

Several types of additive solutions have been licensed for use with stored blood. Some increase red cell levels of 2,3-DPG and/or ATP by adding adenine, inosine, pyruvate, and other compounds to red blood cells nearing the end of their shelf-life. Such "rejuvenated" units can be transfused immediately or stored frozen for transfusion at a later date. This procedure salvages units that might otherwise outdate and be discarded.

Other additive solutions, containing combinations of saline, adenine, glucose and mannitol, are added shortly after phlebotomy to red cells from which maximum amounts of plasma have been removed. Because these additives maintain red cell function without the need for residual plasma, more fresh plasma can be harvested and the less viscous red cell component can more easily be infused.[16]

Leukocyte-Poor Red Blood Cells

Multiparous women and previously transfused patients may develop antibodies to leukocytes and/or platelets.[17] Patients with leukocyte antibodies may sustain febrile reactions after receiving blood containing incompatible leukocytes. Febrile reactions also occur in patients without demonstrable white cell or platelet antibodies. Febrile nonhemolytic reactions do not damage red blood cells, but the symptoms, such as chills, fever, headache, malaise, nausea and vomiting, may be very uncomfortable and may persist for up to 8 hours. These reactions seem to result from immune damage to donor leukocytes, even those that are

not viable when transfused. Some of these symptoms may follow release of C5a when reactions between leukoagglutinins and leukocyte antigens activate complement. The production of C3a may induce vasomotor instability and lead to hypotension, tachycardia or bronchospasm. It is not clear whether mild nonhemolytic reactions result primarily from leukocyte-mediated complement activation or from other causes.

In one study, only 15% of patients who experienced a nonhemolytic febrile reaction had a similar episode with the next blood transfusion.[18] Accordingly, leukocyte-poor preparations should probably be offered only after two or more such reactions. The frequency and severity of febrile reactions are proportional to the number of leukocytes transfused. Tests for defined leukocyte- or platelet-specific antibodies are usually unrewarding.

Several methods effectively remove leukocytes from stored blood. Centrifugation, followed by removal of the buffy coat, is the least efficient way to remove white cells, but does have the advantage of maintaining a closed system. Open system techniques include the use of automated cell washers and manual washing procedures. The washing process removes most of the plasma proteins, microaggregates, platelets and leukocytes.

Microaggregate Filtration

Wenz et al[19] and Schned et al[20] reported that passing citrated blood, stored longer than 5 days, through microaggregate blood filters reduced the incidence of febrile transfusion reactions. The small-pore filter removes unwanted leukocyte and platelet debris. In comparison with more expensive automated cell washing systems, this technique provides an appreciable saving of both cost and time and permits maintenance of a closed system until transfusion. Centrifuging the unit before infusion through the microaggregate blood filter increases the size of the microaggregates and the efficiency of removal, but may not be necessary for units stored over

1 week in which the size of accumulated aggregates does not need enhancement. This technique permits leukocyte removal at the bedside, thus relieving the blood bank of the burden of cell washing. Any of the available microaggregate filters are suitable for this purpose.[21,22]

Deglycerolized Red Blood Cells

Freezing is the ideal form of storage for rare bloods and for long-term storage of blood intended for autologous transfusion. Freezing multiple aliquots from a single unit makes possible numerous small-volume transfusions from a single unit of blood. Freezing can also improve inventory management, in that units of commonly used blood groups drawn in excess of need can be frozen for transfusion in times of shortage. Deglycerolized red blood cells are suitable for transfusing patients who are sensitized to IgA protein[23] or to leukocyte or platelet antigens.

Disease Transmission

Deglycerolized red blood cells, however, do not have some of the advantages initially anticipated. Retrospective studies initially suggested that hepatitis virus was eliminated by the multiple washings used to remove glycerol. Transfusion of deglycerolized frozen and washed red cells, however, has been shown to transmit hepatitis B to chimpanzees,[24] and human transmission of both hepatitis B and non-A and non-B (NANB) hepatitis has been documented.[25]

Immunization

Transfusion with frozen deglycerolized red cells does not improve survival of transplanted kidneys. Indeed, data suggest that transfusion of blood components containing buffy coat actually improves survival of cadaver kidney grafts.[26] Most kidney transplantation protocols now call for multiple transfusions preceding transplantation.

Freezing was initially thought to kill all nucleated blood cells, eliminating viable lymphocytes and thereby preventing graft-versus-host (GVH) reactions in severely immunodeficient recipients. However, viable lymphocytes have been demonstrated after washing[27] even in blood frozen for several years. Irradiating donor units is the only technique that effectively prevents lymphocyte blastogenesis.

Other Considerations

The *Code of Federal Regulations* (21 CFR 610.53) currently limits the postthaw storage of frozen red blood cells to 24 hours because deglycerolization and resuspension occur in an open system.

Cost is another drawback. Requirements for storage equipment, apparatus, solutions and technician time make this component two to three times more expensive than liquid-stored red cell components.

For a more comprehensive discussion of frozen red blood cells, see Chapter 4.

Platelet Transfusion

Effects of Platelet Transfusion

A platelet concentrate prepared from single units of whole blood usually contains a minimum of 5.5×10^{10} platelets. This would be expected to increase the platelet count approximately 5 to 10,000/μl in a hematologically stable adult with 1.8 m^2 surface area.[28] Smaller increments commonly occur, however, depending on the patient's clinical condition. Platelet survival is shortened and incremental platelet count reduced when the patient has fever, infection, disseminated intravascular coagulation, active bleeding or splenomegaly.

In patients with platelet antibodies, such as those with immune thrombocytopenic purpura or alloimmune HLA or platelet antibodies, survival of transfused platelets may be extremely brief, sometimes only a matter of minutes.

Prior transfusion or, less commonly, pregnancy may provoke alloantibodies to platelet-specific or HLA antigens. Platelets collected from unselected donors have shortened survival in patients with alloantibodies and may not be effective in preventing or controlling bleeding. Counting circulating platelets 1 hour posttransfusion detects impaired platelet recovery, and identifies those patients who have become refractory to random-donor platelets.[29] (For further discussion, see "HLA Compatibility," page 273).

Indications for Platelet Transfusion

The decision to transfuse platelets depends upon the clinical condition of the patient, the cause of the thrombocytopenia, the platelet count and the functional ability of the patient's own platelets (Table 15-3).[30] Patients with transient thrombocytopenia from treatment regimens for malignancy constitute the largest group of patients receiving platelet transfusions. There is little risk of serious hemorrhage in these patients when the platelet count is above 20,000/μl.[31]

Prophylactic Platelet Transfusion

Because the risk of immunization increases with exposure to increasing numbers of different antigens, prophylactic administration of random-donor platelets may hasten production of lymphocytotoxic antibodies in susceptible recipients. If lymphocytotoxic antibodies develop, the patient no longer experiences clinical benefit from random-donor platelet concentrates.[32-34]

A study comparing patients given prophylactic platelet transfusions with patients transfused only for clinically significant bleeding[35] found no difference between groups in overall survival or deaths from bleeding, but the prophylactic group required twice as many platelet transfusions. Patients transfused prophylactically have fewer hemorrhagic episodes early in their disease but in the later stages, some experience bleeding that cannot be controlled by platelet transfusions because they have become refractory.[30]

It has been suggested[30] that the commonly used threshold level of 20,000/μl may be too high. When 5000/μl is used instead, minor forms of hemorrhage (eg, petechiae, ecchymosis or epistaxis) occur more often but serious bleeding episodes such as hemorrhagic strokes or major gastrointestinal bleeding appear not to be increased.[36] Utilizing a lower threshold level decreases the overall requirement for platelet transfusion and the incidence of alloimmunization. Bleeding at any level of platelet count may be aggravated by fever, infection or drugs such as aspirin or semisynthetic penicillins.[37]

Table 15-3. Thrombocytopenia and Platelet Transfusions

Cause	Therapy
Amegakaryocytic thrombocytopenia (eg, leukemia, hypoplastic anemia)	Platelets useful in treating hemorrhage and for prophylaxis to prevent bleeding episodes
Immune thrombocytopenia (ITP)	Platelets of little value because of rapid destruction in spleen
Dilutional thrombocytopenia (eg, massive transfusion with stored blood)	Platelets of value in replacement (usually after 15 to 20 units transfused)
Disseminated intravascular coagulation (DIC)	Platelets useful when combined with efforts to stop DIC or treat the cause
Functional platelet abnormalities	Platelets from normal donors may achieve hemostasis during hemorrhage, surgery, and dental extractions

Thrombocytopenias

Platelet counts above 60-70,000/μl may be necessary for adequate hemostasis in patients undergoing major surgery or treatment for severe trauma. After transfusion of 15 to 20 units of whole blood, red blood cells or modified whole blood, platelet counts often fall below this level, and platelet transfusion may be indicated.[13] Stored blood does not correct thrombocytopenia because, at 1 to 6 C storage temperatures, platelets rapidly become dysfunctional because disassembly of the microtubule system prevents the release reaction. The decision to administer platelets should rest on the actual count, however, not on a replacement formula based on number of units transfused.

In patients with immune thrombocytopenic purpura (ITP), transfused platelets quickly disappear from the circulation and provide little benefit. Effective forms of treatment for ITP include steroids or splenectomy. After ligation of the splenic pedicle, platelet transfusion may be effective in controlling serious bleeding during splenectomy.

In drug-induced thrombocytopenia, the offending drug should be discontinued and the patient closely observed. While the drug remains in the circulation, transfused platelets undergo the same damage as the patient's own platelets, so transfusion should be avoided in these patients unless there is significant hemorrhage. Intravenous gamma globulin has been used to treat ITP and other forms of antibody-mediated thrombocytopenia.[38]

ABO and Rh Groups in Platelet Transfusion

ABO antigens are present on the platelet surface; recovery of group A platelets transfused into group O patients is somewhat decreased.[39] Although ABO-incompatible platelets may have slightly diminished 24-hour recovery,[40] prompt administration of available platelets is more important to patient outcome than delay to obtain ABO-matched platelets. When large numbers of patients require platelet transfusions from a limited donor pool, availability becomes the major consideration. If the platelet concentrates contain ABO antibodies incompatible with the recipient's red cells, it may be desirable to remove most of the donor plasma, especially when transfusing children.

Plasma

Platelet concentrates, either single-donor or pooled random-donor, require neither major nor minor crossmatching. The small volume of unexpected antibodies possibly present in plasma is not considered clinically important. Anti-A or anti-B in donor plasma may cause a positive direct antiglobulin test and, rarely, shortened red cell survival or frank hemolysis if the volume of transfused plasma is large relative to the recipient's red cell mass. It may be desirable to remove ABO-incompatible plasma from the pooled platelet concentrates just before they are administered[41] (see page 469), or from single-donor concentrates prepared by thrombocytapheresis.

Red Cells

Platelet concentrates properly prepared from individual units of whole blood contain 0.5 ml or less of red blood cells. Significant hemolysis would not occur even in a recipient with antibodies to antigens on the donor red cells. Single-donor platelets prepared by thrombocytapheresis usually do not contain a significant number of red cells, but if more than 5 ml of red cells are present, compatibility studies should be performed.

The D antigen is not detectable on platelets. Platelets from D-positive donors survive normally in recipients with anti-D and do not induce immunization in a D-negative recipient. D-negative patients may, however, become immunized by red blood cells contaminating the platelet preparation. In one study of D-negative patients being treated for leukemia, 8% of these immunosuppressed patients developed anti-D after transfusion of 80 to 110 units of Rh-positive platelets.[42] Another study, however, found no anti-D alloimmunization in similar patients.[43] Although the risk of immunization is small, it is desirable to avoid giving platelet concentrates from D-positive donors to D-negative girls or women who might, in the future, bear children. When D-negative platelets are not available, the life-threatening nature of most thrombocytopenic conditions justifies transfusing platelet concentrates from D-positive donors to D-negative recipients. Rh Immune Globulin (RhIG) can be given to prevent immunization. If each concentrate contains a maximum of 0.5 ml of red cells, a full dose of RhIG would provide protection against red cells in 30 units of D-positive platelet concentrates. (See page 318.)

HLA Compatibility

Platelets manifest HLA antigens whose expression results from adsorption of plasma antigens onto the platelet surface.[44] In patients refractory to random-donor platelets, HLA matching of patient and donor may result in acceptable post-transfusion increments in platelet count. A single HLA-compatible donor may be able to provide all of a patient's transfusion needs if platelets are obtained by repeated cytapheresis. The most likely source of HLA-identical or HLA-compatible donors would be the patient's blood relatives. Additionally, many centers have files of HLA-typed donors.[45]

Studies of HLA antigens and survival of transfused platelets indicate that: 1) a number of HLA antigens have sufficient serologic similarity (crossreactivity) that platelet survival can be satisfactory even when these antigens are mismatched; 2) mismatching of antigens at the HLA-C locus is usually not important; 3) patients who are negative for the antigen HLA-A2 need not be precisely matched; and 4) mismatching is acceptable for certain HLA-B

locus antigens that are weakly expressed on the platelet surface.[46] Such findings have simplified matching of "compatible" donors for alloimmunized patients, so that hemostatically effective platelets can be supplied for most individuals from a panel of approximately 2000 HLA-typed donors.[45] Patients under consideration for bone marrow transplantation should not receive platelets or other components from family members who are potential marrow donors because pretransplantation exposure to the donor's antigens increases the likelihood of immunization and decreases the chances for successful bone marrow transplant.

Despite intense efforts to develop crossmatch procedures for platelets, there are no tests currently suitable for routine pretransfusion determination of probable platelet survival in recipients immunized to HLA or other antigens.[47]

Autologous Platelet Transfusion

Autologous transfusion is another approach to providing compatible platelets for patients being treated for leukemia. While the patient is in remission, platelets can be collected by thrombocytapheresis and then frozen, using dimethylsulfoxide (DMSO) as the cryopreservative. This procedure gives a postthaw recovery of approximately 55%.[48] These platelets are hemostatically effective and their use reduces exposure to allotypic antigens that might cause immunization or immune-mediated destruction.[48]

Glycerol has not been a successful cryoprotective agent for platelet concentrates. Recent licensure of platelets frozen with DMSO as the cryoprotective agent will probably lead to more widespread use of autologous frozen platelets.

Appropriate Use of Single-Donor Platelets

There is no convincing evidence that single-donor platelets collected by thrombocytapheresis are more beneficial for nonimmunized individuals than random-donor platelet concentrates. Single-donor platelets, which are costly and of limited availability, should only be used for patients demonstrated to be refractory to random-donor platelets.[49] Patients not immunized to platelets after a course of induction chemotherapy often do not develop alloimmunization despite additional platelet transfusions. This is another reason to withhold single-donor platelets until evidence of alloimmunization is obtained.[34]

Granulocyte Transfusion

Transfused granulocytes function normally and, in selected patients, produce clinical benefits.[50] Preparing granulocyte concentrates by cytapheresis requires expensive technology, close professional supervision and 2 to 4 hours of the donor's time. Although granulocyte concentrates given during intensive anti-leukemia therapy reduce somewhat the number of deaths from infection, the ratio of cost to effectiveness is very high.[51] Indications for granulocyte transfusions and the goals of therapy should be clearly defined before a course of therapy is initiated.

Indications and Contraindications

Only patients with documented granulocyte dysfunction, such as those with chronic granulomatous disease, or those with profound neutropenia should receive granulocyte transfusions. An absolute granulocyte count below 500/µl is an important criterion, because patients with higher counts have better intrinsic resistance to infection.[52]

The candidate for granulocyte transfusions should have a good chance of recovering from the episode of neutropenia. Expected eventual recovery of bone marrow function is important because a series of granulocyte transfusions improves the patient's condition only temporarily. The patient whose granulopoiesis does not resume eventually succumbs when transfusions become ineffective because of

alloimmunization or infection with bacteria resistant to standard antibiotics.[53,54]

It is important to evaluate which types of infections can best be treated with granulocyte transfusions. Ideally, septicemia should be documented by cultures to identify the infecting organism and determine antibiotic sensitivity. Granulocyte transfusion has not been proven effective in patients with localized infections or infections with agents other than bacteria. A 24- to 48-hour course of empirically selected antibiotics control many infections without the need for granulocyte therapy. Gram-positive bacteria more often respond to antibiotics than gram-negative organisms.

The recipient of granulocyte transfusions should be one who can, following survival of the acute infection, reasonably expect a period with a satisfactory quality of life. Patients with advanced debilitating malignancies who are refractory to further therapy and have no reasonable chance of survival should not be considered candidates for granulocyte transfusions.

Course of Therapy

Granulocytes should be transfused as soon as possible after collection, but must be infused within 24 hours.[55] If storage is unavoidable, granulocyte function is best preserved at room temperature without agitation.[56] The number of days to continue transfusions is still controversial.[57] Granulocyte concentrates are ordinarily given daily for at least 4 to 6 days unless bone marrow recovery or severe reactions supervene. Granulocyte concentrates should be infused through a standard blood administration set with an in-line filter. Potential bone marrow recipients should not receive granulocytes from the potential transplant donor.

Compatibility Testing

Currently there is no effective in vitro compatibility test for granulocyte transfusion. Typing for granulocyte-specific and HLA antigens does not correlate well with posttransfusion results. If granulocytes and platelets are obtained concurrently, the platelet count increment can be used to evaluate recipient immunization and donor-recipient compatibility.[58]

The extent of pretransfusion testing depends on the quantity of red cells present in the granulocyte concentrate. Components prepared by a method expected to produce less than 5 ml of contaminating red cells need not be crossmatched, although the donor's red cells should be ABO-compatibile with the recipient's plasma.[55] For granulocyte concentrates containing more than 5 ml red cells, standard considerations for red cell compatibility testing apply.[55]

Since the volume of donor plasma is 200 to 400 ml, it should contain no clinically significant antibodies to antigens present on the recipient's red cells. Pretransfusion tests should, if possible, be performed before leukapheresis, to avoid delaying transfusion when the component is available. Concentrates prepared for pediatric patients should have a reduced volume to avoid the risk of fluid overload.

Evaluating Effectiveness

Posttransfusion cell counts, the traditional index of efficacy for other component transfusions, are unreliable for evaluating granulocyte transfusions because the cells rapidly leave the vascular compartment. The best index of effectiveness is clinical improvement, eg, resolution of fever, favorable changes in chest x-rays or stabilization of a previously deteriorating clinical course. Labeling granulocytes with [111]Indium can help evaluate in vivo efficacy by demonstrating sequestration of radiolabeled neutrophils in areas of infection or inflammation.

Pulmonary Reactions

Severe pulmonary reactions may follow granulocyte transfusions, particularly when there is established lung infection. Initial symptoms may include cough, shortness of breath, increased respiratory rate and, usually, fever. A number of events may cause the pulmonary reactions associated with granulocyte transfusions[50,59]: 1) Fluid overload may cause respiratory embarrassment in patients with marginal cardiac function. This rarely causes fever or chills and the patient responds to diuretics. 2) Patients with preexisting bacterial pneumonia may develop lung consolidation from rapid pulmonary localization of transfused granulocytes. 3) Leukoagglutinins in the recipient may react with and agglutinate transfused white cells, often producing degranulation, activation of complement and damage to pulmonary capillaries. 4) In patients with gram-negative septicemia, endotoxemia may cause granulocyte degranulation, complement activation and pulmonary dysfunction.

Febrile Reactions

Febrile reactions often occur in patients receiving granulocyte concentrates. These usually mild reactions, manifest clinically as fever and chills, can usually be treated by administering non-aspirin antipyretics and slowing the rate of infusion. Meperidine injection may be useful to stop shaking chills. Aspirin, which inhibits the release reaction and produces platelet dysfunction, should be avoided in thrombocytopenic patients. Febrile reactions accompanied by dyspnea or cardiovascular changes such as hypotension are clearly more serious. When severe respiratory distress occurs during a granulocyte transfusion, the infusion should be discontinued and intravenous steroids given in addition to other symptomatic treatment. It may be prudent in such cases to give steroids before subsequent granulocyte transfusions, which should be infused very slowly and with careful observation. If no benefit is obtained from these interventions, further use of granulocyte transfusions may be contraindicated.

Other Considerations
Prophylactic Transfusions

Still controversial is giving granulocytes prophylactically to granulocytopenic patients who are not infected.[54] Most investigators believe, however, that routine use of prophylactic granulocyte transfusion is not desirable.

Usage Trends

The status of granulocyte transfusion has changed in the past several years. Granulocytes are no longer collected by filtration leukapheresis because of the high frequency of reactions in both the donor and the recipient.[57,60,61] Much evidence suggests that granulocyte transfusions confer little additional benefit over appropriate use of antibiotic therapy alone, and requests for granulocytes have been declining nationwide. (See Table 15-4.) Prophylactic granulocyte transfusions are more likely to produce problems with transfusion reactions and alloantibody formation than to provide demonstrable clinical benefit.[63-65] In some major medical centers, requests for granulocyte transfusions have almost completly stopped.

Granulocytes produced by neonates perform phagocytosis less effectively than granulocytes from adults.[66] Some workers suggest that granulocyte transfusions are especially appropriate for treatment of septic newborns.[66]

Clinical Problems

A problem specific to granulocyte transfusion is the possibility that simultaneous use of this blood component with amphotericin B causes severe pulmonary infiltrates and respiratory distress.[59,67,68] Although controversy exists as to the cause of this clinical syndrome, many physicians prefer to avoid granulocyte transfusions in patients receiving amphotericin B for treatment of fungal infections. Granulocyte transfusions have not been found useful for treatment of fungal infections.

Granulocyte transfusions are implicated in two important causes of death in recipients of bone marrow transplants. The first is cytomegalovirus infection, which is transmissible by granulocytes[69,70] and causes interstitial pneumonia. The second, graft-versus-host (GVH) disease, results from transfusion of viable lymphocytes to severely immunocompromised recipients. Granulocyte concentrates, which may contain large numbers of lymphocytes, are usually irradiated with at least 1500 rad before transfusion to bone marrow recipients. (See page 340.) Increasingly effective new antibiotic therapy is likely to cause still further declines in granulocyte transfusions.

Treatment of Coagulation Deficiencies

Use of Plasma

Fresh frozen plasma (FFP) contains all the clotting factors including the labile Factors V and VIII. Fresh frozen plasma, stored plasma and cryoprecipitate-poor plasma are all sources of stable clotting factors.

Table 15-4. Use of Granulocyte and Single-Donor Platelet Transfusions. (Data from the American National Red Cross)

	Method of Collection		
Year	Single-Donor Plateletpheresis	Leukapheresis	Leuko-Plateletpheresis
1979	22,949	9,848	6,800
1980	23,041	4,120	11,454
1981	25,881	4,048	9,532
1982	28,628	3,298	6,981
1983	32,312	3,203	5,118

Plasma should not be used to expand blood volume; its proper use is to replace coagulation factors. Transfusing plasma for volume expansion carries a risk of transmitting disease that can be avoided by using crystalloid or colloid solutions such as albumin; cost may be an additional factor. Plasma is not ordinarily a suitable source of immunoglobulins, especially now that intravenous IgG is available and has no hepatitis risk.

Von Willebrand's Disease

The Factor VIII molecule has three parts: Factor VIII:C is the procoagulant activity; Factor VIII:Ag is the immunologically reactive antigen portion; and Factor VIII:vWF is the von Willebrand Factor required for normal platelet function.[71] The most common of the inherited coagulopathies is von Willebrand's disease (vWD), in which platelet function is abnormal and there is partial deficiency of Factor VIII. Levels of Factor VIII antigen and Factor VIII clotting activity are low, as well as Factor VIII:vWF. Laboratory tests usually disclose assay levels of Factor VIII clotting activity from 5-20%, a prolonged template bleeding time and impaired aggregation of platelets in response to ristocetin. VWD is inherited in an autosomal dominant pattern and both sexes are affected; clinical severity of the disease is variable.

Commercial concentrates of Factor VIII raise the patient's Factor VIII:C level but do not correct the platelet function defect of vWD. Cryoprecipitate corrects both defects.[72] The quantity of cryoprecipitate required to treat bleeding episodes or to prepare for surgery varies greatly among patients. Therapy is usually monitored clinically and by Factor VIII assays, although some patients also require monitoring of template bleeding times. Experience with hemophilia A suggests that patients with vWD should be transfused to Factor VIII levels greater than 50% during major surgery and be maintained at 30% levels during convalescence.

Factor VIII Deficiency (Hemophilia A)

Congenital deficiency of Factor VIII:C results from an abnormal gene on the X chromosome. It is a sex-linked disorder manifested in males and transmitted by female carriers. Clinical severity depends upon the patient's level of Factor VIII. Levels of Factor VIII:Ag are normal despite deficient Factor VIII:C, suggesting a defect in the molecular composition of a Factor VIII complex manufactured in normal quantities. Characteristic laboratory studies include prolonged partial thromboplastin time (PTT) with normal values for both prothrombin time (PT) and template bleeding time and a severe deficiency of Factor VIII as determined by clotting assays.

Concentrates of Factor VIII

One unit of Factor VIII equals the Factor VIII clotting activity of 1 ml of fresh pooled plasma. A cryoprecipitate prepared from a single blood donation should contain a minimum of 80 units of Factor VIII activity per bag.[55] Concentrated Factor VIII preparations are made from pools of thousands of individual units of plasma and a high incidence of chronic liver disease occurs in hemophiliacs treated with this product.[73] In some treatment centers the low hepatitis risk of cryoprecipitate makes it the preferred therapy for patients whose mild disease requires infrequent treatment, while concentrates are used only for severe hemophiliacs. Concentrates are supplied in lyophilized form and the quantity of Factor VIII coagulant activity is stated on the label. After reconstitution, Factor VIII concentrate should be filtered and administered by syringe or via an administration set.

Calculating Dosage

The amount of transfused Factor VIII required depends upon the nature of the bleeding episode and the severity of the initial deficiency. For example, treatment for hematuria or hemarthrosis ordinarily requires more Factor VIII than for soft tissue hematomas. Factor VIII levels in hemophilic patients are usually reported as a percentage of normal. Severe hemophiliacs have Factor VIII levels below 1%; moderate hemophiliacs, 1-5%; and mild hemophiliacs, 6-30%. The amount of Factor VIII required for transfusion can be calculated as follows:

1. Weight (kg) × 70 ml/kg = blood volume (ml)
2. Blood volume (ml) × (1.0 − hematocrit) = plasma volume (ml)
3. Plasma volume (ml) × (desired Factor VIII level % − initial Factor VIII level %) = units Factor VIII required.

Example: To raise the Factor VIII level to 50% in a 70-kg patient with a hematocrit of 40% and an initial Factor VIII level of 0%:

70 kg × 70 ml/kg = 4900 ml
4900 ml × (1.0 − 0.40) = 2940 ml
2940 ml × (0.5 − 0) = 1470 units

This dose will give a level of 50% immediately following transfusion.

The half-life of circulating Factor VIII is 8 to 12 hours. It is usually necessary to repeat Factor VIII transfusions at 8- to 12-hour intervals to maintain hemostatic levels. After 12 hours, the above patient would have a 25% level. Therefore, for the next dose of Factor VIII, 2940 ml × (0.50 − 0.25) = 735 units would elevate Factor VIII to 50% again.

Clinical Considerations

Variables that may affect therapeutic results include the distribution of the factor between the intravascular and extravascular spaces and the possible presence of an inhibitor to Factor VIII. About one fourth of transfused Factor VIII enters the extravascular space during prolonged therapy. The duration of treatment with Factor VIII transfusions depends upon the type and location of the hemorrhage and the clinical response of the patient.

Following major surgery or dental extraction, the Factor VIII level should be maintained above 30%. If Factor VIII assays are unavailable, the partial thromboplastin time (PTT) can be used as a rough guide to Factor VIII activity. If the PTT is in the normal range, the Factor VIII level is usually over 30%; if the Factor VIII level is below 30%, the PTT will generally be prolonged.

Inhibitors to Factor VIII

Ten to 20% of patients with hemophilia A develop a detectable inhibitor to Factor VIII, characteristically an antibody that inactivates the portion of the Factor VIII molecular complex necessary for coagulation activity. Patients who develop an inhibitor may become unresponsive to Factor VIII transfusions. Immunosuppressive drugs, exchange plasmapheresis or infusions of moderate to large quantities of Factor VIII have been used to treat these patients, with inconsistent results. Because the inhibitor is an antibody, neutralization of inhibitor activity by administering large Factor VIII doses may induce a subsequent anamnestic increase in inhibitor activity.

Concentrates of Factor IX complex (prothrombin complex, containing Factors II, VII, IX and X) have been hemostatically effective in treating hemophiliacs with Factor VIII inhibitors. It is postulated that the activated Factor X in this preparation bypasses the step in the coagulation cascade that requires Factor VIII, so that clotting occurs. The exact mechanism of action, however, is unknown.

Initial studies have shown prothrombin complex to be effective in about two-thirds of the bleeding episodes treated,[74] but clinical response is unpredictable.[75] Concentrates of Factor IX, like those of Factor VIII, carry a very high risk of hepatitis transmission[76]; they can also induce a state of disseminated intravascular coagulation and have been implicated in thrombotic episodes, including myocardial infarction.

New Products

A recently licensed product is a lyophilized coagulation concentrate intended specifically for treatment of patients with high-titer Factor VIII inhibitors. This material, known as anti-inhibitor coagulation complex (AICC), is prepared from large pools of donor plasma. The exact mechanism of action is unknown but there seems to be Factor VIII inhibitor bypassing activity, presumably activated Factor X.[77,78] Patients receiving this product must be closely monitored for signs of thrombosis. As this product is a pooled plasma derivative the risk of viral transmission is high. Currently this product is more expensive than the standard Factor VIII concentrate.

A new form of Factor VIII concentrate recently available in the United States is heat treated to inactivate the viruses present. Heat treatment, which decreases the risk of virus transmission, also reduces the Factor VIII activity by about 50%. A highly purified Factor VIII concentrate that contains relatively little fibrinogen and other contaminants has also become available, but is still capable of transmitting hepatitis. Concern over the possible transmission of the acquired immune deficiency syndrome (AIDS) has caused some physicians to recommend a shift to the use of cryoprecipitate for treatment of hemophilia. If heat treatment proves successful in eliminating viral infectivity without unacceptable loss of anticoagulant potency, however, prepared concentrates may become safer than single-donor components.

DDAVP (1-deamino-8-D-arginine vasopressin) is a chemical used for in vivo stimulation of Factor VIII in hemophiliacs. The exact mechanism is unknown but may relate to release of Factor VIII from endothelial cells. DDAVP may be a useful adjunct to standard therapy for both hemophilia A and VWD.[79]

Factor IX Deficiency (Hemophilia B)

Factor IX deficiency is clinically indistinguishable from Factor VIII deficiency, in that both are sex-linked disorders that cause a prolonged PTT in the presence of normal prothrombin time and bleeding time. The problem, caused by an abnormal gene on the X chromosome, is defective synthesis of Factor IX. Normal plasma, either stored or fresh, corrects the coagulation deficiency because Factor IX is stable when stored at 4 C or − 20 C, and it remains in plasma after cryoprecipitate removes Factor VIII. No single-donor concentrate, analagous to cryoprecipitate, is available for Factor IX, and achieving therapeutic levels of Factor IX with whole plasma requires use of very large volumes. Commercial preparations containing concentrated Factor IX (II, VII, IX and X complex) are available but this product, prepared from large pools of plasma, carries a high risk of disease transmission.[76] The half-life of transfused Factor IX is 24 hours.

The formulas for calculating Factor VIII dosage (see page 278) can be used to calculate Factor IX dosage, but observed posttransfusion Factor IX increments are often less than half that expected from the calculations, even in patients without inhibitors.

Fibrinogen

Hypofibrinogenemia may occur as a rare isolated inherited deficiency or may be acquired as part of the disseminated intravascular coagulation (DIC) syndrome. Cryoprecipitate is the only concentrated fibrinogen product available. An average unit of cryoprecipitate contains approximately 250 mg of fibrinogen.[80] Fibrinogen preparations formerly available are no longer manufactured because of the high risk of transmitting hepatitis B.

Deficiencies of Multiple Coagulation Factors
Factors II, VII, IX and X

The most common condition involving multiple coagulation abnormalities is deficiency of the vitamin K-dependent factors made by the liver; this usually occurs in patients with liver disease or, more rarely, those with deficiency of fat-soluble vitamin K. Production and absorption of vitamin K requires normal intestinal flora and normal mechanisms for digesting and absorbing fats. Vitamin K deficiency may occur when intestinal flora are reduced, as in normal newborns or in adults receiving certain types of antibiotic therapy; in malabsorption syndromes involving digestion of fats; in biliary disease when bile fails to reach the intestine; or after prolonged periods of starvation.

Defects of vitamin K metabolism are best managed by treating the underlying condition, with or without vitamin K administration. If liver function is adequate, coagulation factors return to effective levels about 12 hours after intravenous administration of vitamin K or 24 to 48 hours after intramuscular injection. When liver function is impaired, production of these coagulation proteins is impaired even when vitamin K levels are adequate. Coumarin anticoagulants produce their effect by inhibiting vitamin K utilization and depressing levels of Factors II, VII, IX and X. Injecting vitamin K neutralizes the effect of coumarins within several hours to a day.

Replacement Therapy

Factors II, VII, IX, and X are stable during storage so plasma of any age provides effective replacement. A general guideline for plasma therapy is that 1 ml of plasma contains one unit of coagulation factor activity. Duration of beneficial effect varies with the patient's condition. Factor levels decline faster in consumption coagulopathy than in the presence of simple hemorrhage. The prothrombin time and partial thromboplastin time provide useful information about the need for additional therapy. These screening tests reach normal values when factor levels are at or above 30%. Specific factor assays are also useful if available.

For most patients with multiple coagulation factor deficiencies, fresh frozen plasma is the usual component of choice. The very high hepatitis risk makes commercial concentrates of Factor IX complex (II, VII, IX, X) inadvisable for treating acquired deficiency of multiple factors. Acquired clotting abnormalities rarely produce factor levels as low as those in congenital deficiency, so plasma infusion usually achieves adequate levels without undue risk of disease transmission.

Clinical Conditions

In patients with liver disease there may be deficiencies of several coagulation factors since almost all factors are made in the liver. Since administering vitamin K has no effect, these patients usually require replacement with fresh frozen plasma. Patients with uremia rarely lack plasma coagulation proteins, but often have bleeding problems apparently associated with some degree of platelet dysfunction. There have been reports that cryoprecipitate shortens the prolonged bleeding time in thrombocytopenic uremic patients, possibly through an effect on Factor VIII:vWF.[81]

DIC is another condition associated with deficiency of multiple coagulation factors. Disseminated intravascular coagulation, resulting in intravascular consumption of fibrinogen, platelets and coagulation Factors V and VIII may result from such diverse conditions as obstetric complications, septicemia, shock, disseminated cancer and many others. Hypofibrinogenemia due to DIC requires treatment of the initiating disorder, although replacement of fibrinogen and other clotting factors is often necessary. Very low levels of fibrinogen in these patients cause all the standard clotting tests, including prothrombin time, partial thromboplastin time and thrombin time, to be prolonged; this is in addition to the effects of procoagulant deficiencies and the possible presence of inhibitory protein fragments.

Administration of Components

Fresh frozen plasma (FFP) should be ABO-compatible with the recipient's red blood cells. As a cell-free product, FFP can be given without regard to Rh group. Compatibility testing (minor crossmatch) is not necessary.

It is preferable but not essential to administer ABO-compatible cryoprecipitate. The volume of each unit is small, but most patients receive many units. With large volumes or with units containing especially potent ABO antibodies, the isoagglutinins may cause a positive direct antiglobulin test (DAT) and, rarely, hemolysis. This is more commonly a problem in children, because of their small blood volume, than in adults. Cryoprecipitate can be administered without regard to Rh group and unexpected antibodies are not usually a problem. Commercial Factor VIII concentrates also contain anti-A and anti-B and a positive direct antiglobulin test can be seen after prolonged use. If the recipient of plasma, cryoprecipitate or coagulation factor concentrate develops a positive DAT, initial investigations should focus on ABO antibodies.

Large doses of cryoprecipitate may elevate the recipient's fibrinogen level. Although this rarely cause clinical problems, elevated fibrinogen levels cause a high erythrocyte sedimentation rate (ESR).

Anaphylaxis, allergic reactions to plasma proteins, fluid overload and other serious reactions can follow transfusion of plasma components or products prepared from plasma. Transfusionists should be aware of these hazards and maintain careful clinical surveillance.

Other Blood Proteins

Several new blood fractions are under investigation as potentially clinically useful. These include antithrombin III, protein C and fibronectin. Antithrombin III (AT III), also known as heparin cofactor,[82,83] is manufactured in the liver. When AT III combines with heparin, an arginine site on the AT III is exposed; this neutralizes the serine on thrombin and inactivates its potent enzymatic activity. In normal plasma, AT III is present in concentrations of 23-40 mg/dl.[83] Patients deficient in AT III do not effectively regulate thrombin activity and are prone to thromboembolic diseases. AT III deficiency can be congenital or acquired, as in DIC. The liver synthesizes AT III, and patients with cirrhosis frequently have low levels of this protein; transfusion of AT III may be beneficial to such patients. Currently no purified concentrate of AT III is available, and single-donor plasma is the only transfusion source. The dosage and endpoint for plasma treatment of patients with AT III deficiency are not well defined.[84]

Protein C has profound anticoagulant effect based on its ability to inactivate Factor V and Factor VIII, and also causes an increase in fibrinolytic activity. Normally present in plasma at about 4μg/ml, it is decreased in patients with disseminated intravascular coagulation.[85] Decreased levels of protein C are associated with recurrent thromboembolic disease. Clinical studies are in progress to determine whether replacement therapy is beneficial and what appropriate dosage and monitoring should be.

Fibronectin is an opsonic glycoprotein thought to play a role in the clearance by the reticuloendothelial system (RES) of blood-borne particulate matter such as bacteria and protein aggregates.[86,87] Fibronectin deficiency may be associated with impaired RES function and development of end-organ failure. Uncontrolled clinical studies suggest that infusing fibronectin may be of value in treating septic, burn or trauma patients.[88] The only concentrated form of fibronectin available is cryoprecipitate. If current studies are confirmed,[89] fibronectin may find limited use primarily for critically ill septic patients. Indications for use and methods of monitoring fibronectin therapy remain undetermined.

Plasma Substitutes

Plasma substitutes, chiefly 5% and 25% albumin solutions and plasma protein fraction (PPF), provide volume expansion and colloid replacement without risk of hepatitis,[90] but are often used when less costly or more widely available products would be more appropriate.[91] Albumin solutions do not correct nutritional deficiencies. In cost per calorie, albumin is the most expensive nutrient supplied in the hospital. Nutritional hypoalbuminemia is best treated by enteric or parenteral alimentation or hyperalimentation. Patients with chronic liver disease, notably cirrhosis, have abnormalities of albumin distribution and production, but transfusion of albumin does not alter these abnormalities.

Daily albumin synthesis in a normal adult is about 16 g. Less than half of the body albumin is in the vascular space, with approximately 60% being extravascular.[92] For each 500 ml of blood lost, a person would lose only 11 g or 3.5% of the total body albumin. Thus, albumin in a four-unit hemorrhage (2000 ml) is entirely replaced by normal synthesis in 3 days.

Clinical Considerations

Albumin infusion is appropriate therapy to correct acute, large scale loss of colloid. Examples include treatment of hypovolemic shock, patients with burns, and patients undergoing retroperitoneal surgery, in which a large volume of protein-rich fluid may pool in the atonic bowel.[93] One study has cast doubt on the need for albumin or other colloid solutions during large-volume transfusion in surgery.[94] Problems associated with colloid therapy include the following:

1. Albumin as the 25% solution rapidly increases intravascular oncotic pressure, drawing large volumes of water from the tissues into the vascular space and causing a risk of cardiac overload and/or interstitial dehydration.
2. Hypotensive episodes may accompany rapid infusion of plasma protein fraction, due to the presence of vasoactive kinins.[95] Plasma protein fraction should not be used for rapid restoration of volume, as in treating hypovolemic shock. No specific indications exist for using plasma protein fraction in preference to albumin.
3. Massive daily infusions of albumin (average 150 g/day) decrease synthesis of alpha, beta and gamma globulins, fibrinogen and other coagulation factors.[96]

Special Situations Involving Transfusion

Autologous Transfusion

See Chapter 19.

Massive Transfusion
Emergency Issue

Massive transfusion is defined as transfusion approximating the patient's blood volume within a 24-hour interval. The medical or surgical problems created by hypovolemia and hypotension pose greater risks to the patient than do the risks associated with the blood transfusions.[11,97] The transfusion service must respond promptly but without sacrificing patient safety. If the patient requires immediate transfusion, blood may be issued before completion of routine testing. Group O, Rh-negative red blood cells may be issued immediately; uncrossmatched group-specific whole blood or red blood cells can be issued if there is time to determine the patient's ABO and Rh groups. When volume replacement is critical whole blood is the preferred component.

If the patient's ABO and Rh groups are unknown, group O D-negative blood should be given as red blood cells to avoid possible problems from anti-A and anti-B isoagglutinins.[55] Issuing group-specific blood is desirable as this practice conserves scarce group O D-negative units. However, ABO and Rh determination require approximately 5 minutes and, without a crossmatch, there is no check on ABO compatibility of the donor unit. A combination of approaches is best if the transfusion requirement continues to be urgent. One or two units of group O D-negative red blood cells can be issued immediately, allowing time to determine the patient's ABO and Rh groups and perform an immediate-spin crossmatch on suitable donor units for subsequent transfusion.[98]

Following large-volume transfusion over a short time period, the composition of circulating blood changes and the proportion of the patient's own cells and plasma diminishes. The pretransfusion specimen ceases to represent the patient's current status and crossmatches using the initial specimen have limited validity. If the pretransfusion specimen contained no unexpected antibodies, it is permissible to perform a saline immediate-spin crossmatch for confirmation of ABO compatibility; if unexpected antibodies were present, the same policy is permissible provided the donor blood administered is known to lack the corresponding antigen. This policy must be set forth in the laboratory procedures manual and must be in compliance with *Standards.*

Changing Blood Groups

A transfusion service should establish guidelines for switching to a different blood group during massive transfusion. The age and sex of the patient are important to consider in this decision. When transfusing a young Rh-negative woman it is usually preferable to switch ABO groups, if feasible, before switching Rh; for example, from group A Rh-negative to O Rh-negative, instead of to A Rh-positive. The clinical situation should also be evaluated. If the estimated transfusion requirement exceeds the available amount of all Rh-negative blood, the change to Rh-positive should be done immediately in order to conserve blood from relatively scarce blood groups. In such situations the blood bank medical director should be consulted.

Coagulation Factors

Massive transfusion is sometimes associated with coagulation abnormalities that have been attributed to dilution, or "washout," of platelets or coagulation factors. The unpredictable occurrence of abnormal bleeding during massive transfusion indicates that simple dilution with platelet-deficient or factor-deficient blood is not the only etiology.[11] Furthermore, abnormal test results do not always correlate with clinical problems.

Patients requiring massive transfusion should receive the volume support of whole blood or modified whole blood. After or during transfusion the patient's platelet count as well as coagulation profile should be monitored. If abnormal bleeding occurs, platelet concentrates or fresh frozen plasma should be given based on the results of laboratory testing. Additional tests may be indicated to evaluate the possibility of DIC. Freshly drawn whole blood is not indicated as a supplement to massive transfusion of stored whole or modified whole blood.

A prospective study[13] of 27 patients receiving massive transfusions of modified whole blood from which platelets and cryoprecipitate had been removed revealed that dilutional thrombocytopenia (five cases) and disseminated intravascular coagulation (three cases) were the common causes of hemostatic failure. The eight patients who developed abnormal bleeding had received a mean of 35 units of blood before the coagulopathy developed. Factor V levels were found to vary independently of the quantity of blood transfused and consistently remained above the 5 to 10% of normal necessary for coagulation. Blood stored for 21 days had a mean Factor V level of 35%.

Factor VIII levels were 1% of normal in whole blood modified by cryoprecipitate removal. In whole blood stored more than 48 hours, the activity of Factor VIII decreased to 30%, which is the minimum required for coagulation. Nevertheless, in all of these massively transfused patients, Factor VIII levels remained above 30% except for two patients who developed disseminated intravascular coagulation

(DIC). This indicates that there is a large physiologic reserve of Factor VIII. Factor VIII is one of the plasma proteins described as "acute phase reactants," whose levels increase after trauma or surgery. The levels of the other coagulation factors varied independently of the quantity of blood transfused.

Platelets

Platelet counts decline in massively transfused patients, falling below $100,000/\mu l$ after infusion of 15 to 20 units of modified whole blood in a carefully observed series.[13] The patients in this study who developed DIC had low platelet counts in addition to decreased levels of Factor V, Factor VIII and fibrinogen.

Six of the eight patients who developed bleeding responded to transfusion of platelet concentrates. Platelet concentrates stored at room temperature for 72 hours have substantial quantities of the labile coagulation factors: 68% of normal Factor VIII, and 47% of Factor V.[99] A pool of eight platelet concentrates, with a volume of about 400 ml, should be considered the therapeutic equivalent of one to two units of fresh frozen plasma.

Bacterial Infection

Many plasma constituents contribute to defense against bacterial infection. This group of plasma proteins, called opsonins, includes IgG, IgM and IgA antibodies; components of the classical and alternative complement pathways; and glycoproteins such as fibronectin. Opsonic activity is stable in CPD blood stored under standard conditions for 28 days.[100] Fibronectin is also stable in stored blood components.[101] Patients receiving massive transfusion with red blood cells, crystalloids or albumin solutions may have diminished circulating opsonins.[102] Massively transfused patients are often critically ill and highly susceptible to infection. Some workers have suggested that raising plasma opsonin levels might be beneficial in these patients, but specific therapeutic recommendations must await controlled clinical studies and further understanding of the role of these proteins in health and disease.

Tissue Oxygenation

In hypovolemic shock, the underlying pathophysiologic defect is inadequate tissue oxygenation. Oxygen supply to the tissues is determined by many factors: blood flow, which is in turn affected by cardiac output and vascular constriction or dilation; hemoglobin concentration; red cell 2,3-diphosphoglycerate (2,3-DPG); and degree to which tissues extract oxygen. There are few clinical data to support the thesis that the low 2,3-DPG level found in stored blood is detrimental to massively transfused patients,[11] although in infants undergoing exchange transfusion or in some patients with severe cardiopulmonary disease, this may be important. The most important factor in supporting tissue oxygenation is maintenance of adequate blood flow and blood pressure, by transfusing enough blood to correct or prevent hypovolemic shock. Transfused red cells regenerate 50% of normal 2,3-DPG levels in 3 to 8 hours.[103]

Hypothermia

Warming blood during massive transfusion avoids adverse effects of hypothermia, such as cardiac arrhythmia, and enhances body homeostatic mechanisms that are being stressed.[11] Warming, however, should not slow the rate of infusion so that resuscitation is impeded. (See below.)

Transfusion for Autoimmune Hemolytic Anemia

For patients with autoimmune hemolytic anemia (AIHA), it is desirable to avoid transfusion if at all possible. Transfusion, if unavoidable, should involve the smallest amount of blood sufficient to achieve the clinical objective. This minimizes the volume of cells given, thereby minimizing possible adverse effects if the transfused red cells are rapidly hemolyzed. Transfusion should not be withheld, however, if the patient's anemia is truly life-threatening. (See Chapter 14 for a more detailed discussion.)

Administration of Blood and Components

Identifying Recipient and Donor Unit

Accurate identification of the donor's blood and the intended recipient may be the single most important step in ensuring transfusion safety. Most fatal hemolytic transfusion reactions occur because ABO-incompatible blood was inadvertently administered.[104] Accurate identification and labeling of donor blood are discussed in Chapter 1; procedures to identify the patient's specimen used for compatibility testing are discussed in Chapter 12. The final steps in safe transfusion practice occur when blood is issued for transfusion and at the patient's bedside when blood is administered.

At the Time of Issue

Both the transfusion service personnel who issue the blood and the clinical representative who receives the unit have responsibility for identifying the blood. Before a unit of blood is released, transfusion service personnel must complete the following steps:
1. The name and identification number of the intended recipient must be recorded on the blood request form, the compatibility form and the transfusion form that will become part of the patient's permanent record. The transfusion form and the attached compatibility label or tie tag may be the same piece of paper, but they need not be.
2. The notation of ABO and Rh groups must be the same on the primary label of the blood bag and on the transfusion form. This information is to be recorded on the attached compatibility label or tag.
3. The donor identification number must be identically recorded on the label of the blood bag, the transfusion form and the attached compatibility tag.
4. The color, appearance and expiration date of the blood or component must be checked before issue, and a record made of this inspection.
5. The name of the person issuing the blood, the name of the person to whom the blood is issued and the date and time of issue must be recorded.

At the Time of Infusion

The transfusionist who administers the blood is the last point at which identification errors can be detected before the patient is subjected to transfusion. Before administering the blood or component, the transfusionist must check all identifying information at the patient's bedside, and record on the transfusion form that this information has been checked and found to be correct. Items to be checked are:

1. The name and identification number on the patient's wrist band must be identical with the name and number on the transfusion form and on the compatibility label or tie tag.
2. The ABO and Rh groups of the patient and of the donor unit must be recorded on the transfusion form. The ABO and Rh groups on the primary label of the donor unit must be the same as those noted on the compatibility label or tie tag, and these must be ABO and Rh compatible with the patient's ABO and Rh groups.
3. The same donor unit identification number must be on the primary label of the bag, the transfusion form, and the attached compatibility tag. The expiration date of the donor unit should be verified before infusion.
4. The compatibility label or tie tag must indicate the identity of the person per-

forming the compatibility tests and the interpretation of the results. If blood was issued before compatibility tests were completed, this must be conspicuously indicated on the label.

5. The blood or component should be checked against the physician's written order, to be sure the correct component is being given.

Before administering the blood, the transfusionist must perform positive identification of the patient. Checking the wrist band is the best means of identification. Even if the patient's name is unknown, there must be some emergency identification number that can be permanently recorded. In addition to the wrist band, the transfusionist should check the identification a second way; this can be done by:

1. Asking the patient to state his name if he is able to respond. It is not a good idea to ask "Are you (name)?" because patients often agree to anything that hospital personnel say, to avoid being uncooperative. If the patient is responsive, it is important to explain what the transfusion procedure involves and how long it is likely to take. The patient should be encouraged to ask questions about the procedure. This is also an opportunity for the transfusionist to inquire whether the patient has experienced adverse effects from previous transfusions, and to warn of symptoms that should prompt the patient to call for clinical assistance.

2. Asking a relative or someone involved with the clinical care to state the patient's name.

Starting the Transfusion

After checking all the identifying information, the transfusionist must sign the transfusion form to indicate that the identification was correct and to document who started the transfusion. The directors of many transfusion services require that a second individual confirm the identity of the blood unit and of the patient. Notation of date and time of transfusion may also be required on the transfusion form. The date and time of transfusion, and the patient's condition at the start of transfusion should be recorded, and name and volume of the component and its identification number must be recorded in the patient's clinical record.

In addition to informing the patient of the procedure and checking all identification steps, the transfusionist should observe and record the patient's vital signs before administering the blood. Knowing the patient's pretransfusion temperature, pulse, respiration and blood pressure is important because the first sign of adverse reaction may be a change in these variables. Alternatively, the patient's posttransfusion vital signs may be abnormal, but if they were abnormal at the start, the transfusion will not necessarily be implicated. Prior to transfusion the patient should be asked about any symptoms, such as dizziness, itching or difficulty breathing, that also might be confused with a transfusion reaction.

Issuing Blood or Components

Blood should be administered as soon as possible after issue. Blood must not be stored in unmonitored refrigerators of the sort commonly found in nursing stations and on wards. If transfusion cannot be initiated within a short time, the blood should be returned to the blood bank. Many blood banks set a time limit past which issued blood will not be accepted back into inventory. This limit is often 30 minutes, which is the time it takes for blood to reach 6 C when exposed to room temperature.[105] Blood remains at room temperature for several hours during transfusion; while this does not harm the red cells, prolonged stay outside the refrigerator makes a unit of blood unsuitable for reissue by the blood bank. An unused unit of blood that has reached 10 C or above cannot be reissued by the blood bank due to the risk of bacterial growth.

If it appears that more than three or four hours will be needed to complete the transfusion, it may be wise to administer the blood in several aliquots so that part of the blood can remain refrigerated while part is slowly infused. The transfusion service can divide any transfusion component into aliquots, although following entry into the container during separation, all the aliquots must be used within 24 hours. If separation is effected without breaking the closed system, the unused portions retain their original expiration date. A new crossmatch sample is needed if more than 2 days elapse after administration of the initial portion of red blood cells or whole blood. It is not permissible to add medication to blood or components.

Transfusion Devices

An increasing number of mechanical devices are available to facilitate administration and storage of blood and components. Individuals involved in transfusion practice should know the proper use of these products.

Blood Warmers

Patients receiving refrigerated blood at rates faster than 100 ml/minute for 30 minutes have had an increased incidence of cardiac arrest as compared with a control group receiving blood warmed to 37 C.[106] Large volumes of rapidly infused cold blood can lower the temperature of the sino-atrial node to below 30 C, at which point ventricular arrhythmias occur. There is no evidence, however, that patients receiving one to three units of blood over several hours are at similar risk for arrhythmias. Routine warming of blood is unnecessary. In addition, blood warming usually slows the rate of infusion.

There are several types of blood warmers: 1) a coil of plastic tubing through which the blood travels; 2) electrically heated plates in contact with a flat plastic blood bag. Microwave devices damage red cells[107,108] and should not be used for blood. Coiled plastic tubing, which warms blood

because the blood is exposed to increased surface area, can be left at ambient temperature or be placed in a monitored waterbath at a temperature no higher than 37 C. Exposure to temperatures above 37 C may cause hemolysis. Electrical blood warmers must have a visible thermometer and should have an audible or visual warning system to notify the transfusionist when temperatures rise above 37 C. Blood warmers should be used only when there is significant risk of transfusion-induced cardiac hypothermia.

Red blood cells or whole blood should not be subjected to warming devices or water baths that warm the entire unit; only the blood passing through the administration set should be warmed. Frozen components placed in a waterbath for thawing must either be protectively wrapped or be positioned so the water does not touch the transfusion ports of the bag.[109]

Electromechanical Infusion Devices

Mechanical pumps that facilitate infusion at controlled rates are useful especially for very slow rates of transfusion to pediatric or neonatal patients. When using these pumps for blood transfusion, the transfusionist must ensure that hemolysis does not occur. Some pumps use a mechanical screwdrive to advance the plunger of a syringe filled with blood; others use roller pumps or other forms of pressure applied to infusion tubing. Although some can be used with standard blood administration sets, most require dedicated software supplied by the manufacturer. Packed cells, with their high hematocrit and therefore high viscosity, are likely to undergo hemolysis when infused under pressure. Whole blood or red blood cells diluted with saline and whole blood have lower hematocrits and therefore lower viscosities, so they experience lower shear forces during pumping and are less likely to undergo hemolysis. The manufacturer should be consulted before transfusing red blood cells with an infusion pump designed for use with crystalloid or colloid solutions. Studies with [111]Indium labeled platelet concentrates administered through a pump showed no loss of in vitro platelet function or in vivo recovery.[110]

Filters

Blood and components must be administered through a filter designed to retain blood clots and other debris. Standard blood filters have a pore size of 170-260 μ and can trap large blood clots. Some administration sets for platelets or cryoprecipitate have filters incorporated in tubing suitable for syringe administration. Filters are not routinely necessary for infusion of commercially prepared plasma products like albumin, but the manufacturer's instructions should be consulted for individual products.

Microaggregate filters have an effective pore size of 20-40 μ, and trap microaggregates composed of degenerating platelets, white cells and fibrin strands which form in blood after 5 or more days of storage. Microaggregates, which range in size from 20-160 μ, can pass through standard blood filters and are thought to accumulate in pulmonary capillaries after transfusion. Whether or not microaggregate debris causes the adult respiratory distress syndrome or other pulmonary dysfunction has been extensively debated.[111-113] Microaggregate blood filters are routinely used during cardiopulmonary bypass. No published data support the routine use of microaggregate blood filters for low-volume transfusions.[113] Some emergency room physicians, surgeons and anesthesiologists consider that the slowed flow that results from use of these filters makes them inappropriate in settings of very rapid massive transfusion.[111,113] There have been recent reports of hemolysis induced by use of a pediatric microaggregate filter,[114,115] due, at least in part, to the small surface area of the pediatric filter. (See Chapter 3 and pages 269-270 for use of microaggregate filters to reduce the transfused load of white cell antigens.)

Platelet Storage

For platelet concentrates, storage at 20-24 C is preferable to refrigerated storage at 1-6 C.[116] The first widely used plastic containers for platelet storage were made of polyvinyl chloride with a 2-diethylhexylphthalate (DEHP) plasticizer; platelets stored in these bags had a 3-day shelf-life. Plastic bags of newer formulas permit a shelf-life as long as 7 days. These are made of polyolefin without any plasticizer (Fenwal Laboratories, PL-732) or of polyvinyl chloride with a non 2-DEHP plasticizer, the most popular being tri(2-ethylhexyl) trimellitate (Cutter, CLX System; Fenwal Laboratories, PL-1240). These plastics permit improved gas exchange during platelet storage and allow maintenance of a more favorable pH. The trimellitate plasticizer does not leach into plasma to the same extent as the diethylhexylphthalate plasticizer. The storage characteristics of the various plastic bags have been evaluated.[117-119]

Platelet concentrates must be gently agitated during room-temperature storage. Platelet agitators come in a variety of types including units with an elliptical axis of rotation at 1 or 6 rpm, a circular axis of rotation at 2 or 6 rpm, or horizontal motion oscillating at 70 cycles per minute.

There are no guidelines specifying the type of agitation to be used for platelet storage. At present, any of the 1 rpm elliptical, or 2 or 6 rpm circular tumblers appear satisfactory for storage of any available 7-day platelet bag. Platelets stored in PL-732, a polyolefin plastic, and agitated on 6 rpm elliptical rotators for 5 days have decreased in vivo survival.[120,121]

Cell Washers

A variety of automated machines are available for washing units of blood. These devices all the use an open system in which blood is washed with large volumes of normal saline. These machines effectively remove plasma, platelets and most white cells, but they increase the cost of transfusion and impose a 24-hour expiration for the washed unit. Washed red cells may be useful for patients who have experienced two or more documented febrile transfusion reactions. There is little justification for routine washing of all units of blood.

Needles

Flow at high pressure or through large-gauge needles may damage red cells.[122,123] For infusing whole blood or red blood cells, an 18- or 19-gauge needle gives good flow rates without excessive discomfort for the patient. For patients with small veins, much smaller needles must be used. A thin-walled, 23-gauge "scalp vein" needle is useful not only in scalp veins but for pediatric transfusions in general, and for adults whose large veins are inaccessible. Blood, especially red cells, flows very slowly through a 23-gauge needle, and applying excessive external pressure to speed infusion may damage the cells. Diluting red cells with saline reduces viscosity and enhances flow, but the added saline may cause unwanted volume expansion. If flow is so slow that transfusion will not be completed within four hours, it may be desirable to separate the unit into aliquots, and keep part of it stored in the blood bank while the first portion is transfused.

Either steel needles or plastic catheters can be used for intravenous infusions. Catheters are more comfortable if infusions are to continue for a long period of time, and are less likely to become dislodged or allow solutions to infiltrate. The risks of infection and of thrombophlebitis increase with the length of time a catheter remains in place. Local procedures manuals should state the maximum time a catheter may remain in a vein, and should outline a surveillance procedure to be sure that catheters are maintained aseptically and changed as often as specified.

Compatible Fluids

Standards is explicit in stating that no medication or intravenous solutions other than normal saline may be added to blood or components.[55] Diluting red blood cells to reduce viscosity is the circumstance to which this most often applies, but intravenous solutions are sometimes used to rinse cryoprecipitate out of the bag. Normal saline is the only acceptable crystalloid fluid. ABO-compatible plasma or 5% (not 25%) serum albumin may be used to dilute red cells or other components.

Standards is not, however, explicit about which fluids may come in contact with blood in infusion sets, stating only that there must be adequate evidence that they are safe. Contraindicated are lactated Ringer's solution, 5% dextrose in water and hypotonic sodium chloride solutions. The dextrose solution causes red cells to clump in the tubing and, more importantly, causes red cells to swell and hemolyze as dextrose and associated water diffuse from the medium into the cells.[124] Lactated Ringer's solution contains enough ionized calcium (3 mEq/l) to overcome the anticoagulant effect of CPDA-1 and allow small clots to develop. When blood follows an electrolyte solution through administration tubing, 25% of the electrolyte solution remains in the tubing after 10 minutes, and 10% persists at 30 minutes.[124] The best solution to use is 0.9% NaCl USP.

Care During Transfusion

The transfusionist should remain with the patient for the initial 5 to 15 minutes of the infusion. Catastrophic events such as anaphylactic reactions or massive hemolysis due to ABO incompatibility usually become apparent after a very small volume of blood enters the patient's circulation. The earlier these catastrophes are detected, the more promptly the infusion can be discontinued and treatment instituted. If no problems occur in the first 5 to 15 minutes, the risk of immediate life-threatening complications declines sharply, although the possibility of adverse effects continues throughout and after the entire process. After the first 15 minutes, the patient's vital signs should be recorded and, if there is no evidence of impending reaction, the rate of infusion can be increased to that specified in the clinical order. Patient-care personnel should observe the patient frequently throughout the transfusion.

Rate of Infusion

The desirable rate of infusion varies with the patient's blood volume, hemodynamic condition and cardiac status. For rapid infusion, external pressure devices make it possible to administer a unit of blood within a few minutes. These should be used only with a large-bore needle. External compression devices should be equipped with a pressure gauge, and the pressure exerted should not be greater than 300 mm Hg. Blood pressure cuffs are not suitable because they do not exert uniform pressure against all parts of the bag, and irregularly applied pressure may cause the bag to leak.

There is no definitive rule for the maximum time a transfusion may take. Most blood bankers believe that infusion of a single unit of blood or component should take no more than 4 hours, although there are no experimental or clinical data on which a specific temporal restriction can be based.

There are also no definitive rules for the length of time an administration set or filter may remain in use. A reasonable maximum time limit for use of a blood filter is 4 hours. Filters trap clumped cells, cellular debris and coagulated protein, resulting in a high protein concentration at the filter surface. If bacteria are present, the combination of room temperature incubation and high protein concentration could allow the bacteria to multiply on the filter more rapidly than they would in refrigerated blood. Accumulated material also slows the rate of flow. Filters can ordinarily be used for two to four units of blood but filters that have remained at room temperature for prolonged periods should not be reused.

If blood flows more slowly than is wished, the filter or the needle may be obstructed, or the component may simply be too viscous for rapid flow through the administration set. Steps to investigate and correct the problem include the following:
1. Elevate the blood container to increase gravitational pressure.
2. Check the patency of the needle.
3. Examine the filter of the administration set for excessive debris.
4. If red blood cells are flowing too slowly, and there is an order permitting addition of saline, add 50 to 100 ml normal saline.

Discontinuing the Transfusion

After each unit of blood has been infused, patient-care personnel should record the time, the volume and type of component given, the patient's condition and the identity of the person who stopped the transfusion and observed the patient. Many transfusion services require that a copy of the completed transfusion form be returned to the transfusion service. Returning the empty blood bag after uncomplicated transfusions serves no useful purpose, and creates a serious risk of contamination to personnel who handle and sort through these opened, often leaking, containers. The patient should remain under observation for at least an hour after the transfusion is completed, and posttransfusion vital signs should be recorded according to the protocol established in the institution's procedures manual.

Part of good transfusion practice is posttransfusion observation to ensure that the desired clinical goal has been achieved. This includes obtaining posttransfusion hematocrit, platelet count or coagulation factor level, as indicated for the component transfused. The possibility of delayed hemolytic reactions, usually occurring 3 to 14 days after transfusion, should also be kept in mind. Posttransfusion hepatitis can develop as early as 2 weeks or as late as 6 months after transfusion and there should be some form of follow-up to determine whether liver damage has occurred.

Use of Rh Immune Globulin

When Rh-positive red cells are given to an Rh-negative recipient, either intentionally or accidentally, the patient's physician should be advised that treatment with Rh Immune Globulin (RhIG) may prevent sensitization. One full dose of RhIG is required for each 15 ml of Rh-positive red cells transfused. Thus 15 to 20 vials of RhIG would be needed after transfusion of one unit of Rh-incompatible red blood cells or whole blood. The blood bank director and the patient's physician should decide jointly on undertaking prophylaxis. Issues to consider include the discomfort of injecting large volumes of gamma globulin, the cost of the RhIG, the consequences of possible immunization on subsequent transfusions or pregnancies and the possibility that the RhIG immunosuppression may be unsuccessful. Since platelet and granulocyte concentrates contain sufficient red cells to immunize an Rh-negative patient if the cells are D-positive, consideration should be given to administering RhIG after tranfusing these components. (See page 273 for more detailed discussion.) Fresh frozen plasma and cryoprecipitate may be transfused without regard to Rh group, although one case was reported in which anti-D developed after exchange transfusion involving 24 liters of plasma.[125]

References

1. Mollison PL. Blood transfusion in clinical medicine. 7th ed. Oxford: Blackwell Scientific Publications, 1983:114.

2. Orlina AR, Josephson AM. Comparative viability of blood stored in ACD and CPD. Transfusion 1969;9:62-69.

3. Zuck TF, Bensinger TA, Peck RK, et al. The in vivo survival of red blood cells stored in modified CPD with adenine. Transfusion 1977;17:374-382.

4. Gollub S, Svigals R, Bailey CP, Hirose T, Schaefer C. Electrolyte solutions in surgical patients refusing transfusion. JAMA 1971;215:2077-2083.

5. Rigor B, Bosomworth P, Rush BF, Jr. Replacement of operative blood loss of more than 1 liter with Hartmann's solution. JAMA 1968;203:399-402.

6. Rawstron RE. Preoperative haemoglobin levels. Anaesth Intensive Care 1976;4:175-183.

7. Graves CL, Allen RM. Anesthesia in the presence of severe anemia. Rocky Mt Med J 1970;67:35-40.

8. Czer LSC, Shoemaker WC. Optimal hematocrit value in critically ill postoperative patients. Surg Gynecol Obstet 1978; 147:363-368.

9. Friedman BA, Oberman HA, Chadwick AR, Kingdon KI. The maximum surgical blood order schedule and surgical blood use in the United States. Transfusion 1976;16:380-387.

10. Rouault C, Gruenhagen J. Reorganization of blood ordering practices. Transfusion 1978;18:448-453.

11. Collins JA. Problems associated with massive transfusion of stored blood. Surgery 1974;75:274-295.

12. Schmidt PJ. Red cells for transfusion. N Engl J Med 1978;299:1411-1412.

13. Counts RB, Haish C, Simon TL, Maxwell NG, Heimbach DM, Carrico CJ. Hemostasis in massively transfused trauma patients. Ann Surg 1979;190:91-99.

14. Milner LV, Butcher K. Transfusion reactions reported after transfusions of red blood cells and of whole blood. Transfusion 1978;18:493-495.

15. Friedman BA. An analysis of surgical blood use in United States hospitals with application to the maximum surgical blood order schedule. Transfusion 1979;19:268-278.

16. Heaton A, Miripol J, Aster R, et al. 49 to 56 day storage of high hematocrit red cell concentrates using ADSOL preservation solution. (abstract) Transfusion 1982;22:432

17. Thulstrup H. The influence of leukocyte and thrombocyte incompatibility on non-haemolytic transfusion reactions. Vox Sang 1971;21:233-250.

18. Menitove JE, McElligott MC, Aster RH. Febrile transfusion reactions: what blood component should be given next. Vox Sang 1982;42:318-321.

19. Wenz B, Gurtlinger KF, O'Toole AM, Dugan EP. The preparation of granulocyte poor red blood cells by microaggregate filtration. Vox Sang 1980;39:282-287.

20. Schned AR, Silver H. The use of microaggregate filtration in the prevention of febrile

transfusion reactions. Transfusion 1981;21:675-681.

21. Hughes ASB, Brozovic B. Leucocyte depleted blood: an appraisal of available techniques. Br J Haemat 1982;50:381-386.

22. Grunnet N, Rasmussen NJ. Production of leukocyte poor blood - a comparison of five different methods. Scand J Urol Nephrol 1981; Suppl 64:106-111.

23. Yap PL, Pryde EAD, McClelland DBL. IgA content of frozen-thawed-washed red blood cells and blood products measured by radioimmunoassay. Transfusion 1982; 22:36-38.

24. Alter HJ, Tabor E, Meryman HT, et al. Transmission of hepatitis B virus infection by transfusion of frozen-deglycerolized red blood cells. N Engl J Med 1978;298:637-642.

25. Haugen RK. Hepatitis after the transfusion of frozen red cells and washed red cells. N Engl J Med 1979;301:393-395.

26. Opelz G, Terasaki PI. Dominant effect of transfusions on kidney graft survival. Transplantation 1980;29:153-158.

27. Kurtz SR, Van Deinse WH, Valeri CR. The immunocompetence of residual lymphocytes at various stages of red cell cyropreservation with 40% W/V glycerol in an ionic medium at − 80 C. Transfusion 1978;18:441-447.

28. Freireich EJ, Kliman A, Gaydos LA, Mantel N, Frei E. Response to repeated platelet transfusion from the same donor. Ann Intern Med 1963;59:277-287.

29. Daly PA, Schiffer CA, Aisner J, Wiernik PH. Platelet transfusion therapy. JAMA 1980;243:435-438.

30. Slichter SJ. Controversies in platelet transfusion therapy. Ann Rev Med 1980;31:509-540.

31. Gaydos LA, Freireich EJ, Mantel N. The quantitative relationship between platelet count and hemorrhage in patients with acute leukemia. N Engl J Med 1962;266:905-909.

32. Howard JE, Perkins HA. The natural history of alloimmunization to platelets. Transfusion 1978;18:496-503.

33. Dutcher JP, Schiffer CA, Aisner J, Wiernik PH. Alloimmunization following platelet transfusion: the absence of a dose-response relationship. Blood 1981;57:395-398.

34. Dutcher JP, Schiffer CA, Aisner J, Wiernik PH. Long-term follow-up of patients with leukemia receiving platelet transfusions: Identification of a large group of patients who do not become alloimmunized. Blood 1981;58:1007-1011.

35. Solomon J, Bofenkamp T, Fahey JL, Chillar RK, Beutler E. Platelet prophylaxis in acute non-lymphocytic leukemia. (letter) Lancet 1978;1:267.

36. Slichter SJ, Harker LA. Thrombocytopenia: mechanisms and management of defects in platelet production. Clin Haematol 1978;7:523-539.

37. Weiss HJ. Platelets—pathophysiology and antiplatelet therapy. New York: Alan R. Liss; 1982.

38. Junghans RP, Ahn YS. High dose intravenous gamma globulin to suppress alloimmune destruction of donor platelets. Am J Med 1984;76(3A):204-208.

39. Aster RH. Effect of anticoagulant and ABO incompatibility on recovery of transfused human platelets. Blood 1965;26:732-743.

40. Duquesnoy RJ, Anderson AJ, Tomasulo PA, Aster RH. ABO compatibility and platelet transfusions of alloimmunized thrombocytopenic patients. Blood 1979;54:595-599.

41. Moroff G, Friedman A, Robkin-Kline L, Gautier G, Luban N. Reduction of the volume of stored platelet concentrates for neonatal use. (abstract) Transfusion 1982;22:427.

42. Goldfinger D, McGinniss MH. Rh incompatible platelet transfusion—risks and consequences of sensitizing immunosuppressed patients. N Engl J Med 1971;284:942-944.

43. Lichtiger B, Surgeon J, Rhorer S. Rh-incompatible platelet transfusion therapy in cancer patients. Vox Sang 1983;45:139-143.

44. Lalezari P, Driscoll AM. Ability of thrombocytes to acquire HLA specificity from plasma. Blood 1982;59:167-170.

45. Schiffer CA, Keller C, Dutcher JP, Aisner J, Hogge D, Wiernik PH. Potential HLA-matched platelet donor availability for alloimmunized patients. Transfusion 1983;23:286-289.

46. Aster RH. Matching of blood platelets for transfusion. Am J Hematol 1978;5:373-378.

47. Menitove JE, Aster RH. Transfusion of platelets and plasma products. Clin Haematol 1983; 12:239-266.

48. Schiffer CA, Aisner J, Wiernik PH. Frozen autologous platelet transfusion for patients with leukemia. N Engl J Med 1978;299:7-12

49. Schiffer CA, Slichter SJ. Platelet transfusions from single donors. N Engl J Med 1982;307:245-247.

50. Higby DJ, Burnett D. Granulocyte transfusions: current status. Blood 1980;55:2-8.

51. Rosenshein MS, Farewell VT, Price TH, Larson EB, Dale DC. The cost effectiveness of therapeutic and prophylactic leukocyte transfusion. N Engl J Med 1980;302:1058-1062.

52. Bodey GP, Buckley M, Sathe YS, Freireich EJ. Quantitative relationships between circulating leukocytes and infection in patients with acute leukemia. Ann Intern Med 1966;64:328-340.

53. Pflieger H, Arnold R, Bhaduri S, et al. Granulocyte transfusions in acute leukemia. Scand J Haematol 1981;26:215-220.

54. Dahlke MB, Keashen M, Alavi JB, Koch PA, Eisenstaedt R. Granulocyte transfusions and outcome of alloimmunized patients with gram-negative sepsis. Transfusion 1982;22:374-378.

55. Schmidt PJ, ed. Standards for blood banks and transfusion services, 11th ed. Arlington, VA: American Assocation of Blood Banks, 1984.

56. McCollough J. Liquid preservation of granulocytes. Transfusion 1980;20:129-137.

57. Buchholz DH, Blumberg N, Bove JR. Long term granulocyte transfusion in patients with malignant neoplasms. Arch Intern Med 1979;139:317-320.

58. Schiffer CA. Some aspects of recent advances in the use of blood cell components. Br J Haematol 1978;39:289-294.

59. Karp DD, Ervin TJ, Tuttle S, Gorgone BC, Lavin P, Yunis EJ. Pulmonary complications during granulocyte transfusions: incidence and clinical features. Vox Sang 1982;42:57-61.

60. Aisner J, Schiffer CA, Wiernik PH. Granulocyte transfusions: evaluation of factors influencing results and a comparison of filtration and intermittent centrifugation leukapheresis. Br J Haematol 1978;38:121-129.

61. Dahlke MB, Shah SH, Sherwood WC, Shafer AW, Brownstein PK. Priapism during filtration leukapheresis. Transfusion 1979;19:482-486.

62. Winston DJ, Ho WG, Gale RP. Therapeutic granulocyte transfusion for documented infections. Ann Int Med 1982;97:509-515.

63. Ford JM, Cullen MH, Roberts MM, Brown LM, Oliver RTD, Lister TA. Prophylactic granulocyte transfusions. Transfusion 1982;22:311-316.

64. Strauss RG, Connett JE, Gale RP, et al. A controlled trial of prophylactic granulocyte transfusions during initial induction. N Engl J Med 1981;305:597-603.

65. Winston DJ, Ho WG, Gale RP. Prophylactic granulocyte transfusions during chemotherapy of acute nonlymphocytic leukemia. Ann Int Med 1981;94:616-622.

66. Laurenti F, Ferro R, Isacchi G, et al. Polymorphonuclear leukocyte transfusion for the treatment of sepsis in the newborn infant. J Ped 1981;98:118-123.

67. Dana BW, Durie BGM, White RF, Heustis DW. Concomitant administration of granulocyte transfusions and amphotericin B in neutropenic patients: absence of significant pulmonary toxicity. Blood 1981;57:90-94.

68. Wright DG, Robichaud KJ, Pizzo BS, Deisseroth AB. Lethal pulmonary reactions associated with the combined use of Amphotericin B and leukocyte transfusions. N Engl J Med 1981;304:1185-1189.

69. Hersman J, Meyers JD, Thomas ED, Buckner CD, Cleft R. The effect of granulocyte transfusions on the incidence of cytomegalovirus infection after allogeneic marrow transplantation. Ann Intern Med 1982;96:149-152.

70. Winston DJ, Pollard RB, Ho WG, et al. Cytomegalovirus immune plasma in bone marrow transplant recipients. Annals Int Med 1982;97:11-18.

71. Hoyer LW. The Factor VIII complex: structure and function. Blood 1981;58:1-13.

72. Perkins HA. Correction of the hemostatic defects in von Willebrand's disease. Blood 1967;30:375-380.

73. Preston FE, Triger DR, Underwood JCE, et al. Percutaneous liver biopsy and chronic disease in haemophiliacs. Lancet 1978;2:592-594.

74. Buchanan GR, Kevy SV. Use of prothrombin complex concentrates in hemophiliacs with inhibitors: Clinical and laboratory studies. Pediatrics 1978;62:767-774.

75. Lusher JM, Shapiro SS, Palascak JE, et al. Efficacy of prothrombin-complex concentrates in hemophiliacs with antibodies to Factor VIII. N Engl J Med 1980;303:421-425.

76. Food and Drug Administration. Factor IX complex and hepatitis. FDA drug bulletin 1976;6:22.

77. Hilgartner MW, Knatterud GL, FEIBA Study Group. The use of factor eight inhibitor by-passing activity (FEIBA IMMUNO) product for treatment of bleeding episodes in hemophiliacs with inhibitors. Blood 1983;61:36-40.

78. Abildgaard CF, Penner JA, Watson-Williams J. Anti-inhibitor coagulant complex (Auto-

plex) for treatment of Factor VIII inhibitors in hemophilia. Blood 1980;56:978-984.

79. Warrier AI, Lusher JM. DDAVP: a useful alternative to blood components in moderate hemophilia-A and von Willebrand's disease. J Pediatrics 1983;102:228-233.

80. Ness PM, Perkins HA. Cryoprecipitate as a reliable source of fibrinogen replacement. JAMA 1979;241:1690-1691.

81. Janson PA, Jubelirer SJ, Weinstein MS, Deykin D. Treatment of bleeding tendency in uremia with cryoprecipitate. N Engl J Med 1980;303:1318-1322.

82. Schipper HG, Ten Cate JW. Antithrombin III transfusion in patients with hepatic cirrhosis. Br J Haematol 1982;52:25-33.

83. Seegers WH. Antithrombin III. Therapy and clinical applications. Am J Clin Pathol 1978;69:367-374.

84. Liebman HA, McGehee WG, Patch MJ, Feinstein DI. Severe depression of antithrombin III associated with disseminated intravascular coagulation in women with fatty liver of pregnancy. Ann Intern Med 1983;98:330-333.

85. Griffin JH, Mosher DF, Zimmerman TS, Kleiss AJ. Protein C, an antithrombotic protein, is reduced in hospitalized patients with intravascular coagulation. Blood 1982;60:261-264.

86. Saba TM, Jaffe E. Plasma fibronectin (opsonic glycoprotein): its synthesis by vascular endothelial cells and role in cardiopulmonary integrity after trauma as related to reticuloendothelial function. Am J Med 1980;68:577-594.

87. Mosher DF. Fibronectin. Prog Hemost Thromb 1980;5:111-151.

88. Scovill WA, Saba TM, Blumenstock FA, Bernard H, Powers SR, Jr. Opsonic α_2 surface binding glycoprotein therapy during sepsis. Ann Surg 1978;188:521-529.

89. Snyder EL, Barash PG, Mosher DF, Walter SD. Plasma fibronectin level and clinical status in cardiac surgery patients. J Lab Clin Med 1983;102:881-889.

90. Gerety RJ, Aronson DL. Plasma derivatives and viral hepatitis. Transfusion 1982;22:347-351.

91. Alexander MR, Ambre JJ, Liskow BI. Trost DC. Therapeutic use of albumin. JAMA 1979;241:2527-2529.

92. Beattie HW, Evans G, Garnett ES, Regoeczi E, Webber CE, Wong KL. Albumin and water fluxes during cardiopulmonary bypass. J Thorac Cardiovasc Surg 1974;67:926-931.

93. Snyder E. Clinical use of albumin, plasma protein fraction and isoimmune globulin products. In: Silvergleid A, Britten A, eds. Plasma products: use and management. Arlington, VA: American Association of Blood Banks; 1982:87-107.

94. Virgilio RW, Rice CL, Smith DE, et al. Crystalloid vs colloid resuscitation: is one better? Surgery 1979;85:129-139.

95. Alving BM, Hojima Y, Pisano JJ, Mason BL, Buckingham RE, Mozen MM, et al. Hypotension associated with prekallikrein activator (Hageman-factor fragments) in plasma protein fraction. N Engl J Med 1978;299:66-70.

96. Lucas CE, Bouwman DL, Ledgerwood AM, Higgins R. Differential serum protein changes following supplemental albumin resuscitation for hypovolemic shock. J Trauma 1980;20:47-51.

97. Sohmer PR, Dawson RB. Transfusion therapy in trauma: a review of the principles and techniques used in the MIEMS program. Am Surg 1979;45:109-125.

98. Barnes A. The blood bank in hemotherapy for trauma and surgery. In: Hemotherapy for trauma and surgery. Washington, DC: American Association of Blood Banks; 1979:77-87.

99. Simon TL, Henderson R. Coagulation factor activity in platelet concentrates. Transfusion 1979;19:186-189.

100. McClellan MA, Alexander JW. The opsonic activity of stored blood. Transfusion 1977;17:227-232.

101. Snyder EL, Ferri PM, Mosher DF. Fibronectin level in liquid and frozen stored blood components. Transfusion 1984;24:53-56.

102. Alexander JW. Hemotherapy and antibacterial defense mechanisms. In: Collins JA, Lundsgaard-Hansen P, eds: Surgical hemotherapy (Bibliotheca haematologica 46). New York: S. Karger; 1980:26-36.

103. Beutler E, Muel A, Wood LA. Depletion and regeneration of 2,3-diphosphoglyceric acid in stored red blood cells. Transfusion 1969;9:109-114.

104. Honig CL, Bove JR. Transfusion-associated fatalities. Transfusion 1980;20:653-661.

105. Pick P, Fabijanic J. Temperature changes in donor blood under different storage conditions. Transfusion 1971;11:213-215.

106. Boyan CP, Howland WS. Cardiac arrest and temperature of bank blood. JAMA 1963;183:58-60.

107. Staples PJ, Griner PF. Extracorporeal hemolysis of blood in a microwave blood warmer. N Engl J Med 1971;285:317-319.

108. Linko K, Hynynen K. Erythrocyte damage caused by the Haemotherm microwave blood warmer. Acta Anaesth Scand 1979;23:320-328.

109. Rhame FS, McCullough J. Follow up on nosocomial *Pseudomonas cepacia* infection. Mort Morbid Week Rep 1979;28:409.

110. Snyder EL, Ferri P, Smith E, Ezekowitz M. Study of in vitro damage and in vivo survival of stored platelet concentrate after passage through an electromechanical infusion pump. Transfusion 1984;24:524-527.

111. International Forum. Does a relationship exist between massive blood transfusions and the adult respiratory distress syndrome? If so, what are the best preventive measures? Vox Sang 1977;32:311-320.

112. Durtschi MB, Haisch CE, Reynolds, et al. Effect of micropore filtration on pulmonary function after massive transfusion. Am J Surg 1979;138:8-14.

113. Snyder E, Bookbinder M. Role of microaggregate blood filtration in clinical medicine. Transfusion 1983;23:460-470.

114. Schmidt WF, Kim HC, Tomassini N, Schwartz E. Red blood cell destruction caused by a micropore blood filter. JAMA 1982;248:1629-1632.

115. Longhurst DM, Gooch W, Castillo RA. In vitro evaluation of a pediatric microaggregate blood filter. Transfusion 1983;23:170-172.

116. Murphy S, Sayar SN, Gardner FH. Storage of platelet concentrates at 22C. Blood 1970;35:549-557.

117. Snyder EL, Koerner TAW, Kakaiya R, Moore P, Kiraly T. Effect of mode of agitation on storage of platelet concentrates in PL-732 containers for 5 days. Vox Sang 1983;44:300-304.

118. Snyder EL, Bookbinder M, Kakaiya R, Ferri P, Kiraly T. Five day storage of platelet concentrates in CLX containers: effect of type of agitation. Vox Sang 1983;45:432-437.

119. Holme S, Vaidya K, Murphy S. Platelet storage at 22C: effect of type of agitation on morphology, viability and function in vitro. Blood 1978;52:425-435.

120. Murphy S, Kahn R, Holme S, et al. Improved storage of platelets for transfusion in a new container. Blood 1982;60:194-200.

121. Snyder EL, Ferri P, Smith E, Pope C, Ezekowitz M. In vivo survival of Indium-111 labeled platelet concentrates: lack of correlation with in vitro release of lactic dehydrogenase and thromboglobulin. (abstract) Transfusion 1983;23:425.

122. Wilcox GJ, Barnes A, Modanlou H. Does transfusion using a syringe infusion pump and small gauge needle cause hemolysis? Transfusion 1981;21:750-751.

123. Herrera AJ, Corless J. Blood transfusions: effect of speed of infusion and of needle gauge on hemolysis. J Pediat 1981;99:757-758.

124. Ryden SE, Oberman HA. Compatibility of common intravenous solutions with CPD blood. Transfusion 1975;15:250-255.

125. McBride JA, O'Hoski P, Barnes CC, Spiak C, Blajchman MA. Rhesus alloimmunization following intensive plasma exchange. Transfusion 1983;23:352-354.

16

Neonatal and Obstetrical Transfusion Practice

The neonatal period is generally considered to extend from birth to four months. Newborn infants present unique problems in transfusion therapy. Indications for transfusion of infants differ with weight, gestation, circumstances of delivery and with subsequent maturation. Appropriate transfusion practice requires knowledge of neonatal physiology and astute clinical observation. Supplying blood banks should be capable of providing components tailored to satisfy the specific requirements of these tiny recipients whose small blood volumes provide little margin of safety. The fact that ill newborn infants are more likely to receive transfusions than hospitalized patients of any other age[1] testifies to the importance of this aspect of blood banking.

Fetal and Neonatal Erythropoiesis

As the embryo develops, the predominant site of hematopoiesis shifts, at about the 9th week of gestation, from the wall of the yolk sac to the liver, and at about the 24th week from the liver to the bone marrow.[2] Hematopoiesis is regulated by gradually increasing erythropoietin levels stimulated by low oxygen tensions during intrauterine life. At 40 weeks (term), normal infants have a cord blood hemoglobin of 19 ± 2.2 g/dl. Neonates of lower birth weight have lower normal hemoglobin levels (Table 16-1). Fetal red cells present at birth have a life span of 45 to 70 days[3] and contain 53 to 95% hemoglobin F.[4] Hemoglobin F is physiologically well-adapted to low intrauterine oxygen tensions; its high oxygen affinity allows fetal red cells to acquire oxygen from maternal erythrocytes throughout pregnancy, but the high oxygen affinity results in poor tissue oxygenation in the extrauterine circumstances following birth. As hemoglobin A replaces hemoglobin F during extrauterine maturation, oxygen delivery to the tissues increases progressively. The oxygen dissociation curve shifts to the right (Fig 16-1), reflecting improving oxygen delivery to tissue. Premature infants have lower hematocrits and a greater percentage of hemoglobin F in their red cells than term newborns.

As tissue oxygenation in the newborn improves, levels of erythropoietin decline and erythropoiesis diminishes. This decline in red cell production, combined with short survival of fetal red cells, produces a "physiologic anemia of infancy". Hemoglobin concentration at 1 week approximates that of cord blood and thereafter declines over the next 1 to 3 months (Table

Table 16-1. Serial Hemoglobin Values* in Low-Birth-Weight Infants

Birth Weight (grams)	Age in Weeks				
	2	4	6	8	10
800–1000	16.0(14.8–17.2)	10.0(6.8–13.2)	8.7(7.0–10.2)	8.0(7.1– 9.8)	8.0(6.9–10.2)
1001–1200	16.4(14.1–18.7)	12.8(7.8–15.3)	10.5(7.2–12.3)	9.1(7.8–10.4)	8.5(7.0–10.0)
1201–1400	16.2(13.6–18.8)	13.4(8.8–16.2)	10.9(8.5–13.3)	9.9(8.0–11.8)	9.8(8.4–11.3)
1401–1500	15.6(13.4–17.8)	11.7(9.7–13.7)	10.5(9.1–11.9)	9.8(8.4–12.0)	9.9(8.4–11.4)
1501–2000	15.6(13.5–17.7)	11.0(9.6–14.0)	9.6(8.8–11.5)	9.8(8.4–12.1)	10.1(8.6–11.8)

(Reproduced with permission[1])
*Values are mean figures, in gm/dl, with range in parentheses.

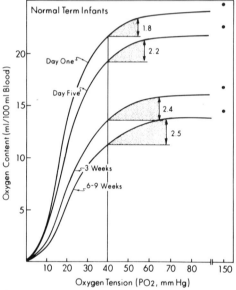

Figure 16-1. Oxygen equilibrium curves in blood from term infants at different postnatal ages. Arrows indicate the capacity to unload oxygen at given arterial and venous PO₂ levels. Reproduced, with permission, from Delivoria-Papadopoulos M, et al.[5]

16-1). Despite hemoglobin levels that would indicate anemia in older children and adults, the normally developing infant usually maintains adequate tissue oxygenation. Arterial PO₂ rises with the increase in hemoglobin A and red cell content of 2,3-diphosphoglycerate (2,3-DPG).[5] Physiologic anemia should not be confused with anemia later in infancy, which may result from dietary inadequacy. Physiologic anemia requires treatment only if the degree or timing of the anemia deviates significantly from normal, and the infant is symptomatic. Although transfusion is rarely indicated for the newborn who is feeding, growing and developing normally, evaluation of anemia is important in infants known to have other problems or to be especially at risk.

Unique Aspects of Neonatal Physiology

Differences between newborns and adults may dictate differences in transfusion practice. Newborns are small and physiologically immature. Those requiring transfusion are often premature, sick and unable to tolerate minimal stresses.

Infant Size

Full-term newborns have a blood volume of approximately 85 ml/kg; prematures average 100 ml/kg. It is important to calculate transfusion needs on an individual basis. As survival rates improve for infants weighing 1500 g or less at birth, blood banks are increasingly asked to provide blood components for patients whose total blood volume is less than 150 ml. The small blood volumes of neonates and the need for frequent laboratory tests makes replacement of iatrogenic blood loss the most common indication for transfusion of these patients.

Hypovolemia

The newborn does not compensate for hypovolemia as well as an adult. A newborn responds to a 10% volume depletion by diminishing the stroke volume ejected by the left ventricle, without increasing heart rate. Peripheral vascular resistance increases to maintain systemic blood pressure and this, combined with the diminished cardiac output, results in poor tissue perfusion, low tissue oxygenation and metabolic acidosis.[6]

Marrow Response to Anemia

The infant's bone marrow responds more slowly than mature marrow to anemia. A hemolytic episode that would elicit a reticulocyte response within 4 to 6 days in adults may elicit little or no increased erythropoiesis for 2 to 3 weeks in the newborn.[7]

Cold Stress

Hypothermia in the newborn causes exaggerated effects, including increased metabolic rate, hypoglycemia, metabolic acidosis and a tendency to apneic episodes that may lead to hypoxia, hypotension and cardiac arrest. Exchange transfusions utilizing blood at room temperature may decrease the newborn's rectal temperature 0.7 to 2.5 C. Consideration should be given to using an in-line blood warmer for exchange transfusion. Warmers are unnecessary for small volume transfusions that equilibrate to room temperature fairly rapidly. A small quad pack or syringe placed in the isolette reaches room temperature in approximately 20 minutes.

Immunologic Status

Infants have immature antibody-producing mechanisms, and antibodies present in their plasma originate almost entirely from the maternal circulation. IgG is the only immunoglobulin class that crosses the placenta, through mechanisms more complex than simple diffusion. Antibody concentrations are higher in cord blood than maternal blood, suggesting an active placental transport mechanism; in addition, catabolism of IgG occurs more slowly in the fetus than in the mother.[8] Thus passively acquired antibody is conserved during the neonatal period. Infants exposed to an infectious process in utero or shortly after birth may produce small amounts of IgM detectable by sensitive techniques, but they rarely form red blood cell antibodies during the neonatal period.

The cellular immune system of neonates is similarly immature. Graft-versus-host (GVH) disease has been reported in newborns who received intrauterine transfusion followed by postnatal exchange transfusion.[9] The lymphocytes given during intrauterine transfusion may have induced host tolerance, so that the lymphocytes given in the subsequent exchange transfusion were not rejected in the normal way. GVH has not been reported in immunologically normal newborns who receive multiple exchange transfusions. For exchange transfusion, irradiation of blood to prevent GVH is probably unnecessary, but blood for intrauterine transfusion is usually irradiated.[10]

Metabolic Problems

Because immature kidneys have reduced glomerular filtration rate and concentrating ability, the newborn may have difficulty excreting potassium, acid and/or calcium loads. Acidosis or hypocalcemia may also occur because the immature liver metabolizes citrate inefficiently. Although plasma potassium increases rapidly in stored packed red cells, simple transfusions have little effect on serum potassium concentration in newborn infants. A study of sick newborns who received a total of 11 transfusions of 10 ml/kg stored packed red cells revealed a posttransfusion drop in mean serum potassium levels from 5.1 to 4.9 mEq/l.[11] Serum potassium may rise after exchange transfusion, depending upon the plasma potassium levels in the blood used for exchange.

2,3-Diphosphoglycerate (2,3-DPG)

Tissue oxygenation is poor in sick newborns. Newborns have a high percentage of fetal hemoglobin, which delivers oxygen to tissues less well than does adult hemoglobin. Infants with respiratory distress syndrome or septic shock have decreased levels of 2,3-DPG, and alkalosis and hypothermia can further increase the oxygen affinity of hemoglobin, shifting the dissociation curve to the left and making oxygen less available to the tissues. Respiratory distress syndrome or other pulmonary disease compromises arterial oxygenation. Mechanisms that compensate for hypoxia in adults, such as increased heart rate, are limited in newborns. If transfused blood constitutes a large proportion of the infant's blood volume, transfusion of 2,3-DPG-depleted blood to newborns may cause problems that would not affect older children or adults. Since 2,3-DPG levels decrease in stored blood, newborns should be given the freshest blood conveniently available, certainly less than 7 days old, to ensure that red cells have adequate 2,3-DPG.[12]

Cytomegalovirus Infection

Infection by cytomegalovirus (CMV) may occur in the perinatal period. Viral infection can occur in utero or during the birth process. Newborn infants can be infected by close contact with mothers or nursery personnel.[13] CMV may also be transmitted by transfusion. The virus seems to be associated with leukocytes in blood and components.

Infection in newborns is extremely variable in its manifestations, ranging from asymptomatic seroconversion to death. Symptomatic infection may produce pulmonary, hepatic, renal, hematologic and/or neurologic dysfunctions.

Epidemiology and prevention of posttransfusion CMV in neonatal recipients are under investigation. Some conclusions are emerging:
1. The overall risk of symptomatic posttransfusion CMV infection seems to be inversely related to the incidence of seropositivity in the community. That is, where many adults are positive for CMV antibodies, there is a low rate of symptomatic CMV infection.[14]
2. Infants born of seropositive mothers are unlikely to develop symptomatic infections during the neonatal period.
3. Premature infants who are born of seronegative mothers, weigh less than 1250 grams and require multiple transfusions are at some risk for symptomatic posttransfusion infections.[14,15]
4. The infective component of blood appears to be associated with the leukocytes and the cumulative amount of transfusions correlates directly with the risk of acquired CMV infection.
5. The risk of transmission of CMV by blood and cellular blood components can be reduced or eliminated by transfusing blood from seronegative donors or by transfusing components processed to eliminate viable CMV-containing leukocytes. Deglycerolized red cells have been used successfully,[16,17,18] and studies are in process to determine whether the use of washed cells reduces CMV transmission.

The 11th edition of *Standards* urges that, in geographic areas where posttransfusion CMV transmission is a problem, blood with minimal risk of transmitting CMV be used for newborns weighing less than 1250 grams, born to mothers who lack CMV antibodies or whose antibody status is unknown.

Hemolytic Disease of the Newborn

Pathophysiology

In hemolytic disease of the newborn (HDN), red cells of the fetus and newborn become coated with IgG antibody of maternal origin, directed against antigen present on the fetal cells. These IgG-coated cells undergo accelerated destruction, both before and after birth. Clinical severity of the disease is extremely variable, ranging from intrauterine death to a condition that can be detected only by serologic tests on blood from a healthy baby.[19]

Shortened red cell survival causes fetal hematopoietic tissue to increase production of new red cells, many of which enter the circulation prematurely as nucleated cells. Organs containing hematopoietic tissue increase in size, particularly liver and spleen. If red cell production adequately replaces lost cells, oxygen-carrying capacity is adequately maintained. If increased hematopoiesis cannot compensate for the immune destruction, anemia becomes progresively more severe. The severely affected fetus may develop high output cardiac failure with generalized edema, the condition called hydrops fetalis, and death may occur in utero. If live-born, the severely affected infant exhibits heart failure and profound anemia. Less severely affected infants continue to experience accelerated red cell destruction, which generates large quantities of bilirubin.

Before birth severs the communication between maternal and fetal circulation, fetal bilirubin is excreted by the mother's liver, but after birth the infant must excrete large quantities of unconjugated bilirubin, a substance toxic to the developing central nervous system. The immature liver is deficient in the enzyme necessary to conjugate bilirubin for excretion, and accumulation of bilirubin constitutes a severe threat to the infant. For the live-born infant with HDN, rising bilirubin levels are a greater clinical problem than the loss of oxygen-carrying capacity resulting from continuing hemolysis. The decision of when or whether to undertake exchange transfusion rests primarily on bilirubin accumulation and on anemia and severity of hemolysis only to a lesser degree.

Mechanisms of Maternal Immunization

HDN may be classified into three categories based on serologic specificity of the causative IgG antibody. In descending order of severity these are:

1. Rh hemolytic disease, due to anti-D alone or in combination with anti-C or anti-E.
2. "Other" HDN, due to antibodies against other antigens in the Rh system, such as anti-C or anti-E, or to antigens in other systems, such as anti-K, anti-Fy^a, and many others.
3. ABO HDN, due usually to anti-A,B in a group O woman, but rarely to anti-A or anti-B.

In HDN other than ABO, maternal antibodies result from immunization by previous pregnancy or transfusion. Rising titers of antibody can be documented during pregnancy, and the baby may be symptomatic at birth. In ABO HDN the immunizing stimulus is seldom known; the condition cannot be diagnosed during pregnancy and the disease is rarely symptomatic at birth.

Pregnancy

Immunization during pregnancy occurs when fetal red cells possessing an antigen foreign to the mother enters her circulation. The antigen that most frequently induces immunization is D, but any red cell antigen present on fetal cells and absent from the mother can, in theory, stimulate antibody production. Small numbers of fetal cells enter the mother's circulation during the last half of pregnancy, but this quantity is rarely sufficient to induce immunization. Most immunizations result from the fetomaternal hemorrhage that occurs during placental separation at delivery. In approximately half of all recently delivered women, small quantities of fetal cells are detectable in a post-delivery blood specimen.[20] Immunization to D can occur with volumes of fetal blood less than 0.1 ml. The incidence of immunization to D correlates with the volume of Rh-positive red cells entering the Rh-negative mother's circulation.[21] Although the usual immunizing event is delivery, primary immunization does occasionally occur during the last half of pregnancy.

Transfusion

In Rh-negative women who receive transfusions of Rh-positive red cells, subsequent pregnancies with an Rh-positive fetus run a high risk of HDN as a complication. It is extremely important to avoid transfusing Rh-positive whole blood or red blood cells to Rh-negative girls or women who might subsequently become pregnant. The red cells in platelet or granulocyte concentrates can constitute an immunizing stimulus, and Rh-negative girls or women who receive platelet therapy should be considered candidates for Rh prophylaxis if the donors are Rh-positive. See page 273.

ABO Antibodies

The IgG antibodies that cause ABO HDN nearly always occur in the mother's circulation with no history of prior immunization by foreign red cells. ABO HDN can develop in any pregnancy including the first, but it is restricted almost entirely to group A or B babies born to group O mothers. This seems to be because the pathogenic antibody is anti-A,B, which is present only in group O individuals.

Natural History Without Immunoprophylaxis

Before the availability of successful prophylaxis for Rh sensitizaton, the incidence of anti-D formation in Rh-negative women who had had Rh-positive, ABO-compatible babies was approximately 8%.[22] An additional 8% developed detectable anti-D during their next Rh-positive pregnancy. The latter group of women probably experienced primary immunization during delivery of their first Rh-positive child but did not produce detectable levels of antibody. The small numbers of Rh-positive fetal cells entering their circulation during the next pregnancy constituted a secondary stimulus sufficient to elicit overt production of IgG anti-D. In susceptible women not immunized during their first two pregnancies, subsequent pregnancies might cause immunization, but

the frequency diminished. Once immunization had occurred, successive Rh-positive pregnancies usually manifested HDN of increasing severity.

Rh immunization occurred in untreated Rh-negative women less frequently after delivery of an ABO-incompatible Rh-positive baby than when the fetal cells were ABO-compatible with the mother. ABO incompatibility between mother and fetus has a substantial but not absolute protective effect against maternal immunization.

Prenatal Tests

Serologic Studies

Alloimmunization that could result in HDN can be diagnosed during pregnancy with suitable serologic tests. Initial studies on all pregnant women should include tests for ABO and D, and a screen for unexpected antibodies. If the woman's cells are not agglutinated by anti-D, a D^u test should be done. When the patient is D^u, some physicians then request testing for C. When the D^u phenotype results from the presence of a *C* gene in *trans* position (see page 133), the patient is not susceptible to immunization with D. Individuals whose D^u has other causes do sometimes produce anti-D (see page 134), and HDN has been reported in the fetus of one such individual.[23]

All positive antibody screening tests require identification of the antibody.[24] The presence of an antibody does not indicate that HDN will inevitably occur. IgM antibodies existing without known red cell stimulation, notably anti-Le and anti-I, are relatively common during pregnancy but do not cross the placenta. Treating the serum with 2-mercaptoethanol or dithiothreitol will aid in distinguishing IgM antibodies from IgG. (See Special Methods, page 454.) The results of prenatal antibody studies should be reported with sufficient additional information to alert the obstetrician to the relative risk to the fetus of specific antibodies identified.

When the woman has anti-D, some obstetricians test the father to determine the likelihood of his being homozygous or heterozygous for alleles determining the presence of the D antigen. A homozygote will always transmit a gene for D to the offspring, whereas in the mating of an Rh-negative woman and a heterozygous Rh-positive man, half the offspring are expected to be Rh-negative. This information may be useful in counseling a couple when anti-D is known to be present.

Amniotic Fluid Analysis

During gestation, the clinical history and amniotic fluid analysis can be used to assess the probable severity of HDN. Anti-D HDN rarely occurs in the first pregnancy but once a woman has anti-D, HDN tends to get worse with each succeeding pregnancy. Information about the severity of the disease in the previous infant is somewhat helpful in predicting severity in subsequent infants. In a woman with anti-D, the severity of fetal HDN correlates modestly with the maternal antibody titer.[25] A better index of intrauterine hemolysis and fetal well-being is the level of bile pigment in the amniotic fluid, obtained by amniocentesis. Amniocentesis is usually undertaken in Rh-negative women with a history of previously affected pregnancies or with anti-D titers at or above 16.

Amniotic fluid is obtained by inserting a long needle through the mother's abdominal wall and uterus into the uterine cavity. The aspirated fluid is scanned spectrophotometrically for a change in optical density at 450 nm, the figure that indicates concentration of bile pigments. This value is plotted on a semilogarithmic graph against the estimated age of gestation, because bile pigment concentration has different clinical significance at different gestational ages. In general, the higher the pigment concentration, the more severe the intrauterine hemolysis. The risk of allowing a severely affected pregnancy to continue must be weighed against the risk of premature delivery and the problems of fetal lung immaturity. Respiratory distress syndrome may result when there is inadequate surfactant lecithin and other pulmonary lipids to maintain stable pulmonary alveolar structures in the newborn. Maturity of the fetal lung is assessed by determining the ratio of lecithin to sphingomyelin (L/S ratio) in the amniotic fluid.[26] If the change in optical density at 450 nm indicates severe HDN but the L/S ratio indicates the lungs are not sufficiently mature to prevent respiratory distress syndrome, intrauterine transfusion may be indicated.

Amniocentesis may be complicated by fetomaternal hemorrhage, which can cause immunization of susceptible mothers. If amniocentesis has been performed on an Rh-negative woman for some indication other than the presence of anti-D, Rh immunoprophylaxis should be given. In most such cases the Rh status of the fetus will be unknown, but the likelihood is high that the fetus is Rh-positive, and the bleeding induced by amniocentesis could induce anti-D in a woman not previously immunized.

Intrauterine Transfusion

Intrauterine transfusion carries a high risk to the fetus[27] and should be performed only after careful clinical evaluation. Intrauterine transfusion is seldom feasible before the 24th to 26th week of gestation. Once initiated, the series of transfusions is usually administered every 2 weeks until delivery. Intrauterine transfusion is performed through a needle passed, with radiographic monitoring, through the mother's abdominal and uterine wall into the fetal abdominal cavity. The transfused red cells enter the fetal circulation by absorption from lymphatic channels draining the peritoneal cavity.

For maximum survival of the transfused cells, intrauterine transfusion usually requires red cells less than 5 days old. Because deglycerolized frozen red cells have normal electrolyte levels; contain no anticoagulant, plasma or platelets; and have very low levels of leukocytes, this component is preferred by many physicians. A hematocrit of 80% or greater is desirable to minimize the chance of volume overload in the fetus. The red cells should be group O, Rh-negative and compatible with the mother's serum. The volume transfused ranges from 75 to 175 ml depending on the fetal size and age. Blood for intrauterine transfusions probably should be irradiated because of the potential risk of graft-versus-host disease.[28]

Newborns who have had successful intrauterine transfusions often type at birth as Rh-negatve or very weakly Rh-positive, because at birth over 90% of their circulating red cells may be those of the donor. Similarly, the ABO grouping and direct antiglobulin test may give misleading results.

Laboratory Investigation During the Neonatal Period

A sample of cord blood, preferably collected by needle and aspiration, should be obtained on every newborn. This tube should be identified as cord blood and be labeled in the delivery suite with the mother's name, baby's identification, hospital number and date. Samples should be stored in the blood bank for at least 7 days. The cord sample is then available for testing if the mother is Rh-negative or if the newborn develops signs and symptoms suggestive of HDN.

Samples of both cord and maternal blood should be tested as shown in Table 16-2. When the mother is known to have antibodies capable of causing HDN, the cord blood should be tested for hemoglobin or hematocrit and for serum bilirubin. Tests on the mother's blood present no special problems and can be done with routine techniques. Testing cord blood may present some special problems, which are described below.

ABO Testing

ABO testing on newborns relies entirely on cell grouping because alloantibodies present in cord serum are of maternal origin. If maternal alloantibodies are present, they will be IgG and, unless present at high levels, may not agglutinate reverse grouping cells on immediate spin. No useful information will be gained from routine serum grouping tests, although in investigating possible HDN due to ABO incompatibility, tests for antiglobulin-reactive ABO antibodies may be helpful.

Rh Testing

Accurate Rh testing can be difficult if red cells are heavily coated with IgG antibodies. Either false-positive or false-negative results may occur. Rh-negative cells heavily coated with any antibody or contaminated by Wharton's jelly may appear Rh-positive if the anti-D serum contains potentiators of agglutination that cause nonspecific aggregation. The problem should become apparent from positive results in the tube containing reagent diluent control. If there is agglutination in the control system, saline or chemically modified anti-D can be used to determine the Rh group.

False-negative or very weakly positive results sometimes occur with the saline anti-D when the newborn is Rh-positive and the red blood cells are so fully saturated with maternal anti-D that no D sites are available to react with the reagent serum, a condition sometimes called "blocked D." This should be suspected when the immunized mother is Rh-negative and the baby's cells give a strongly positive direct antiglobulin test and negative or ambiguous results with saline anti-D. Maternal anti-D can be removed from these cells by gentle heat elution (see page 417) and the anti-D test repeated. Chloroquine should not be used to remove antibody from the baby's cells because this method causes apparent destruction of the Rh antigen. Chloroquine treatment is helpful when using non-Rh blood group antisera that react only by the indirect aniglobulin technique to test cells with a positive direct antiglobulin test.

Table 16-2. Laboratory Studies Recommended for Maternal and Cord Bloods in Cases of Suspected HDN

Maternal Blood

ABO group
Rh group
D^u, if apparently Rh-negative
Antibody screening test
Identification of antibody, if present

Cord Blood

ABO group
Rh group
D^u, if apparently Rh-negative
Direct antiglobulin test
Eluate from red cells, if direct antiglobulin test positive and clinical circumstances warrant
Identification of antibody in eluate

Antiglobulin Testing

The direct antiglobulin test (DAT) usually gives strongly positive results in HDN due to anti-D or antibodies in other blood groups; reactions are much weaker or negative in HDN due to ABO. If the DAT on cord cells is positive, the antibody can be eluted from the cells and tested for specificity. In most cases the antibody from cord cells is also present in the maternal serum and this establishes the cause of the HDN.

If the direct antiglobulin test is positive and the maternal serum has a negative antibody screening test, suspicion falls on ABO HDN or HDN due to antibody against a low-incidence test antigen not present on reagent test cells. If the mother's serum is ABO-incompatible with the baby's cells, the presence of antiglobulin-reactive IgG antibody in the baby's serum points strongly to ABO HDN. Testing the eluate from the cord cells against A and B cells, in addition to the usual O cells, confirms the diagnosis but need not be done on samples from asymptomatic infants.

ABO hemolytic disease may be suspected on clinical grounds even though the direct antiglobulin test is negative. In many cases it is possible to elute anti-A or anti-B from the infant's cells despite a negative DAT; if elution is performed, the eluate should be tested against A$_1$, B and O cells, using antiglobulin technique. If transfusion is required, group O blood will be transfused, whether or not the diagnosis has been serologically confirmed.

If ABO hemolytic disease is ruled out, antibody against a low-frequency antigen should be suspected, and the eluate should be tested against the father's red cells, using antiglobulin technique. The diagnosis can be confirmed by testing the mother's serum against the father's red cells, if they are ABO-compatible. If either or both of these tests are positive, it indicates that the father has transmitted an antigen to the offspring that has elicited an IgG antibody in the mother. Since antibody to a low-incidence antigen causes no difficulty in obtaining compatible blood, these studies can be performed after initial clinical concerns have been resolved.

If the DAT is positve and all attempts to characterize the coating antibody are consistently negative, causes of a false-positive direct antiglobulin test should be considered. (See page 97.)

Treatment

See section on exchange transfusion, pages 310-316.

Components Used for Neonatal Transfusion

Newborns may need any or all of the blood components available in other transfusion settings, but special problems exist in achieving the small volumes needed, the adjusted hematocrits and narrow acceptable ranges of pH and electrolyte values.

Red Cell Components

The uniquely small transfusion volume requirements of neonatal recipients make it possible to provide several aliquots from a single donor unit, thus limiting donor exposure and decreasing donor-related risks such as hepatitis. Several technical approaches are available to realize this advantage and to minimize wastage.

Quadruple Packs

In a quadruple pack (quad pack) system, a single unit of blood can be apportioned into four integrally attached containers of 125 ml. Since the original seal remains intact, each container has a normal shelf-life until entered. The contents of individual quad packs can be transferred to smaller containers providing two to four smaller aliquots, each with a 24-hour shelf-life. Hematocrit can be adjusted at either division step. For example, most of the plasma (approximately 220 ml) can be removed as fresh frozen plasma shortly after drawing. The remaining packed red cells can be divided into each of the other attached bags without altering the shelf-life of the cells. If each quad pack is apportioned, at the time of use, into four pediatric transfer packs that outdate in 24 hours, a single unit can provide twelve 20 ml aliquots of packed red cells and a unit of fresh frozen plasma.[29] Alternatively, whole blood in the original container can be expressed into the satellite bags, which can be entered for subsequent removal of plasma or subdivision into smaller aliquots. Each aliquot must be fully labeled as it is prepared, including the time of outdating. Records must be kept of the origin and disposition of each aliquot.

Multi-Portion System

A multi-portion system is useful in settings where large numbers of infants receive small-volume transfusions given with syringe pumps. Blood is collected either into single or multiple packs. If triple or quadruple bag sets are used, hematocrit can be adjusted initially and fresh frozen plasma may be prepared if the resulting hematocrit is acceptable. An alternative method of red cell concentration uses gravity sedimentation for 12 hours. This results in a hematocrit of approximately 65%, which many workers consider ideal

for transfusion to neonates.[30] Bags are hung in an inverted position in the refrigerator so that sedimented cells can be carefully drawn through one of the access ports into a syringe.

A resealable sampling or injection site coupler inserted into the access port permits repeated entry. Once the coupler is inserted, the contents of the bag have a 24-hour shelf-life. The precise volume of blood requested can be aspirated into a syringe through a large bore needle inserted through the sampling site coupler. If desired, the packed or sedimented red cells can be drawn through an in-line filter when loading the syringes. If blood is not filtered during loading, a filter is required in the infusion set. Aseptic technique should be used and the sampling site coupler covered with sterile gauze when not in use. The sterile cap should be replaced on the filled syringe, which must be appropriately labeled for the recipient. The distribution to individual recipients of aliquots as filled syringes must be recorded. The system's flexibility in volume of component prepared minimizes wastage.

Deglycerolized Red Cells

After glycerolization and before freezing, a unit of red cells can be divided into three or four aliquots. A single unit may be designated for repeated transfusion to a single recipient, or aliquots can be assigned to different infants. Each aliquot can be thawed as needed, with a 24-hour shelf-life after thawing and deglycerolization. Aliquots may be further divided for small-volume transfusions. This is an expensive system, but it provides a product with 2,3-DPG levels of freshly drawn blood and, after the postthaw wash, with much reduced content of plasma proteins, electrolytes, anticoagulant, white cells and platelets.[31] Alternatively, entire group O units can be thawed and deglycerolized, and aliquots removed as needed during the permitted 24-hour shelf-life. Rejuvenation (see page 41) prior to freezing offers two additional advantages: outdated units can be salvaged, and red blood cells with greater than normal levels of 2,3-DPG can be provided.

Half-Unit Donations

The need for small-volume neonatal and pediatric transfusions provides an opportunity to utilize blood donors who weigh less than the 50 kilograms required for donation of a 450 ml unit. It is possible to draw less than the usual volume from a small but otherwise acceptable donor. After excess anticoagulant is expressed into a satellite bag, approximately 225 ml of blood can be collected into a triple pack. Separated plasma can be expressed into the same bag, which is then discarded. The remaining red cells can be apportioned between the primary container and the remaining satellite bag; this provides two units of red cells of approximately 60 ml volume. An alternative application of this approach is to draw 225 ml monthly from a group O donor of a desirable phenotype, rather than 450 ml every 8 weeks.

Individual Small Units

Units containing approximately 30 to 60 ml of whole blood can be obtained by collecting blood into a container with an extra satellite bag. A unit intended for use as whole blood would be collected in a double bag; a unit intended for division into red cells, platelets and fresh frozen plasma would be collected in a quadruple set instead of a triple set. It is permissible to draw 450 ml ± 10% from a donor. If there is an accurate means of measuring volume drawn, it is possible to draw 495 ml of whole blood into the primary bag. Removing 30 to 60 ml into the extra satellite bag leaves a satisfactory volume in the primary bag and provides an extra small-volume unit with normal shelf-life. The hematocrit of these small units can be adjusted by removing plasma prior to transfusion.

Walking Donor Program

Ambulatory donors, often hospital employees, have blood drawn directly into heparinized syringes for immediate infusion into neonatal recipients. This approach, a relic of less sophisticated times, is mentioned only to itemize the hazards: no labeling or routine pretransfusion testing of donor blood; generally poor record keeping; no donor sample available to work up reactions; risk of excess heparin; potential contamination through faulty technique; and risk of hepatitis from untested blood drawn from donors working in proximity to patients and blood.

Fresh Frozen Plasma (FFP)

Group AB plasma, which lacks anti-A and anti-B and has been found to lack unexpected antibodies, is often used to dilute packed group O red cells to the desired hematocrit, either for predelivery preparation for a fetus whose blood type is unknown, or for transfusion without crossmatching to newborns of any blood group. Since FFP must be frozen within 6 hours of phlebotomy, it is an excellent source of labile coagulation factors, if transfused within 24 hours after thawing. Thawed plasma stored more than 24 hours at l-6 C provides stable coagulation factors and other plasma proteins. A thawed unit of FFP can be divided into aliquots for small-volume transfusions; these aliquots must be used within 24 hours of entering the primary bag.

Small volumes of FFP appropriate for neonates may be prepared by aliquoting 20 ml of freshly drawn plasma under sterile conditions into sterile pyrogen-free evacuated vials. If frozen within 6 hours after the primary bag was entered, the aliquots can be stored frozen for up to 1 year. Pharmaceutical vials have injectible caps through which aliquots of thawed plasma can be aspirated by syringe and needle. By this technique, a single donor can provide about 12 neonatal FFP transfusions. Laminar air flow hoods, commonly available in a hospital pharmacy, provide ideal conditions for preparing multiple aliquots. Appropriate labeling procedures and quality control of sterility and coagulation factor levels are essential.

Platelet Concentrates

A platelet concentrate prepared from a single donation of blood contains approximately 5.5×10^{10} platelets and should raise the platelet count of an average full-term newborn 75,000 to 100,000/mm³.[32] Platelet concentrates should be group-specific if possible. Transfusion of incompatible plasma is more dangerous in neonatal recipients than adults. The plasma volume of stored platelet concentrates can be reduced without adversely affecting platelet properties.[33] Incompatible plasma should be removed to the maximum extent possible (see Special Methods page 469), and the platelets resuspended in compatible plasma.

Granulocyte Concentrates

Optimum use of granulocyte transfusion for neonatal recipients is under investigation. Granulocytes may be harvested by standard apheresis techniques or, for newborns, smaller quantities of granulocytes can be harvested from the buffy coat of units of freshly donated blood by gravity sedimentation or by a cell washing process.[34] Clinical trials using buffy coat concentrates have not yet been published. Because granulocyte concentrates contain large numbers of lymphocytes, it may be desirable to irradiate granulocyte concentrates for neonatal transfusion to prevent graft-versus-host disease.

Compatibility Testing

Because the immunologic system of the newborn is immature and relatively unresponsive to antigenic stimulation during the first 4 months of life, standards for compatibility testing are different from those for adults. In a report of 65 neonates who received 572 transfusions from different donors, the predicted incidence of antibodies was 6.4 whereas the observed incidence, even with very sensitive detection techniques, was zero.[35]

The most common indication for transfusion of sick neonates is to replace blood drawn for laboratory studies[36]; samples drawn for repeated compatibility testing contribute to this iatrogenic blood loss. Since infants seem not to produce antibodies despite multiple transfusions and since repeated blood bank testing causes demonstrable harm through blood loss, *Standards* permits pronounced reduction in serologic tests on neonates. Initial testing must include ABO and Rh testing of a neonatal recipient's red cells and an antibody screening test, which may be done on the newborn's or the mother's serum or plasma.[37] If the antibody screen is negative and if all red cells transfused during the neonatal period are type O and are either Rh-negative or the same Rh group as that initially found, compatibility testing and further typing may be omitted during the first 4 months of life.

If unexpected antibody is detected in the initial sample from the infant, or the mother's serum contains clinically significant antibody, then compatibility testing is necessary for as long as maternal antibody persists in the infant. If transfusions are to continue for several days or longer, the antibody screening test should be repeated on each sample of the baby's blood received with a request for transfusion. Once a negative result is obtained, subsequent crossmatches and antibody screening tests are unnecessary.

If the infant is to receive red cells of an ABO group incompatible with the mother's serum, it is necessary to crossmatch the cells, using an antiglobulin technique, to demonstrate that no maternal antibodies are in the baby's serum. This should be continued for as long as maternal antibodies remain. A compatible crossmatch indicates that maternal antibodies are not present. Once a compatible crossmatch has been obtained, subsequent group-specific units need not be crossmatched.

A special group of recipients are infants who will inevitably receive regular or frequent transfusions—for example, children with thalassemia, sickle cell disease or aplastic anemia. It is desirable to test their red cell antigens as completely as possible before beginning transfusion therapy because transfusions will give them a mixed population of red cells unsuitable for antigen testing. These patients are liable to develop complex combinations of antibodies, and knowing their initial phenotype can be helpful in selecting compatible blood. Records of this testing should be retained indefinitely.

Transfusion Administration

Vascular access is often difficult in the tiny newborn and in any infant requiring long-term or repeated intravenous infusions. The umbilical artery may be cannulated in newborns. Thereafter, a vein large enough to accommodate a 23- or 25-gauge needle or a 22- or 24-gauge vascular catheter should be chosen for blood administration. It is not usually necessary to warm small-volume transfusions that are given slowly.

Constant rate syringe delivery pumps have been shown to be satisfactory for transfusion of red cells through small gauge needles.[38,39] Hemolysis increases with cells stored longer than 7 days and with slow rates of infusion.

The length of the plastic tubing used can add significantly to the amount of blood required for a transfusion. Platelet or component infusion sets have much less dead space than standard transfusion sets because they have short tubing and a 170 micron blood filter of the needle type. All blood components must be filtered before or during infusion. Microaggregate filters (40 or 20 micron) are superfluous, since microaggregates do not accumulate significantly in blood stored less than 1 week,[10] and blood transfused to infants is usually less than 7 days old. There has been a report[11] of hemolysis occuring when stored blood was infused through a 20 micron stainless steel mesh filter.

Indications for Red Cell Transfusions

Because the tissue need for oxygen cannot be measured directly, and so many variables determine oxygen availability, no universally accepted criteria exist for transfusion of premature or term infants. The decision to transfuse a newborn for anemia should include evaluation of expected hemoglobin levels ascertained from references (Table 16-1) and the patient's clinical status. Other potentially useful considerations include the presence or absence of reticulocytes as an index of bone marrow erythroid function, and development of adaptive mechanisms, such as the increased intracellular 2,3-DPG occurring in physiologic anemia of infancy. Table 16-3 lists representative criteria for replacement transfusion in a high-risk newborn.[42] Because the neonate in respiratory distress is hypoxic and more vulnerable to cerebral hemorrhage, red cell transfusions are given more aggressively.

Iatrogenic Blood Loss

Although specialized care in neonatal intensive care units requires close laboratory monitoring, unnecessary laboratory testing should be avoided. Repeated blood sampling to measure blood gases, pH and electrolytes often results in anemia. The volume of blood removed from infants must be carefully recorded. When blood loss equals 10% of the infant's calculated blood volume, it is usual practice to replace with packed or sedimented red cells on a volume-for-volume basis. If an anemic infant develops congestive heart failure, it may be better to remove aliquots of dilute blood from the infant and replace with packed red cells. This is sometimes called a "partial exchange" transfusion.

Causes of Blood Loss

A variety of acute or chronic problems occurring prenatally, during delivery or postnatally may lead to anemia. Causes of prenatal blood loss include spontaneous

Table 16-3. Criteria for Replacement Transfusion in the High Risk Infant

With Respiratory Distress, Transfusion Should Be Given When:

1. The hematocrit is less than 40%, or
2. Hypovolemia is present as judged by:
   pallor
   pulse rate greater than 160/minute
   systolic blood pressure less than 50 mm Hg
   (BW greater than 1000 g)
3. More than 10% of the blood volume has been removed within 48 hours and the hematocrit is less than 45%

In the Absence of Respiratory Distress, Transfusions Should Be Given When:

1. The hematocrit is less than 30% in the first week of life, or
2. The pulse rate is greater than 160/minute, the respiratory rate is greater than 60/minute, or cardiomegaly exists by X-ray

(Reproduced with permission[42])

fetomaternal or fetoplacental hemorrhage, traumatic amniocentesis, complications of intrauterine transfusion, or twin-twin transfusion, when monozygotic twins share a monochorionic placenta. Clinically significant twin-twin transfusion causes a hemoglobin difference of at least 5 g/dl; if twin-twin transfusion continues chronically, the infants will differ markedly in birth weight and organ size. The smaller, anemic twin is at risk of congestive heart failure; the larger, plethoric twin is at risk for hyperbilirubinemia or hyperviscosity, but the condition of the smaller twin is nearly always more dangerous.

The fetus may lose blood into the placenta if the cord is wrapped tightly around the neck, or if the infant is placed above the placenta before the cord is clamped. Obstetric accidents, umbilical cord rupture, abruptio placentae, placenta previa and other cord and placenta abnormalities can also result in hemorrhage and an anemic, hypovolemic newborn.

Postnatal anemia may result from internal hemorrhage, usually the result of traumatic delivery. This may not become apparent until 24 to 72 hours of age. Common bleeding sites include the brain, liver, lungs, spleen, adrenal glands and scalp.

Failure to Thrive

An indication for transfusion unique to this age group is absence of expected weight gain in the absence of other known causes of failure to thrive. Anemia in newborns increases oxygen consumption, probably because anemia increases cardiac workload. Increased oxygen consumption at a fixed caloric intake causes diminished rate of weight gain. A group of premature infants[43] with no other medical problems had an average weight gain of only 21 g, compared with normal average gain of 28 g. Eleven of thirteen of these infants gained weight when transfused from a mean hemoglobin of 8.5 to 11.4 g/dl. There was an associated 11% decrease in oxygen consumption.

Indications for Exchange Transfusion

Exchange transfusion, originally used almost exclusively as treatment for hemolytic disease of the newborn, has recently been advocated as adjunctive therapy for a variety of life-threatening diseases affecting newborns including respiratory distress, disseminated intravascular coagulation and sepsis. The potential risks of exchange transfusion are listed in Table 16-4. The procedure carries a mortality rate of approximately 1% and there may be substantial morbidity.[44] Exchange transfusion is often quantified (eg, two-volume, single-volume) to reflect the effect on the infant's total blood volume.

Hemolytic Disease of the Newborn

Exchange transfusion is the indicated treatment for severe hemolytic disease of the newborn. Removing the baby's plasma not only reduces the load of accumulated bilirubin but also reduces the number of unbound antibody molecules present in the infant. Antibody-coated cells, whose destruction would further raise the bilirubin load, are removed and replaced with red cells compatible with the maternal antibody. For a discussion of hematologic and mechanical considerations of exchange transfusion, see page 315.

Selection of Blood

Unique problems in exchange transfusion for HDN pertain to selecting appropriate blood. In most cases the mother's serum is used for crossmatching and the transfused cells are compatible with her ABO antibodies as well as with whatever antibody or antibodies have caused the hemolytic process. Since the mother and the baby may be of different ABO groups,

Table 16-4. Possible Complications of Exchange Transfusion

Cardiac
Arrhythmias and/or arrest due to hyperkalemia, hypocalcemia, and citrate toxicity
Myocardial infarct
Vascular-Mechanical
Volume overload or depletion
Perforation of vessels
Thrombosis of hepatic or portal veins
Embolization with air or thrombi
Injury to donor cells, mechanical, thermal, osmotic
Perforation of bowel with or without necrotizing enterocolitis
Infectious
Bacterial, eg, sepsis, omphalitis, septic thrombophlebitis, hepatic abscess
Viral, eg, hepatitis, cytomegalovirus
Hematologic-Coagulation
Over heparinization (if heparinized blood is used)
Aggravation of thrombocytopenia in severe disease
Sickling of donor blood
Immunologic
Incompatible erythrocytes or plasma
Graft-versus-host disease
Other
Hypoglycemia
Hypothermia
Retrolental fibroplasia
Intracranial hemorrhage

(Reproduced with permission[2])

this usually means that group O cells are used. In ABO hemolytic disease, the cells used for exchange must be group O. If the antibody is anti-D the cells must, of course, be Rh-negative. Not every exchange transfusion, however, need be with O, Rh-negative blood. If the mother and the baby have the same ABO group, group-specific cells can be used. If the pathogenic antibody is not anti-D, the cells given to an Rh-positive baby may be Rh-positive.

To crossmatch blood for exchange transfusion, the mother's serum is the specimen of choice. It is available in large quantity, has the antibody present in high concentration, and can be accurately and completely analyzed before birth. If the infant is to be transferred to another center from the place where delivery occurred, a carefully labeled specimen of maternal blood should accompany the child.

Problems with Crossmatching

If the maternal blood is not available, or if it is unsuitable for immediate use in crossmatching, either the baby's serum or an eluate from the baby's cells, or both can be used for crossmatching.

Maternal serum may contain antibodies directed against antigens other than those on the baby's cells, or IgM antibodies that have not crossed the placenta. If the mother's serum contains a complex mixture of antibodies, blood for the baby may be selected by crossmatching with the baby's serum or the eluate from cord cells. Neither serum nor eluate alone is ideal for crossmatching. The eluate provides a concentrated preparation of the antibodies responsible for red cell destruction, but will not contain antibodies against antigens absent from the baby's cells. The serum, on the other hand, may not contain a high concentration of antibody if most of the molecules are bound to the red cells. Use of either or both may, however, be preferable to delaying transfusion while a maternal specimen is obtained or while the antibodies in the mother's serum are separated and identified.

Subsequent Transfusion

In severe HDN, bilirubin may reaccumulate rapidly after an initially successful exchange, partly because a large quantity of extravascular bilirubin is available to rebound (see section below) and partly because hemolysis characteristically continues at a reduced but nonetheless significant rate. If rising bilirubin levels make a second or third exchange transfusion necessary, the same considerations of cell selection and crossmatching apply.

Transfusion When Antibody Reacts with a High-Incidence Antigen

Rarely, the mother's serum may contain an antibody to a high-incidence antigen and no compatible blood is available. If this problem is recognized and identified, there will be time to test the siblings of the mother for compatibility and suitability, and to work with the rare donor file to locate compatible donors. If this problem is not recognized until after delivery, three choices are open:

1. Test mother's siblings for compatibility and suitability, if they are available.
2. Collect a unit of blood from the mother, if the obstetrician agrees that this is safe. Centrifuge the whole blood and remove as much plasma as possible. Resuspend her red cells to the desired hematocrit in group AB plasma.
3. Use available donor blood that possesses the antigen and is incompatible. If no compatible blood is available and the clinical situation is urgent, exchange transfusion with incompatible blood is preferred to no transfusion at all. The procedure does remove antibody and bilirubin, but it will almost certainly have to be followed with several additional incompatible exchanges, since the transfused cells will be destroyed and will generate additional bilirubin.

Hyperbilirubinemia

The most common indication for neonatal exchange transfusion is excessive unconjugated bilirubin. Whenever unconjugated bilirubin in serum exceeds the level at which free bilirubin crosses the blood-brain barrier, bilirubin may concentrate in the basal ganglia and cerebellum, causing central nervous system damage of the type called kernicterus. The fetal liver has limited capacity to conjugate bilirubin, but during intrauterine existence unconjugated bilirubin crosses the placenta to be excreted through the mother's hepatobiliary system.

Several mechanisms may cause unconjugated bilirubin to accumulate, in the newborn. Normal newborns rarely develop dangerous hyperbilirubinemia, but there are several processes that lead to rising bilirubin levels. These include:

1. Poor hepatic uptake of bilirubin, due to low levels of the hepatocellular acceptor protein ligandin.
2. Transient deficiency of the hepatic microsomal enzyme, uridine diphosphoglucuronyl transferase, responsible for converting bilirubin from a lipid-soluble form to the water-soluble glucuronide conjugate that is excreted without damage to the CNS.
3. Rapid bilirubin production caused by the shortened life span of fetal red cells.
4. Efficient enterohepatic resorption of bilirubin.

Prematurity amplifies all of the processes listed above. Neonatal patients who require exchange transfusion are usually premature and may also have one or more of the following pathologic processes:

1. Hemolysis secondary to maternal alloantibody, most commonly those of the ABO system and anti-D, but occasionally other antibodies in the Rh system or in systems such as Kidd, Duffy or Kell
2. Hemolysis secondary to:
   a. inherited deficiencies of red cell enzymes, most commonly glucose-6-phosphate dehydrogenase or, less often, pyruvate kinase
   b. congenital red blood cell membrane defects, such as hereditary spherocytosis

c. hemoglobinopathy, associated with shortened red cell survival
3. Hemorrhage into an enclosed space, especially likely in prolonged labor or difficult delivery
4. Increased enterohepatic circulation due to any form of intestinal obstruction or delay in bowel transit time allowing deconjugation and reabsorption
5. Displacement of bound bilirubin from albumin by competing substances, usually drugs given to mother or infant, such as sulfonamides, vitamin K or salicylates.
6. Sepsis

Phototherapy with fluorescent blue lights sometimes avoids the need for exchange transfusion. When bilirubin near the surface of the skin is exposed to light it undergoes photoisomerization to form "photobilirubin." These isomers of bilirubin are transported in the plasma to the liver where they are rapidly excreted in bile without being conjugated.

Effects of Exchange

Exchange transfusion removes unconjugated bilirubin and provides additional albumin to bind residual bilirubin. If there is antibody-mediated hemolysis, exchange transfusion is additionally beneficial in removing free antibody and antibody-coated red cells and providing red cells that will survive normally.

Exchange transfusion should be done before bilirubin rises to levels at which CNS damage occurs. Several factors affect the threshold for toxicity. CNS damage occurs at lower levels if there is prematurity, decreased albumin binding capacity or the presence of such complicating conditions as sepsis, hypoxia, acidosis, hypothermia or hypoglycemia. In infants with very low birth weights, kernicterus may occur at levels of unconjugated bilirubin as low as 6 to 9 mg/dl.[45] The level of hyperbilirubinemia, not the cause, influences the decision to perform exchange transfusion; representative danger levels are listed in Table 16-5.

The rate at which bilirubin rises better predicts the need for exchange transfusion than any single value. Infants with an accumulation rate greater than 0.5 mg/dl/hour and/or significant anemia usually require exchange transfusion.[46] A two-volume exchange transfusion decreases the serum bilirubin to 45-50% of its preexchange value.[45] This observed efficiency is less than the predicted theoretical efficiency (see page 23) because the need for slow exchange of small increments permits reequilibration between bilirubin in plasma and in extravascular tissues. Within the subsequent few hours, more extravascular bilirubin enters the circulation to equilibrate with lowered serum levels. This rebound rise in bilirubin, combined with continued bilirubin production, may restore serum concentration to a level requiring a repeat exchange transfusion. The indications for repeat exchange are similar to those for the initial exchange.

Table 16-5. Bilirubin Values* Indicating the Need for Exchange Transfusion in the Newborn Patient

Birthweight (grams)	<1250	1250–1499	1500–1999	2000–2500	>2500
Uncomplicated	13	15	17	18	20
Complicated†	10	13	15	17	18

(Reproduced with permission[45])
*Bilirubin expressed in mg/dl
†Complicated includes the presence of any of the following:
5 minutes Apgar less than 3; PaO$_2$ less than 40 mg Hg for one hour; pH less than 7.15 for one hour; rectal temperature 35°C or less; serum albumin 2.5 gm/dl or less; signs of CNS deterioration; proven sepsis or meningitis; hemolytic anemia; birth weight less than 1000g;

Respiratory Distress

Exchange transfusion has been shown to improve survival in low birthweight infants with respiratory distress,[5] possibly because substitution of hemoglobin A for hemoglobin F results in a shift of the oxyhemoglobin curve to the right and increases tissue oxygenation. Infants who are hypoxic due to respiratory distress are also more susceptible to intracerebral hemorrhage. Other effects, including improvement in coagulation status, removal of toxic substances and repletion of serum proteins, have been suggested to explain the beneficial effects of exchange transfusion.[12]

Disseminated Intravascular Coagulation

In the neonatal period disseminated intravascular coagulation (DIC) occurs secondary to many conditions, particularly sepsis and necrotizing enterocolitis. In spite of demonstrated severe shortening of both platelet and fibrinogen survival times in these patients, the tests for fibrin degradation products and the routine coagulation screening tests (PT, PTT, TT) may remain normal.[47]

The most important therapy for neonatal DIC is to treat the underlying disease. Exchange transfusion has produced variable results, perhaps due to the fact that only the sickest infants have been selected to receive this therapy.

Sepsis

Newborn infants experience exceedingly high morbidity and mortality from bacterial infections, particularly from group B streptococcus. Treatments with exchange transfusion, transfusion of fresh whole blood, and granulocyte concentrates have been shown to improve survival.[48,49]

Other Toxins

Exchange transfusion is occasionally used to remove other toxins, such as drugs or chemicals given to the mother near the time of delivery, drugs given in toxic doses to the infant or substances such as ammonia that accumulate in the newborn because of prematurity or inherited metabolic diseases.

Partial Exchange Transfusion for Polycythemia

A venous hematocrit greater than 65% or hemoglobin in excess of 22 gm/dl any time in the first week of life is considered polycythemia. As hematocrit rises above 50%, the viscosity of blood increases exponentially and oxygen transport decreases.[50] The infant has limited ability to increase cardiac output to compensate for hyperviscosity and may develop congestive heart failure.

Polycythemia in the newborn, which may have a variety of causes, requires treatment whether or not it produces symptoms.[51] If untreated, the resulting hyperviscosity can produce sludging of blood flow, hyperbilirubinemia, reduced tissue oxygenation and increased incidence of microthrombi. Many organs may be affected resulting in CNS signs, pulmonary or renal failure or necrotizing enterocolitis. Newborn polycythemia may be due to maternal-fetal transfusion, placental-to-fetal transfusion, twin-to-twin transfusion or intrauterine hypoxia. At increased risk are males, infants small for gestational age and infants of diabetic mothers.[51]

The goal of partial exchange with plasma is to lower the hematocrit to 60%. Whole blood is removed and replaced with an equal volume of 5% albumin or fresh frozen plasma. This procedure lowers the hematocrit while maintaining blood volume.[4] A formula for the volume of plasma required for the exchange is:

$$\text{Volume of plasma} = \frac{\text{blood volume} \times (\text{observed hemoglobin} - \text{desired hemoglobin})}{\text{observed hemoglobin}}$$

Example: Calculations for volume of plasma needed for a partial exchange to achieve a hemoglobin of 20 gm/dl in a 2 kg infant who has a hemoglobin of 24 gm/dl.

Blood volume $= 2 \times 85 = 170$ ml

Volume of plasma needed $=$
$$\frac{170 \text{ ml} \times (24 - 20 \text{ gm/dl})}{24 \text{ gm/dl}} = 28 \text{ ml}$$

Technique of Exchange Transfusion

Vascular Access

Exchange transfusions in the newborn period are usually accomplished via catheters in the umbilical vessels. Catheterization is easiest within hours of birth, but it may be possible to achieve vascular access at this site for several days. The catheters should be radiopaque to facilitate radiographic monitoring of placement. Once placed, they should be secured with sutures and should not be covered from sight, although they should not be open to the air. Holes should be at the end, as side holes allow thrombus formation in the dead space at the end, and the catheter should be kept filled with solution at all times. If umbilical catheters are not available for exchange transfusion, small central venous or saphenous catheters may be used.

Choice of Components for Exchange Transfusion

Many different combinations of blood components have provided safe and effective exchange transfusion; no single product or combination is unequivocally best. Most frequently used are red blood cells or deglycerolized red blood cells. These can be used alone, with 5% albumin or with fresh frozen plasma. Heparinized blood has been used in the past but is not recommended. Whole blood collected in CPDA-1 appears satisfactory for exchange transfusion in term infants.[52] Blood components of the infant's ABO and Rh groups are generally used, except in hemolytic disease due to maternal alloantibodies (see page 311). In infants who are hypoxic or acidotic, it is desirable that blood selected for exchange transfusion be known to lack hemoglobin S.[53]

Supplemental Materials

Traditionally, calcium has been administered to infants receiving blood anticoagulated with citrate, to offset the calcium-binding effects of citrate. There is little documentation to support this practice. In one study, posttransfusion levels of ionized calcium did not differ significantly between infants given 100 mg of calcium gluconate after each 100 ml of blood exchanged and a similar group receiving no supplemental calcium.[54] If used, calcium should never be infused through the same IV line as blood because it will cause clots to form.

Albumin binds unconjugated bilirubin. Increasing intravascular binding is thought to enhance diffusion of bilirubin from the extravascular compartment into the circulation, thereby increasing the total quantity of bilirubin removed during the exchange and protecting the infant's brain from bilirubin toxicity. Some physicians give 25% serum albumin, either 1 hour prior to the exchange (1 g/kg) or at 100-ml intervals during exchanges intended to reduce hyperbilirubinemia. However, in a study comparing 15 hyperbilirubinemic infants given albumin with 27 who received none, the efficiency of bilirubin removal was the same in both groups.[55] Because infusing albumin raises the colloid osmotic pressure and increases intravascular volume, it should be given cautiously, if at all, to severely anemic infants, those in congestive heart failure or those with increased central venous pressure.

Volume and Hematocrit

An exchange transfusion equal to twice the patient's blood volume is typically recommended for newborns. Rarely is more than one full unit of donor blood needed during an exchange transfusion, since bilirubin, antibody, sensitized cells or toxins are removed with progressively less efficiency in the late stages of the exchange. The blood volume of a full-term newborn is approximately 85 ml/kg. The volume of whole blood required for a two-volume exchange equals weight in kg × 85 × 2. If red blood cells and fresh frozen plasma are combined, the following formula will give the infant a hematocrit of 50% at the end of a two-volume exhange:

1. Total volume (ml) needed = weight in kg × 85 × 2.
2. Absolute volume of red cells needed to give hematocrit of 50% = result of #1 divided by 2.
3. Actual volume (ml) of packed red blood cells needed = the result of #2 divided by 0.7 (approximate hematocrit of packed red blood cells).
4. Actual volume (ml) of fresh frozen plasma needed = #1 − #3.

Example: Calculations for two-volume exchange for a 2 kg infant, to have a final hematocrit of 50%:

2 × 85 × 2 = 340 ml = total volume of blood needed

340/2 = 170 ml = absolute volume of red cells needed to give 50% hematocrit

170/0.7 = 243 ml = volume needed of red cell component at 70% hematocrit

340 − 243 = 97 ml = volume of FFP needed for two-volume exchange

It is important to keep the donor blood mixed during the exchange. If whole blood is allowed to settle in the container, the final aliquots will not have the intended hematocrit. Samples should be obtained from the last aliquot removed in the exchange for determination of the infant's hematocrit and bilirubin.

Methods Used

Two methods of exchange transfusion are in common use. The isovolumetric method requires vascular access through two catheters of identical size. Withdrawal and infusion occur simultaneously, regulated by a single peristaltic pump. The umbilical artery is usually used for withdrawal, the umbilical vein for infusion. The push-pull technique can be accomplished through a single vascular access if necessary. A three-way stopcock joins the unit of blood, the baby and an extension tube that leads to the graduated discard container. A maximum of 5 ml/kg is used for each withdrawal and infusion.

An in-line blood warmer and a standard blood filter should be incorporated in the administration set.

The following additional considerations may apply to exchange transfusion in newborns:

1. The infant's oxygenation, ventilation and acid-base balance should be monitored frequently; it is often necessary to increase the inspired oxygen concentration during the procedure.
2. If the postexchange platelet count is less than 25,000/mm³, it may be desirable to administer platelets.
3. Hypoglycemia may occur as a rebound phenomenon after exchange or secondary to the hyperinsulinism that may accompany severe hemolytic disease. Infusion of 10% dextrose solution after the exchange is completed may be desirable.
4. If the initial exchange transfusion was performed for hyperbilirubinemia, phototherapy using fluorescent blue light bulbs should be instituted when the exchange is completed.

Platelet Transfusion

The normal range of the platelet count in newborns is similar to that in adults. A platelet count less than 100,000/mm³ in a full-term or premature infant is abnormal and requires evaluation. In the absence of other coagulopathy, however, the thrombocytopenic infant rarely bleeds unless the platelet count is less than 10,000/mm.³ Premature infants, or those with other complicating illnesses, may bleed at higher platelet counts and thus require platelet transfusion. When platelet transfusions are given, a 1-hour posttransfusion platelet count should be obtained to evaluate efficacy.

Neonatal thrombocytopenia may result from decreased platelet production, increased platelet destruction or both.[56] Decreased production occurs in congenital megakaryocytic hypoplasia, an entity usually associated with skeletal deformities; in congenital leukemia or systemic histiocytosis; and in rare, genetically determined thrombocytopenias. Platelet transfusion is indicated if bleeding occurs with these forms of thrombocytopenia. Increased platelet destruction occurs in conditions such as immune thrombocytopenia, large cavernous hemangioma or disseminated intravascular coagulation.

Neonatal Immune Thrombocytopenia

Maternal IgG antibodies can cross the placenta and damage fetal platelets, causing severe antenatal thrombocytopenia. The stress of labor and delivery can cause petechiae to develop in the first few hours postpartum, followed by hemorrhages with severe morbidity. Two categories of immune thrombocytopenia are recognized, and the distinction between them is therapeutically important.

Secondary to Maternal ITP

Profound thrombocytopenia will be present in 50% of infants born to mothers with active idiopathic (autoimmune) thrombocytopenic purura (ITP).[56] The circulating antiplatelet antibody is usually IgG, which readily crosses the placenta. Some women with systemic lupus erythematosus have similar circulating antiplatelet antibodies. If maternal ITP is in remission throughout gestation and delivery, fetal risk declines, but any antiplatelet antibodies that persist in the mother's circulation may affect the infant. Occasionally, delivery of a severely thrombocytopenic infant has led to the diagnosis of previously unsuspected ITP in a moderately affected mother (platelet count 75,000 to 100,000/mm^3 postpartum).

The antiplatelet antibody of ITP has broad reactivity against all platelets. Transfusions of platelets from random donors, the mother or other family members have uniformly short survival in the infant and are therefore used only as emergency therapy for hemorrhage. Exchange transfusion may be used to remove circulating antibodies and to provide platelets. Heparinized blood should be avoided, since it may increase the risk of hemorrhage.

Alloimmune Neonatal Thrombocytopenia

A fetus whose platelets possess an antigen absent from maternal platelets may immunize the mother during gestation or delivery, in a pathogenic process similar to hemolytic disease of the newborn. The result is formation of maternal IgG alloantibody that crosses the placenta, usually in a subsequent pregnancy, and causes neonatal thrombocytopenia. The maternal platelet count remains normal. Although the infant's thrombocytopenia is self-limited, usually persisting less than 3 weeks, transfusion therapy is indicated if there is birth trauma, progressive purpura or hemorrhage.

Several dominantly inherited platelet antigens have been implicated in alloimmune neonatal thrombocytopenia.[56] The most commonly involved antigen is Pl^{A1}, present in homozygous or heterozygous state in 98% of unselected individuals. Platelets from random donors are usually positive for Pl^{A1} and are ineffective because of rapid destruction by the alloantibody. Only 2% of the population is Pl^{A1} negative. Often the most readily available source of compatible platelets is the mother. It is usually safe to draw platelets from the mother by thrombocytapheresis (see page 21), even in the postpartum period. Before the platelets are transfused, the mother's antibody-containing plasma should be removed and replaced by group-compatible fresh frozen plasma. A woman who has given birth to a similarly affected infant would also be expected to have compatible platelets.

Granulocyte Transfusion

Compared to those of adults, neutrophils from newborns have diminished levels of chemotaxis, phagocytosis and bacterial killing. Newborns also have deficient reserves of bone marrow neutrophils. Newborn infants are especially susceptible to overwhelming bacterial sepsis. The clinical course of group B streptococcal sepsis may be death within 24 hours despite vigorous antibiotic therapy.

Two preliminary studies have shown that granulocyte transfusions may benefit septic newborns. A group of 16 neonates with neutropenia and sepsis due to various bacteria were studied.[58] All had demonstrated depletion of bone marrow neutrophil reserves. Seven received granulocyte transfusions, irradiated to prevent graft-versus-host disease, and all seven survived, compared to survival of only one of nine nontransfused control infants.

Another series studied 38 neonates with sepsis due to predominately klebsiella or pseudomonas organisms that were resistant in vitro to most antibiotics.[59] Mortality in the 20 transfused infants was only 20% compared to 72% in the nontransfused group.

Because septic neonates have such a rapid clinical course and poor prognosis, granulocyte transfusion for them must be regarded as an emergency procedure. A prolonged regimen of transfusions may be unnecessary. Irradiation of the granulocyte concentrates before transfusion is recommended because of the large quantity of lymphocytes that they also contain. Donors should be ABO- and Rh-compatible with the infant.

Other Blood Products

Hemorrhagic disease of the newborn, caused by deficiency of vitamin K-dependent coagulation factors (II, VII, IX, X), may result in significant cutaneous, gastrointestinal or CNS hemorrhage at 2 to 4 days of age. This disease is now rare because intramuscular vitamin K is routinely given at birth. If vitamin K therapy is omitted, and especially if the infant is breast fed, hemorrhagic disease may occur. If there is life-threatening hemorrhage, the treatment is fresh frozen plasma.

Because maternal clotting factors do not cross the placenta, hereditary deficiencies of coagulation factors may be apparent in the newborn. Significant bleeding, however, is rare. If hemorrhage occurs, therapy is fresh frozen plasma and local thrombin for small superficial bleeds and specific factor concentrates for life-threatening hemorrhage.[60] Patients with hemophilia A may have severe bleeding following circumcision. This can usually be treated with cryoprecipitate.

Obstetrical Considerations

Rh Immune Globulin

Rh Immune Globulin (RhIG) is a concentrated solution of IgG anti-D derived from human plasma. A 1-ml dose, containing 300 μg, is sufficient to counteract the immunizing effects of 15 ml of Rh-positive red cells; this corresponds to 30 ml of fetal blood. RhIG, like other immune serum globulin preparations, does not transmit hepatitis. The immunosuppressive effect of RhIG on Rh-negative individuals exposed to Rh-positive cells probably results from interference with antigen recognition in the induction phase of primary immunization.

Antenatal Administration

The Rh-negative mother of an Rh-positive, ABO-compatible infant, who receives no protection, has a 7 to 8% chance of developing anti-D. When 300 μg RhIG is administered postpartum, the risk of immunization decreases to about 1%. A further decrease in risk, to 0.1%, is achieved if RhIG is given antepartum at 28 weeks gestation, in addition to the postpartum dose.[61] No adverse effects have been observed in infants of mothers who have received up to two antenatal doses of RhIG.[62] The American College of Obstetrics and Gynecology has recommended RhIG antenatal prophylaxis.[63] When there is antenatal RhIG administration, there must be good communication between the patient's physician and the blood bank staff of the hospital where the patient will be delivered, so that laboratory tests made at the time of delivery will be correctly interpreted.

Testing at Delivery

Standards[37] does not require that blood from Rh-negative women be tested at the time of delivery for the presence of unexpected antibodies. It does require ascertainment of Rh status on all women admitted for delivery, abortion or amniocentesis; neither the pre- nor postdelivery specimen need be tested for antibodies, provided there is not a request for red cell transfusion. The Rh test on the mother must include D^u if there is not immediate agglutination with anti-D.

Cord blood from infants born to Rh-negative mothers should be tested for D; ABO testing is not required but is desirable. The mother's antibody status and the baby's clinical condition dictate whether or not a DAT should be done. In some hospitals it is routine to perform ABO testing and a DAT on cord blood from all infants born to group O mothers, but in other centers these tests are performed only if symptoms develop.

The following women are not candidates for RhIG:
1. Rh-negative women who have Rh-negative babies.
2. Rh-positive women. Controversy exists over administration of RhIG to women with a D^u phenotype. Most of these women are also C-positive, and the D^u results from the suppressive effect of C in *trans* position. Individuals with this kind of D^u cannot be immunized to D. Individuals with D^u of other origins have produced anti-D and one case of HDN has been reported.[23] However, this is extremely rare and probably does not justify routine RhIG prophylaxis in women of the D^u phenotype.[64]
3. Rh-negative women known to be immunized to D. Since the presence of anti-D in the postpartum specimen does not prove active immunization, postpartum RhIG is indicated unless an accurate history is available.

Anti-D in a Postpartum Specimen

The woman who has received antenatal RhIG often has anti-D present in an antibody screening test done at delivery. Such a woman should receive postpartum RhIG. Only if the anti-D present at delivery is known to be the result of active immunization can administration of RhIG be omitted. There are some laboratory clues that may help distinguish the origin of the antibody. Passively administered RhIG is IgG. If a woman's anti-D is saline-reactive or can be inactivated by treating the serum with 2-mercaptoethanol or dithiothreitol, it probably represents active immunization. Passively acquired anti-D is usually weakly reactive, rarely achieving a titer above 4. High-titered anti-D is likely to be of maternal origin. However, confirmation should always be sought from the physician's records. RhIG should be given whenever there is doubt that cannot be resolved.

Administration of RhIG

The antenatal dose of RhIG is given between 28 and 30 weeks of gestation, a recommendation based on the fact that, of women who develop anti-D during pregnancy, 92% do so at 28 weeks or later.[65] A sample for laboratory testing should be obtained before injection of RhIG. Tests on the specimen drawn at 28-30 weeks should include:
1. ABO group
2. Rh group and D^u if anti-D does not cause immediate agglutination
3. Antibody screen
4. Identification of antibody, if present

The presence, in an Rh-negative woman, of antibodies other than anti-D does not preclude giving RhIG.

The anti-D from an injected dose of RhIG may remain detectable for as long as 5 months. The half-life of an injected dose is approximately 23 days; of 300 μg of antibody given at 28 weeks, 20 to 30 μg should remain at the time of delivery 12 weeks later. At delivery antibody may not be detectable in the maternal serum, yet in 1-2% of cases the cord red cells will have a positive DAT due to anti-D.[65] Some data suggest that the presence of antibody at levels around 20 μg may enhance the likelihood of immunization if fetomaternal hemorrhage occurs.[66] Postpartum RhIG should be injected within 72 hours of delivery, whether or not RhIG has been given during pregnancy. It is extremely important that RhIG administration not be omitted or delayed because of uncertainty in interpreting an antibody screening test. If for some reason RhIG was not given within 72 hours, later administration should not be withheld.

The "Utilization Gap"

Administration of RhIG is indicated, but sometimes inadvertently omitted, after several common events: abortion, ectopic pregnancy, antepartum hemorrhage or fetal death. If pregnancy in an Rh-negative woman terminates before 13 weeks gestation, a dose of 50 μg ("microdose") is adequate to cover the small fetal blood volume during the first trimester. From 13 weeks until term, the standard 300 μg dose should be given. To ensure complete ascertainment of RhIG candidates, the medical staff of a hospital may direct the surgical pathology service to report to the blood bank staff the name of all patients from whom products of conception or decidual or gravid endometrium are examined.

Amniocentesis

Since fetomaternal hemorrhage may accompany amniocentesis, the procedure can cause Rh immunization.[67] The Rh-negative woman who has amniocentesis at 16-18 weeks for genetic analysis should receive a 300 μg dose of RhIG. A second dose should be given 12 weeks later or at 28 weeks gestation and a third dose given after delivery if the baby is Rh-positive. Amniocentesis performed in the second or third trimester of pregnancy on the nonimmunized Rh-negative woman should be followed by the injection of 300 μg RhIG. If a subsequent amniocentesis is done more than 21 days later, an additional injection of 300 μg RhIG should be given. A mother who delivers within 21 days of receiving a 300 μg dose of RhIG probably does not need a postpartum injection unless there is evidence of a massive fetomaternal hemorrhage.

Amniocentesis is frequently performed near term to assess fetal maturity. If delivery is then scheduled electively and occurs within 48 hours of the amniocentesis, the 300 μg RhIG can be withheld until after the baby is confirmed to be Rh-positive. If amniocentesis precedes delivery by more than 48 hours, the patient should receive 300 μg RhIG following amniocentesis, and no additional RhIG need be given if delivery occurs within 21 days and there is no evidence of a massive fetomaternal hemorrhage.

Detection and Quantitation of Fetomaternal Hemorrhage
Screening Procedures

Postpartum Rh immunization can occur despite RhIG administration if the quantity of Rh-positive fetal red cells entering the mother's circulation exceeds the 30 ml of whole blood covered by a single 300 μg dose of RhIG. The incidence of transplacental hemorrhage greater than 30 ml has been estimated as only about 0.3%, but large fetomaternal hemorrhage is an important and preventable cause of failure of immunoprophylaxis.[68] *Standards*[37] states that a postpartum specimen from all Rh-negative women at risk of immunization should be examined to detect the presence of fetomaternal hemorrhage larger than that for which one dose of RhIG provides protection. Until recently a microscopic examination of the D^u test was the best available method to screen for Rh-positive red cells in the maternal circulation, but it is not very sensitive. In a survey of laboratories, 12% failed to detect Rh-positive cells in a specimen simulating hemorrhage of approximately 30 ml.[69]

Although the Kleihauer-Betke acid elution technique is sensitive for detecting and quantifying small volumes of fetal cells in the maternal circulation, the difficulty of performance and interpretation make it unsuitable as a screening procedure.[69]

The Rosetting Test

The erythrocyte rosetting test[70] is more sensitive than the microscopic examination of the D^u test and gives more reproducible results.[71] The rosette test utilizes D-positive indicator red cells to form easily identified rosettes around any individual D-positive fetal cells that may be present in the maternal circulation. (Special Methods page 481). This method will detect fetomaternal hemorrhages of approximately 10 ml. Such sensitivity provides a margin of safety that is desirable for a screening test. The rosette test gives only qualitative results, and positive results must be followed by the quantitative Kleihauer-Betke acid elution test to quantify the hemorrhage. D^u positive cells from the infant do not react as strongly in the rosette procedure as normal D-positive cells. If the newborn has a D^u phenotype, then a Kleihauer-Betke acid elution test should be done routinely. If the mother's blood is D^u, the rosette test may be strongly positive, but the Kleihauer-Betke test, which detects fetal hemoglobin and not the presence of the D antigen, will be negative.

Acid Elution

Results of the Kleihauer-Betke acid elution test are reported as percentage of fetal cells, but the precision of the procedure is poor, even in highly experienced hands. To calculate the volume of fetomaternal hemorrhage, this percentage of fetal cells is multiplied by 50.[72] Since one 300 μg dose of RhIG will protect against a transplacental hemorrhage of 30 ml of Rh-positive fetal blood, the volume of fetal blood should be divided by 30 to determine the number of doses of RhIG required.

For example: 1. Kleihauer-Betke reported as 1.3%

2. $1.3 \times 50^* = 65$ ml of fetal blood

3. $\dfrac{65}{30} = 2.2$ doses of RhIG required

*5000 ml (mother's arbitrarily assigned blood volume) $\times \dfrac{1}{100}(\%) = 50$

Because quantification by this procedure is inherently imprecise and because the consequences of undertreatment can be so serious, it is important to provide a safety margin in calculating RhIG dosage. One approach is as follows:

When the number to the right of the decimal point is less than 5, round down and add one dose of RhIG.
Example: 2.2 doses—give 3 doses

When the number to the right of the decimal point is 5 or greater, round up to the next number and add one dose of RhIG.
Example: 2.8 doses—give 4 doses

A more conservative approach uses the dose schedule shown in Table 16-6, which embodies both a wider range of enumeration error and a wider margin for inconsistency in absorption or efficacy. Suggested dose exceed those of the preceding formula by 1 or 2 vials.

Table 16-6. RhIG Dosage for Massive Fetomaternal Hemorrhage, Based on the Acid Elution Test[73]

% Fetal Cells	Fetomaternal Hemorrhage Volume (ml whole blood)		Vials of RhIG to Inject
	Average	Range*	
0.3–0.5	20	<50	2
0.6–0.8	35	15– 80	3
0.9–1.1	50	22–110	4
1.2–1.4	65	30–140	5
1.5–2.0	88	37–200	6
2.1–2.5	115	52–250	6

*The range provides for the poor precision of the acid elution test. These recommendations are based upon 1 vial needed for each 15 ml red blood cells or 30 ml whole blood.

Not more than five doses of RhIG should be injected at one time into each buttock. If more than 10 doses are required, the injections may be spaced over a 72-hour period; however, the optimum time sequence for these injections has not been established.

References

1. Stockman JA, III. Red cell transfusions in the newborn. Am J Pediatr Hem/Onc 1981;3:205–211.

2. Gray JM. The use of blood components in fetal and neonatal medicine. In: Umlas J, Silvergleid AJ, eds. Transfusion for the patient with selected clinical problems. Arlington, VA: American Association of Blood Banks, 1982:117–179.

3. Batteby L, Garby L, Wadman B. Studies on erythro-kinetics in infancy:XII. Survival in adult recipients of cord blood cells labeled in vitro with di-isopropyl fluoro-phosphate (DF[32]P). Acta Paediatr Scand 1968;57:305–310.

4. Oski FA, Naiman JL. Hematologic problems in the newborn. 3rd ed. New York: WB Saunders, 1982.

5. Delivoria-Papadopoulos M, Roncevic NP, Oski FA. Postnatal changes in oxygen transport of term, premature and sick infants: the role of red cell 2,3-diphosphoglycerate and adult hemoglobin. Pediatr Res 1971;5:235–245.

6. Wallgren G, Hanson JS, Lind J. Quantitative studies of the human neonatal circulation. Acta Paediatr Scand (suppl) 1967;179:43–54.

7. Gairdner D, Marks J, Roscoe JD. Blood formation in infancy—Part IV. The early anemia of prematurity. Arch Dis Child 1955;30:203–211.

8. Pollock JM, Bowman, JM. Placental transfer of Rh antibody (anti-D IgG) during pregnancy. Vox Sang 1982;43:327–334.

9. Parkman R, Mosier D, Umansky I, Cochran W, Carpenter CB, Rosen FS. Graft-versus-host disease after intrauterine and exchange transfusions for hemolytic disease of the newborn. N Engl J Med 1974;290:359–363.

10. Holland PV. Other adverse effects of transfusion. In: Petz LD, Swisher SN, eds. Practice of blood transfusion. New York: Churchill Livingstone, 1981;783–803.

11. Batton DG, Maisels MJ, Shulman G. Serum potassium changes following packed red cell transfusions in newborn infants. Transfusion 1983;23:163–164.

12. Delivoria-Papadopoulos M, Martens RJ, Anday EK, Kumar SP. Neonatal oxygen transport: the role of exchange transfusion. In: Sherwood WS, Cohen A, eds. Transfusion therapy: the fetus, infant, and child. New York: Masson, 1980;63–74.

13. Stagno S, Pass RF, Dworsky ME, et al. Congenital cytomegalovirus infection: the relative importance of primary and recurrent maternal infection. N Engl J Med 1982;306:945–949.

14. Smith D, Wright P, Krueger L, et al. Posttransfusion cytomegalovirus infection in neonates weighing less than 1250 grams (abstract). Transfusion 1983;23:420.

15. Yeager AS, Grumet FC, Hafleigh EB, Arvin AM, Bradley JS, Prober C. Prevention of transfusion-acquired cytomegalovirus infections in newborn infants. J Pediatr 1981;98:281–287.

16. Lang DJ, Ebert PA, Rodgers BM, Boggess HP, Rixse RS. Reduction of postperfusion cytomegalovirus-infections following the use of leukocyte depleted blood. Transfusion 1977;17:391–395.

17. Brady M, Anderson D, Milam J, Hawkins E, et al. Prevention of posttransfusion cytomegalovirus infection in neonates by the use of frozen-washed red blood cells. Clinical Research 1982;30:895A.

18. Simon T, Johnson J, Koffler H, Aldrich M, et al. Impact of previously frozen deglycerolized red blood cells on cytomegalovirus transmission to newborn infants (abstract). Blood 1983;62(Suppl):238a.

19. Polesky HF. Diagnosis, prevention, and therapy in hemolytic disease of the newborn. In: Myhre BA, ed. Clinics in laboratory medi-

cine. Philadelphia: WB Saunders, 1982;2:107–122.

20. Cohen F, Zuelzer WW. Mechanisms of isoimmunization: II. Transplacental passage and postnatal survival of fetal erythrocytes in heterospecific pregnancies. Blood 1967;30:796–804.

21. Ascari WO, Levine P, Pollack W. Incidence of maternal immunization by ABO compatible and incompatible pregnancies. Br Med J 1969;1:399–401.

22. Woodrow JC, Donohue WTA. Rh-immunization by pregnancy; results of a survey and their relevance to prophylactic therapy. Br Med J 1968;4:139–144.

23. Lacey PA, Caskey CR, Werner DJ, Moulds JJ. Fatal hemolytic disease of a newborn due to anti-D in an Rh-positive Dᵘ variant mother. Transfusion 1983;23:91–94.

24. Tregellas WM. Serological evaluation of the prenatal patient. In: Tregellas WM, Wallas CH, eds. Prenatal and perinatal immunohematology. Washington, DC: American Association of Blood Banks, 1981;1–16.

25. Goldsmith KLG, Mourant AE, Banghan DR. The international standard for anti-Rho(D) incomplete blood typing serum. Bull Wld Hlth Org 1967;36:435–445.

26. Gluck L. Fetal maturity and amniotic fluid surfactant determinations. In: Spellecy WN, ed. Management of the high risk pregnancy. Baltimore: University Park Press, 1976;189–207.

27. Bowman JM. Rh erythroblastosis fetalis 1975. Semin Hematol 1975;12:189–207.

28. Norman JL, Punnett HH, Lischer HW, Destine ML, Arey JB. Possible graft-versus-host reaction after interauterine transfusion in Rh erythroblastosis fetalis. N Engl J Med 1969;281:697–701.

29. Konugres AA. Transfusion therapy for the neonate. In: Bell CA, ed. A seminar on perinatal blood banking. Washington, DC: American Association of Blood Banks, 1981;93–107.

30. White KJ, Wilson JK, Barnes A: Sedimented red cells (letter). Transfusion 1980;20:476.

31. Valeri CR, Valeri DA, Gray A, et al. Cryopreserved red blood cells for pediatric transfusion: frozen storage of small aliquots in polyvinyl chloride (PVC) plastic bags. Transfusion 1981;21:517–536.

32. Hathaway WE. The bleeding newborn. Semin Hematol 1975;12:175–188.

33. Moroff G, Friedman A, Robkin-Kline L, Gautier G, Luban NLC. Reduction of the volume of stored platelet concentrates for use in neonatal patients. Transfusion 1984;24:144–152.

34. Goldfinger D, Connelly M, McPherson J, Medici M. Preparation of granulocyte concentrates for transfusion to neonates using the IBM 2991 Blood Processor (abstract). Transfusion 1982;22:434.

35. Ludvigsen C, Swanson J, Thompson T, McCullough J. Failure of neonates to form red cell alloantibodies following transfusion (abstract). Transfusion 1982;22:405.

36. Cohen AR, Schwartz E. Transfusion in the newborn period. In: Sherwood WS, Cohen A, eds. Transfusion therapy: the fetus, infant and child. New York: Masson, 1980;37–50.

37. Schmidt PJ, ed. Standards for blood banks and transfusion services. 11th ed. Arlington, VA: American Association of Blood Banks, 1984.

38. Gibson JS, Leff RD, Roberts RJ. Effects of intravenous delivery systems on infused red blood cells. Am J Hosp Pharm 1984;41:468–472.

39. Wilcox GJ, Barnes A, Modanlou H. Does transfusion using a syringe infusion pump and small-gauge needle cause hemolysis? Transfusion 1981;21:750–751.

40. Solis RT, Goldfinger D, Gibbs MB, Zeller JA. Physical characteristics of micro-aggregates in stored blood. Transfusion 1974;14:538–550.

41. Schmidt WF, Kim HC, Tomassini N, Schwartz E. RBC destruction caused by a micropore blood filter. JAMA 1982;248:1629–1632.

42. Lubin B. Neonatal anaemia secondary to blood loss. Clin Haematol 1978;7:19–34.

43. Stockman JA III, Clark DA, Levin EA. Weight gain, a response to transfusion in preterm infants (abstract). Pediatr Res 1980;14:612.

44. Bowman JM. Rh erythroblastosis fetalis. Semin Hematol 1975;12:189–207.

45. Lee K, Gartner LM, Eidelman AI, Ezhuthachan S. Unconjugated hyperbilirubinemia in very low birth weight infants. Clin Perinatol 1977;4:305–320.

46. Maisels MJ. Jaundice in the newborn. Pediatrics in Review 1982;3:305–319.

47. Feusner JH, Slichter SJ, Harker LA. Acquired hemostatic defects in the ill newborn. Br J Haemat 1983;53:73–84.

48. Tollner U, Pohlandt F, Heinze F, Henrichs I. Treatment of septicemia in the newborn infant: choice of initial antimicrobial drugs and role of exchange transfusion. Acta Paediatr Scand 1977;66:605–610.

49. Shigeoka AO, Hall RT, Hill HR. Blood transfusion in group B streptococcal sepsis. Lancet 1978;1:636–638.

50. Erslev AJ, Clinical manifestations of erythrocyte disorders. In: Williams WJ, Beutler E,

Erslev AJ, Lichtman MA, eds. Hematology. 3rd ed. New York: McGraw-Hill, 1984:58–63.

51. Ramamurthy RS, Brans YW. Neonatal polycythemia: criteria for diagnosis and treatment. Pediatrics 1981;68:168–174.

52. Kreuger A. Adenine metabolism during and after exchange transfusions in newborn infants with CPD-adenine blood. Transfusion 1976;16:249–252.

53. Murphy RJC, Malhotra C, Sweet AY. Death following an exchange transfusion with hemoglobin SC blood. J Pediatr 1980;96:110–120.

54. Gershanik JJ, Levkoff AH, Duncan R. Serum ionized calcium values in relation to exchange transfusion. J Pediatr 1973;82:589–593.

55. Chan G, Schoff D. Variance in albumin loading in exchange transfusions. J Pediatr 1976;88:609–613.

56. Pearson HA, McIntosh S. Neonatal thrombocytopenia. Clin Haematol 1978;7:111–122.

57. Christensen RD, Anstall HB, Rothstein G. Review: deficiencies in the neutrophil system of newborn infants, and the use of leukocyte transfusions in neonatal sepsis. J Clin Apheresis 1982;1:33–41.

58. Christensen RD, Rothstein G, Anstall HB, Bybee B. Granulocyte transfusions in neonates with bacterial infection, neutropenia, and depletion of mature marrow neutrophils. Pediatrics 1982;70:1–6.

59. Laurenti F, Ferro R, Isacchi G, et al. Polymorphonuclear leukocyte transfusion for the treatment of sepsis in the newborn infant. J Pediatr 1981;98:118–123.

60. Gill M. Transfusion therapy for coagulation disorders in the newborn infant. In: Sherwood WC, Cohen A, eds. Transfusion therapy: the fetus, infant and child. New York: Masson, 1980:75–94.

61. Bowman JM, Chown B, Lewis M, Pollock JM. Rh isoimmunization during pregnancy: antenatal prophylaxis. Can Med Assn J 1978;118:623–627.

62. Jennings ER, Dibbern HH, Hodell FH, Monroe CH, et al. Prevention of Rh hemolytic disease of the newborn. Calif Med 1969;10:130–133.

63. American College of Obstetrics and Gynecology: Prevention of Rho(D) isoimmunization, technical bulletin number 79, August 1984.

64. Konugres A, Polesky H, Walker R. Rh immune globulin and the Rh positive, D^u variant mother. Transfusion 1982;22:76–77.

65. Frigoletto FD Jr. Risk perspectives of Rh sensitization. In: Frigoletto FD Jr, Jewett JF, Konugres AA, eds. Rh hemolytic disease: new strategy for eradication. Boston: GK Hall, 1982;103–110.

66. Contreras M, Mollison PL. Rh immunization facilitated by passively-administered anti-Rh? Br J Haematol 1983;53:153–159.

67. Lele AS, Carmody PJ, Hurd ME, O'Leary JA. Fetomaternal bleeding following diagnostic amniocentesis. Obstet Gynecol 1982;60:60–64.

68. Zipursky A, Israels LG. The pathogenesis and prevention of Rh immunization. Can Med Assn J 1967;97:1245–1257.

69. Polesky HF, Sebring ES. Evaluation of methods for detection and quantitation of fetal cells and their effect on RhIgG usage. Am J Clin Pathol 1981;76:525–529.

70. Sebring ES, Polesky HF. Detection of fetal maternal hemorrhage in Rh immune globulin candidates. Transfusion 1982;22:468–471.

71. Taswell HF, Reisner RK. Laboratory medicine: prevention of Rho hemolytic disease of the newborn: the rosette method - a rapid, sensitive screening test. Mayo Clin Proc 1983;58:342–343.

72. Walker RH. A summary, detection of fetomaternal hemorrhage. In: Detection of fetomaternal hemorrhage. Washington, DC: The American Association of Blood Banks, 1972.

73. Walker RH. Relevancy in the selection of serologic tests for the obstetric patient. In: Garratty G, ed. Hemolytic disease of the newborn. Arlington, VA: American Association of Blood Banks, 1984.

17

Adverse Effects of Blood Transfusion

Transfusion of blood and components is ordinarily a safe and effective way of temporarily correcting hematologic deficits, but untoward results do occur. Some of these adverse effects are commonly called transfusion reactions, but the potentially deleterious results of administering blood include a range of events and problems broader than the limited connotations usually evoked by the term "transfusion reaction" (Table 17-1). Some adverse effects can be prevented; others cannot. Health care providers should know the risks of blood transfusion and consciously evaluate these risks against potential therapeutic benefits.

Suspected Hemolytic Transfusion Reactions

The time between suspicion of a transfusion reaction and the investigation and initiation of appropriate therapy should be as short as possible. Responsibility for recognizing a reaction rests with the transfusionist, who is often a nurse, physician or other member of the clinical team. The presenting events of fever and chills may be the same for life-threatening hemolytic transfusion reactions and less serious febrile or allergic reactions. Any adverse symptoms or physical signs occurring during transfusion of blood or its components should be considered potentially a part of a life-threatening reaction and the following actions must be taken immediately:

1. Stop the transfusion to limit the amount of blood infused. Notify a responsible physician.
2. Keep the intravenous line open with infusion of normal saline or other suitable intravenous solution.
3. Check all labels, forms and patient identification to determine if the patient received the correct blood or component.
4. Report the suspected transfusion reaction to blood bank personnel immediately.
5. Send required blood samples, carefully drawn to avoid mechanical hemolysis, to the blood bank as soon as possible, together with the discontinued bag of blood, the administration set, attached IV solutions and all the related forms and labels.
6. Send other samples for evaluation of acute hemolysis as directed by the blood bank director or patient's physician. A suggested outline for laboratory investigation of a suspected hemolytic transfusion reaction follows.

Suggested Outline for Laboratory Investigation

When a suspected hemolytic transfusion reaction is reported to the blood bank, the technologist should:

Table 17-1. Immediate and Delayed Adverse Effects of Transfusion

Immediate Effects

Immunologic Effects	Usual Etiology
Hemolysis with symptoms	Red cell incompatibility
Febrile nonhemolytic reaction	Antibody to leukocyte antigens
Anaphylaxis	Antibody to IgA
Urticaria	Antibody to plasma proteins
Noncardiac pulmonary edema	Antibody to leukocytes or complement activation
Nonimmunologic Effects	
Marked fever with shock	Bacterial contamination
Congestive heart failure	Volume overload
Hemolysis with symptoms	Physical destruction of blood, eg, freezing or overheating
	Mixing nonisotonic solutions with red blood cells

Delayed Effects

Immunologic Effects	Usual Etiology
Hemolysis	Anamnestic antibody to red cell antigens
Graft-vs-host disease	Engraftment of transfused functional lymphocytes
Posttransfusion purpura	Development of antiplatelet antibody (usually Pl^{A1})
Alloimmunization to RBC or WBC antigens, platelets or plasma proteins	Exposure to antigens of donor origin
Nonimmunologic Effects	
Iron overload	Multiple transfusions (100 +)
Hepatitis	NANB, occasionally B (rarely A)
Acquired immune deficiency syndrome	Host response to agent in donor blood
Protozoal infection	Malaria parasites

1. Check identification of patient and of donor blood. If there is a discrepancy, immediately notify the patient's physician or other responsible health-care professional and search appropriate records to find if other patient samples or donor units have been misidentified or incorrectly issued. After ascertaining if other patients are at risk, and after performing appropriate diagnostic and therapeutic procedures, trace each step of the transfusion process to find the error.

2. Compare the patient's prereaction specimen and postreaction specimen for:
   a. Color of serum or plasma
      Pink or red discoloration present in the postreaction specimen but not in the pretransfusion specimen usually indicates the presence of free hemoglobin and destruction of red cells. Intravascular hemolysis of as little as 5 ml of red cells can produce visible hemoglobinemia. Mechanical hemolysis occurring during blood sample collection can produce pink or red-tinged serum. If this is suspected, a repeat specimen should be requested but a slightly hemolyzed sample can still be used for the direct antiglobulin test. In samples drawn 4 to 10 hours after transfusion, yellow or brown discoloration, from increased bilirubin and other hemoglobin breakdown products, may indicate recent hemolysis.

   b. Direct antiglobulin test
      If antibody- or complement-coated transfused incompatible cells are not immediately destroyed, the direct antiglobulin test on the postreaction specimen will be positive, with a mixed-field appearance. Since circulating antibody- or complement-coated cells may be very rapidly

destroyed, the direct antiglobulin test may be negative if the specimen is drawn several hours after the suspected reaction. Nonimmune hemolysis, (eg, from thermal damage or mechanical trauma from the roller pumps used in cardiac bypass systems) can produce hemoglobinemia without a positive direct antiglobulin test. These and other causes of nonimmune hemolysis should be considered whenever hemoglobinemia occurs without an obvious immune etiology. (See below.)

Interpretation of Laboratory Evaluation

Negative results on observations for hemoglobinemia and the presence of antibody or complement on the transfused cells usually indicate that there has not been an acute immune hemolytic reaction. Positive results from any of these procedures require additional investigation. If any findings are positive or doubtful, some or all of the tests described below should be done and the results and interpretations must be recorded. If the patient's clinical condition strongly suggests a hemolytic reaction, further investigation is warranted despite negative results in preliminary testing.

Investigation for Possible Alloantibodies

To determine if an antibody has caused the reaction and to identify the antibody:

1. Repeat ABO and Rh tests on patient's prereaction sample and on blood from the bag or from a segment still attached to the unit. Test the postreaction sample for ABO and Rh; a mixed-field pattern suggests the presence of incompatible donor cells.

   If ABO and Rh typing on the patient's two samples do not agree, there has been an error in either patient indentification, typing or blood drawing. Another patient's blood may have been drawn at the same time and may have been correspondingly mislabeled, so it is especially important to check records of all specimens received at approximately the same time.

   If the donor blood specimen is not of the ABO group noted on the bag label, there has been an error in labeling and, thus almost certainly, an error in the crossmatch as well.

2. Repeat the crossmatch, testing both the prereaction serum sample and the postreaction serum sample against a sample of red blood cells from the bag or from a segment still attached to the unit.

   If results are incompatible with both the prereaction and postreaction specimens, an error was made during prereaction testing. The donor specimen used for the crossmatch may have been taken from a different unit. Whenever possible the crossmatch should be repeated against cells from the segment actually used in the initial crossmatch. If the crossmatch is incompatible with the postreaction specimen but compatible with the prereaction sample, suspect an anamnestic antibody response. This is most likely if the reaction has occurred, or if the postreaction sample was drawn, several days after transfusion. If only a short time has elapsed after transfusion, check the patient's previous transfusion history. It is possible that an antibody has developed to red cells transfused in the preceding few days. Less likely, antibody might have been present in a transfused blood component.

   If both crossmatches are compatible and there is strong clinical reason to believe an acute immune hemolytic reaction has occurred, further testing is necessary. Check the records and performance of the original crossmatch. For other investigations, see section on special testing later in this chapter on page 329.

3. Repeat the antibody detection tests on the prereaction and postreaction samples and on the donor blood. If any tests are positive, identify the antibody (see Chapter 13). Test donor units for the presence of the corresponding antigen. If the patient's prereaction sample or the donor blood has an unexpected antibody not previously reported, check records to see how the discrepancy occurred. If the donor blood proves to have a previously overlooked antibody, do a minor crossmatch against the patient's prereaction sample. If the postreaction specimen has an antibody not present before transfusion, suspect an anamnestic reaction or passive administration of antibody in a transfusion component recently infused.

If antibody is identified, phenotype the patient's cells from the prereaction sample to be sure that the patient lacks the corresponding antigen. Check transfusion records to determine whether there might be recently transfused cells in the prereaction specimen. Such cells would give a mixed-field or weak reaction with typing reagents, and could confuse the interpretation of results. Such cells could also be the stimulus for an anamnestic antibody response.

Investigation for Other Problems

To evaluate the possibility of nonimmunologic hemolysis:

1. Consider bacterial contamination of the donor unit if 1) the cells or plasma have brownish or purple discoloration, 2) there are clots or abnormal masses in the liquid blood, 3) the delineation between cells and plasma in a spun sample is fuzzy or blurred, 4) the plasma is opaque or muddy looking, or 5) there is a peculiar odor.
   a. Before manipulating the bag excessively, take specimens from the bag for cultures at 4 C, 20-24 C and 35-37 C, as bacterial contaminants will grow at a variety of temperatures.
   b. Examine a smear of the blood stained with gram stain or acridine orange, which stains DNA.[1]

2. Examine the supernatant plasma of the blood from the donor blood container for presence of free hemoglobin.

   If present, the unit may have been damaged by improper temperatures in shipping or storage or at the time of administration, by the injection of drugs or hypotonic solutions, or by bacterial contamination.

3. Examine the blood remaining in administration tubing for presence of free hemoglobin.

   If the administration set had previously been used for hypotonic solutions or dextrose solutions, there could be hemolysis in the tubing but not in the bag.

   Excessive heat from a faulty in-line blood warmer could also damage the infused blood without causing abnormalities of the blood container. This would not ordinarily be obvious in the returned administration set tubing but the possibility should be pursued if the patient has posttransfusion hemoglobinemia with no other apparent cause.

4. Consider the possibility that the patient has an intrinsic red cell defect. Patients with glucose-6-phosphate dehydrogenase (G-6-PD) deficiency or sickle cell anemia may experience intravascular hemolysis because of medical problems not necessarily related to the transfusion. Paroxysmal nocturnal hemoglobinuria (PNH) is a rare problem but, when present, may produce severe hemoglobinemia and hemoglobinuria as a result of transfusion.

5. Consider the possibility of mechanical hemolysis. Mechanical red cell lysis can occur with the use of roller pumps such as those used in cardiac bypass surgery, pressure infusion pumps, pressure cuffs or small-bore needles (see Chapter 15).

6. Consider osmotic hemolysis due to inadvertent entry into the circulation of hypotonic fluids, such as distilled water used for postprostatectomy bladder irrigation.
7. Exclude myoglobinemia by use of ammonium sulfate precipitation or electrophoretic studies.[2,3] (See Special Methods, page 491.)

Clinical Evaluation

To follow the patient's clinical condition when hemolysis is proven or strongly suspected:
1. Examine postreaction urine specimens for the presence of free hemoglobin.

   Intact red cells in the urine (hematuria) are a sign of hemorrhage into the urinary tract; hemolytic transfusion reactions do not cause red cells to enter the urine. Following hemolysis, hemoglobin released by intravascular hemolysis enters the urine, but the cells do not. The test for hemoglobin should be done on the supernatant of a centrifuged specimen of freshly collected urine. If the urine does contain red cells that hemolyze in vitro, however, the results will be misleading.

   If there has been a delay of several days before diagnosing hemolysis or before obtaining a urine sample, it may be preferable to test for hemosiderin in the urine. (See Special Methods, page 490.)
2. Test postreaction serum samples for unconjugated bilirubin but keep the time of such testing in mind. The rate and magnitude of bilirubin rise are very variable. Rising bilirubin may be detectable as early as 1 hour postreaction. Peak levels occur at 4 to 6 hours and disappear within 24 hours if bilirubin excretion is normal.
3. Measure serum haptoglobin in pre-reaction and postreaction specimens.

   If there is visible hemoglobinemia, there is little point in measuring haptoglobin, because visible hemoglobi-nemia develops only after haptoglobin depletion.

   Haptoglobin levels are so variable that the postreaction values must be compared against the prereaction level. Even after the uneventful administration of several units of blood, the recipient's haptoglobin level may fall substantially, although rarely to levels below 50% of the initial concentration.[4] Haptoglobin levels are stable in serum, and analysis is not affected by in vitro hemolysis. Documenting a decline in haptoglobin has most diagnostic value in demonstrating subtle or chronic hemolysis. Serum haptoglobin rarely provides useful information in acute hemolytic transfusion reactions. Haptoglobin is an acute phase reactant that may regenerate rapidly after depletion; if studies are performed several days after a hemolytic episode, normal levels may be restored.

Special Tests to Diagnose Red Cell Incompatibility

If routine tests are uninformative and if immune hemolysis continues to be strongly suspected:
1. Perform antibody detection tests and compatibility tests with more sensitive techniques. (See Chapter 13.) Previously undetected antibody in the pre-transfusion specimen may become apparent by using low ionic strength solution (LISS), Polybrene® or enzyme techniques, or by increasing the ratio of serum to cells.[5-7]
2. Perform direct antiglobulin and antibody detection tests on several postreaction specimens at daily or other frequent intervals.

   The immediate postreaction specimen may have a negative direct antiglobulin test if all the antibody-coated cells were removed from the circulation. Similarly, the serum may contain no free antibody because all of it reacted with the transfused cells. Under these circumstances antibody concentration usually rises rapidly, so detection and identification become possible within a few days.

3. Measure hematocrit or hemoglobin at frequent intervals posttransfusion to document whether the transfused cells have or have not produced the expected therapeutic rise, or to demonstrate that a drop in hematocrit has occurred after an initial rise.

A unit of red blood cells is expected to increase hemoglobin level by approximately 1 g/dl (see Table 15-2) and the hematocrit by about 3% when administered to a hemodynamically stable 70 kg recipient.

4. Type the cells of the recipient and of the donor unit under suspicion to find antigens present in the donor and absent in the recipient, and examine the patient's postreaction blood for the presence of cells bearing these antigens. The recipient's specimen must be a prereaction sample that contains only the patient's cells. This may be difficult if the patient has recieved transfusions within the previous several weeks. For a technique to obtain truly autologous cells, see page 419.

If an antigen can be found that is present on the donor cells and absent from the patient's cells, its presence or absence in postreaction samples indicates the degree to which the transfused cells have survived and remain in the circulation.

Acute Hemolytic Transfusion Reaction

An acute hemolytic transfusion reaction is triggered by an antigen-antibody reaction and mediated by neuroendocrine responses and by activation of the complement and coagulation systems. Clinically catastrophic events that may occur include shock, disseminated intravascular coagulation (DIC) and acute renal failure. Life-threatening hemolytic transfusion reac-

tions are almost always due to ABO mismatch attributable to an identification error that results in the recipient receiving the wrong blood. Incompatibility in other blood groups may also cause acute hemolysis in a recipient with alloantibodies stimulated by previous transfusions or pregnancy. These reactions, however, are rarely as severe as those involving ABO incompatibility. Clinically serious nonimmunologic causes of hemolysis include bacterial contamination of the unit of blood, infusion of hypotonic solutions or transfusion of donor blood damaged by excessive pressure, freezing or overheating.

Diagnosis

Initial signs and symptoms that may occur with an acute hemolytic transfusion reaction are listed in Table 17-2. The most common initial symptom noted in recipients is fever, frequently accompanied by chills.[8] Reactions may occur when as little as 10-15 ml of incompatible blood have been infused. The onset of symptoms may be misleadingly mild, such as vague uneasiness or an aching back. The first sign the patient observes may be red urine, which may or may not be accompanied by back pain. The severity of initial symptoms is often related to the amount of blood transfused and may presage the severity of the ensuing clinical problems. In unconscious or anesthetized recipients the only manifestations of an acute hemolytic transfusion reaction may be bleeding at the surgical site (due to DIC), hypotension or the presence of hemoglobinuria. It is critical that whenever a hemolytic, or indeed

Table 17-2. Signs and Symptoms that May Accompany Hemolytic Transfusion Reactions

Fever	Hemoglobinuria
Chills	Shock
Chest pain	Generalized bleeding
Hypotension	Oliguria or anuria
Nausea	Back pain
Flushing	Pain at infusion site
Dyspnea	

any, transfusion reaction is suspected the transfusion be stopped immediately, before any other action is taken. The intravenous line should be maintained with normal saline to treat the reaction if one has occurred.

Investigation of a possible hemolytic transfusion reaction should begin at the patient's bedside with a check of the name and hospital number on the patient's wristband against the same data on the compatibility label or the tag of the donor unit. Since patient or blood sample identification errors may involve two patients, it is imperative to determine if another patient is also in danger of receiving incompatible blood.

The postreaction blood samples should be used for further diagnostic testing and for a baseline against which evolving clinical findings can be compared. Laboratory tests that may be useful in evaluating acute hemolysis have been outlined above and are listed in Table 17-3.

Pathophysiology

Interaction of antibody with antigen initiates the pathophysiologic events of immunologically mediated acute hemolytic reactions, through activation of the following three interrelated mechanisms.[9]

The Neuroendocrine Response

Antigen-antibody complexes can activate Hageman factor (Factor XIIa), which, in turn, acts on the kinin system to produce bradykinin. Bradykinin increases capillary permeability and dilates arterioles. Because of resulting hypotension, and/or as a direct effect of the complexes, the sympathetic nervous system is stimulated and norepinephrine and other catecholamine levels rise. These catecholamines produce vasoconstriction in organs with a vascular bed in which α-adrenergic receptors are highly concentrated, largely renal, splanchnic, pulmonary and cutaneous capillaries. Coronary and cerebral vessels have few α-adrenergic receptors and these vascular beds participate very little in the reaction.

Table 17-3. Tests for Red Cell Destruction in Hemolytic Transfusion Reactions

Immediate

Visual or photometric determination of free hemoglobin (pink) or bilirubin (yellow-brown) in serum of prereaction and postreaction specimens

Direct antiglobulin test on postreaction sample

As Indicated

Repeat ABO and Rh determinations on pre- and postreaction samples and unit of blood

Crossmatch prereaction and postreaction samples with red blood cells from unit or stored, sealed segment

Measure unconjugated bilirubin, preferably on specimen drawn 5 to 7 hours after transfusion

Look for urine free hemoglobin (rule out intact red blood cells)

Look for urine hemosiderin (delayed)

Perform routine and/or especially sensitive tests for unexpected antibody in donor and patient

Evaluate response to transfusion with hemoglobin and hematocrit results (in a 70-kg recipient 1 g/dl hemoglobin or 3% hematocrit per unit of blood or packed cells transfused)

Make gram stain of blood smear from unit

Culture unit at 4°C, 22°C, and 35–37°C

Look for free hemoglobin in plasma or donor unit

Measure serum haptoglobin on both prereaction and postreaction samples

In addition, antigen-antibody complexes activate the complement system (see below), resulting in anaphylatoxic stimulation of mast cells, which release histamine and serotonin. Serotonin and histamine are also released from platelets, stimulated by antigen-antibody complexes or through initiation of clotting (DIC). These vasoactive amines mediate many of the clinical signs and symptoms of the reaction. Once these substances have been released, their regeneration requires time; this explains the occasional deceptive observation that the transfusion of a second unit of incompatible blood does not elicit another dramatic pathophysiologic response.

The Complement System

Antigen-antibody complexes can activate complement on the red cell membrane.

When complement is activated and the enzymatic cascade proceeds to completion, intravascular hemolysis results. If complement activation does not proceed to completion, red cells coated with C3b are removed following interaction with phagocytes, which have receptors for C3b. In some instances C3b inactivator and β_1-microglobulin convert C3b to C3d. Cells coated with C3d survive normally, since macrophages do not have C3d receptors. In an ABO mismatch, complement activation proceeds to completion with activation of C9. When the C5-C9 membrane attack complex binds to the red cell, osmotic red cell lysis occurs within the intravascular space, causing both free hemoglobin and red cell stroma to enter the plasma. Free hemoglobin was formerly thought to play a major role in renal ischemia, but current thought attributes renal vasoconstriction, acute tubular necrosis and renal failure largely to the presence of antibody-coated cell stroma. With most other (non-ABO) blood group antibodies, complement activation is, at most, partial. For a more complete discussion of the actions of complement, see Chapter 5.

The Coagulation System

The intrinsic clotting cascade may be activated by antigen-antibody complexes through Hageman factor activation or directly by the presence of incompatible red cell stroma. Disseminated intravascular coagulation, thus initiated, may cause: 1) formation of thrombi within the microvasculature; 2) consumption of fibrinogen, platelets, and Factors V and VIII; 3) activation of the fibrinolytic (plasmin) system; 4) generation of fibrin split products; and, possibly, 5) uncontrolled bleeding.[10]

The cumulative effect of systemic hypotension, renal vasoconstriction, and formation of intravascular thrombi compromises the blood supply to the kidney. This renal ischemia may be transient or may progress to acute tubular necrosis and, possibly, bilateral renal cortical necrosis.

Therapy

Vigorous treatment of hypotension and promotion of adequate renal blood flow are the cornerstones of therapy for hemolytic transfusion reactions. If shock can be prevented or adequately treated, renal failure can usually be avoided. Adequacy of renal perfusion can be monitored by assessing urine flow. Fluid therapy should be directed at maintaining urine flow rates at or over 100 ml/hour in adults for at least 18-24 hours. The presence of underlying cardiac and/or renal disease, however, may complicate therapy. To improve blood flow to the kidneys and increase urine output, osmotic or diuretic agents should also be administered. Administering intravenous furosemide both improves renal blood flow and produces diuresis.[9,11] Mannitol is an osmotic diuretic that increases blood volume but may not increase renal blood flow. Accordingly, some workers believe that mannitol should not be used for treatment of acute hemolytic transfusion reactions, while others consider mannitol a useful agent.[9]

Vasopressor agents that decrease renal blood flow are contraindicated, but dopamine, which in low doses ($<5\mu g/kg/min$) dilates the renal vasculature while increasing cardiac output, may be useful in treating the acute phase of hemolytic transfusion reactions.[12] Dopamine must be diluted and given intravenously in a metered dose while the patient's urine flow, cardiac output and blood pressure are carefully monitored. High doses of dopamine ($>15\mu g/kg/min$) are vasoconstrictive and may decrease renal blood flow.[12]

DIC with resulting bleeding is the predominant clinical problem in some hemolytic transfusion reactions. Heparin treatment of DIC is controversial because heparin itself can cause bleeding and may be hazardous in patients who have recently undergone surgery. The severity of the reaction and the patient's clinical status must influence the decision whether or not to heparinize. Heparin is probably indicated only when the reaction is due to an ABO mismatch and the patient has received more than 200 ml of blood. For adults, a loading dose of 4000 units of heparin given intravenously followed by continuous IV infusion of 1500 units/hour for 6 to 24 hours, has been recommended.[9]

Prevention

Total prevention of hemolytic transfusion reactions is impossible because hemolysis may occur even when the crossmatch is compatible.[8,11,13,14] Errors in identifying samples, donor units or recipients are the most common causes of severe, acute hemolytic transfusion reactions.[15,16] Human error of this sort is difficult to prevent, but opportunities for error can be minimized through careful delineation, in a readily available procedures manual, of every step in transfusion procedure; and careful adherence to detail by every member of the transfusion service and clinical team, from phlebotomist to medical technologist to transfusionist.

Starting a transfusion is a critical step because the transfusionist has the last opportunity to prevent misidentification and the first opportunity to detect a transfusion reaction. Transfusion errors are especially likely if administering transfusions is one of the many demands and responsibilities undertaken by large numbers of nursing personnel, house staff, medical students and other health care personnel. Having a hospital infusion team start all transfusions provides significant safety advantages. In this system, transfusions are given by relatively few people, all of whom are well-trained, well-motivated, and have relatively few unrelated responsibilities to distract them.

Other Immediate Adverse Effects

Febrile Nonhemolytic Reactions

A febrile nonhemolytic (FNH) reaction is a temperature rise of 1 C or more occurring in association with transfusion and without any other explanation. FNH reactions are thought to be caused by cytotoxic or agglutinating antibodies in recipient plasma reacting against antigens present on the cell membranes of transfused lymphocytes, granulocytes, or platelets.[17] The cause of many FNH reactions remains obscure, and it is seldom rewarding to pursue a search for leukocyte antibodies. Transfusion of leukocyte-poor products may minimize the occurrence of fevers.[18] (See Chapter 15.) The temperature rise may be mild to severe and may begin any time, from early in the transfusion to the time when most of the unit has been transfused or even an hour or two after the transfusion has finished. The fever usually responds to antipyretics. FNH reactions tend to occur in recipients who have been repeatedly transfused or who have had multiple pregnancies.

Fever may be the initial manifestation of several types of transfusion reaction, some of which are potentially fatal. Although true FNH reactions are seldom dangerous, it is important to establish as soon as possible the cause of a fever occurring during transfusion. For example, fever may be the first sign of an acute hemolytic transfusion reaction, or of a patient's response to infusion of a unit of bacterially contaminated blood. FNH reactions are often more uncomfortable and frightening than they are life-threatening; the fever (38-39 C) and chill symptoms are usually self-limiting. Subcutaneous or intravenous meperidine promptly controls severe shaking chills that occasionally accompany FNH reactions.

True rigors, which may be a sign of bacteremia, are clinically much more severe and are often associated with cardiovascular collapse as well as high fevers over 40 C. The diagnosis of a febrile nonhemolytic reaction is a diagnosis of exclusion; other causes of fever must be ruled out first. These usually benign FNH reactions are very common and usually can be prevented or ameliorated by giving antipyretics or leukocyte-poor blood components. Observation has shown that only one patient in eight who experiences a single FNH reaction will have a similar reaction to the next blood transfusion.[11,19] Thus, it seems reasonable to recommend use of leukocyte-poor preparations only after a patient has had two or more FNH reactions.[19,20] Antipyretics such as aspirin or acetaminophen can be given before the transfusion to patients with a history of previous FNH reactions. Aspirin, however, alters platelet function by inhibiting the release reaction and should not be given to thrombocytopenic patients or those with qualitative platelet disorders (thrombocytopathy).

Bacterial Contamination

Bacteria may enter the blood or component containers or contaminate the port of the bag during phlebotomy or component preparation.[21] Bacteria are more likely to multiply in products stored at room temperature but multiplication can occur in refrigerated components. With sterile disposable equipment, bacterial contamination of blood and components is very rare, especially when there is strict adherence to appropriate protocols during donor phlebotomy and scrupulous attention to maintenance of a closed system during component preparation and storage.

Bacteria present in blood, platelet concentrates or other components can cause a devastating septic transfusion reaction. Such reactions are usually due to endotoxin produced by psychrophilic (cold-growing), gram-negative bacteria, most commonly *Pseudomonas* species, *Citrobacter freundii*, and *Escherichia coli*.[22-24] The reaction is characterized by high fever, shock, hemoglobinuria, DIC and renal failure. Clinically, this type of shock is the "warm" type with flushing and dryness of skin. Abdominal cramps, diarrhea, vomiting, and generalized muscle pain also may occur.

If bacterial contamination is suspected, the transfusion should be halted immediately and the unit examined for signs of bacterial growth. A purple color, clots in the bag or hemolysis suggest contamination, but the appearance of the blood bag is often unremarkable. A gram stain of the product revealing bacteria is confirmatory, but absence of visible organisms does not rule it out. The patient's blood, the suspect component and all IV solutions used should be cultured for aerobic and anaerobic organisms at refrigerator, room and body temperatures.[25]

Bacterial contamination is very rare but such reactions are often fatal. Treatment includes immediate intravenous administration of steroids and antibiotics combined with therapy for shock with vasopressor drugs such as dopamine. Prevention depends upon careful preparation of the phlebotomy site when blood is drawn, maintenance of sterility during component preparation, attention to prescribed storage conditions and inspection of blood and components prior to issue.

Anaphylactic Reactions

Features that distinguish anaphylactic reactions from other immediate reactions are: 1) occurrence after infusion of only a few milliliters of blood or plasma and 2) absence of fever. Onset is characterized by some of all of the following symptoms: coughing, bronchospasm, respiratory distress, vascular instability, nausea, abdominal cramps, vomiting, diarrhea, shock and loss of consciousness.

Some of these reactions occur in IgA-deficient patients who have developed anti-IgA antibodies after immunization through previous transfusion or pregnancy,[19,26] although sometimes the immunizing event cannot be identified. Although IgA deficiency occurs in about 1 person per 700, anaphylactic reactions due to anti-IgA are very rare.[11] IgA-deficient individuals may have antibodies against the alpha heavy chain, called class-specific antibodies, or type-specific antibodies directed against light chain specificity (ie, kappa or lamda). Individuals with normal IgA levels can have type-specific antibodies but not class-specific. Some workers believe that IgA-deficient blood components should only be given if prior anaphylactic reactions have occurred. Indeed, unless there has been large-scale population screening or there is a family history of IgA deficiency, individuals with anti-IgA antibodies will be detected only if they have an anaphylactic transfusion reaction and the investigation reveals the presence of antibody.

Treatment and Prevention

Immediate treatment of any anaphylactic transfusion reaction is to: 1) stop the transfusion; 2) keep the I.V. open with normal saline to allow administering pressor agents; and 3) immediately give epinephrine, 0.4 ml of a 1:1000 solution subcutaneously. Steroid therapy, such as 100 mg of hydrocortisone given intravenously, may also be useful. Under no circumstances should the transfusion be restarted. Treatment is initiated on the basis of clinical impression of anaphylaxis; diagnosis is made retrospectively. Demonstration of antibody to IgA remains primarily a research procedure, not readily available in most laboratories, but suggestive evidence can be obtained by documenting absence of serum IgA by immunodiffusion or immunoelectrophoresis.

Sensitized IgA-deficient patients must be transfused with blood components that lack IgA.[26] Files of such donors are maintained by the AABB Rare Donor File, the Irwin Memorial Blood Bank in San Francisco, the American National Red Cross in Washington, DC, and the Canadian Red Cross in Toronto, Ontario. Deglycerolized red cells and/or washed units of liquid stored red blood cells may be used if the only therapeutic need is for red cells.[27]

For components that contain plasma, IgA-deficient donors will be needed.

It may be possible to collect and store frozen autologous components for patients known to experience anaphylactic reactions. There are, of course, other causes of anaphylactic reactions. These have been

attributed to antibodies to soluble plasma antigens or to drugs contained in transfused blood components such as penicillin.[28] Immediate treatment is the same as for reactions due to anti-IgA, and prevention requires identifying the antibody and avoiding exposure to the antigen.

Urticaria

Urticarial allergic reactions are characterized by local erythema, hives and itching, usually without fever or other adverse effects. If localized urticaria is the only manifestation, it is usually not necessary to discontinue transfusion. Indeed, the risk of hepatitis from a replacement unit of blood poses a greater threat to the patient than does continuation of the original unit once the urticaria has resolved following use of an antihistamine. The infusion can be interrupted while 25-50 mg of antihistamine such as diphenhydramine is administered orally or parenterally. After relief of symptoms, the transfusion is continued slowly. Recipients who have frequent urticarial reactions may be pretreated with an antihistamine.

Because mild urticaria is rarely a prodome to hemolytic or anaphylactic reaction, and reactions limited to mild urticaria carry no risk to the patient, isolated urticarial reactions do not require extensive serological investigation.

The etiology of these limited cutaneous reactions is unknown; allergy to a soluble product in donor plasma is suspected. Transfusion of washed or deglycerolized frozen red cells prevents urticarial reactions but is rarely necessary unless the patient has repeated and/or severe reactions. Urticarial reactions that accompany cardiovascular instability should be treated as described above under anaphylactic reactions and not as a simple skin hypersensitivity reaction. If a patient develops extensive urticaria or a confluent total body rash during transfusion, it is probably best to discontinue the transfusion completely and not restart the unit after symptoms have responded to antihistamine administration.

Circulatory Overload

Hypervolemia due to excessive volume or speed of infusion must be considered if congestive heart failure, dyspnea, severe headache or peripheral edema occur during or soon after transfusion. Rapid increases in blood volume are poorly tolerated by patients with compromised cardiac or pulmonary status and/or those with chronic anemia and an expanded plasma volume. Transfusion of even a limited amount of blood may cause problems in infants who have small blood volumes. Infusion of 25% albumin, which attracts large volumes of interstitial fluid into the vascular space, may also cause circulatory overload.

Symptoms of circulatory overload include coughing, cyanosis and difficulty in breathing. A rapid increase in systolic blood pressure of 50 mm Hg or more supports the diagnosis. Symptoms usually improve when the infusion is stopped and the patient is placed in a sitting position and given diuretics and oxygen. If symptoms are not relieved, phlebotomy may be necessary.

Prevention

Patients susceptible to circulatory overload should receive red blood cells, not whole blood, in small volumes, slowly infused. It is often desirable to divide a donor unit into aliquots, so that part of the unit can be stored at 1 to 6 C while the remainder is slowly administered. Subsequent aliquots can be issued as needed during a 24-hour period so that the rate of infusion does not exceed 1 ml/kg of body weight/hour.[29] Giving diuretics before the transfusion may be helpful. For some patients with hematocrits in the 15-20% range, phlebotomy followed by transfusion may be useful in increasing oxygen-carrying capacity without expanding blood volume. The blood removed may be discarded and replaced with allogeneic red blood cells with a higher hematocrit, or the blood removed can be centrifuged and the autologous cells reinfused after removal of supernatant plasma. Caution must be exercised before phlebotomy, however, to ensure that the patient's cardiovascular system can tolerate an acute volume loss of up to 450 ml of blood.

The blood bank director and members of the medical staff must agree on protocols for these situations, and the blood bank procedures manual should have detailed instructions for the approved procedures. Among the concerns to be addressed are: the ratio of blood to anticoagulant if the cells are to be reinfused, proper labeling of the blood bag, sterile phlebotomy technique, and proper patient identification.

Noncardiogenic Pulmonary Reactions

Rare transfusion recipients experience clinically apparent pulmonary edema without concurrent changes in cardiac pressures.[30,31] The chest x-ray is typical of pulmonary edema and there is acute respiratory insufficiency but no evidence of heart failure. Symptoms of respiratory distress occur after infusion of volumes too small to produce hypervolemia and may be accompanied by chills, fever, cyanosis and hypotension. At least two mechanisms have been postulated. One is a reaction between donor leukoagglutinins and recipient leukocytes to produce white cell aggregates that are trapped in the pulmonary microcirculation, where they produce pronounced changes in vascular permeability.[32,33] During transfusion of granulocyte concentrates, the reverse is also possible, ie, leukoagglutinins in the recipient aggregate the transfused granulocytes.[34] An alternative pathogenic mechanism may be activation of complement to generate the anaphylatoxins C3a and C5a, which affect histamine and serotonin in tissue basophils and platelets, and also directly aggregate granulocytes to produce leukoemboli that lodge in the microvasculature of the lungs.[35,36]

As with all acute transfusion reactions the transfusion should be stopped immediately. Treatment includes intravenous steroids and respiratory support as required. If subsequent transfusions are needed, washed red cells may prevent such reactions. Donors whose blood has been found to contain leukoagglutinins should have any future donations restricted to use as washed or frozen red blood cells.

Delayed Adverse Effects

Hemolytic Transfusion Reactions

There are two different types of delayed hemolytic transfusion reactions. The first is mild, occurs several weeks after transfusion, and is the result of primary alloimmunization. The overall risk of immunizing a recipient to a red cell antigen other than the D antigen has been estimated as 1 to 1.6% for each unit of blood transfused.[37] Antibody production, when it occurs, begins no earlier than 7-10 days after receipt of the stimulating transfusion and usually several weeks or months later. As the antibody increases in titer and avidity, it can react with transfused cells that are still circulating. The degree of shortened red cell survival depends on the quantity of antibody produced and the quantity of transfused cells remaining. Primary immunization rarely causes hemolysis of transfused red cells, and such delayed immune interactions are usually unsuspected clinically. Diagnosis might be suggested by an unexplained fall in hemoglobin coupled with a positive direct antiglobulin test and/or the appearance in the serum of red blood cell alloantibody.

Anamnestic Responses

The second type of delayed hemolytic transfusion reaction occurs in a previously immunized recipient who experiences an anamnestic, or secondary, response to transfused red cell antigens. Some alloantibodies formed after primary immunization may diminish to levels undetectable in serum. Antibodies in the Kidd system (anti-Jk^a and anti-Jk^b) typically behave in this manner. Pretransfusion testing reveals no unexpected antibody and no serologic incompatibility. After transfusion, however, generally within 3 to 7 days, an anamnestic response leads to rapidly increasing levels of IgG antibodies that react with the transfused cells. The combination of high antibody levels and large numbers of transfused cells in the circulation may produce readily apparent manifestations. The most common presenting signs are fever, an unexplained fall in the patient's hemoglobin and mild jaundice, but associated clinical problems are infrequent. Acute renal failure is a rare complication.[38] Treatment is rarely necessary, but the patient's urine output and renal function should be followed.

It is often the blood bank that diagnoses delayed hemolytic reaction, through serologic findings in patients with no clinical symptoms. If more transfusions are ordered, the new blood specimen may prove to have a positive direct antiglobulin test. In addition, positive antibody detection tests and crossmatch incompatibilities might be noted. AABB *Standards* requires that the specimen used for compatibility testing be no more than 2 days old at the time of transfusion if the patient has been transfused or pregnant within the past 3 months. This is to detect rapidly developing antibodies that, if missed, might cause acute hemolytic transfusion reaction upon subsequent transfusion. If a direct antiglobulin test is performed at this time, or is part of a routinely performed autologous control, the presence of antibody-coated transfused cells may be detected even though there is not yet detectable antibody in the serum.

Elution and identification of the antibody is critical when the direct antiglobulin test becomes positive in a patient who has been transfused within the previous 2-3 weeks.[39] In cases where the direct antiglobulin test is positive but results on testing the patient's serum are negative or equivocal, crossmatching with the red blood cell eluate may be useful.

Viral Hepatitis
Incidence

Transfusion-associated hepatitis remains the most frequent serious infectious complication of blood transfusion. Transmission of hepatitis A virus by transfusion is extremely rare, because with this virus there is apparently only a short period of viremia and no carrier state. Hepatitis B transmission has been significantly reduced by mandatory testing for hepatitis B surface antigen (HBsAg) in donor blood and by eliminating the use of paid blood donors. If, however, transfusion recipients are carefully followed with tests for the liver-associated enzyme alanine aminotransferase (ALT, previously called SGPT), some degree of liver damage is found to occur in approximately 7 to 10% of transfused patients.[40,41] For at least 90% of these cases, no known viruses can be identified as the etiologic agent, and these cases have been termed non-A, non-B (NANB) hepatitis.[42] Although initial illness is mild, with about 75% of infections being anicteric, the long-term effects of NANB hepatitis may be more serious. About half of the patients have abnormal liver function tests for 6-12 months after transfusion. This is thought to indicate chronic active hepatitis which in some cases may progress to cirrhosis.[43,44]

Hepatitis Risk of Blood and Components

All blood components and products carry a risk of transmitting hepatitis except those for which the manufacturing process eliminates infectivity. Albumin and plasma protein fraction (PPF) are exposed to high temperatures that kill the virus. Immune globulin preparations, although not heat-treated, carry no risk of hepatitis transmission when manufactured by the Cohn cold ethanol fractionation procedure.

The degree of risk for non-heat-treated products depends on the number of donors for each product. Products prepared from pools of donor plasma, such as coagulation factor concentrates, have the highest risk.

Prevention

Because there is no reliable test to detect NANB hepatitis, prevention depends upon careful screening of donors and careful follow-up of recipients to detect transfusion-associated hepatitis and discover potentially dangerous donors. Screening all donors for elevated ALT has been suggested, but this test is so nonspecific that many safe donors would be excluded. In addition many cases of NANB hepatitis are associated with blood from donors whose serum ALT levels are within normal limits. Compared with blood from paid donors, blood from volunteer donors has repeatedly been shown to have a lower risk of transmitting both hepatitis B and NANB.[45,46]

Physicians and other hospital staff must be made aware of the necessity of reporting all cases of hepatitis in patients who have received blood transfusion. The hospital epidemiologist or other responsible person should routinely investigate all known hepatitis patients for a history of blood transfusion in the preceding 6 months. The blood bank should be given the names of all hepatitis patients so that their records can be checked for recent transfusion. For further discussion of hepatitis, incuding the hepatitis B vaccine, see Chapter 18.

Other Transfusion-Associated Diseases
Cytomegalovirus

Cytomegalovirus (CMV) infection has been implicated in the "postperfusion syndrome," a self-limiting condition developing after cardiopulmonary bypass surgery.[47] Immunosuppressed patients are at high risk for more severe forms of transfusion-induced CMV infections. For example, patients who have undergone bone marrow transplantation may develop fatal CMV interstitial pneumonitis.[48] CMV is known to be transmissible by viable leukocytes in peripheral blood. The carrier rate for this virus is reported to be 6 to 12% in the general population.[49,50] At present, there is no test to detect infectivity.

Significant morbidity and mortality attributable to CMV infection may occur in low birth weight premature infants born of CMV seronegative mothers. In one study a group of these infants transfused with 50 ml or more of CMV seropositive blood developed CMV infections, whereas no mortality or morbidity occurred in a comparable group who received only blood with titers of CMV antibody below 8, by indirect hemagglutination assay.[51] This suggests that blood from some CMV seropositive donors is infectious and that such blood may be dangerous if given to low birth weight neonates born of CMV seronegative mothers. Infants born of CMV seropositive mothers do not show the same rate of seroconversion as do infants born of seronegative mothers.

Another group examined the feasibility of screening blood donors to find CMV seronegative units for neonatal transfusion.[52] Of 561 consecutive O negative blood donors tested, 23.9% were seronegative. CMV seronegative blood was most likely to be found in males under 20 years of age; it was not useful to screen donors over the age of 30. The small percentage of males under 20 years of age who donate blood, coupled with the need to retest donors at each donation to identify those donors who have undergone seroconversion, makes this a formidable task.

Further studies are needed to confirm whether transfusing CMV seropositive units to low birth weight infants poses a substantial hazard,[53] and whether different levels of risk exist in different geographic areas. Use of deglycerolized red blood cells may be an effective alternative to screening.[54] Recent work involving prevention of cytomegalovirus infection by cytomegalovirus immune globulin as well as by a cytomegalovirus vaccine has shown promising results.[55,56] Additional studies are needed, however, before conclusions can be drawn.

Malaria

There are no practical laboratory screening tests for malaria. Although still quite rare, the number of cases of transfusion-associated malaria has increased to the highest level in the past 25 years, according to recent reports.[57,58] Travel and immigration are among the factors responsible for this increase. Exclusion of donors at high risk of harboring parasites is the only effective preventive measure. This requires careful questioning of donors for a history of immigration from or travel in areas where malaria is endemic.

Syphilis

Transmission of syphilis by transfusion is possible, but requires that blood be drawn during the rather brief period of spirochetemia, and that the organisms remain viable at the time of transfusion. The treponemal spirochete cannot survive more than 72 hours at 4 C so only components stored at room temperature (platelet concentrate) or transfused very promptly after donation have any risk of transmitting syphilis.[59] Performing an STS on donor blood does not prevent transmission of syphilis because this test does not become positive until well after the brief period of potential infectivity. The test is characteristically negative in infectious individuals and most positive STS results occur in donors whose reactions are unrelated to syphilitic infection, so-called biological false-positive reactions. AABB *Standards* has dropped the requirement for serologic tests for syphilis (STS) on donor blood. However, the STS is still required by Federal regulations and by some states.

Acquired Immune Deficiency Syndrome

In late 1979 the Centers for Disease Control became aware of the increased incidence of an atypical form of Kaposi's sarcoma and of *Pneumocystis carinii* pneumonia and other opportunistic infections in gay males.[60] Later investigations disclosed the occurrence of lymphopenia and a change in the ratio of helper (OKT4 or Leu 3a positive) to suppressor (OKT8 or Leu 2a positive) T lymphocytes in these individuals.[61] This combination of Kaposi's sarcoma and/or opportunistic infections with alterations in T helper and T suppressor lymphocytes without known cause has been called Acquired Immune Deficiency Syndrome (AIDS). Over 7000 cases have been reported, of which almost 50% have been fatal. Except for cases occuring in persons of Haitian origin (4%), most have been associated with intimate personal contact among gay males (72%) or illicit intravenous drug use (17%).[62] Over the past several years these percentages have not changed.

AIDS has occurred in hemophiliacs (1% of AIDS cases) who have been treated with large quantities of commercial Factor VIII concentrates.[62,63] AIDS developed in a neonate who received blood components from 19 donors, one of whom later developed AIDS. The transmission of AIDS by blood transfusion is now known to occur, with about 1% of AIDS cases associated with blood transfusion.[62,65,66]

AIDS occurs most frequently in promiscuous gay males, but both heterosexual and homosexual transmission are known to occur. The incubation period appears to be 6 to 24 months; in cases of suspected transfusion-associated AIDS, transfusion within the preceding 5 years should be considered relevant.[62] Hemophiliacs who have received Factor VIII concentrates have a higher incidence of AIDS and of altered T cell ratios than those who have received only cryoprecipitate[67] but cryoprecipitate can also be involved in AIDS transmission. Current work with heat-treated Factor VIII concentrates and with screening cryoprecipitate and plasma donors for antigens of or antibodies to the implicated virus should make future treatment options more definitive.

The suspected AIDS agent has been identified as a Type III retrovirus called HTLV-III, for Human T-cell Lymphotropic Virus. It is an RNA virus with a Mg^{++} dependent reverse transcriptase. The RNA is retrocopied into DNA and the latter is then inserted into the host's genome.[68-70] A test for the HTLV-III antibody has recently become available. Many persons in high risk categories for developing or transmitting AIDS have antibodies to HTLV-III. The role of antibody testing in selecting blood donors is under intense investigation.

The AABB, ARC, CCBC and the FDA have made recommendations, which can be summarized as follows, to reduce the potential spread of AIDS through blood transfusion: 1) transfusions of blood, components or products should be given only for clear medical indications; 2) blood donors should be carefully screened (see Chapter 1) and individuals in high risk groups should be educated to abstain from donation; 3) autologous transfusion should be employed as widely as possible; and 4) cryoprecipitate should be used to treat newly diagnosed or mild hemophiliacs, pending availability of components or products with less risk of disease transmission.

Graft-Versus-Host Disease

Graft-versus-host disease (GVH) occurs relatively commonly in patients receiving bone marrow transplants, and very rarely following transfusion to patients who are severely immunosuppressed, such as those being intensively treated with chemotherapy and irradiation.[71] Patients at risk include those with lymphopenia (absolute count less than 500/μl lymphocytes), and bone marrow suppression.[72,73] GVH has occurred in infants who received intrauterine transfusions followed by exchange transfusion for hemolytic disease of the newborn.[74]

GVH occurs if immunocompetent donor lymphocytes engraft and multiply in a severly immunodeficient recipient. These engrafted donor cells react against the "foreign" tissues of the host-recipient. The clinical syndrome of GVH may include fever, skin rash, hepatitis, diarrhea, bone marrow suppression and infection, usually progressing to a fatal outcome.[75] Pretransfusion irradiation of all blood components containing lymphocytes will prevent GVH.[76] A radiation dose of 1500 to 5000 rad renders 85-95% of the lymphocytes in a unit of blood, granulocyte or platelet concentrate incapable of replication. The function of red blood cells, granulocytes and platelets is not affected by such irradiation.[77]

Posttransfusion Purpura

Posttransfusion thrombocytopenic purpura is a rare event, occurring almost exclusively in women. A precipitous fall in platelet count produces generalized purpura about a week after a blood transfusion. Some patients have been shown to have developed a platelet-specific alloantibody, anti-Pl^{A1} (in Europe: anti-Zw$_a$).[78] This antigen has a prevalence of 98.3% in the population, so only 1.7% of recipients are at risk of developing the alloantibody. The antibody destroys not only the transfused Pl^{A1}-positive platelets but also the patient's own Pl^{A1}-negative platelets. It is thought that initial reaction of alloantibody with transfused Pl^{A1}-positive platelets causes formation of antigen-antibody complexes that attach nonspecifically to the patient's own platelets, which are subsequently destroyed. The thrombocytopenia is usually severe,[79] and if treatment is needed exchange plasmapheresis has been suggested as possible therapy.[80] The thrombocytopenia is usually self-limiting and platelet transfusions are usually not beneficial.

Transfusion Hemosiderosis

Every unit of red cells contains approximately 250 mg of iron. For chronically transfused patients, such as thalassemics with persistent hemolysis, progressive and continual accumulation of iron can be dangerous. When patients have received more than 100 transfusions, iron deposition may interfere with function of the heart, liver or endocrine glands. Treatment is directed at removing iron without unduly reducing the patient's circulating hemoglobin.[81] Metered subcutaneous infusion of desferrioxamine, an iron-chelating agent, has shown promise for reducing body iron stores in such patients.[82] Use of neocytes is being investigated as well. These young red blood cells should remain longer in the circulation and thereby decrease the number of transfusions needed.

Records of Transfusion Complications

Records must be kept of all reports of transfusion complications. Cases of transfusion-associated hepatitis (including but not confined to those confirmed as type B) must be reported to the center that drew the blood. Fatalities resulting directly from transfusion complications, eg, hemolytic reactions, must be reported to the FDA, Office of Biologics Research and Review. Suspected cases of transfusion-associated AIDS should be reported to the Centers for Disease Control, for epidemiologic investigation.

References

1. McCarthy LR, Senne JE. Evaluation of acridine orange stain for detection of microorganisms in blood cultures. J Clin Microbiology 1980;11:281-285.

2. Blondheim SH, Margoliash E, Shafrir E. A simple test for myohemoglobinuria (myoglobinuria). JAMA 1958;167:453-454.

3. Brodine CE, Vertrees KM. Differentiation of myoglobinuria from hemoglobinuria. In:

Sunderman FW and Sunderman FW Jr, eds. Hemoglobin—its precursors and metabolites. Philadelphia: JB Lippincott; 1964: 90-93.

4. Fink DJ, Petz LD, Black MD. Serum haptoglobin: a valuable diagnostic aid in suspected hemolytic transfusion reactions. JAMA 1967;199:615-618.

5. Langley JW, McMahan M, Smith N. A nine-month transfusion service experience with low-ionic strength saline solution (LISS). Am J Clin Pathol 1980;73:99-103.

6. Lalezari P. Serologic profile in autoimmune hemolytic disease: pathophysiologic and clinical interpretations. Sem Hematol 1976;13:291-310.

7. Lalezari P, Jiang AF. The manual polybrene test—a simple and rapid procedure for detection of red cell antibodies. Transfusion 1980;20:206-211.

8. Pineda AA, Brzica Jr SM, Taswell HF. Hemolytic transfusion reaction: recent experience in a large blood bank. Mayo Clin Proc 1978;53:378-390.

9. Goldfinger D. Acute hemolytic transfusion reactions—a fresh look at pathogenesis and considerations regarding therapy. Transfusion 1977;17:85-98.

10. Bick RL. The clinical significance of fibrinogen degradation products. Sem Thrombosis Hemostasis 1984;8:302-330.

11. Mollison PL. Blood transfusion in clinical medicine. 7th ed. London: Blackwell Scientific Publications; 1983.

12. Goldberg LI. Cardiovascular and renal actions of dopamine: potential clinical application. Pharm Reviews 1972;24:1-29.

13. Stewart JW, Mollison PL. Rapid destruction of apparently compatible cells. Br Med J 1959;1:1274-1275.

14. Fudenberg HH, Allen FH. Transfusion reactions in the absence of demonstrable incompatibility. N Engl J Med 1957;256:1180-1184.

15. Myhre BA. Fatalities from blood transfusion. JAMA 1980;244:1333-1335.

16. Honig CL, Bove JR. Transfusion-associated fatalities: a review of Bureau of Biologics reports 1976-1978. Transfusion 1980; 20:653-661.

17. Brittingham TE, Chaplin H. Febrile transfusion reactions caused by sensitivity to donor leukocytes and platelets. JAMA 1957;165:819-825.

18. Thulstrup H. The influence of leukocyte and thrombocyte incompatibility on non-haemolytic transfusion reactions: a retrospective study. Vox Sang 1971;21:233-250.

19. Kevy SV, Schmidt PJ, McGinniss MH, Workman WG, Febrile, non-hemolytic transfusion reactions and the limited role of leukoagglutinin in their etiology. Transfusion 1962;2:7-16.

20. Menitove JE, McElligott MC, Aster RH. Febrile transfusion reaction: what blood component should be given next? Vox Sang 1982;42:318-321.

21. Braude AI. Transfusion reactions from contaminated blood: their recognition and treatment. N Engl J Med 1958;258:1289-1293.

22. Tabor E, Gerety RJ. Five cases of pseudomonas sepsis transmitted by blood transfusions. Lancet 1984;1:1403.

23. Blajchman MA, Thornley JH, Richardson H, Elder D, Spiak C, Racher J. Platelet transfusion-induced Serratia marcescens sepsis due to vacuum tube contamination. Transfusion 1979;19:39-44.

24. Buchholz DH, Young VM, Friedman NR, Reilly JA, Mardiney MR Jr. Detection and quantitation of bacteria in platelet products stored at ambient temperature. Transfusion 1973;13:268-275.

25. Elin RJ, Lundberg WB, Schmidt PJ. Evaluation of bacterial contamination of blood processing. Transfusion 1975;15:260-265.

26. Vyas GN, Holmdahl L, Perkins HA, Fudenberg HH. Serologic specificity of human anti-IgA and its significance in transfusion. Blood 1969;34:573-581.

27. Yap PL, Pryde EAD, McClelland DBL. IgA content of frozen-thawed-washed red blood cells and blood products measured by radioimmunoassay. Transfusion 1982;22:36-38.

28. Wells JV, King MA. Adverse reactions to human plasma proteins. Anaesth Inten Care 1980;8:139-144.

29. Marriott HL, Kekwick A. Volume and rate in blood transfusion for relief of anemia. Br Med J 1940;1:1043-1046.

30. Ward HN. Pulmonary infiltrates associated with leukoagglutinin transfusion reactions. Ann Int Med 1970;73:689-694.

31. Dubois M, Lotze MT, Diamond WJ, Kim YD, Flye MW, Macnamara TE. Pulmonary shunting during leukoagglutinin-induced noncardiac pulmonary edema. JAMA 1980;244:2186-2189.

32. Thompson JS, Severson CD, Parmely MJ, Marmorstein BL, Simmons A. Pulmonary "hypersensitivity" reactions induced by transfusion of non-HLA leukoagglutinins. N Engl J Med 1971;284:1120-1125.

33. Kernoff PBA, Durrant IJ, Rizza CR, Wright FW. Severe allergic pulmonary edema after plasma transfusion. Br J Haematol 1972;23:777-781.

34. Higby DJ, Burnett D. Granulocyte transfusions: current status. Blood 1980;55:2-8.

35. Jacob HS, Craddock PR, Hammerschmidt DE, Moldow CF. Complement-induced granulocyte aggregation. N Engl J Med 1980;302:789-794.

36. Hammerschmidt DE, Weaver J, Hudson LD, Craddock PR, Jacob HS. Association of complement activation and elevated plasma-C5a with adult respiratory distress syndrome. Lancet 1980;1:947-949.

37. Lostumbo MM, Holland PV, Schmidt PJ. Isoimmunization after multiple transfusions. N Engl J Med 1966;275:141-144.

38. Holland PV, Wallerstein RO. Delayed hemolytic transfusion reaction with acute renal failure. JAMA 1968;204:1007-1008.

39. Judd WJ, Butch SH, Oberman HA, Steiner EA, Bauer RC. The evaluation of a postive direct antiglobulin test in pretransfusion testing. Transfusion 1980;20;17-23.

40. Aach RD, Kahn RA. Posttransfusion hepatitis: current perspectives. Ann Intern Med 1980;92:539-546.

41. Alter HJ, Purcell RH, Feinstone SM, Holland PV, Morrow AG. Non-A/Non-B hepatitis: a review of interim report of an ongoing prospective study. In: Vyas GN, Cohen SN, Schmid R, eds. Viral hepatitis. Philadelphia: The Franklin Institute Press; 1978:359-369.

42. Seeff LB, Wright EC, Zimmerman HJ, McCollum RW, and Members of VA Hepatitis Cooperative Studies Group. VA cooperative study of post-transfusion hepatitis, 1969-1974: incidence and characteristics of hepatitis and responsible risk factors. Am J Med Sci 1975;270:355-362.

43. Aach RD, Lander JJ, Sherman LA, et al. Transfusion transmitted viruses: interim analysis of hepatitis among transfused and nontransfused patients. In: Vyas GN, Cohen SN, Schmid R, eds. Viral hepatitis. Philadelphia: The Franklin Institute Press; 1978;383-396.

44. Knodell RG, Conrad ME, Ishak KG. Development of chronic liver disease after acute non-A, non-B posttransfusion hepatitis: role of γ-globulin prophylaxis in its prevention. Gastroenterology 1977;72:902-909.

45. Gerety RJ. Based on your analysis of the benefits and costs of routine donor screening for ALT-GPT to reduce the incidence of post-transfusion non-A, non-B hepatitis in your blood services region, what action would you recommend on this matter? Vox Sang 1983;44:52-54.

46. Aach RD, Szmuness W, Mosely JW, et al. Serum alanine aminotransferase of donors in relation to the risk of non-A, non-B hepatitis in recipients. N Engl J Med 1981;304:989-994.

47. Foster KM, Jack I. A prospective study of the role of cytomegalovirus in posttransfusion mononucleosis. N Engl J Med 1969;280:1311-1316.

48. Weller TH. The cytomegaloviruses: Ubiquitous agents with protean clinical manifestations. N Engl J Med 1971;285:203-214.

49. Perham TGM, Caul EO, Conway PJ, Mott MG. Cytomegalovirus infection in blood donors— a prospective study. Br J Haematol 1971;20:307-320.

50. Drew WL. The far-reaching effects of cytomegalovirus infection. Diagnostic Medicine 1983;6:61-66.

51. Yeager AS, Grumet FC, Hafleigh EB, Arvin AM, Bradley JS, Prober CG. Prevention of transfusion-acquired cytomegalovirus infection in newborn infants. J Pediat 1981;98:281-287.

52. Silvergleid AJ, Kott TS. Impact of cytomegalovirus testing on blood collection facilities. Vox Sang 1983;44:102-105.

53. Sandler G. Posttransfusion cytomegalovirus infection—updated. Amer Red Cross Blood Services Letter #82-26 March 26, 1982.

54. Lang DJ, Ebert PA, Rodgers BM, Boggess HP, Rixse RS. Reduction of postperfusion cytomegalovirus infection following the use of leukocyte depleted blood. Transfusion 1977;17:391-395.

55. Meyers JD, Leszczynski J, Zaia JA, Flournoy N, Newton B, Snydman DR. Prevention of cytomegalovirus infection by cytomegalovirus immune globulin after marrow transplantation. Ann Inter Med 1983;98:442-446.

56. Balfour HH. Cytomegalovirus disease: Can it be prevented? Ann Inter Med 1983;32:544-546.

57. Johnson B, Brown JH, Yoedino R, et al. Transfusion malaria: serologic identification of infected donors. MMWR 1983;32:222-229.

58. Wyler DJ. Malaria-resurgence, resistance and research. N Engl J Med 1983;308:875-878.

59. Chambers RW, Foley HT, Schmidt PJ. Transmission of syphilis by fresh blood components. Transfusion 1969;9:32-34.

60. Friedman-Kien AE, Laubenstein LJ, Rubinstein P, et al. Disseminated Kaposi's sarcoma in homosexual men. Ann Int Med 1982;96:693-700.

61. Fauci AS, Macher AM, Longo DL, et al. Acquired immunodeficiency syndrome: epidemiologic, clinical, immunologic, and therapeutic considerations. Ann Intern Med 1984;100:92-106.

62. CDC Update: Acquired immunodeficiency syndrome (AIDS)—United States. MMWR l984;33:661-664.

63. Ehrenkranz NJ, Rubini J, Gunn R, et al. Pneumocystis carinii pneumonia among persons with hemophilia A. MMWR 1982;31:365-367.

64. Ammann A, Cowan M, Wara D, et al. Possible transfusion associated acquired immune deficiency syndrome (AIDS)—California. MMWR 1982;31:652-654.

65. Curran J, Lawrence DH, Jaffe H, et al. Acquired immunodeficiency syndrome (AIDS) associated with transfusion. N Engl J Med 1984;310:69-75.

66. Bove JR. Transfusion associated AIDS—A cause for concern. N Engl J Med 1984;310:115-116.

67. Menitove J, Aster RH, Casper JT, et al. T-lymphocyte subpopulations in patients with classic hemophilia treated with cryoprecipitate and lyophilized concentrates. N Engl J Med 1983;308:83-86.

68. Popovic M, Sarngadharan MG, Read E, Gallo RC. Detection, isolation, and continuous production of cytopathic retroviruses (HTLV-III) from patients with AIDS and pre-AIDS. Science 1984;224:497-500.

69. Schupbach J, Popovic M, Gilden RV, Gonda MA, Sarngadharan MG, Gallo RC. Serological analysis of a subgroup of human T-lymphotropic retroviruses (HTLV-III) associated with AIDS. Science 1984;224:503-505.

70. Sarngadharan MG, Popovic M, Bruch L, Schupbach J, Gallo RC. Antibodies reactive with human T-lymphotropic retroviruses (HTLV-III) in the serum of patients with AIDS. Science 1984;224:506-508.

71. Brubaker DB. Human posttransfusion graft-versus-host disease. Vox Sang 1983;45:401-420.

72. Woods WG, Lubin BH. Fatal graft-versus-host disease following a blood transfusion in a child with neuroblastoma. Pediat 1981;67:217-221.

73. Schmidmeier W, Feil W, Gebhart W, et al. Fatal graft-versus-host reaction following granulocyte transfusions. Blut 1982;45:115-119.

74. Parkman R, Mosier D, Umansky I, Cochran W, Carpenter CB, Rosen FS. Graft-versus-host disease after intrauterine and exchange transfusion for hemolytic disease of the newborn. N Engl J Med 1974;290:359-363.

75. Glucksberg H, Storb R, Fefer A, et al. Clinical manifestations of graft-versus-host disease in human recipients of marrow from HLA-matched sibling donors. Transplantation 1974;18:295-304.

76. Sandler G. Irradiated blood products. Amer Red Cross Blood Services Letter 82-55, July 1, l982.

77. Von Fliedner V, Higby DJ, Kim U. Graft-versus-host reaction following blood product transfusion. Am J Med 1982;72:951-961.

78. Shulman NR, Aster RH, Leitner A, Hiller MC. Immunoreactions involving platelets. V. Posttransfusion purpura due to a complement-fixing antibody against a genetically controlled platelet antigen. A proposed mechanism for thrombocytopenia and its relevance in "autoimmunity." J Clin Invest 1961;40:1597-1620.

79. Farboody GH, Clough JD, Hoffman GC. Posttransfusion purpura. Clev Clin Q 1978;45:241-246.

80. Abramson N, Eisenbert PD, Aster RH. Posttransfusion purpura: immunologic aspects and therapy. N Engl J Med 1974;291:1163-1166.

81. Jacobs A. Iron chelation therapy for iron loaded patients. Br J Haematol 1979;43:1-5.

82. Hoffbrand AV, Gorman A, Laulicht M, et al. Improvement in iron status and liver function with long-term subcutaneous desferrioxamine. Lancet 1979;1:947-949.

18

Hepatitis

Hepatitis is inflammation of the liver; many forms are caused by viruses. The form of disease acquired during epidemics is usually due to the hepatitis A virus. Sporadic cases may also occur. Sometimes called "infectious" hepatitis, hepatitis A is very rarely transmitted by blood components, but is spread by the fecal-oral route. Hepatitis acquired after parenteral exposure to infective blood or body fluids, or to needles or equipment contaminated with infective blood, is usually due to the hepatitis B virus or to an undefined agent which causes non-A, non-B (NANB) hepatitis. Hepatitis B is the condition formerly called "serum" hepatitis. Table 18-1 lists hepatitis-related terms and abbreviations in current use.

Hepatitis B and NANB can occur after transfusion of any blood components or products except immune globulin preparations, heat-treated albumin and plasma protein solutions. Unexplained acute liver dysfunction, with or without jaundice, developing 15 to 180 days after the transfusion of blood or blood components must be evaluated as a possible case of posttransfusion viral hepatitis.

Hepatitis Markers

Individuals can appear perfectly healthy yet be carriers of hepatitis viruses. For at least one cause of posttransfusion hepati-

tis, hepatitis B virus (Fig 18-1), laboratory tests are available to identify markers of infectivity (viral antigens) and evidence of prior exposure to the virus (viral antibodies). Since blood from individuals with proven circulating HBsAg can potentially transmit hepatitis B virus (HBV), these persons must not donate blood for any transfusion purpose. The recipient of HBsAg-positive blood has a substantially higher risk of developing hepatitis than recipients of blood without detectable HBsAg.[1] The presence of HBsAg in blood may indicate a chronic carrier state for HBV, or the incubation phase of acute hepatitis B or the presence of chronic hepatitis B. Testing donor blood for hepatitis B surface antigen (HBsAg) does not, however, disclose all bloods that may transmit hepatitis.

Figure 18-1 illustrates the usual sequence of laboratory findings in acute HBV infection. Individuals with circulating HBsAg usually have simultaneous circulation of antibody to hepatitis B core antigen (anti-HBc) and either of two additional HBV markers, the hepatitis Be antigen (HBeAg) or its antibody (anti-HBe). The presence of anti-HBc with no detectable HBsAg or anti-HBs may, in some individuals, indicate the presence of hepatitis B virus in the liver or the blood.[2-4] This phase of anti-HBc circulating after the disappearance of HBsAg and before the appear-

Table 18-1. Hepatitis Terms and Abbreviations

HBV Hepatitis B virus (formerly "serum" hepatitis virus and also called the Dane particle)

HBsAg Hepatitis B surface antigen (excess viral coat protein of the HBV detectable in blood of carriers of HBV) previously called the Australia and hepatitis-associated antigens (Au and HAA respectively)

Anti-HBs Antibody to HBsAg

HBcAg Hepatitis B core antigen (determinant of the capsid of the HBV, containing deoxyribonucleic acid) enveloped by HBsAg and hence not usually detectable in blood

Anti-HBc Antibody to HBcAg

HBeAg Hepatitis Be antigen

Anti-HBe Antibody to HBeAg

HAV Hepatitis A virus (formerly "infectious" hepatitis virus)

Anti-HAV Antibody to HAV

Non-A, Non-B (NANB) Hepatitis Viral hepatitis not due to either HBV, HAV, cytomegalovirus (CMV), or Epstein-Barr virus (EBV), ie, no serologic markers of these other viruses. It is probably due to more than one virus.

IG Immune globulin (purified human gamma globulin prepared by cold ethanol fractionation)

HBIG Hepatitis B immune globulin, a preparation with a high titer of anti-HBs, used for HBV prophylaxis

Hepatitis B vaccine Vaccine prepared from noninfectious hepatitis B surface antigen particles. Produces immunity in over 90% of vaccinees.

---

ance of anti-HBs is sometimes called the core antibody "window." The observation that occasional donors have these findings and that their blood can be infectious has been used to support the testing of donor blood for anti-HBc as well as for HBsAg. The simultaneous presence of HBeAg with HBsAg may indicate that a donor is especially infectious for HBV; the presence of anti-HBe in a donor with HBsAg indicates a relatively low level of infectivity, but cannot be considered evidence that the blood is noninfectious.[4]

Clinical Manifestations of Hepatitis

Most individuals who acquire viral hepatitis, whether type A, B or NANB, have a subclinical infection without significant symptoms or physical evidence of disease. Certainly in asymptomatic patients, but also in patients with clinically evident hepatitis, serologic studies are the only reliable way to discriminate among the different hepatitis viruses; clinically, pathologically and biochemically, the effects of these viruses are similar. In general, hepatitis A is less clinically severe than NANB, which tends, in turn, to be milder than hepatitis B. This generalization, based on epidemiological observations, cannot be applied to any individual case.

Infection with hepatitis virus occurs in three phases: an incubation period, an acute phase and a convalescent phase. The clinical course may additionally be complicated by such sequelae as fulminant hepatitis, relapsing or recrudescent illness, chronic hepatitis or hepatocellular carcinoma. A brief description of the typical clinical picture of infection with hepatitis B and NANB is given below. Hepatitis A, because it so rarely accompanies transfusion, is not described in any detail.

Incubation Period

The incubation period is defined as the interval between the time of exposure and either the onset of symptoms (clinical hepatitis) or the first appearance of laboratory abnormalities (subclinical hepatitis). The mean incubation period for NANB hepatitis is approximately 50 days, with a range of 15-180 days. For hepatitis B, the average incubation period is 90 days, with a range of 15-180 days. In hepatitis B, the length of the incubation period is inversely proportional to the amount of hepatitis B virus (HBV) to which the individual is exposed. The route of exposure also affects incubation period, with parenteral exposure causing a shorter incubation period than oral exposure, presumably because

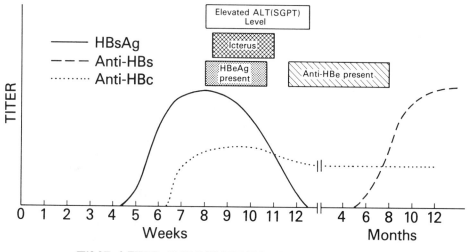

Figure 18-1. Laboratory findings associated with an idealized case of type B viral hepatitis to illustrate the appearance and disappearance of abnormal chemical and serological findings.

different concentrations of virus are transmitted.

Acute Phase

In patients who develop jaundice (icterus), the acute phase can be subdivided into two stages: a prodromal or preicteric phase, and the icteric stage. Only 20-30% of patients with hepatitis B or NANB become jaundiced; anicteric hepatitis is 3-4 times more common than icteric hepatitis.

The earliest prodromal symptoms are nonspecific and flu-like; prominent complaints include anorexia, nausea, extreme fatigue, severe weakness, abdominal discomfort and headache. Approximately 10% of patients with hepatitis B may have a prodrome that resembles serum sickness, characterized variously by skin rash including urticaria, angioneurotic edema, arthralgias or arthritis. This syndrome presumably results from the circulation and deposition in the skin and joints of immune complexes containing HBV and antibodies to HBV. During the prodromal phase there are relatively few physical findings. A tender and enlarged liver, or splenomegaly (in 10-15% of patients), may

be detected. Diagnosis during this phase can only be made on the basis of elevated levels of aspartate aminotransferase (AST or SGOT) and/or alanine aminotransferase (ALT or SGPT), and/or positive serologic tests for virus markers.

The icteric phase is heralded by the retention of the bile pigment, bilirubin, usually first manifest in the urine. Clinical jaundice develops soon thereafter, usually visible first in the sclerae and subsequently the skin. With the onset of jaundice, the constitutional symptoms of the prodromal phase usually diminish, although anorexia and weakness may linger. During this phase patients may experience intense itching from retention of bile salts. The feces frequently lack bile pigment; these whitish-grey stools are described as acholic. Physical examination is remarkable only for jaundice and tender hepatomegaly. Most patients lose 5-15 pounds, primarily as a result of anorexia, during this time.

Laboratory studies during the icteric phase reveal a gradual decrease in aminotransferase levels, which generally peak just before jaundice begins, followed by a similar decline in the serum bilirubin. The duration of this phase is variable, generally lasting 1-6 weeks.

Convalescent Phase

This phase begins when the patient demonstrates sustained clinical improvement. During this phase the patient's appetite is excellent, lost weight is regained, strength and energy return to normal, jaundice is no longer evident and hepatomegaly resolves. In uncomplicated cases the convalescent phase ends with complete clinical recovery, including resolution of all laboratory abnormalities. Convalescence is generally complete within 4 months of the onset of illness, though in some cases it may be delayed 6 months or longer.

Clinical Variants
Fulminant Hepatitis

This complication of hepatitis infection is fortunately rare, occurring in approximately 1% of patients with type B infection. Its incidence in NANB is unknown, but apparently lower than in type B. Clinical manifestations, which begin early in the acute phase, include mental confusion, deepening jaundice, fluid retention, coagulation disturbances, severe abdominal pain and coma. The mortality rate among patients who develop fulminant hepatitis is 75-95%. Younger patients usually fare somewhat better than older or debilitated individuals.

Relapsing Hepatitis

This pattern of hepatitis infection is quite common in, and may well be characteristic of, NANB posttransfusion hepatitis. It consists of one or more distinct clinical or biochemical flares of hepatitis before complete recovery from the primary infection. Neither the cause nor the precipitating factors for the recrudescence are understood. In some cases the apparent relapses may actually represent distinct episodes of hepatitis caused by different viruses; substantiation of this hypothesis awaits the development of serologic tests for NANB hepatitis.

Chronic Hepatitis

Chronic hepatitis exists when laboratory evidence of hepatic inflammation persists for more than 6 months. This complication is seen in approximately 5-10% of patients with hepatitis B,[5] and in perhaps as many as 10-50% of patients with NANB posttransfusion hepatitis.[6-8] Chronic hepatitis may assume either a nonprogressive form, called *chronic persistent hepatitis*, or a progressive form, called *chronic active hepatitis*. Chronic persistent hepatitis, characterized by minimal clinical symptoms and mild biochemical alterations, rarely progresses to cirrhosis. Chronic active hepatitis often leads to increasing liver cell necrosis and fibrosis, and in many cases ultimately to cirrhosis. Liver biopsy is required to distinguish between persistent and active hepatitis.

Hepatoma

There is increasing evidence that hepatocellular carcinoma (hepatoma) is causally related to chronic hepatitis B infection.[9] Hepatoma, a rare malignancy in North America and Western Europe, is the most common malignancy in Asia and sub-Saharan Africa, where carrier rates for hepatitis B virus approximate 5-15%.

Chronic HBsAg Carrier State

Individuals whose serum remains HBsAg-positive for prolonged periods following infection by HBV are designated as carriers. Some carriers have chronic hepatitis, either persistent or active, but others lack evidence of ongoing inflammation. Epidemiologic evidence suggests that there are 200 million HBsAg carriers worldwide. In the United States the carrier prevalence, calculated from results of donor blood screening, varies from 0.1 to 0.5%,[10] or approximately 500,000 to 800,000 carriers. Higher prevalence rates may be found in certain subpopulations, including Asian immigrants, homosexual men, parenteral drug abusers, dialysis patients, and institutionalized individuals with Down's syndrome. The factors that predispose to a carrier state seem to include: exposure early in life, male gender, impaired immunological responsiveness and a postulated genetic susceptibility.

Risk from Transfusion

Transfusion-associated hepatitis B has decreased since blood banks switched to predominantly volunteer blood and adopted mandatory HBsAg screening of all donors.[11,12] However, despite the most sensitive tests for HBsAg detection, occasional cases of hepatitis B continue to occur after transfusion.[13-15] Prospective studies[13-15] of serum aminotransferase levels in transfusion recipients have shown as many as 10% to have posttransfusion elevations of this liver enzyme, leading to the conclusion that HBsAg screening has not affected the frequency of NANB hepatitis; more casual surveillance of transfusion recipients reveals disease incidence much lower than 10%. The true clinical significance of posttransfusion elevation of serum aminotransferase levels requires additional study.

Selection of Prospective Blood Donors

History

A review of some of the donor selection criteria given in Chapter 1 follows. Specific questions should be designed to detect a history of past or present viral hepatitis. Donors must be asked specifically if they have ever had a positive test for hepatitis B surface antigen, as well as a history of illnesses diagnosed as or thought to be hepatitis. While a history of hepatitis regardless of causation is reason for permanent deferral, liver inflammation associated with infectious mononucleosis or cytomegalovirus is not. To determine whether a potential donor may be in the incubation phase of hepatitis, he or she

must be questioned about transfusion and direct exposure, within the past 6 months, to tissue grafts; potentially contaminated needles or other equipment; and to blood, including components and products known to transmit the disease.

Contact with Patients

Prospective donors in close contact with individuals with viral hepatitis (eg, their spouses, or others with whom they share kitchen and bathroom facilities) must be deferred from donating blood until 6 months after the last exposure. The type of patient contact most physicians, nurses and technical personnel have in their routine work is not considered "close contact" and such work is not a cause for donor exclusion. Medical, technical and nursing staff who work in renal dialysis units may be at increased risk of acquiring viral hepatitis from their patients and should be questioned about the ways HBsAg-positive patients are identified and treated. If all patients on such units are tested, and appropriate handling procedures observed for potentially infectious patients, then staff members from such units may be acceptable donors. Although the usual incubation period is 6 months or less, administration of Hepatitis B Immune Globulin (HBIG) may delay the onset of manifest infection.[16] Persons who have received HBIG must not donate blood until 12 months have passed since their last injection.[17] On the other hand, individuals who have been, or are in the process of being, vaccinated need not be deferred from donating, provided the vaccine was not given because of specific exposure to hepatitis B virus.

Physical Findings

Physical examination must include inspection of both forearms for evidence of needle tracks or sclerotic veins suggestive of intravenous drug abuse, as this is associated with an increased incidence of both type B and NANB hepatitis. Such evidence permanently excludes a prospective donor. Tattooing within 6 months imposes temporary deferral because of the risk of hepatitis from blood-contaminated tattoo needles. Ear piercing or acupuncture within 6 months may be cause for deferral, unless sterilized or disposable single-use instruments were used.

Payment of Blood Donors

The risk of posttransfusion hepatitis increases following transfusion of blood from commercial sources when compared to blood from voluntary donors.[11,12] Payment per se does not affect the safety of the blood; but, in most places, payment or other inducement attracts donors in whom there is increased risk of viral hepatitis, either type B or NANB. Testing for HBsAg reduces, but does not eliminate, the risk; despite testing with third-generation tests for HBsAg, blood drawn from paid donors still has an excessive risk of transmitting both HBV and NANB disease.[18] In New Jersey, for example, the introduction of HBsAg testing and a switch to predominantly volunteer blood donors decreased the incidence of posttransfusion hepatitis requiring hospitalization from 1 in 117 blood recipients to 1 in 734.[18] Measures to decrease further the incidence of posttransfusion hepatitis must be directed toward judicious utilization of blood, surveillance of transfusion recipients to identify infective blood donors, procurement of blood from volunteer donors only and further research on the etiology and prevention of NANB posttransfusion hepatitis.[1]

Blood Products with a High Hepatitis Risk

Certain blood products derived from pooled human plasmas have an especially high risk of transmitting hepatitis. These include prothrombin-complex concentrates (Factors II, VII, IX, X; "Factor IX Complex"), AHF concentrates (Factor VIII) and specifically activated factor concentrates designed to bypass Factor VIII

inhibitor activity. Use of these and other pooled products should be restricted to patients whose specific indications for their use justify exposing them to the increased risk.

Testing for Hepatitis B Surface Antigen (HBsAg)

The AABB *Standards*[17] state that:

"A sample of blood from each donation shall be tested for HBsAg. Whole Blood and blood components shall not be used for transfusion unless the test is nonreactive. In an emergency, blood may be transfused before completion of the test for HBsAg but a notation to the effect that HBsAg testing is not completed shall appear conspicuously on an attached label or tag. If the test is subsequently reactive, the recipient's physician must be notified."

Both *Standards*[17] and the Office of Biologics Review and Research (OBRR) require that HBsAg testing be performed using reagents and techniques licensed by FDA,[19] such as radioimmunoassay (RIA), enzyme-linked immunosorbent assay (ELISA) or reversed passive hemagglutination (RPHA). However, the *Code of Federal Regulations* (21 CFR 610.40a) allows the use of certain less sensitive tests (eg, the abbreviated RIA), in emergency situations. *Standards*[17] allows testing after transfusion in emergency situations. The requirement for HBsAg testing applies to blood drawn for any purpose: for transfusion, for production of derivatives for transfusion, for stimulation of antibody(ies) in donors or for use in the manufacture of reagents for technical procedures. The interpretation of HBsAg testing must be included on the label of all units of blood and blood components. There must, in addition, be a statement that the agent(s) of viral hepatitis may be present despite the existence of a negative test for HBsAg (21 CFR 606.1206b).

Each unit of blood or hemapheresis unit must be tested by the collecting facility or in an approved independent laboratory and be found negative before it is released for routine transfusion. Transfusion services that obtain blood from another facility need not repeat testing for HBsAg.

Radioimmunoassay and Enzyme-Linked Immunoassay

Radioimmunoassay and enzyme-linked immunoassay are two of the widely used types of third-generation tests for HBsAg. Both RIA and ELISA employ a solid support (eg, bead, tube, column) coated with unlabeled anti-HBs. The general principles of these techniques are outlined below. The reader is referred to the manufacturer's package insert for specific instructions on each commercially available RIA or ELISA test for HBsAg.

1. Add the sample to be tested to the coated solid support and incubate at the specified temperature for the specified time. NOTE: If plasma is incubated above room temperature it may coagulate.
2. Aspirate the excess sample and wash the solid support. Washing removes extraneous protein and fluid but HBsAg present in the test specimen combines specifically with the anti-HBs attached to the solid support and is not removed by washing.
3. Add a specified amount of radioactively labeled (^{125}I) or enzyme-linked anti-HBs and incubate with the solid support. Radiolabeled or enzyme-linked antibody is usually designated anti-HBs*.
4. Aspirate and wash the mixture to remove all labeled anti-HBs* that has not bound to solid phase.
5. Measure the amount of bound anti-HBs* either with a gamma counter or, if enzyme-labeled antibody is used, a spectrophotometer.
6. Run replicate known positive and known negative controls with each set of donor blood samples. Calculate the mean for the negative controls. For RIA testing, a positive result is usually any value more than 2 to 2.5 times the mean count of the negative controls; for ELISA, it is an absorbance value that exceeds the negative results by more than the level specified by the manufacturer.
7. Check values for the replicate positive control specimens. If the known positive controls are not all greater than the cutoff value, repeat the whole run.

False-positive reactions for HBsAg are known to occur with the RIA and ELISA.[20] Before a donor is designated HBsAg-positive, a status that permanently excludes him from donating and carries significant clinical and social consequences, it is important to perform repeat and/or confirmatory testing for HBsAg reactivity on the original specimen. This caution is usually included in the manufacturer's package insert. If repeating the initial test reveals a reproducibly positive result, a confirmatory neutralization test can be performed, although this is not specifically required by AABB *Standards*. If the positive test result is inhibited by incubation with human serum containing anti-HBs, but not inhibited by incubation with a human serum lacking anti-HBs[20] the specificity of the result is confirmed. Confirmatory neutralization test kits are available for all commercial HBsAg tests.

1. Add presumed positive serum to each of two labeled tubes, in the standard manner for the test in use, RIA or ELISA.
2. Add to one tube the same volume of a human serum known to contain anti-HBs and to the other tube that volume of a human serum that does not contain anti-HBs.
3. Incubate for 30 minutes at 37 C.
4. Add the incubated serum mixtures to each of two standard supports (bead, tube, column) with unlabeled anti-HBs.
5. Perform the test as specified by the manufacturer's directions.

If incubation with human serum containing anti-HBs reduces the counts or absorbance by more than 50%, when compared to the specimen incubated with human serum lacking anti-HBs, the positive initial result is considered specific for HBsAg.

Some of the commercially available tests for HBsAg can also be performed with abbreviated incubation times. These are not usually as sensitive as the longer procedures but can be useful in urgent transfusion situations. Samples screened by abbreviated procedures should later be tested by the standard technique.

Reversed Passive Hemagglutination

The reversed passive hemagglutination test (RPHA) for HBsAg has sensitivity comparable to that of RIA and ELISA. RPHA utilizes red cells coated with anti-HBs. Addition of serum that contains HBsAg alters the settling pattern of these antibody-coated cells. As with RIA and ELISA results, it is desirable to confirm all positive reactions. Uncoated control red cells can be run to rule out false-positive agglutination.

Special Notes on Hepatitis Tests

1. Quality assurance is important in HBsAg testing as with all areas of the blood bank or transfusion service. *Standards* requires participation in a proficiency test program as part of quality assurance for HBsAg tests. The American Association of Blood Banks and the College of American Pathologists jointly sponsor such a program.
2. All blood products and samples should be regarded as potentially infectious whether or not they are known to be HBsAg-positive. Current tests may miss minute amounts of HBsAg and associated hepatitis B virus; blood from persons with negative HBsAg test results may transmit hepatitis B after transfusion or following accidental inocula-

tion of personnel. In addition, NANB viruses may be present; these are unrelated to HBV so would not be detected by HBsAg testing.
3. All HBsAg-positive blood should be retested and confirmed as specifically HBsAg-positive, since all test methods can give false-positive results on occasion.

   Before a donor is told that he or she is HBsAg-positive, the test should be demonstrated to be reproducibly and specifically positive.[20]
4. When red cells are used to stimulate antibody production, the HBsAg status of the donor must be negative at the time of each donation.
5. Routine testing of intended transfusion recipients for HBsAg is not recommended. The patient should be tested for HBsAg only when the results are directly related to that patient's diagnosis or care.
6. The presence of anti-HBs in blood from unvaccinated donors is not associated with an increased risk of hepatitis B in recipients.[21] Routine testing for anti-HBs in donors is not recommended, especially since increasing numbers of donors now have vaccine-stimulated anti-HBs. There is some suggestion that the isolated presence of anti-HBc without simultaneous anti-HBs or HBsAg may, in occasional cases, identify otherwise undetectable HBV carriers[2,3]; arguments against routine anti-HBc testing include increased cost and the need to discard a far higher percentage of donor units than is suggested by the apparent level of hepatitis B transmission.
7. It has been reported that an elevated level of alanine aminotransferase in donor blood indicates an increased risk of transmitting NANB hepatitis.[14] The ALT test may possibly be a useful, albeit nonspecific, method to identify carriers of this major cause of transfusion-associated hepatitis. Before measurement of ALT levels can be considered

for routine use, however, difficulties in standardizing the test will have to be resolved. In addition, prospective trials are needed to determine what ALT level best discriminates between possible carriers of NANB hepatitis viruses and innocuous donors with nonspecifically elevated ALT, and whether exclusion of all donors with elevated ALT levels will result in a decrease in transfusion-associated hepatitis.

Posttransfusion Hepatitis

It is imperative that the source blood bank be notified of every patient who develops hepatitis within 2 weeks to 6 months following transfusion. The incubation period may be more prolonged if the recipient received Hepatitis B Immune Globulin (HBIG) after a known exposure.[16] Recipients, their families and their physicians all tend to underreport the occurrence of viral hepatitis. The blood bank can improve its case-finding rate by consulting additional sources to detect occurrence of possible cases of posttransfusion hepatitis. Potentially useful sources include:

1. The hospital's medical records, especially discharge diagnosis.
2. Gastroenterology service records.
3. Laboratory records, especially the hepatitis testing and chemistry laboratories.
4. The hospital's social service and business offices personnel.
5. The hospital's infection control officer.
6. The local public health service director.

All reported cases of unexplained acute liver dysfunction occuring 2 weeks to 6 months after transfusion of blood or blood components must be investigated as possible posttransfusion hepatitis.

Necessary Records

A system for recording and reporting all cases of known or suspected posttransfusion hepatitis is required by AABB *Standards*. When a case of posttransfusion hepatitis is confirmed, records of all blood or components given to the patient must be reviewed. Any components still in storage from implicated donors should be located and quarantined until the donor's status is decided. It must be possible to trace a unit of blood and its components from final disposition (transfused to specific recipient, shipped or discarded) back to the donor source and to recheck the laboratory records applying to each component of the unit. Blood-collecting facilities should have some system to record and retrieve reports on donors implicated in hepatitis cases.

The *Code of Federal Regulations* (21 CFR 606.170b) requires that fatalities attributed to transfusion complications (eg, hepatitis and hemolytic reactions) be reported to the Office of Biologics Review and Research within 7 days. Transfusion services and collecting facilities must keep records of the number of cases of reported transfusion-associated hepatitis, including those confirmed as HBsAg-positive. Collecting facilities must record the number of donors found to be HBsAg-positive, and must keep a permanent record of their identity.

Implicated Donors

If hepatitis occurs in the recipient of blood or components from only a single donor, that donor must be permanently excluded from giving blood subsequently. This should be noted on the individual's donor record and that name should be placed in a file of donors who have been permanently rejected. Such a file should also include those with a history of viral hepatitis and those known to have been positive for HBsAg.

If a patient gets hepatitis after exposure to multiple units of blood and/or blood components, it is not necessary to exclude all of the involved donors. A note should be made on the donor records that the donor was one of several donors (specify the number) involved in a case of transfusion-associated hepatitis. The names should be placed in a special file for hepatitis-implicated donors. The blood bank director may want to evaluate such donors for an interim history of hepatitis. A donor implicated for the first time need not be rejected as a future blood donor, if there were two or more donors. If, on the other hand, a donor is found to have been implicated in one or more other cases of transfusion hepatitis, the blood bank physician should decide if permanent rejection is warranted.

Calculating Probability

Some centers routinely exclude donors implicated in two cases of posttransfusion hepatitis[22]; other centers prefer a policy of calculating probability values.[23] This tends to protect frequent donors whose components or blood are given to patients who develop liver dysfunction and have received large numbers of transfusions. The probability value for a multiply-implicated donor is calculated as the sum of the fraction of the total donor pool he or she represents for each hepatitis case. For example, if a donor is 1 of 12 donors in one case, 1/12 (0.08), and 1 of 9 donors in another, 1/9 (0.11), the probability value is 0.19. When pooled concentrates (eg, Factor VIII) are administered along with other blood components, at least 10,000 donors may be implicated, but an arbitrary figure of 100 donors is assigned for including the pool in the calculation. Permanent exclusion would occur only when a donor reaches a designated probability value, eg, 0.3 or 0.4. The probability approach avoids automatic exclusion of regular donors, who are likely to become implicated in more than one case. A modification of this approach has been described,[24] in which considering the specific history of each multiply-implicated donor permits more accurate estimation of possible donor responsibility.

Notifying the Donor. The excluded donor must be notified of the exclusion and its cause. The donor must be made to understand clearly that he/she is precluded from future blood donations and that he/she has a potentially hazardous condition, but this should be handled with concern and tact. A repeat donor examination, follow-up laboratory tests and a private discussion with the donor and the personal physician would constitute optimal management of blood donors placed on the permanent exclusion list.

Use of Gamma Globulin with Transfusion

It is not recommended that gamma globulin, either immune globulin (IG) or Hepatitis B Immune Globulin (HBIG), be given to transfusion recipients to prevent viral hepatitis.[25,26] IG and HBIG have not been shown to prevent posttransfusion hepatitis B. The little available evidence is conflicting as to whether IG or HBIG can reduce the frequency or severity of NANB viral hepatitis, the most common form of transfusion-related hepatitis occurring today.[23]

Laboratory Safety

In handling any human blood specimen, personnel must be aware of the risk of hepatitis as well as any other virus infection. Blood bank and transfusion service personnel should routinely follow safety precautions.[27] The following measures are appropriate for a hepatitis testing area, as well as any part of the blood bank, transfusion service or clinical laboratory, and apply to the handling of any donor or patient specimen that could be contaminated with blood or other body fluids.

1. Eating, drinking and smoking in the laboratory, or wherever blood is handled, are prohibited.
2. Mouth pipetting is forbidden.
3. Personnel with open cuts or sores on their hands should wear disposable gloves when handling specimens.
4. Hands should be washed before leaving any area in the laboratory.

5. All blood specimens should be centrifuged only in covered carriers.
6. HBsAg testing should be done in a separate area.
7. HBsAg reagents and HBsAg-positive blood should be segregated if placed in refrigerators that contain blood or blood products for transfusion. Using different and suitably labeled shelves or secondary containers is appropriate segregation.
8. HBsAg-positive material and disposable equipment used in testing for HBsAg should be placed in leak-proof containers. They should be labeled as infectious, handled carefully and autoclaved or incinerated. Appropriate disposal methods must be used with all radioactive waste material used in hepatitis testing.
9. Bench tops in test areas should be constructed with nonabsorbent materials and should be free of such extraneous items as forms, reports and slips. It is good practice to clean surfaces with a 1 in 5 dilution of bleach (undiluted bleach equals 5% hypochlorite) each work day or after completion of each batch of tests. Spills of blood, sera or HBsAg-positive materials can be treated with undiluted bleach. Liquid waste can be treated with equal volumes of either 5% hypochlorite or 2% formaldehyde. Allow 30 minutes for effective decontamination.[28]
10. Care should be exercised when entering reagent or specimen vials with needles to prevent accidental parenteral exposure to potentially infectious material. Avoid resheathing needles, as this is frequently associated with inadvertent needlesticks.
11. If HBsAg-positive blood or secretions are accidentally inoculated into potentially susceptible individuals (those lacking HBsAg and anti-HBs), prophylactic injections of HBIG should be given[29,30] (see next section for dosage and timing). After prophylactic HBIG, the individual should be observed for 1 year for evidence of hepatitis B.[16]

Preventing Viral Hepatitis

Official guidelines for the immunoprophylaxis of viral hepatitis are prepared by the Public Health Service (PHS) Advisory Committee on Immunization Practices. The PHS recommendations for the use of IG and HBIG to prevent or modify viral hepatitis are summarized below.

Hepatitis A Prophylaxis

1. After close personal contact with an individual with hepatitis A, give 0.02 ml/kg of body weight of IG intramuscularly.
2. For foreign travel to areas endemic for hepatitis A, give 0.02 ml/kg of IG. Travelers planning to stay more than 3 months should receive 0.06 ml/kg of IG every 5 months.

Hepatitis B Prophylaxis

1. After accidental needlestick exposure or contamination of mucosal surfaces or open cuts with HBsAg-positive blood products, give HBIG in a dose of 0.05-0.07 ml/kg of body weight immediately, or within 24 hours of exposure, and again 25-30 days later. Individuals who are already HBsAg-positive or who have anti-HBs need not be given HBIG; but, if these tests cannot be performed within the 7 days after exposure, draw a blood sample for the tests and give HBIG. If HBIG is not available, give IG.

   HBV-susceptible health workers who sustain a needlestick injury should also be considered candidates for hepatitis vaccine (see below).[31,32] The vaccine will provide long-term protection against future accidental needlestick. If HBIG and vaccine are utilized in combination, only a single dose of HBIG need be given and this should be administered as soon as possible after exposure. Vaccination can be initiated simultaneously or within 1 week. HBIG and vaccine do not interfere with each other, but should be injected at separate sites.The usual second dose of HBIG can then be omitted and additional vaccine given at 1 and 6 months after the initial dose.

2. For infants born to mothers with acute hepatitis B in the third trimester or with HBsAg at the time of delivery, give 0.5 ml HBIG intramuscularly as soon after birth as possible and no later than 24 hours; give an additional 0.5 ml at 3 months and 6 months of age. Such infants may also be candidates for hepatitis B vaccine.

Hepatitis B Vaccine

In 1982 the first vaccine against hepatitis B was licensed and marketed.This vaccine is prepared from isolated and concentrated HBsAg particles that have been inactivated with formalin, pepsin and urea. These procedures are capable of effectively inactivating hepatitis B virus as well as viruses from every known group, including agents of human NANB hepatitis.[32] In large clinical trials the vaccine was found to be 95% successful in stimulating antibodies to HBsAg.[33,34] The presence of these antibodies was found to be consistent with immunity to hepatitis B virus infection. The vaccine must be given on three separate occasions; initial dose is 20 μg, followed by 20 μg at 1 and 6 months after the primary injection. Side effects are rare and mild, and include fever, tenderness over the injection site and arthralgias.

Individuals at high risk of contracting hepatitis B are technologists and pathologists who handle large numbers of patient blood specimens. Donor center personnel are not at increased risk unless they are exposed to patient, as well as donor, blood specimens. Some feel that the high cost of this vaccine makes it desirable to prescreen for the presence of serologic markers of hepatitis B virus prior to vaccinating individuals in groups with a high prevalence of infection.[35]

Frozen Red Cells and Viral Hepatitis

Transfusion of red blood cells that have been frozen, thawed and deglycerolized has been suggested as a possible means to reduce the risk of posttransfusion hepatitis.[36] An experimental study in chimpanzees did not substantiate this for type B viral hepatitis.[37] A subsequent clinical study similarly failed to justify the use of frozen or washed red blood cells to reduce the risk of NANB hepatitis.[38] Until additional studies provide evidence that frozen and washed red blood cells are noninfective, the use of unpaid blood donors and the maintenance of careful blood bank records to identify and interdict hepatitis-implicated donors will remain the best means to reduce the risk of transfusion-associated hepatitis.

References

1. Alter HJ, Holland PV, Purcell RH. Current status of post transfusion hepatitis. In: Ioachim HL, ed. Pathobiology Annual 1980. New York:Raven Press, 1980:135-136.

2. Hoofnagle JH, Seeff LB, Bales ZB, et al. Type B hepatitis after transfusion of blood containing antibody to hepatitis B core antigen. N Engl J Med 1978;298:1379-1383.

3. Lander JJ, Gitnick GL, Gelb LH, Aach RD. Anticore antibody screening of transfused blood. Vox Sang 1978;34:77-80.

4. Okada M, Kamiyama I, Inomata M, et al. e antigen and anti-e in the serum of asymptomatic carrier mothers as indicators of positive and negative transmission of hepatitis B virus to their infants. N Engl J Med 1976;294:746-749.

5. Nielsen JO, Dietrichson O, Elling P, et al. Incidence and meaning of persistence of Australia antigen in patients with acute viral hepatitis:development of chronic hepatitis. N Engl J Med 1971;285:1157-1160.

6. Koretz RL, Suffin SC, Gitnick GL. Post-transfusion chronic liver disease. Gastroenterology 1976;71:797-803.

7. Knodell RG, Conrad ME, Ishak KG. Development of chronic liver disease after acute non-A, non-B posttransfusion hepatitis: Role of γ-globulin prophylaxis in its prevention. Gastroenterology 1977;72:902-909.

8. Alter HJ, Purcell RH, Feinstone SM, et al. Non-A, non-B hepatitis: its relationship to cytomegalovirus, to chronic hepatitis, and to direct and indirect test methods. In: Szmuness W, Alter HJ, Maynard JE, eds.Viral hepatitis. Philadelphia: The Franklin Institute Press, 1982:279-294.

9. Beasley RP, Lin CC, Hwang LY, et al. Risk of hepatocellular carcinoma in hepatitis B virus infections: A prospective study in Taiwan. In: Szmuness W, Alter HJ, Maynard JE, eds.Viral hepatitis. Philadelphia: The Franklin Institute Press, 1982:261-272.

10. Holland P, Golosova T, Szmuness W, et al. Viral hepatitis markers in Soviet and American blood donors. Transfusion 1980;20:504-510.

11. Seeff LB, Zimmerman HJ, Wright EC, et al. A randomized, double blind controlled trial of the efficacy of immune serum globulin for the prevention of posttransfusion hepatitis. A Veterans Administration cooperative study. Gastroenterology 1977;72:111-121.

12. Alter HJ, Holland PV, Purcell RH, et al. Posttransfusion hepatitis after exclusion of commercial hepatitis-B antigen-positive donors. Ann Intern Med 1972;77:691-699.

13. Alter HJ, Purcell RH, Feinstone SM, Holland PV, Morrow AG.Non-A/non-B hepatitis: a review and interim report of an ongoing prospective study. In: Vyas GN, Cohen SN, Schmid R, eds. Viral hepatitis. Philadelphia: Franklin Institute Press, 1978:359-369.

14. Aach RD, Lander JJ, Sherman LA, et al. Transfusion transmitted viruses: interim analysis of hepatitis among transfused and non-transfused patients. In: Vyas GN, Cohen SN, Schmid R, eds. Viral hepatitis. Philadelphia: Franklin Institute Press, 1978:383-396.

15. Seeff LB, Wright EC, Zimmerman HJ, et al. Posttransfusion hepatitis, 1973-1975: a Veterans Administration cooperative study. In: Vyas GN, Cohen SN, Schmid R, eds. Viral hepatitis. Philadelphia: Franklin Institute Press, 1978:371-381.

16. Grady GF, Lee VA, Prince AM, et al. Hepatitis B immune globulin for accidental exposures among medical personnel: final report of a multicenter controlled trial. J Infect Dis 1978;138:625-638.

17. Schmidt PJ, ed. Standards for blood banks and transfusion services. 11th ed. Arlington, VA: American Association of Blood Banks, 1984.

18. Goldfield M, Bill J, Colosimo F. The control of transfusion-associated hepatitis. In: Vyas GN, Cohen SN, Schmid R, eds. Viral hepa-titis.Philadelphia: Franklin Institute Press, 1978:405-414.

19. Code of federal regulations, 21 Food and Drugs, 610.40b, April 1, 1982.

20. Alter HJ, Holland PV, Purcell RH, Gerin J. The Ausria test: critical evaluation of sensitivity and specificity. Blood 1973;42:947-957.

21. Aach RD, Alter HJ, Hollinger FB, et al. Risk of transfusing blood containing antibody to hepatitis B surface antigen. Lancet 1974;2:190-193.

22. Walker RH, Inclan AP. Utilization of the biologic test in posttransfusion hepatitis for the detection of carriers. South Med 1965;58:1131-1134.

23. Polesky HF, Hanson MR. Transfusion-associated hepatitis. ASCP Check Sample. Immunohematology 1-107 (1979). Chicago, American Society of Clinical Pathologists, 1980.

24. Ladd DJ, Hillis A. A new method for evaluating the hepatitis risk of the multiply-implicated donor. Transfusion 1984;24:80-82.

25. Maynard JE. Immunoprophylaxis for viral hepatitis (editorial). Gastroenterology 1979;77:190-192.

26. Seeff LB, Hoofnagle JH. Immunoprophylaxis of viral hepatitis.Gastroenterology 1979;77:161-182.

27. Schmidt N, Lennette E. Safety precautions for performing tests for hepatitis-associated "Australia" antigen and antibodies. Am J Clin Pathol 1972;57:526-530.

28. Cossart Y. Epidemiology of serum hepatitis. Brit Med Bull 1972;28:156.

29. Immune globulins for protection against viral hepatitis. Morb Mort Weekly Report 1977;26:425-429.

30. Mosley JW. Immunoprophylaxis for viral hepatitis. (editorial) Gastroenterology 1979;77:189-190.

31. Schwartz JS. Health and public policy committee ACP: hepatitis B vaccine. Ann Intern Med 1984;100:149-150.

32. Gerety RJ, Tabor E. New licensed hepatitis B vaccine. JAMA 1983;249:745-746.

33. Szmuness W, Stevens CD, Harley EJ, et al. Hepatitis B vaccine: demonstration of efficacy in a controlled clinical trial in a high-risk population in the United States. New Engl J Med 1980;303:833-841.

34. Francis DP, Hadler SC, Thompson SE, et al. The prevention of hepatitis B with vaccine: report of the Centers for Disease Control

multi-center efficacy trial among homosexual men. Ann Intern Med 1982;97:362-366.

35. Krugman S. The newly licensed hepatitis B vaccine: characteristics and indications for use. JAMA 1982;247:2012.

36. Tullis JL, Hinman J, Sproul MT, Nickerson RJ. Incidence of post transfusion hepatitis in previously frozen blood. JAMA 1970;214:719-723.

37. Alter HJ, Tabor E, Meryman H, et al. Transmission of hepatitis B virus infection by transfusion of frozen-deglycerolized red blood cells. N Engl J Med 1978;298:637-642.

38. Haugen RK. Hepatitis after the transfusion of frozen red cells and washed red cells. N Engl J Med 1979;301:393-395.

19

Autologous Transfusion

When a recipient serves as his own donor, he receives the safest possible transfusion. Although this in itself is sufficient justification for autologous transfusion, autologous transfusion provides additional benefits to the donor-patient, the blood donor center and the transfusion service. Some of these are outlined in Table 19-1.[1,2]

The term *autologous transfusion* describes any transfusion of blood or components that have originated with the intended recipient. Two broad categories of autologous transfusion are: 1) predeposit, in which blood withdrawn before expected transfusion is stored until used; and 2) intraoperative, in which blood is both collected and infused during the surgical procedure. Major indications for predeposit are long-term storage of blood with specific or unusual types and presurgical donation for specific planned procedures. Hemodilution with short-term storage and blood salvage are the usual intraoperative indications.

Some indications for autologous transfusion are listed in Table 19-2. Potential problems associated with autologous transfusion are listed in Table 19-3.

Autologous transfusion supplements the community's blood supply in several ways. First, the autologous donor has less need for homologous blood. In one report, predeposited blood was sufficient to meet the transfusion requirements of 54% of patients undergoing cardiovascular surgery.[3] In another, predeposited blood provided over 85% of transfusions given to patients undergoing elective plastic and/or orthopedic procedures.[4] Second, unused predeposited autologous blood can be put into the regular inventory if the donor-patient met standard donor criteria. Finally, one study[4] suggests that physicians transfuse less blood to patients who have autologous blood available, rarely transfusing more than the amount previously donated and thus sparing the total supply.

Patients with Rare Blood Types

Persons at risk of immunization to high-incidence antigens absent from their red cells, and persons with multiple antibodies to several antigens should be encouraged to donate blood for prolonged, frozen storage, even if no immediate transfusion needs are foreseen. Finding crossmatch-compatible or nonimmunizing homologous blood would be difficult or impossible at a time of acute need. A supply of 4-6 units is considered appropriate for individuals with no major foreseeable transfusion needs. Above that level the donor-patient should be encouraged to make units available for other patients who require that particular rare blood and, if possible, to continue donating as units are used.

Table 19-1. Benefits of Autologous Transfusion

1. For the donor-patient
   a. No transmission of infectious disease (hepatitis, syphilis, cytomegalovirus or HTLV-III)
   b. No risk of alloimmunization to erythrocyte, leukocyte, platelet or protein antigens
   c. No risk of hemolytic, febrile or allergic reactions due to alloimmunization
   d. No risk of graft-versus-host reactions
   e. Stimulation of erythropoiesis by repeated preoperative phlebotomy
   f. May reduce costs, if pretransfusion testing is curtailed
   g. May reduce quantity of homologous blood given in a procedure
2. For the blood center and transfusion service
   a. Ready availability of blood for patients for whom compatible blood is not easily available
   b. Provision of additional homologous blood supply, if autologous units are not used
   c. Reduction (often) of overall transfusion levels for patients involved
   d. Provision of blood for surgical procedures in remote areas in which blood supplies are unpredictable
   e. Increase in the donor base and the community's blood supply

Table 19-2. Indications for Autologous Transfusion

1. Requirement for rare blood types
2. Prevention of alloimmunization
3. History of previous severe transfusion reactions
4. Presence of alloantibodies
5. Religious beliefs*
6. Difficulty in maintaining blood supply in isolated or remote communities
7. Improvement of selected surgical procedures (hemodilution with short-term storage and/or intraoperative blood salvage)
8. Massive hemorrhage in clean wound (intraoperative blood salvage)
*Some Jehovah's Witnesses will accept autologous transfusions,
but others refuse.[23,24]

Table 19-3. Potential Problems Associated with Autologous Transfusion

1. Presurgical donation and storage
   a. Anemia and hypovolemia
   b. Loss of working time to donate
   c. Possible clerical errors in recipient identification, labeling, and storage
   d. Increased cost: professional time, paperwork, donor reactions
   e. Units lost when surgery is delayed or cancelled, or during thawing or deglycerolization
2. Hemodilution and short-term storage
   a. Possible hypoxemia
   b. Incorrect processing or storage, causing damage to blood
3. Intraoperative blood salvage
   a. Consumption of coagulation factors and platelets
   b. Cancer dissemination
   c. Sepsis from contaminated wounds

The American Association of Blood Banks maintains a national Rare Donor File as a 24-hour-a-day, no-fee service. The file lists name and location of rare blood donors and also provides a liaison with the Rare Donor Registry of the American Red Cross. Any autologous donor of rare blood who gives permission for homologous use of his/her blood should be registered with the AABB Rare Donor File. (See page 414 in Special Methods headed "Procedure for Using AABB Rare Donor File.")

Presurgical Donation and Storage

Although many patients undergoing elective surgery are capable of donating blood prior to their operation, and despite its advantages to patient and blood centers, autologous transfusion is not widely used.[5] This may be due partly to ready availability of homologous blood, but most such apathy stems from lack of enthusiastic promotion by blood bankers and lack of information in the general medical community. One early problem was the 21-day limit for liquid storage of autologous blood. The prolonged shelf life possible with newer anticoagulant-preservative solutions permits greater flexibility in scheduling phlebotomies and the collection of more units without resorting to frozen storage or salvage protocols. If the collecting facility can freeze red blood cells and plasma, the predeposit process may be extended as long as necessary to collect the needed number of units.[6]

Recruitment

Since requests for presurgical autologous donations usually originate with the surgeon or other attending physician, the primary focus of autologous recruitment efforts should be the medical community. Blood bank physicians can be especially effective by initiating physician education programs. Hospital staff conferences, medical society meetings, blood bank newsletters and brochures are useful for informing physicians about autologous transfusion. The following information may be contained in the educational materials:

1. Advantages of autologous transfusion
2. Types of patients for whom autologous transfusion may be particularly appropriate (eg, patients anticipating elective plastic or orthopedic surgery)
3. Medical requirements for donation
4. The recommended interval between donations and from last donation until operation
5. Importance of oral iron supplementation for selected patients
6. Descriptions of other autologous transfusion programs
7. Directions for contacting the donor facility to make an appointment
8. A telephone number to request further information

Physician Responsibility

Although predeposit phlebotomy may be performed only at the written request of the patient's physician, the medical director of the drawing facility is responsible for determining, prior to each donation,

the suitability of drawing blood from the patient. It is important that the patient's physician and the blood bank physician establish good communication; if the blood drawing facility is separate from the transfusing facility, it is essential that the transfusion service know that predeposit autologous blood is available. A card signifying that autologous blood is available can be provided to the donor-patient, who presents it to hospital personnel at the time of admission.

Donor Consent and Release

The patient must give written consent for the procedure. If the donor-patient is a minor, a parent or guardian must give consent. Medical risks of predeposit phlebotomy are, in most cases, the same as those for regular blood donation, and the patient must be informed in the usual way of possible adverse reactions to donation. If the predeposited blood or blood components could appropriately be used for homologous transfusion, a release for such use should be included. An example of a consent form is shown in Fig 19-1.

Criteria for Phlebotomy

Candidates for autologous donation need not meet all the usual criteria for homologous blood donations. When donors do not meet those criteria established to protect the recipient, units must be labeled "For Autologous Use Only" and must be segregated while in storage and discarded if not used by the patient. Bacteremia is an absolute contraindication to autologous donation because bacteria may proliferate in stored blood even at temperatures of 1 to 6 C.

Age

There is no upper age limit for autologous donation. The lower age limit is determined by the capacity of the child to understand and cooperate. Children who have adequate veins can tolerate the physiologic effects of phlebotomy as well as adults, but the volume withdrawn must be

1. The advantages, nature and purposes of autologous transfusions, the risks involved, and the possibility of complications have been explained to me by _____M.D. I acknowledge such counseling. Among those specific aspects of autologous transfusion which were discussed with me were:

   a. That blood drawn from me for later transfusion to me is the safest blood for me to receive.
   b. That a mild anemia and/or decrease in my blood volume may result from frequent blood donation for autologous transfusion. That because of these possible changes, I should refrain from strenuous athletic events and hazardous occupations or endeavors between the time the first unit is drawn and the scheduled use of predeposited units.
   c. That I should contact either the blood bank or my personal physician, should I feel faint, weak, giddy, lightheaded or dizzy.
   d. That if the scheduled procedure is delayed for any reason it may be necessary to transfuse an older unit back to me, and withdraw a fresh unit to prevent expiration and discarding of the older unit.
2. I consent to withdrawal of blood by authorized members of the staff of the blood bank for autologous transfusion purposes, and further consent to such additional procedures pursuant to autologous transfusion as may be necessary or desirable. Should I not require transfusion of the blood withdrawn for autologous transfusion, I further consent to the use or disposal of my blood in any manner deemed appropriate.
3. Authorized Signatures:

_____   _____
Date   Donor-Patient Signature

_____   _____
Witness   Authority to Consent if Not Patient's Own
                                         Signature

_____

Donor-Patient
Identification (eg. Birth-
date, SS #, Hosp. #, or
Donor-Patient
License #)

_____
                        Address of Donor-Patient

Figure 19-1. Statement of consent for autologous transfusion.

appropriate for the patient's blood volume. In general, most patients suitable for elective surgical procedures will be suitable candidates for predeposit phlebotomy. If a patient has special medical problems that might make phlebotomy hazardous, a knowledgeable physician should be on the premises or readily available during the donation. Although certain high-risk patients can successfully participate in a hospital-based autologous transfusion program,[7] it may be inappropriate for such patients to donate at a community blood center, unless there are provisions for the active support of patients who experience a medical emergency.

Weight

There are no specific weight requirements. Not more than 450 ± 45 ml or 12% of estimated blood volume (whichever is less) should be withdrawn at a single donation. A handy guideline for patients weighing less than 50 kg (110 pounds) is to decrease the volume of blood drawn by 8 ml for every kg under 50 (4 ml for every pound under 110). The volume of anticoagulant must be reduced proportionately if the amount of blood to be drawn is below the allowable limits of a standard bag. The proper volume of anticoagulant to be left in the blood-collection container may be calculated as follows:

$$V_1 = V_o \times \frac{\text{weight of patient}}{50 \text{ kg or } 110 \text{ pounds}}$$

V_1 = ml anticoagulant to be left in blood collection container
V_o = ml anticoagulant normally used for 450 ml blood. Example: If anticoagulant volume is 63 ml CPDA-1 and the patient weighs 73 pounds,

$$V_1 = 63 \times \frac{73}{110}$$
$$V_1 = 42 \text{ ml}$$

Therefore, 21 ml (63 − 42) anticoagulant should be removed from the primary container. This is most easily done with a double-pack donor set, transferring the excess into the satellite container and sealing the integral tubing. Because blood will be drawn into only a small amount of anticoagulant, it is especially important to mix the contents of the bag frequently during phlebotomy.

Pregnancy

Phlebotomy for predeposit of autologous blood is not contraindicated during the second trimester of an uncomplicated pregnancy. Limited experience with predeposit phlebotomies in pregnant patients suggests that it may be best to avoid drawing blood from pregnant women in either the first or third trimester.[7] Autologous donations are extremely valuable in managing pregnancies in women with antibodies against high-incidence antigens, both to treat potential hemolytic disease of the newborn and to provide adequate supplies of blood for the mother, should she require transfusion.

Hemoglobin

Except in special circumstances, the hemoglobin concentration at each phlebotomy should be 11 g/dl or greater. Hematocrit, if used, should be 34% or greater. Below these levels phlebotomies should not be done, except with approval of the patient's physician and the blood bank physician.

Frequency of Donation

The frequency of bleeding for autologous transfusion should be determined by the medical director of the collecting facility in consultation with the patient's physician. Since 72 hours is required for synthesis and mobilization of protein and return of plasma volume to normal,[8] donations should be no more frequent than every three days, and the last phlebotomy should be at least 72 hours before an operation.

Iron Supplementation

The patient's ability to replace lost red cells and maintain adequate hemoglobin levels is a potential source of concern.[9] The rate of erythropoiesis is limited by body iron stores. When an autologous donor undergoes frequent phlebotomy, iron supplementation may be necessary to replenish iron stores. Either the blood bank physician or the referring physician may prescribe the iron, but communication should be adequate to ensure that the prescription has been made. Oral iron is as effective as parenteral iron in supporting intensive phlebotomy.[10] The usual adult dose is ferrous sulfate, 325 mg three times daily, taken with meals to prevent gastric upset. Iron supplementation should be started at least one week before the first donation and continued for several months after the last donation. With adequate iron supplementation, up to eight units of blood have been drawn within a 20-day period without causing unacceptable anemia.[10]

Initially, the hemoglobin decreases 1.0 to 1.5 gm/dl per unit donated, and reticulocyte count increases. Then the hematocrit stabilizes and may actually increase slightly in spite of continued donations.With intense stimulation and in the presence of adequate iron, the normal bone marrow can increase red cell production five to six times its normal level.

Techniques for Prolonged Storage

With prolonged liquid storage permissible with newer anticoagulant-preservative solutions, the "leapfrog" technique for multiple phlebotomies has become virtually obsolete. With this technique, autologous units approaching their expiration date were returned to the donor just after drawing a fresh unit. This exchange, or "leapfrog," technique[11] provided more and fresher units than could be achieved with serial phlebotomies and 21-day liquid storage. With a single venipuncture and a manual plasmapheresis set, the oldest unit was reinfused through the Y-connector of the set after one unit was drawn, and then a second unit drawn after reinfusion.

To preserve labile plasma proteins, units may be drawn into a double pack; the plasma can be expressed into the satellite container and frozen while still fresh, and the liquid packed cells stored under refrigeration. Cryoprecipitate or platelet concentrate could be prepared if desirable. All components prepared from autologous donations must be appropriately identified, and storage and expiration requirements are those dictated by *Standards* for that component.

Records

Complete donation records must be maintained for all autologous predeposited units (Chapter 21), as well as records for components, if these have been prepared.

Serologic Tests

Autologous blood products must be tested for ABO and Rh; for blood intended only for autologous use, testing for HBsAg and

unexpected antibodies is optional. These tests must be done and appropriate labels applied before unused autologous blood can be placed in the general inventory.

Accession procedures for autologous units should be similar to those for homologous units. Clerical and technical errors are less likely to occur when established and familiar procedures are followed. This may be particularly true when the number of autologous units processed is small.

Labeling

Blood for autologous transfusion should be labeled to reflect all testing that has been done. All routine tests may be done, but testing for HBsAg and for unexpected antibodies are not required. If a test has not been done, the label pertaining to that determination must not be applied. In many blood banks, specially colored tags (the uniform labeling code suggests green) are designated exclusively for autologous units. The following information must appear on special tags attached to the blood container[12]:

1. The patient's name
2. The patient's hospital registration number, or, if this is not available, the donor-patient's social security number, birthdate or other unique identification number. In some hospitals, patients can be preadmitted in order to be assigned the patient identification number that they will have during their hospitalization.
3. ABO and Rh group
4. Date of expiration of the donated unit

If the blood is subsequently made available for homologous transfusion, the special tag may be removed or obliterated, and the unit must be labeled with all information required by *Standards*.

Transfusing Autologous Blood

Identification

Before autologous blood is transfused, it is essential to identify the intended recipient as the donor of the predeposited units.

Transfusion to the wrong patient may result in an acute hemolytic transfusion reaction, or any of the adverse effects of homologous transfusion.

Pretransfusion Testing

Standards requires only that the potential recipient of autologous blood be tested for ABO and Rh before the expected transfusion. Most transfusion services find it desirable to treat the donor-recipient of autologous blood like every other potential transfusion recipient, and to perform pretransfusion antibody screening. This permits consistent application of standard procedures and ensures proper testing if the patient subsequently needs homologous blood.

The ABO group of the labeled autologous unit must be confirmed by the transfusing facility. Performing a crossmatch is optional, although many transfusion services perform an immediate-spin crossmatch before issuing the blood as a final precaution against catastrophic labeling or identification errors.

Records of Transfusion and Adverse Reactions

Transfusion records for autologous units should be identical to those required for homologous transfusions, except for the statement of compatibility if this test was not done. The transfusionist must verify that all identification procedures were done. In cases of exchange infusion for freshness ("leapfrogging"), a complete transfusion record, including the transfusionist's verification of identity, must be maintained for each unit reinfused.

Adverse effects following transfusion of autologous blood products must be investigated appropriately and the results documented. In addition to the possibility of mistaken identity, there could be contamination or physical damage to the stored blood, or altered therapeutic or immunologic conditions in the recipient. A patient may receive both autologous and homologous blood products, and maintaining identical transfusion records for both types of transfusion is desirable.

Release of Unused Autologous Blood

Unused autologous blood can be put into the regular inventory if the donor-patient meets all donor criteria intended to protect the recipient and has given given permission for such disposition of unused autologous blood. Questions about hepatitis exposure, travel in malarial areas and other requirements should be asked and the answers recorded at the time of phlebotomy. To ensure that unused autologous units do not outdate needlessly, transfusion service personnel should check with the physicians of autologous transfusion patients 48 hours after the operation. If a patient will not require additional transfusions, the physician should be asked to release the remaining autologous units. This release should be recorded. Upon release, autologous blood must be tested and labeled as *Standards* requires for homologous blood. Unused units unsuitable for release to routine inventory must be discarded in an appropriate manner.

Hemodilution and Short-Term Storage

For some operations, notably those involving cardiopulmonary bypass (CPB), one, or occasionally two, units of blood may be withdrawn just after induction of anesthesia. The patient's blood volume is restored with a hemodiluent, usually a combination of crystalloid and colloid solutions, to produce a state of normovolemic anemia. The extensive monitoring and, often, accompanying hypothermia permit substantial hemodilution without adverse effect. One advantage of the hemodilution technique is that fewer red cells are lost in a given volume of operative blood loss, so the requirement for subsequent homologous blood transfusion may be decreased.[13] After completion of the surgical procedure, diuretics are administered to reduce plasma volume and the autologous units infused to restore the patient's red cell mass. This blood, stored only a few hours, contains viable platelets and may elevate the patient's postoperative platelet count.[13,14] The blood, if properly collected, may be kept at room temperature for up to 6 hours. Careful monitoring is essential to minimize the intraoperative risks of hemodilution and avoid fluid overload when the procedure ends. Since the units are drawn and remain stored in the operating room, personnel from the tranfusion service are not directly involved but can contribute by helping develop protocols for appropriate labeling and storage.

Sometimes blood is drained from the extracorporeal circuit and sent to the blood bank for processing. The red cells can be washed to remove heparin and excess diluting fluid and resuspended in saline as a red cell concentrate.[15] Precise identification and labeling with transfusion service accession number, patient's name and hospital number, date and hour are important when blood is processed in the blood bank and then (or later) returned to the operating suite or recovery room to be infused. Infusion must be within 24 hours and storage must be at temperatures of 1 to 6 C.

Complete written protocols should be developed for autologous transfusion procedures even if they are performed entirely in the surgery suite. The techniques prescribed should be safe and aseptic, and should ensure accurate identification of all blood collected.

Intraoperative Blood Salvage

During intraoperative blood salvage, blood is aspirated from the operative site, processed in various ways depending on the equipment used, and reinfused, usually immediately. This procedure makes large volumes of blood immediately available during massive bleeding but is contraindicated if there is gross contamination of the blood by microorganisms from, for example, intestinal contents or if there is a strong likelihood that malignant tumor cells are present. Blood collected by intraoperative salvage may not be transfused to any patient other than the autologous donor.

At least four autotransfusion devices have been used clinically and their advantages and disadvantages reported.[1,16,17] Indications for intraoperative salvage and reinfusion depend on the system used. Possible complications include: hemolysis; thrombocytopenia, hypofibrinogenemia and DIC; and if pressurized rather than gravity flow is utilized, air embolism. As equipment for collection, microfiltration, washing and concentration improves, intraoperative autologous transfusion is achieving some popularity. Its use in trauma and ruptured ectopic pregnancy has already proved acceptable.[18,19]

A written protocol is required for intraoperative blood salvage procedures. The protocol should include criteria for dosage of ancillary agents used and for the prevention and treatment of patient reactions.[12] The medical director of the transfusion service should assist in preparing the protocol, which should be approved by the appropriate hospital committee.

Use of Other Autologous Components

Although most autologous transfusion programs involve collecting, storing and transfusing red cells, other components may also be predonated for subsequent use. Among these are fresh frozen plasma, platelets, granulocytes and stem cells. Autologous platelet transfusion is useful in two clinical situations. Platelets may be collected by hemapheresis immediately prior to surgery, stored at room temperature and infused at the end of the procedure to aid in hemostasis. In leukemic patients, platelets may be collected by apheresis during remission, and stored frozen until the patient relapses, at which point they may be thawed and used to support remission induction.[20] Since some transfused patients ultimately become refractory to random-donor and, sometimes, HLA-matched platelets, their own platelets harvested during remission can be important in replacement therapy.

Although it is difficult to preserve granulocyte function after frozen storage, recent reports suggest that it may be possible to cryopreserve granulocytes in a manner analogous to preservation of platelets.[21] Granulocytes thus harvested from leukemic patients in remission, or from patients with other malignancies scheduled to receive high-dose chemotherapy, could be used to sustain the patient during a period of bone marrow aplasia associated with granulocytopenia and sepsis.

An area of intense investigation has been techniques for cryopreserving hematopoietic stem cells for autologous bone marrow transplantation or reconstitution.[22] This is particularly well-suited to treatment of tumors that rarely invade the bone marrow, so there is minimal possibility of cryopreserving and reinfusing malignant cells along with marrow stem cells. Another approach is to incubate the stem cell preparation with tumor-specific monoclonal antibodies prior to storage and/or reinfusion. The availability of autologous stem cells should enable clinicians to administer extremely high-dose chemotherapy to individuals with refractory tumors, without fear of inducing irreversible bone marrow aplasia.

References

1. Brzica SM, Pineda AA, Taswell HF. Autologous blood transfusion. CRC Crit Rev Clin Lab Sci 1979;10:31-55.

2. Newmann MM, Hamstra R, Block M. Use of banked autologous blood in elective surgery. JAMA 1971;218:861-63.

3. Cuello L, Vasquez E, Perez V, Raffucci FL. Autologous blood transfusion in cardiovascular surgery. Transfusion 1967;7:309-315.

4. Silvergleid AJ. Autologous transfusions, experience in a community blood center. JAMA 1979;241:2724-2725.

5. Sandler, SG. Overview. In: Sandler SG, Silvergleid A, eds. Autologous transfusion. Arlington, VA: American Association of Blood Banks, 1983:8.

6. Fleming AW, Green DC, Radcliffe JH, St. James DM, Fleming EW. Development of a practical autologous blood transfusion program. Am Surg 1977;43:794-801.

7. Mann M, Sacks HJ, Goldfinger D. Safety of autologous blood donation prior to elective surgery for a variety of potentially "high-risk" patients.Transfusion 1983;23:229-32.

8. Adamson J, Hillman RS. Blood volume and plasma protein replacement following acute blood loss in normal men. JAMA 1968;205:609-612.

9. Finch CA, Cook JD, Labbe RF, Culala M. Effect of blood donation on iron stores as evaluated by serum ferritin. Blood 1977;50:441-448.

10. Zuck TF, Bergin JJ. Adequacy of oral iron to support erythropoiesis during intensive phlebotomy for autologous transfusion. XIII International Transfusion Congress, Washington, DC (abstract) 1972:49.

11. Ascari WQ, Jolly PC, Thomas PA. Autologous blood transfusion in pulmonary surgery. Transfusion 1968;8:111-115.

12. Schmidt PJ, ed. Standards for blood banks and transfusion services of the American Association of Blood Banks, 11th ed. Arlington, VA: American Association of Blood Banks, 1984.

13. Silver H. Banked and fresh autologous blood in cardiopulmonary bypass surgery. Transfusion 1975;15:600-603.

14. Ochsner JL, Mills NL, Leonard GL, Lawson N. Fresh autologous blood transfusions with extracorporeal circulation. Ann Surg 1973;177:811-816.

15. Milam JD, Austin SF. Red cell salvage in open heart surgery. In:Hemotherapy in trauma and surgery. Washington, DC: American Association of Blood Banks, 1979:67-75.

16. Gilcher RO, Orr M. Intraoperative blood salvage. In: Hemotherapy in trauma and surgery, Washington, DC: American Association of Blood Banks, 1979:57-66.

17. Silvergleid AJ. Reviving an old technique: Autologous transfusion.Diagnostic Medicine, November/December, 1981.

18. Mattox KL, Walker LE, Beall AC, Jordan GL. Blood availability for the trauma patient—autotransfusion. J Trauma 1975;15:633-639.

19. Merrill BS, Mills DL, Rogers W, Weinberg PC. Autotransfusion intraoperative use in ruptured ectopic pregnancy. J Reprod Med 1980;24:14-16.

20. Schiffer CA, Aisner J, Wiernik PH. Frozen autologous platelet transfusion for patients with leukemia. N Engl J Med 1978;299:7-12

21. Zaroulis CG, Leiderman IZ, Lee SC. Freeze-preservations of human granulocytes for transfusion therapy, abstracted. Clin Res 1979;27:310A.

22. Dicke KA. Autologous bone-marrow transplantation in relapsed adult leukemia. Lancet 1979;1:514.

23. Dixon JL, Smalley MG. Jehovah's Witnesses. The surgical/ethical challenge. JAMA 1981;246:2471-2472.

24. Findley LJ, Redstone PM. Blood transfusion in adult Jehovah's Witnesses. A case study of one congregation. Arch Intern Med 1982;142:606-607.

The best guarantee of safe transfusion is careful adherence to standard procedures. Most transfusion disasters result from carelessness, specifically from inaccurate identification of the donor, donor specimen, donor unit, patient, patient's blood specimen or requisition forms.[1] Meticulous accuracy is essential in all aspects of clinical contact, laboratory technique and record keeping. Quality assurance programs monitor whether equipment and procedures fulfill their expected functions, and whether personnel perform these procedures in approved, reproducible fashion. Quality assurance programs must be practical and realistic. Testing should not be excessively time-consuming nor should it result in the accumulation of unnecessary data.

General Considerations

Procedures Manual

Each blood bank and transfusion service must prepare and maintain an up-to-date procedures manual containing directions for all procedures performed, including all quality assurance procedures. It is desirable to include examples of forms on which test results and interpretations are recorded, and directions for the maintenance and disposition of these records. This manual should also contain written and/or pictorial descriptions of how to read,

score and record all test results and interpretations. When procedures are added to or replaced in the manual, the new instructions should be marked with the date they went into effect; material removed from the manual should be retained for at least 5 years, and the date of removal should be recorded. It is desirable to devise a system to document that all personnel are aware of changes in the procedures manual.

Checking Results and Records

When the consequences of erroneous testing or interpretations are potentially catastrophic, it is often desirable to have two different people perform the tests independently and then compare the results and interpretations. This is most effectively done with ABO and Rh testing on donors and patients, and with labeling procedures. Unfortunately, even repeated checking does not guarantee that discrepancies will be detected. Once an error slips through the initial check, it tends to be perpetuated. All personnel should be instructed in the importance of confirming all data.

Checking results previously obtained on the same individual helps monitor accurate identification and also allows observation of significant changes in serologic status. *Standards*[2] requires that, for potential transfusion recipients, current findings be checked against records of ABO and Rh tests done in the preceding 12 months and records of significant antibodies, transfusion reactions or difficulties in typing within at least the preceding 5 years. Checking previous results on donors is not required, but is a desirable form of quality assurance.

Proficiency Testing

Standards requires that each blood bank and transfusion service participate in a proficiency testing program. Independently administered programs such as those of the American Association of Blood Banks, the College of American Pathologists or governmental agencies, allow comparison among many participating laboratories and help evaluate the procedures, equipment, materials and personnel of the individual blood bank or transfusion service. Specimens tested as part of proficiency testing should not receive special handling; testing should be rotated among all personnel who routinely perform the specific procedure. There must be a record that supervisory personnel have reviewed the results and evaluations, and that appropriate corrective actions are taken if needed. Periodic replicate, independent or blind testing is helpful in ensuring that all personnel adhere to testing standards and apply them uniformly.

Review Committee and Adverse Effects

It is required by *Standards* and by regulations of other inspecting agencies that transfusion services establish a means to review transfusion practices and record conclusions and recommendations. This is discussed in more detail in Chapter 22. Appropriate topics for review include usage of blood and components, reports of adverse reactions and reports of disease transmission.

There must be a mechanism to obtain reports of adverse transfusion reactions, including posttransfusion hepatitis. Doc-

umented posttransfusion hepatitis must be reported to the facility that collected the transfused units. Transfusion services should establish guidelines for identifying units implicated in posttransfusion hepatitis. Some medical directors report the identification numbers of individual units if the patient received 10 or fewer donor units. If hepatitis develops in the recipient of huge numbers of components, it is not necessary to identify and report every donor identification number. Fatalities resulting directly from transfusion, notably hemolytic transfusion reactions, must be reported to the Office of Biologics.[3] Cases of AIDS suspected of association with transfusion should be reported to the Centers for Disease Control.

Reporting Abnormal Findings

Standards requires that donors be informed of clinically significant abnormal results found in predonation examination and laboratory testing. It is mandatory to inform the donor of positive results on HBsAg testing. The procedures manual of each blood center should include policy on what additional information is to be given to the donor or the donor's physician, and how the information is to be conveyed.

Continuing Education

Standards requires that there be ". . . an adequate and competent staff." One way to document this is to establish a check list of the procedures required for each position, and then document that each individual hired into or occupying the position demonstrate satisfactory performance of each procedure. Appropriately written position descriptions should be available for each category of employment, but the general information in a position description does not substitute for evidence of competence in specific procedures.

Personnel should participate in some form of continuing education. This should include individuals on all shifts and those who work only part-time in the blood bank, not just fulltime daytime employees. Continuing education may include many activities beyond attendance at outside meetings. In-house activities can include reading assignments, written exercises or formal presentations by staff members or by invited guests. Records should be kept for each individual to document the nature of the activity, the subject matter and the date.

Equipment

Properly functioning equipment is essential for accurate testing. All instruments must be properly maintained, cleaned and monitored. Temperature-regulated equipment must be checked for correct temperature each day of use and the results and interpretations recorded and kept for at least 1 year. Corrective action must be documented when temperatures are outside prescribed ranges or instruments fail to function as expected.

Centrifuges for Serologic Testing

Centrifuges are used in serologic testing to enhance red cell antigen-antibody reactions and to wash cell suspensions. Two types of table-top centrifuge are in common use. One has fixed speed and variable time; the other can vary both speed and time. The number of rotations per minute (rpm) must be checked periodically with an optical or electronic device and the results recorded. The time of centrifugation, which includes the time of acceleration but not deceleration, can be checked with a stopwatch.

Continuous Observations

For washing cell suspensions and for enhancing agglutination, centrifugation should bring the cells together in a well-defined button, but should not pack the cells so tightly that unagglutinated cells cannot be resuspended with gentle manipulation. A clearly delineated cell button is a small round dot surrounded by clear supernatant fluid. The periphery of the cell button should be sharply defined,

not fuzzy. The best quality control mechanism is careful observation of results obtained in daily use. Each time the centrifuge is used the technologist should observe red cell buttons for any departure from the usual pattern. If deterioration or inconsistencies are noted, the centrifuge may need recalibration or repair.

Many variables affect the results of centrifugation. The automatic timer may be poorly aligned or the set screw not tightened properly. The set screw can be tightened and the timer set correctly to match preexisting time intervals marked on the face of the timer, or timing can be checked with a stopwatch and the correction marked on the face of the timer. The time of acceleration varies from one centrifuge to another and depends on the load on the head. The viscosity of the medium also affects sedimentation of the suspended cells; red cells suspended in 30% albumin, for example, require longer or faster centrifugation than cells in normal saline to achieve a similar degree of packing.

Specific Testing

Optimum speed and time of centrifugation for different procedures should be marked on the outside of the centrifuge. All observations should be recorded permanently in the quality assurance records. Each centrifuge should be calibrated on receipt and after repairs to find the speed and time that maximally enhance agglutination without causing false-positive reactions. A calibration procedure that may be used for either fixed-speed or variable-speed serologic centrifuges is in the Special Methods section, page 475.

Automatic Cell Washers

Because antiglobulin serum is inactivated so readily by unbound immunoglobulin, the antiglobulin test must be done on red cells washed free of all proteins and suspended in a protein-free medium. Properly functioning cell washers must add large volumes of saline to each tube, resuspend the cells adequately, centrifuge cleanly and decant the saline to leave a dry cell button. Automatic cell washers may be monitored as follows:

1. To each of 12 tubes (10 × 75 mm or 12 × 75 mm) add two drops of bovine albumin, 2 or 3 drops of donor or patient serum, and 1 drop of presensitized red blood cells that give a 1 to 2 + reaction in antiglobulin testing.
2. Place tubes in centrifuge carrier and seat carrier in the cell washer. Start wash cycles.
3. After addition of saline in second cycle, stop cell washer. Observe all tubes. There should be an equal volume of saline in all tubes. (Check manufacturer's directions for correct amount of saline.) Tubes should not be more than 80% full to avoid cross-contamination by splash.
4. Observe all tubes to see that the red cell button has been completely resuspended. Cells should not stream on the sides of the test tubes.
5. Continue washing cycle.
6. After third wash and decant cycle, stop cell washer and observe all tubes to see that saline has been completely decanted, leaving a dry cell button. The size of the cell button should be the same in all tubes and should be the same size as at the start of the wash cycle.
7. Complete wash cycle. Add antiglobulin serum according to manufacturer's directions, centrifuge and read all tubes for agglutination. If the cell washer is functioning properly, all tubes should show agglutination.

Further investigation is needed if:

1. There is variation in the amount of saline.
2. The red cell button is not resuspended completely.
3. There is not agglutination in the antiglobulin phase.
4. There is a significant decrease in the size of the red cell button.

Cell washers that automatically add antiglobulin serum should be checked further to be sure that they are adding antiglobulin serum. In step 7 above, the antiglobulin serum would be added automatically, and failure of addition would be apparent by absence of agglutination. The volume of antiglobulin serum should be inspected and found to be equal in all tubes. Many manufacturers market antiglobulin serum colored with green dye for use in these cell washers so that it will be obvious immediately if the reagent has not been added. The volume of antiglobulin serum delivered by these cell washers should be checked periodically to see that the volume delivered is that specified in the manufacturer's directions and that delivery is uniform in all tubes.

If the cell washer is used for other serologic procedures and if the cycles for timing and speed are adjustable, it can be calibrated with the procedure (see page 475) for variable-speed and fixed-speed serologic centrifuges.

Rh Viewboxes

When Rh testing is done on a slide, the reaction mixture should be subjected to a temperature approximating 37 C. Lighted viewboxes provide this added warmth and make reading easier. The surface of the viewbox should remain between 40 C and 50 C.[4] The temperature should be read and recorded daily.

Waterbaths, Heat Blocks and Incubators

Tests to detect warm-reactive antibodies must be incubated at 37 C, unless appropriate alternative methods have been adopted. Tubes may be incubated either in waterbaths or heat blocks. For most tests, the incubation time can be the same in waterbaths and heat blocks because the small volumes used in serologic testing achieve the desired temperatures so rapidly. It may be desirable to measure how long it takes a standard volume to achieve

37 C and to determine whether changes in volume or incubation time appreciably alter the test results. It may prove necessary to vary the incubation time with the volume incubated and the equipment used. Incubation times should be posted on each incubation device used.

Heat blocks occasionally show a difference in temperature between individual cells. This should be determined when the equipment is received and should be monitored thereafter. The functioning temperature of each piece of heat-regulated equipment must be tested at a single point each day of use. These observations and any corrective action must be recorded.

Waterbaths used to thaw frozen components must have the temperature noted and recorded daily; immediately before each use, the technologist should check the temperature to ensure that temperatures are not unexpectedly high or low. Temperatures may drop if several frozen units are incubated in a small volume of water. If the same waterbath is used for thawing components and for incubating serologic tests, it is important to ensure that the temperature has returned to 37 C before tubes are incubated. A schedule for regular cleaning of the waterbath is recommended.

There must be a means to prevent contact between the entry ports of the blood container and water which may contain bacteria. Use of an overwrap or of a device to keep the partially submerged bags upright will accomplish this.

Thermometers

Thermometers should be monitored on receipt for accuracy and consistency at the temperature of intended use. If available, a thermometer certified by the National Bureau of Standards (NBS) should be used for comparison. Thermometers described as traceable to an NBS thermometer may be the only ones available. It is desirable, if this is the case, to test such thermometers on receipt for consistent temperature

indication, even if it is not possible to determine accuracy. The greatest amount of information can be obtained with the least effort if many thermometers are tested at once.

1. Tag each thermometer with an identifying number, including the NBS thermometer if available.
2. Place all the thermometers in a vessel containing water at a temperature approximately 4 C below the temperature of intended use. For the temperature range 1-6 C, add salt and ice to the water to bring the temperature below 0 C.
3. Observe and record the temperature shown on each thermometer.
4. Slowly warm the water, stirring appropriately, into the range of intended use and up to about 4 C above the expected upper limit.
5. At intervals of 1-2 C, observe and record the temperature shown on each thermometer.

Interpretation: All thermometers should be within ± 1 C of the NBS thermometer or the thermometer traceable to an NBS thermometer. Return to the supplier any that do not meet this expectation. If individual thermometers show a consistent deviation from the standard, label them with a permanent tag stating the magnitude and direction of the deviation; for example, "add 0.5 C." If a thermometer shows an inconsistent deviation of more than 1 C from the standard or from the readings of the other thermometers, it should be returned to the supplier.

Blood Warmers

There must be surveillance of blood warmers used in a transfusion service. It is not necessary for transfusion service personnel to perform this testing; employees of a consulting service or personnel in the departments of anesthesia, surgery, maintenance or biomedical engineering may do the tests and record the results. The director of the blood bank or transfusion service must, however, ensure that this is done and that the records are available. If this is not possible, there must be explicit documentation from the responsible body of the hospital, stating in writing that the transfusion service director is not to have responsibility for the operation and performance checks of the blood warmers.

Blood warmers must have a visible thermometer and should have an audible alarm that sounds if the temperature of the blood approaches unacceptably high levels. The actual temperature of the warming unit should be checked with a thermometer applied to the warming surface or with a thermocouple probe, and the temperature reading on the built-in thermometer should be checked against the reading on the monitoring thermometer.

It is desirable to simulate a warmed transfusion by passing fluid through the instrument and measuring its temperature as it leaves the unit. At flow rates usually used for infusion, refrigerated blood or even blood that has been at room temperature during the infusion process seldom reaches 37 C. With very slow flow or during a temporary interruption of infusion, however, the blood may undergo prolonged contact with the warming surface. Allowing the test fluid to remain stationary in the unit for 10 or 15 minutes will give some idea of the maximum warming that could occur.

The alarm system is ordinarily activated by the temperature of the warming device, not by the temperature of the fluid; it is not possible or desirable to raise the temperature of the heating unit in order to test the alarm. In some units, the alarm can be checked by slowly running through the unit fluid heated to approximately 40 C.

Irradiators

If a device is used to irradiate blood or components, it must be monitored to ensure accurate delivery of the designated dose and to prevent radiation leakage. This testing is usually performed by the institution's radiation safety department, at approximately 6-month intervals. The director of the blood bank or transfusion service should ensure that this testing is done and that the records are available.

Refrigerators and Freezers

There must be a system to monitor temperatures of blood bank refrigerators and freezers as well as an alarm system to warn personnel before storage temperatures reach unacceptable limits. There must be continuous surveillance of temperature, but intermittent recording is permissible. With standard recorders, a continuous written record is generated, but electronic systems that generate periodic printouts are acceptable, provided temperatures are recorded at least every 4 hours. Pronounced temperature fluctuations shown on the written records must be explained, in writing, on the record sheet (eg "alarm check," "cleaned"). Chapter 3 presents a detailed discussion of storage requirements, and procedures for checking alarms are on pages 478–480.

Reagents

Since commercial antisera and reagent red blood cell products are licensed by the Office of Biologics, the manufacturer must demonstrate that they meet minimum standards for specificity and potency before they are licensed. It is neither necessary nor meaningful for individual users to test reagent antisera for titer or avidity. The essential fact that each laboratory must confirm is that each reagent on each day of use reacts as expected when used as described in the facility's procedures manual. If the local procedure differs from that recommended by the manufacturer, there should be documentation that the modification gives satisfactory results.

For nonlicensed reagents that are locally produced, there must be records of reactivity and specificity. IgG-coated red cells and A and B cells for reverse grouping may be prepared locally, with records documenting only their reactivity and specificity. Reagents for all other required tests must be shown to meet or exceed FDA criteria, a requirement that precludes local preparation of most reagents except at very well-equipped centers.

Records of quality assurance testing must include identification of the personnel involved, the source and identification numbers of all reagents tested, the date of testing, and the source and nature of controls, when used.

Antisera

The manufacturer's directions should be reviewed for changes with each new lot number and the package inserts saved from every lot in use. Procedural modifications used in individual blood banks or transfusion services must not conflict with the directions of the manufacturer. Antisera may lose potency or specificity or both, due to poor storage or shipping conditions. Contamination during preparation or use can also impair reactivity. Admixture with other antisera or blood products or contamination with microorganisms are the usual offenders. Reagents should be observed at each use for abnormal appearance, cloudiness or turbidity and should be refrigerated when not in use.

Frozen Storage

Freezing is not recommended for storing most commercially prepared reagents, which often contain additives adversely affected by freezing. Antibody-containing sera and other materials prepared locally without preservatives are often frozen for extended storage. Because repeated freezing and thawing damages proteins, sera should be frozen in aliquots of the volume appropriate for individual use. Frozen sera should be thawed at 37 C and mixed thoroughly before use. Frozen reagents, like any other reagent that is not subjected to daily quality assurance surveillance, should be monitored at the time

of use by testing against appropriately selected controls.

Testing Specificity

Antisera must be tested each day of use, preferably before use or concomitantly with the first tests. Since direct and reverse ABO grouping constitute a built-in check on specificity, it is not necessary to perform additional tests on these sera and cells, provided that an adequate number of consistent results have been observed with those reagent lots on the previous day, and that the observation and interpretation are suitably recorded. In small laboratories, it may not be possible to accumulate a sufficient number of test results, and direct testing should then be done.

Seldom-used antisera should be monitored with control cells at the time the test is performed. Positive and negative controls are usually employed, but controls should be used with discretion to preserve rare sera and cells. If several samples are being tested with antibody against a high-incidence antigen, a negative control is important because positive results are expected and would serve as their own control. Similarly, a positive control but not a negative one is indicated for antibodies against low-incidence antigens. Red blood cells with a weakly reactive example of the antigen provide a better test of antibody potency and specificity than cells with the antigen strongly expressed. If control cells are selected from a pretested panel of group O cells it is best to use a cell heterozygous for the antigenic determinant.

Reagent Red Cells

Red cells used for ABO grouping and for antibody identification may be obtained from commercial suppliers or may be prepared locally from selected donors of known red cell phenotypes. *Standards* requires that cells used for antibody detection tests meet or exceed FDA criteria. Cells used for antibody identification are not subject to specific criteria, and in many laboratories locally available cells are used to confirm or amplify results obtained with commercially available cell panels.

Suspensions of reagent red cells should be inspected visually for evidence of hemolysis each day of use. If the degree of hemolysis is such that a single wash removes the hemoglobin-stained supernatant fluid, the cells can be used satisfactorily as a freshly prepared saline suspension.

When not in use, all reagent red cells should be refrigerated.

Red Cells for Antibody Detection and Identification

It is not feasible to test each cell each day for each antigen. Each cell used in the antibody detection test should be tested daily for reactivity of one antigen. The test may be in any phase of the test procedure, but should simulate as closely as possible clinical conditions with patients' sera; use of actual serum specimens is ideal, but it may be necessary to use diluted reagent antisera. The degree of desired reactivity should be 1 to 2 +. Antibodies that give stronger reactions will not detect minor changes in cell behavior. Maximum information can be obtained with minimum effort if at least one cell is tested with an antibody reactive only in the antiglobulin phase. This documents the reactivity of the antiglobulin serum as well as the integrity of the reagent cell. If antibody-containing serum from a donor or patient is used, it should be stored as small frozen aliquots for individual use.

Serum to Cell Ratio

Personnel in most blood banks use disposable Pasteur-type pipettes to deliver serum in antibody and compatibility testing. These pipettes vary greatly in the size of the drop delivered. A recent study[5] showed that the number of drops delivered per ml serum varied from 21 to 43. The same study showed that the droppers in commercial vials of reagent red cells delivered between 18 and 28 drops per ml. The ratio of serum to cells affects the sensitivity of antibody detection, the optimum ratio being 80:1. (See page 83 for more detailed discussion.)

It is not necessary to test each pipette for volume delivered, but personnel in each laboratory should determine the average drop size and volume delivered by the transfer pipettes and red cell droppers in local use. Once the average delivery volume has been determined, the directions for antibody detection and compatability testing should designate volumes that assure the optimum 80:1 serum-to-cell ratio. Cell suspensions should be consistently prepared and all personnel should use the same techniques once the local reagents and equipment have been standardized.

Antiglobulin Testing

Most unexpected antibodies that cause red cell destruction are IgG; it is the anti-IgG in polyspecific antiglobulin serum that detects most clinically significant antibody activity in antibody detection tests and crossmatching. Anticomplement activity is most useful in detecting immune coating of circulating red blood cells (direct antiglobulin test), although anticomplement may provide the only means of detecting occasional weakly reactive examples of complement-binding antibodies, especially in the Kidd blood group system.

Antiglobulin Serum

In daily quality assurance testing it is sufficient to test antiglobulin serum for anti-IgG only. Anticomplement activity can be checked, if desired, against complement-coated cells prepared as described in steps 1-4 on page 457, but this need not be a routine procedure. *Standards* requires that IgG-coated cells be added as the final check on negative results obtained when antiglobulin serum is used in antibody screening tests or crossmatches. These cells should be lightly coated, to give no more than 2 + macroscopic reactions. In daily quality assurance testing, adding antiglobulin serum to the IgG-coated cells provides a simultaneous check for both reagents. Heavily coated cells may not detect subtle loss of anti-IgG activity. For example, a difference in reactivity between 4 + macroscopically and 2 + macroscopically is not as readily apparent as a difference between 2 + macroscopically and a negative result.

Opened vials of antiglobulin serum should be tested each day of use to ensure their activity. Loss of potency may result from inadvertent contamination with human serum or other reagents, or, less often, from deterioration during storage.

Checking Negative Results

Negative results in antiglobulin procedures can be confirmed by adding red cells lightly coated with IgG antibody, repeating centrifugation and reading. Agglutination at this point indicates that antiglobulin serum present in the test was not inactivated by unbound globulins or diluted by excess residual saline, and that the negative results reflect true absence of reactivity in the test. Using green antiglobulin serum does not substitute for this control. The presence of dye in the tube merely indicates that antiglobulin serum was added, and does not ensure antiglobulin activity.

Donor Processing

Interview, physical examination and other screening of prospective donors should be performed in suitably private conditions by skilled, well-trained personnel. Guidelines for conducting the donor screening and physical examination are described in Chapter 1.

Hemoglobin or Hematocrit

Hemoglobin or hematocrit can be determined by a variety of standard methods. Estimation of acceptable hemoglobin by use of copper sulfate solutions is imprecise but simple, quick and adequate. The microhematocrit is simple and accurate, but noisy, time-consuming and requires special equipment. Very few donor operations employ the most accurate test, which is quantitative measurement of hemoglobin.

Microhematocrit Centrifuge

The microhematocrit centrifuge should be calibrated when first placed in service, after repairs and annually thereafter. The timer and speed should be checked more often, perhaps every 3 months to 6 months. A calibration method that provides quality surveillance and allows selection of optimum centrifugation times is to examine replicate specimens of red cell suspensions within, below and above the acceptable hematocrit range. The time selected for routine use should be the minimum time at which maximum packing occurs. Deviation of 2% between replicate tubes is acceptable.

1. Thoroughly mix anticoagulated samples of blood from individuals with known hematocrits, one within the normal range, one below, and one above. The hematocrit can be raised by removing plasma from an anticoagulated specimen.
2. For each sample, fill replicate microhematocrit tubes to within ½ inch of the top and seal. Fill sufficient tubes to allow testing at a range of centrifugation times between 2 and 10 minutes.
3. Place one pair from each sample in the microhematocrit centrifuge and spin for 2 minutes.
4. Observe color of packed red cells and plasma. The red cell column should be uniform, the plasma clear and transparent, and the line of demarcation sharp.
5. Measure and record the hematocrits.
6. Repeat steps 3 through 5 for times up to and including 10 minutes and compare hematocrit values for each specimen at each time of spin.
7. For routine use choose the shortest centrifugation time that leads to the lowest measured hematocrit.

Copper Sulfate Procedure

Adequacy of a donor's hemoglobin level is often determined indirectly by demonstrating a minimum specific gravity of the donor's whole blood, tested with a copper sulfate solution. This procedure is subject to more variation and intrinsic error than the microhematocrit method, but is widely used because large numbers of donors can be processed in minimal time with very little equipment. Solutions should be changed daily or after 25 tests. Before use, the solutions should be mixed thoroughly and be at room temperature. The solution used to test females has a specific gravity of 1.053, equivalent to 12.5 gm/dl hemoglobin; that for males, 1.055, equivalent to 13.5 gm/dl hemoglobin. The containers should be clearly and conspicuously marked. Copper sulfate solutions should not be frozen or exposed to very high temperatures and stock solutions should be tightly sealed during storage. Specific gravity may change due to contamination or evaporation. The specific gravity should be checked periodically with a calibrated hydrometer. Functional monitoring of the test method can be performed as follows:

1. Obtain anticoagulated samples of blood from individuals with known hemoglobin values. Use several specimens that fall in the lower 0.5 to 1.0 gm/dl of the allowable range for male and female donors and several that are 0.5 to 1.5 gm/dl below each cutoff point. Testing bloods with high hemoglobin does not give useful information.

2. Add one drop of blood from the acceptable samples to each solution, from a height of about 1 cm. If the specific gravity of the copper sulfate is satisfactory, the drop will sink within 15 seconds. If not, the sinking drop will hesitate, remain suspended or rise to the top of the solution.

3. If the drop of blood does not sink, repeat the test on a fresh aliquot of copper sulfate solution.

4. Repeat step 2 for the samples that are below the allowable range. All these drops should remain suspended or rise to the top.

If there is not clear distinction between permissible and unacceptable donors, the solutions should be changed, or a different method of screening donors should be considered. Copper sulfate screening is not a quantitative procedure. Specific measurement of hemoglobin or hematocrit may indicate that a donor rejected by the copper sulfate procedure is, after all, acceptable.

Volume of Blood Drawn

The volume of blood collected must be controlled to protect the donor from excessive loss of blood and to maintain the correct proportion of anticoagulant and blood in the transfusion components. Several kinds of equipment may be used:

1. A trip balance that constricts the tubing to stop blood flow when the phlebotomy bag reaches the desired weight.

2. A vacuum-assisted mechanical agitator calibrated to shut off when the desired weight is achieved.

3. A platform scale that must be kept under observation so that the phlebotomist can stop the blood flow manually when sufficient blood has been drawn.

Weight of Whole Blood

All these methods use weight to indicate the volume of blood drawn. This is the weight of the final product, including bag, tubing and anticoagulant-preservative solution, as well as the fluid blood. The volume of blood must be 450 ± 45 ml. One milliliter of blood weighs not less than 1.053 gm, the weight of blood from a female donor with a hemoglobin of 12.5 gm/dl, so the final container should weigh no less than 426 gm (1.053 gm/ml × 405 ml) plus the weight of the container and its anticoagulant. It is recommended that this weight be determined and posted for the brand of bag in use as products from different manufacturers can vary considerably. The maximum weight is harder to specify, since donors may have variably high hematocrits. Since anticoagulant effectiveness declines with increasing hematocrit and increasing volumes of blood, a practical maximum is 522 gm (1.055 gm/ml × 495 ml) plus the weight of the container and anticoagulant.

Note: some 500 ml bags are in use. The volume they contain must be 500 ± 50 ml.

Monitoring Weight

A simple method to determine if the equipment used in blood collection is functioning properly is to record the weight, determined on a scale or balance, of the first one or two units of blood collected each day with each scale or agitator. This fulfills the requirement that donor scales or other such devices be checked each day of use. If a scale or vacuum-assisted agitator consistently overdraws or underdraws or consistently produces units at one end of the allowable range, it should be recalibrated to bring it nearer to the mean acceptable drawing volume. A procedure for calibrating vacuum-assisted devices may be found in the Special Methods section, page 477.

The performance of platform scales and trip balances can be checked with prefilled bags of known weight. A bag of correct weight should activate the constrictor and register the accurate weight on the scale, while one that weighs less than the minimum should not activate the trip mechanism.

Donor Reactions

The number, type and severity of reactions before, during and after phlebotomy must be recorded and should be evaluated by supervisory personnel and the responsible physician. Any follow-up investigations and actions taken should also be made a part of the record. If reactions increase at certain times of the year, the donor room temperature may need improving. If a higher percentage of donor reactions

can be attributed to one or two phlebotomists, it may be necessary to work with these people individually to improve their techniques and/or confidence.

Labeling

Among the most important steps in safe transfusion practice is careful identification and proper labeling of the donor unit and its associated processing tubes. The crossmatch must be done on cells from a sealed segment of tubing originally attached to the unit of blood itself, but blood samples in tubes numbered and filled at the time of phlebotomy are used in tests for ABO and Rh groups, and for detection of unexpected antibodies and hepatitis B surface antigen. The laboratory that processes donor blood must ensure that the unique number assigned to the donor appears on the donor card, the primary collection bag, all satellite collection bags and all tubes used for processing. This allows prompt identification of the relevant specimen if any processing tests reveal abnormalities or discrepant results.

Blood Components

Quality assurance for component preparation includes in vitro assays to document the effective collection of specific elements or coagulation factors. Observations of posttransfusion effectiveness are often helpful, if available, but are not required. Considerations of donor selection, volume of blood drawn, and accuracy of scales and anticoagulant volume apply to component preparation as well as to whole blood.

Platelets
Calibrating Centrifuges

Centrifuges should always be level. Special attention to leveling is necessary when centrifuges are installed at mobile drawing facilities. Each centrifuge should be calibrated to determine the optimum times and speeds of centrifugation. A procedure may be found in the Special Methods section, page 476.

After the centrifuge has been calibrated, tachometer readings at the selected speed setting should be recorded. If possible, the centrifuge lid should be closed during measurement. After initial calibration, revolutions per minute can be measured every 6 months. If the reading does not vary, and quality assurance testing of the product is satisfactory, the centrifuge need not be recalibrated, but calibration must be performed after repairs. Records must be maintained of calibration data, tachometer readings, temperature, maintenance and repairs.

Testing Platelets

Facilities that regularly prepare platelets should evaluate at least four concentrates monthly for platelet count, volume and pH. Samples should be selected to represent each centrifuge in use. This testing must be done when the platelets are at the end of the allowable storage period and the concentrate should be well mixed before a sample is withdrawn. The temperature at which the pH is measured must be the same at which the concentrate is stored. A volume statement must be on the label and the actual volume must be ± 10% of that stated volume.

The following formula is used to determine the number of platelets in each concentrate:

Platelet count/mm^3 × 1000 × volume (ml) = number of platelets in the platelet concentrate.

FDA regulations[6] and AABB *Standards* require that there be at least 5.5×10^{10} platelets in 75% of platelet concentrates tested at the end of the allowable storage period. The platelets must be suspended in sufficient plasma that pH determined at the temperature of storage is 6.0 or greater in all units, tested at the end of the storage period. The facility in which platelets are prepared, not that in which they are transfused, is responsible for measuring platelet numbers and pH. The FDA and AABB require that both the preparing facility and the transfusing facility observe and record the temperature in the vicinity of storage. This should be between 20 and 24 C, unless the platelets are prepared for refrigerated storage.

Excessive temperature fluctuations or inadequate gas and plasma movement during storage are the most usual causes when pH determinations are below 6.0. Consistently low pH determinations suggest the need to store the platelets either in a part of the laboratory with better temperature control, or in an environmental chamber manufactured especially for platelet storage. If temperature control is not the problem, and if stored units are kept in gentle movement with adequate exposure of container surfaces to air, it may be necessary to increase the volume of plasma in which the platelets are suspended.

Cryoprecipitated Factor VIII

In facilities that regularly prepare cryoprecipitate, in vitro recovery of Factor VIII should be assayed on at least four bags of cryoprecipitate each month. There must be an average of 80 international units of Factor VIII per container in 100% (FDA) or at least 75% (AABB) of units tested.[2,6] Factor VIII assays are difficult to perform accurately and reproducibly. These tests should be performed in a coagulation laboratory that employs an established method on a routine and regular basis.

Red Blood Cells

Red blood cells prepared from whole blood collected in CPDA-1 and intended for 35-day storage should have a final hematocrit no higher than 80%. This is best achieved by removing a standard volume of plasma, usually 225 to 250 ml (232-258 grams), from units that have been collected accurately. The hematocrit can be measured on a representative sample obtained during component preparation.

% RBC recovery =

$$\frac{\text{hematocrit after processing} \times \text{volume of final product after processing}}{\text{hematocrit before processing} \times \text{volume of initial product before processing}} \times 100$$

Note: Preprocessing hematocrit refers to that of the original unit, not after the addition of glycerol.

Figure 20-1. Formula for postthaw recovery of RBC.

1. After plasma has been expressed into the satellite bag, seal tubing well away from the red blood cell bag, leaving a segment of tubing in communication with the red cells.
2. Strip plasma back into red blood cell bag several times, mixing bag well each time. Allow tubing to fill with red blood cells representative of the bag contents.
3. Seal close to red blood cell bag and disconnect.
4. Measure hematocrit on the contents of the segment. Be sure to mix the sample well before determining hematocrit.

Red Blood Cells, Deglycerolized

The final wash solution should be tested periodically by colorimetric or spectrophotometric measurement to ensure acceptably low levels of free hemoglobin, and by osmometry to ensure residual glycerol below 1%. In each center there should be a standard, either in mg/ml or as a color comparator, to designate the allowable level of supernatant hemoglobin. *Standards* does not require each center to monitor red cell recovery and posttransfusion viability of the deglycerolized cells, provided the center adheres strictly to a method known to produce acceptable results. Postthaw recovery of red blood cells can be calculated using the formula shown in Fig 20-1.

Leukocyte-Poor Red Blood Cells

Standards does not require testing individual units of leukocyte-poor red blood cells provided the method used is one that has been shown to remove at least 70% of the white cells and to retain at least 70% of the original red cells. The FDA, however, requires that, if leukocyte-poor red cells are prepared by washing, at least 4 units be tested monthly, or every unit be tested if fewer than 4 are prepared. To calculate white cell removal:

1. White cells in original component = white count (per mm³) × 1000 × vol(ml) of component
2. White cells in WBC-poor component = white count (per mm³) × 1000 × vol(ml) of WBC-poor component
3. Percent residual cells = result #2 divided by result #1

This value should be below 30%.

References

1. Honig CL, Bove JR. Transfusion-associated fatalities: a review of Bureau of Biologics reports 1976-1978. Transfusion 1980;20:653-661.
2. Schmidt PJ, ed. Standards for blood banks and transfusion services. 11th ed. Arlington, VA: American Association of Blood Banks; 1984.
3. US Department of Health and Human Services, Food and Drug Administration. The code of federal regulations, 21 CFR 606.170(b), Washington, DC: US Government Printing Office.
4. Peters RW, Myhre BA. Studies on the variables in Rh slide testing. Am J Clin Pathol 1973;60:729-734.
5. Beattie KM. Control of the antigen-antibody ratio in antibody detection/compatibility tests. Transfusion 1980;20:277-284.
6. US Department of Health and Human Services, Food and Drug Administration. The code of

federal regulations, 21 CFR 600.3. Washington, DC: US Government Printing Office.

Recommended Reading

Hoppe PAH, Kaczmarski GR, Schmidt RP, Ellisor SS. Considerations in the selection of reagents. Washington, DC: American Association of Blood Banks; 1979.

Myhre BA. Quality control in blood banking. New York: Wiley and Sons; 1974.

Taswell HF, Saeed SM, eds. Principles and practice of quality control in the blood bank. Washington, DC: American Association of Blood Banks; 1980.

Hoppe PAH, Tourault MA. Quality control and regulatory requirements. In: Pittiglio D, ed. Modern blood banking and transfusion practices, Philadelphia, PA: FA Davis Co; 1983:283-322.

21

Records

Basil the Great, a fourth century cleric, once observed that "memory is the cabinet of imagination, the treasury of reason, the registry of conscience and the council chamber of thought." Basil, however, did not operate a blood bank or transfusion service, in which it might be surely observed that memory is ephemeral and no substitute for the written word.

Few organizations exist that do not boast of a valued and trusted employee upon whose recollections rest the history of that organization. But, if dependence upon recollection replaces careful record keeping, blood bank operation falters. For this reason, the need to maintain adequate records is a firm tenet of blood banking.

Standard Operating Procedures Manual

Perhaps the most essential record that all blood banks maintain is the Standard Operating Procedures (SOP) manual. This describes in detail the specific procedures and techniques that the laboratory staff use to fulfill the general requirements imposed by various standards and regulations. The SOP manual translates the meaning of all other processing records and must speak for itself. It must be complete, clear, up-to-date and, most importantly, accessible to and followed by the staff.

Standards and regulations usually define adequate performance while allowing choice of specific methods and procedures appropriate for each facility. If the AABB *Technical Manual* serves as a part of the SOP manual, the facility manual must define the edition and pages, and state exactly which procedures are to be used. For example, the *Technical Manual* includes more than one method of preparing the skin for blood collection; the SOP manual must clearly identify which procedure is to be applied.

SOP Elements

Procedural details, such as reagent volumes, times and temperatures of incubation or techniques of observation must be presented in a way that processing records for that procedure will be meaningful. The processing record for antibody detection tests, for example, would include a record of reagent lots employed, the positive or negative results observed, the date and the operator's initials. These data are useless without detailed instructions about how the test was performed.

An adequate procedures manual should provide enough information that any trained person could read it and be able to perform all the procedures used in that facility. By combining the information in the SOP manual and the processing records, one should be able to reconstruct completely each test performed in the individual facility. The SOP manual must present in an accessible, understandable fashion, the instructions and the indications for performing each test.

Under a general heading, such as "Pretransfusion Testing," the following specific information should be given:

1. The kinds of specimens needed and how they are obtained, including the directions for identifying patients and labeling samples
2. The way of recording specimen receipt and identity of the personnel involved
3. The need to compare the request forms and the labels on specimen tubes for accuracy of information before accepting the samples
4. The need to search for previous blood bank records for the patient.
5. Reagents and equipment necessary to perform the tests
6. Detailed instructions for performing and recording each test routinely performed, for performing and evaluating control tests, and for determining when additional tests are indicated
7. Instructions for labeling the blood or component and for completing necessary paperwork

The criteria for interpreting and recording observed results must be documented, and directions for managing possible problems should be included in readily accessible form. The SOP manual should include definitions of symbols used in record keeping and instruction to ensure uniform use of criteria and symbols. For example, agglutination reactions may be recorded as positive or be graded or scored, but this should be consistent for all employees performing all applicable tests. The SOP manual is also the most suitable place to maintain the list of names, identifying initials and inclusive dates of employment of all personnel who make entries in blood bank records.

Review and Revision

The procedures manual should undergo continual review and revision. Whenever problems arise with a procedure, corrective measures or alternative techniques should be considered and, if approved, be made part of the manual. Whenever a new procedure or policy is implemented, or a new regulation or standard becomes applicable, the existing manual should be reviewed and appropriate emendations made. After publication of each new edition of AABB *Standards*[1] and, additionally, before each scheduled inspection, the SOP manual should be examined page by page for conformance with requirements. The medical director must review the SOP manual at least annually and the date of review be documented. If there is a schedule for review of several pages or sections at a time, the review will usually be more complete than if the responsible persons review the entire manual at one time.

Individuals who use the manuals, forms, and labels should participate in drafting and reviewing them. This not only brings the results of their experience to bear on the instructions, but also heightens employees' awareness of problems in writing instructions and keeping good records. Minor revisions may be noted, with date and initials, on the appropriate pages of the master copy; photocopies of amended pages may then be placed in other copies of the manual. For major revisions, a newly typed page, dated and initialed, should be inserted in the master manual and all copies. Pages removed from the master copy should be dated at the time of removal and be retained in a file for at least 5 years, or longer if required by local laws. This allows documentation of the procedures used during the time period covered by statutes of limitations for legal actions. The SOP manual can most easily be revised and modified if it is in looseleaf format. Revised pages and forms must be initialed and dated by the physician responsible for the facility. Alternatively, it is acceptable to list revisions and the approval dates on an index page signed by the responsible physician.

Categories of Records

Two categories of records deserve comment:

1. Processing records, which contain the observations and interpretations at the time of testing
2. Statistical or summary records, which are analyses of the processing records

Processing records document the many operations of the facility and include test results and interpretations, observations of temperatures, distribution of blood components and maintenance of schedules. Statistical records summarize one or more of these operations during a defined time span and provide information useful for evaluating service demands, production, adequacy of personnel, inventory control and other variables.

Professional and governmental organizations have historically placed primary emphasis on processing records, but current trends in evaluating and reviewing medical practice suggest that summary records will achieve increasing importance, especially as computerization makes it easier to prepare statistical summaries. Manual record-keeping systems designed with efficient and rapid summarization in mind, can also allow assembly and surveillance of statistical records.

The Need for Records

Without question, the deficiences most frequently cited in inspection or survey programs are record-keeping violations. This fact has created two widespread misconceptions:

1. The main reason for keeping records is to satisfy inspection programs.
2. The volume of required recordkeeping interferes with the flow of work.

Do inspection programs lead to greater record-keeping demands? Probably so, especially in facilities in which maintaining records was never a priority. Inspections, by their very nature, require records as proof of satisfactory performance, because many procedures cannot be directly observed by the inspector and the nature of past performance can only be inspected through records.

Records reflect the history of operation and provide valuable insights about direction and supervision, and prevalent attitudes and working conditions. Sloppy, inaccurate, illegible, incomplete or missing records suggest imprecision, haste, disorder and error.

Summary of General Requirements

Records must be made concurrently with performance; they must be legible and indelible, must identify the person immediately responsible, must include the dates of performance, and must be as detailed as necessary for clear understanding. Because these principles apply to every record, they will not be repeated as separate items in the following sections listing individual requirements.

Many laboratory procedures are optional but, if they are performed, there must be complete records of these procedures. The *Standards* and the *Code of Federal Regulations*[2] provide additional optional aspects of procedures listed in the following sections.

If it is necessary to alter or correct any record, the change must be dated and initialed. The original recording must not be obliterated; it may be circled or crossed out, but it should remain legible.

There must be a permanent list that coordinates all initials and signatures with the typed or printed names of all personnel, including physicians, that are involved in record keeping. This record should include dates of employment. The record may be kept in personnel department records or the laboratory.

Rubber stamps, brackets or ditto marks are not acceptable means of identifying responsible personnel. Record format should be designed to eliminate the need for repetitive signing by the same individual.

Use of Records

Results of each test must be recorded as observations are made. Interpretation, if separate from results, must be recorded upon completion of testing. If results and interpretation are synonymous, no additional record is needed. Records of each patient's blood group must be kept available for immediate reference for at least 12 months. In addition, *Standards* requires that records of difficulties in ABO grouping, clinically significant antibodies and serious adverse reactions be kept for at least 5 years. These records must be reviewed before blood is issued for transfusion.

Reviewing previous records as part of pretransfusion testing provides some confirmation of the identity of the current sample. It is highly desirable to keep permanent records on problem patients readily available. Knowing whether unexpected antibodies have previously been noted and identified often speeds the procurement of compatible blood, and may prevent delayed hemolytic reactions in patients whose antibodies are weak or undetectable.

Confidentiality

Blood bank records, like all medical information, must not be released or made available to unauthorized persons.

Record Design

To be effective, record systems must meet the need and be used in a manner that satisfies this need. Interference with work flow generally results from imperfectly designed records and poor understanding of their purpose. Each form should have a title that explains its intended use and includes the name of the facility and enough of the address to distinguish it from other institutions with a similar name. Well-designed forms include as much preprinted information as possible, to minimize the number of manual entries needed.

One major concern in records is identification, for legal or investigational purposes, of persons responsible for performing operations. For example, the component preparation log should have entries that correspond with each of the main procedural steps. In a large laboratory in which several persons may prepare components concurrently, the log should make it possible to identify the persons involved in preparation of each group of products. It is not required, however, that each person initial the log for each step of component preparation. The SOP manual may indicate that the supervisor assumes the overall responsibility by initialing each day's records. This obviously requires that the supervisor attend the work area closely and have confidence in subordinate staff.

Significant Steps

The number of records maintained varies according to the facility's methods of operation. Each significant step must be recorded in a manner that permits tracing a blood component or patient specimen and all related procedures from the first step through final disposition. It is often difficult to distinguish the significant from the insignificant. An adequate processing record is one that makes it possible for the reader to reconstruct, from the record alone, the procedures performed. Records of phlebotomy, for example, must include results of examining both arms for signs of illegal drug use, but should not include documentation of each step in the arm preparation. The arm preparation is a single significant step in blood collection; if fully described in the SOP manual, performance is adequately documented when the phlebotomist initials the donation record. Similarly, it is sufficient to record the identity of persons involved in preparing blood containers for use, without recording each step of the process. Assessing the quality of performance requires good supervision rather than tediously detailed records.

Record-Keeping Requirements

Important in deciding the necessary depth of documentation is the adverse effect that an error in each step would produce. If a specific error could adversely affect patient safety or component purity, potency, safety or effectiveness, a record is needed to ensure fulfillment of the requirements of good practice. For example, inappropriately warm storage temperature may render cryoprecipitate useless for its intended purpose; consequently, records of storage temperature are essential. On the other hand, volumes of red cell components are usually not critical, and no routine records of these are required.

In designing records, it is helpful to scrutinize the inspection checklists used by the AABB and the other inspecting agencies to determine whether the procedures and the records comply with published requirements. These checklists summarize the records that are considered necessary. In the component preparation sections of FDA inspection forms, for example, there are lists of critical steps for each product. Records must include personnel identification and performance date of each critical step in preparation.

Retention of Records

Standards requires that records relevant to the operation of a blood bank or transfusion service be kept for not less than 5 years or the applicable state requirement, whichever is longer.[1] There is a federal requirement that records for source plasma be retained for 10 years and 6 months. Records must be kept indefinitely when there is no dating period for the product.

Like recordkeeping, the act of retention is not self-fulfilling. Records of the facility's operation should be accessible in direct proportion to their frequency of use. Records of donors deferred for permanently significant medical reasons must be consulted each time blood is collected and must be maintained until the prospective donor dies or exceeds the maximum age for blood donation. Records of a patient's ABO and Rh groups must be kept immediately available for 1 year, to permit comparison with results subsequently observed, and must be retained for at least 5 years or as required by applicable laws. It must be possible to check current observations against the records for the preceding 5 years of all patients with difficulty in blood typing, clinically significant unexpected antibodies, or severe adverse reactions to transfusion. Records about compatibility testing, issue of transfusion components and therapeutic procedures must be kept for at least 5 years, but do not need to be immediately available. Records of refrigerator temperatures or of the disposition of blood components, on the other hand, may be stored in a location from which retrieval will take much longer. *Standards* requires only 12-month retention for records of temperature, blood inspection and proficiency testing.

Record Storage

The method and location of record storage depends on the volume of records and on available storage space. Some large blood banks use microfilm or microfiche, not only to reduce storage costs but also to enhance ready access to important documents. Such records legitimately replace original documents that may be stored elsewhere or destroyed, but there must be documentation that the transformed records are true copies of the material they replace. The facility must properly index and organize the records, and must have a properly functioning viewer available on the premises. During inspection, the facility personnel must be able to produce legible "hard copy" of the record, if requested.

A designated responsible person must review and, by means of a signed, dated certification record, ensure authenticity and completeness of each group of documents copied. If color-coded records lose meaning in black-and-white reproduction, or if the original document is altered, for example, by erasure or retyping, the original copies should also be retained.

Computers

For records maintained in a computer, there must be a method of verifying accuracy. It is advisable to maintain a second disk or tape against the possibility of unexpected electronic loss of information from the storage medium. While microfilm or microfiche may adequately fulfill requirements for retaining records, computer systems requiring transfer of results may not replace certain required original reords, such as the results of ABO testing. The FDA and the AABB accept magnetically coded employee badges and other computer-related identifying methods in lieu of written signatures, but controls must be established to prevent misuse. All recorded information must be available for hardcopy reproduction. When records are maintained by electronic data processing, there must be a secure means of identifying changes or corrections made in the original records.

Summary Records

In general, summary records are not required. It is very useful, however, to review at least an annual summary of all blood bank errors and accidents. Such a summary provides an overview of operation and may identify procedures that need clarification or personnel who need retraining. Advances in adapting automated data processing equipment to all phases of operation facilitate review of processing records and compilation of summary statistics. Strict adherence to the facility's procedures manual and uniform notation among staff are critical if useful data are to be obtained with a minimum of effort.

Specific Record Requirements

Laboratory Tests on Patient or Recipient Blood

The test performed, results observed and final interpretation of results must be recorded.
1. First and last names and identification
2. Date of testing
3. Results of ABO and D grouping, including control for autoagglutinins and D^u testing, if performed
4. Interpretation of ABO and D tests
5. Results and interpretation of tests for unexpected antibodies

Compatibility Tests
1. Patient's ABO and D group
2. Identification of number of donor unit
3. ABO and D group of donor unit
4. Results and, if appropriate, interpretation of compatibility tests

Transfusion Requests
1. Recipient's first and last name
2. Recipient's identification number (hospital, admission, emergency room or other). Optional but helpful information includes: age, diagnosis, hospital location, clinical history including recent transfusions and pregnancy, drug therapy and name of requesting physician.
3. Number of units of blood or component required; optional but recommended are date and time units are to be available.

Blood Donors

At each blood donation, there must be a record that identifies the donor and gives pertinent information; either single-use or multiple-donation forms are acceptable. These records may be filed either by donor name or donor unit number, with appropriate cross references. Records required for laboratory tests on donor blood are considered in a later section. Information required in the donation record is as follows:
1. Number of donor unit, if assigned

2. First and last name and middle initial
3. Address and phone number
4. Date of birth
5. Date of donation
6. Date of last donation
7. Record of physical examination (temperature, blood pressure, pulse, hemoglobin or hematocrit, arm examination) and identification of the examiner. In addition, the record must include documentation that the donor weighs at least 50 kg (110 pounds).
8. Medical history with answers recorded as "yes" or "no" for each question, with any pertinent explanation. Identification of interviewer.
9. Record of whether accepted, and whether bleeding was satisfactory or unsatisfactory. If donor is deferred, the reason should be given, with notation about temporary or permanent deferral. The names of donors permanently rejected should be entered in a readily accessible file.
10. Release form: Consent to have blood drawn, permission for blood bank to use blood as it deems fit, and signatures of donor and a witness. Legal advice may be helpful in designing this portion of the form.
11. Identification of phlebotomist
12. Record of any donor reaction; symptoms, treatment, condition on release and notation about whether donor can be accepted again; identification of person caring for donor, time released and notation if donor refuses treatment or advice. This record may be kept on a separate form designed for this purpose.
13. ABO and D group
14. Supplementary records: There are additional record requirements for donors in special categories. These records may be included in the donor form, may be attached to it, or may be filed separately.
    a. Over-age donors: Blood bank physician's approval. This may be given on an individual basis, or there may be documentation that the individual donor belongs to a category designated as acceptable by the blood bank physician in the SOP manual.
    b. Under-age donors: Permission from parent or guardian
    c. Therapeutic bleedings: A record that the patient's physician has ordered phlebotomy; records of the disease and whether or not the unit may be used for transfusion purposes; volume of blood drawn.
    d. Autologous bleedings: Written consent of patient's physician, the blood bank physician, and the patient, or, if indicated, the patient's parent or guardian.

Optional Donor Information

1. Identification, such as social security number, driver's license number, or picture
2. Name of patient or donor group to be credited
3. Results of tests for antibody detection and HBsAg. These results are a required part of the processing record but recording results on the donor record is optional except for confirmed positive results of HBsAg testing. Results of abnormal findings may be useful for reference at future donation.
4. Disposition of the unit is required information that may optionally be recorded on the donation form.
5. Race
6. The name of the manufacturer and lot number of container/anticoagulant. This required information is optional on the donation form.

Hemapheresis, Therapeutic Plasma Exchange and Cytoreduction

If no component is prepared, only those records necessary to ensure donor protection are necessary. If transfusion components are prepared, the records of these procedures must include all required information for blood donors and in addition must include the following as part of a separate file on each donor[2]:

1. All initial and periodic physical examinations by a physician, including medical history interviews. The physician's acceptance or rejection of the donor, based on the accumulated laboratory data. In the case of therapeutic procedures, the prescribing physician's order may substitute for all of the above.
2. The results of all laboratory tests to determine donor suitability
3. The explanation of the procedures that will be performed and the patient's or donor's informed consent
4. All positive HBsAg test results
5. A record of any whole blood, red cell, leukocyte or platelet loss, including planned donations of those products
6. For hemapheresis donors who are given medications or hyperimmunization injections, there must be a separate informed consent as well as complete information on drug or antigen source; the schedule, dosage, and route of administration; adverse reactions; and response to the stimulating agent as measured by laboratory tests.
7. The name of the manufacturer and the lot numbers and volumes of all solutions, software and drugs used. This is a required record but it is optional in the individual donor record file.
8. For automated procedures, the time procedure begins and ends, the number of "passes" or the volume of blood processed, the volume of each component harvested, the estimated blood cell loss and any adverse reactions.

Laboratory Processing of Donor Blood

The type of test, the results observed and a final interpretation of results must be recorded for all tests.[1,2] Entries must be made as work is done, using symbols that clearly indicate positive or negative results. The symbols must be defined and used

uniformly by all personnel. Most required records can be incorporated in one worksheet to facilitate labeling and the review of records before release of each batch of blood components. One of the most critical steps in processing donor blood is identification and quarantine of all units unsuitable for distribution. Because an error at this point may result in transfusion of HBsAg-reactive components, it is strongly recommended that labeling procedures include a double check of units to be quarantined before the rest of the group is released for distribution.

Tests Required for Donor Blood Samples
1. Donor unit number
2. Results of ABO and D cell grouping, including D^u if indicated
3. Results of serum or plasma tests for expected antibodies in the ABO system
4. Interpretation of ABO and D groups
5. Results of tests for the detection of unexpected antibodies, if indicated, including use of IgG-coated control cells
6. Results of serologic test for syphilis. Although this test is not required by *Standards*, it is a federal requirement.
7. Results of tests for HBsAg and relevant calculations to define positive results. The record of these calculations may be kept separately from the results on donor samples but must be referable to the sample records.
8. Reagents used, manufacturer, lot number, expiration date and evidence that reagents have been subjected to performance checks

Optional Laboratory Tests
1. Control tests on anti-D serum
2. Identification of unexpected antibodies

Component Preparation
1. Donor unit number
2. Date and, if appropriate, time drawn
3. Name and volume of anticoagulant
4. Name of component
5. Date and, if appropriate, time(s) prepared. If the preparation involves multiple steps such as separation, freezing,

thawing and others, each step must be documented.

6. Date and time of expiration. The time of expiration is required only if the dating period is 72 hours or less.
7. Volume of component, except for Cryoprecipitated AHF and Red Blood Cells prepared in a routine manner from 450 ml of whole blood.

Similar records must be kept when separating and pooling recovered plasma for further manufacture. For any pooled product, records must indicate the identity of each donor contributing to the pool.

Blood and Components Received from Other Facilities

1. Name and address of shipping facility. It is not necessary to record address with each unit if this information is readily available.
2. Name of blood component
3. Donor unit number assigned by collecting facility
4. Accession or inventory number, if any, assigned by receiving bank
5. ABO and Rh blood group
6. Expiration date and time, if indicated
7. Date received
8. For blood received already crossmatched, the name and identification number of the intended recipient and interpretation of results of compatibility tests
9. Results and interpretation of tests done by receiving facility

Storage and Inspection of Blood Components

1. Recording charts for refrigerator and freezer temperatures, with inclusive dates, explanation of abnormal temperatures and action taken, and initials of certifying personnel
2. Records of periodic testing of alarm systems
3. Records of temperatures observed daily and compared against automated temperature recordings. Centralized elec-

tronic temperature recording and alarm systems can replace records of daily observations but *Standards* requires that temperature results be printed at least every 4 hours.

4. Notation of quarantine of unsatisfactory units, record of any tests performed and final disposition of unit

Disposition of Blood and Components

It must be possible to follow every unit of blood or component from records of the donor and the required tests to disposition by transfusion, shipment or discard. When destruction is necessary, the reason for destruction, date and method of destruction must be recorded. When units are shipped, the shipping facility must record the following information:

1. Name and address of receiving facility
2. Date and time of shipment
3. A list of each donor unit number, blood group and expiration date
4. Name of each blood component
5. Final inspection of Whole Blood or Red Blood Cell units
6. Name of person filling order
7. Periodic tests documenting that shipping containers maintain acceptable temperature range

Issue for Transfusion

1. Time and date of issue or reissue. For reissued Whole Blood or Red Blood Cells, a record that proper temperature has been maintained, that container and closure are intact and that inspection for abnormal color or appearance has been satisfactory.
2. Donor unit number of blood or component, or lot number of product

Infusion

1. Signed statement that the information on the container label and the compatibility record has been matched with the intended recipient, item by item, prior to infusion

2. Time and date transfusion is started
3. Optional but desirable is information about the time transfusion is completed, the volume infused and the patient's condition.

Some or all of the compatibility, issue and transfusion records can be combined on one multipart form. After termination of transfusion, one copy of the form is attached to the patient's chart, a record is filed in the blood bank and another copy may be sent to accounting.

Emergency Issue of Blood or Components

Blood components may be issued before completion of routine tests in situations in which delay in providing blood might unduly jeopardize the patient.[1,2] The label or tie-tag must clearly identify those required tests that have not been completed. The records must contain a statement of the requesting physician indicating that the clinical situation is sufficiently urgent to require release of blood before completion of testing. In transfusion services where the SOP manual distinguishes between performing a full antiglobulin crossmatch and performing type and screen, the requesting physician's statement is not required before issuing blood to a patient on whom type and screen has been performed. In these cases, the blood bank director assumes the responsibility for transfusion without individual antiglobulin crossmatch. In all other cases, the compatibility label must clearly state that tests routinely performed in that facility have not been completed, but this need not be part of the permanent record. All other record requirements apply as usual.

Quality Assurance Records

1. Dated and signed or initialed temperature recording charts for each refrigerator and freezer or central monitor record

2. Record of quality assurance tests performed on anti-human globulin, blood grouping serum and reagent red blood cells as specified by the SOP manual
3. Results of tests to evaluate the performance of other reagents (eg, copper sulfate) and equipment, as required by the AABB National Committee on Inspection and Accreditation
4. Log of personnel signatures and inclusive dates of employment. If signature abbreviations or employee codes are used in record keeping, these must be identified.
5. Record of participation in a proficiency testing program
6. Record of quality assurance tests of components prepared
7. Record of periodic checks on sterile technique if products are prepared in an open system (FDA requirement)
8. Record of sterilization of supplies and reagents prepared within the facility, including date, time interval, temperature and mode (FDA requirement)
9. Record of disposition of rejected supplies or reagents used in collection, processing, and compatibility testing of blood and blood components (FDA requirement)
10. Record of supplies and reagents used, including manufacturer, lot numbers, date received, date put in use and expiration date (FDA requirement)
11. Record of employee participation in job-related education or training with inclusive dates, subjects and evaluation, if appropriate

Errors, Accidents and Adverse Reactions

Good practice dictates that records be kept of errors, accidents and adverse reactions. *Standards* and the *Code of Federal Regulations* require records of adverse reactions in donors or patients.[1,2]

Standards requires that each facility have a system for detecting, reporting, and evaluating suspected adverse reactions to transfusion. Chapter 17 outlines the recommended tests for evaluating reported transfusion reactions. The report form and the results of all tests must be retained for at least 5 years, or as required by local statutes of limitations, whichever is longer. When a transfusion error or accident occurs, the following information is recommended for records required by FDA:

1. A description of the error or accident
2. The name of the blood component(s) or product(s) involved
3. The donor unit number(s) of the blood component(s) or lot numbers of the blood product(s) implicated
4. The date of discovery
5. The date of occurrence
6. Whether or not the blood component or product was transfused
7. Whether or not the patient's physician was made aware of the error or accident, if the blood or blood product was transfused
8. The category of personnel responsible for the error or accident (eg, nurse, technologist, shipping personnel or others) and identity of the individual
9. An explanation of how the error or accident occurred
10. The actions taken to prevent a recurrence of the error or accident
11. The name of the manufacturer, lot number and expiration date of the product if defective reagents or supplies were implicated
12. A copy of the notification of appropriate authorities when applicable

The record system should include a method for reporting cases of suspected posttransfusion hepatitis or other serious disease resulting from blood transfusion. It is imperative to make a careful and complete record of all investigations to ensure adequate care of patients, to prevent subsequent errors and to provide legal evidence if this is needed.

FDA Required Reports

Fatalities related to blood collection or transfusion must be reported promptly to the Director, Office of Biologics Research and Review, Center for Drugs and Biologics. An immediate report should be made by telephone (301-443-7381) and a written report should be submitted within 7 days (21 CFR 606.170b).[2] The report should include a description of any new procedures implemented to avoid a recurrence of the error or accident.

If HBsAg-reactive components are transfused, the patient(s) must be followed for 6 months and the final report must indicate whether the patient(s) contracted hepatitis. If plasma from an HBsAg-reactive unit is shipped for further manufacture, both the manufacturer and the Office of Biologics Research and Review should be notified immediately. Reports concerning the infusion of incorrectly identified red cells during a plasmapheresis procedure should also include the approximate volume of red cells infused, the blood groups of the donor and the infused cells, a description of the effect on the donor and the care given to the donor.

References

1. Schmidt PJ, ed. Standards for blood banks and transfusion services. 11th ed. Arlington, VA: American Association of Blood Banks, 1984.
2. Code of federal regulations. Current edition. Title 21, parts 600-799. Washington, DC: U.S. Government Printing Office.
3. Pittiglio, DH, ed. Modern blood banking and transfusion practices. Philadelphia: F. A. Davis Company; 1983:283.

22

The Hospital Transfusion Committee

Requirements for Review

Peer review of transfusion practice is required by the Joint Commission for Accreditation of Hospitals (JCAH) as a prerequisite for hospital accreditation; by the *Code of Federal Regulations* (CFR) for a hospital to qualify to receive Medicare reimbursement; by most states for Medicaid reimbursement; and by the College of American Pathologists (CAP) and the American Association of Blood Banks (AABB), as part of their inspection and accreditation processes. The JCAH standards state, in part: "The medical staff shall provide a mechanism that insures review of blood transfusion for proper utilization ... not less than quarterly. Particular attention shall be given to ... use of whole blood vs. components . . . amount of blood requested vs. amount transfused . . . amount of wastage." The CFR states, "A committee of the medical staff . . . reviews all transfusions of blood or blood derivatives and makes recommendations concerning policies governing such practices. The review committee investigates all transfusion reactions occurring in the hospital and makes recommendations to the medical staff regarding improvements in transfusion procedures."

These regulations specify functions that can be met by mechanisms other than a hospital transfusion committee, such as a tissue committee or a laboratory utilization committee. However, the specified functions are so demanding that most hospitals have found it expedient to have a staff committee concerned solely with blood transfusion.

Results of Review

Is monitoring transfusion practice necessary? Several reports have suggested that many blood transfusions are given without valid indications. In 1962 a blood conservation program was described that is remarkably similar to current "model" peer review programs.[1] A hospital staff adopted in its bylaws "indications for blood transfusions" which were: 1) for replacement of needed whole blood volume; 2) for oxygen transport in: a) an anemic patient having a 7 gm/dl hemoglobin or less, or b) an anemic patient with complications affecting oxygenation or undergoing anesthesia, who could be transfused if hemoglobin was less than 10 g/dl; 3) for exchange tranfusion of infants; and 4) for replacement of labile coagulation factors, a rare indication for use of fresh whole blood. Emphasizing these simple indications, a hospital staff education program produced a drop in use factor (units of blood transfused divided by the number of patients hospitalized) from 0.237 to 0.110, a decrease of more than 50%.

A prospective study[2] of blood transfusion practice in a large general hospital during a 2-month period when 675 units of blood were transfused, revealed that 17% of the units transfused on the surgical service, 25% on the medical service and 38% on the obstetric and gynecologic service did not meet criteria similar to those described above. Comparison of single unit transfusions with multiple unit transfusions showed far more single units than multiple units to be considered unnecessary.

In a study[3] of patients admitted at 300 hospitals located throughout the United States, 401 nonsurgical patients were analyzed who had a diagnosis of anemia and a recorded hemoglobin equal to or greater than 10 gm/dl. These patients received a mean of 2.5 units of blood, yet most physicians would agree that most of these patients did not require transfusion. One possible exception might be severe coronary artery disease causing liability to angina at hemoglobin levels below 10 gm/dl, but 14% of these patients were women between the ages of 20 to 49 years, a group known not to be subject to coronary artery disease. This group received a mean of 2.4 units of blood transfused even though the diagnosis was iron deficiency anemia. The unnecessary transfusions exposed the recipients to the hazards of transfusion, increased cost and imposed an extra burden on donor recruitment and blood collection. The necessity for peer review of transfusion practice is obvious.

Organization of the Transfusion Committee

The transfusion committee may be a standing committee, or its functions may be carried out by a hospital committee with a broader scope of responsibility, such as "tissue and transfusion." The transfusion committee members and its chairman are generally appointed by the hospital chief of staff upon the recommendations of department chairmen. Representation should include all major medical departments that routinely order blood: surgery, anesthesiology, medicine, obstetrics and pediatrics. In addition, the high blood-use subspecialties should be represented, such as cardiovascular surgery, hemodialysis, oncology, hematology and neonatology. Other members are also desirable: a hospital administrator; a nurse, to represent the service that administers most of the transfusions; a medical records department representative, because most reviews are done using patient records; and a blood bank technologist, to provide practical and technical information to the committee.

Members should be knowledgeable and experienced in one or more aspects of transfusion therapy and blood banking. Tenure on the committee should be long enough that skills acquired by new members can be used and shared. In small hospitals with few specialists on the staff, individual staff member interest and commitment may be the criteria for appointment. In such cases it may be useful to have a medical or technical representative from the supplying blood center as a consultant to the committee. Observers, such as SBB students or interested staff and residents, are usually welcome to attend committee meetings.

The medical director of the transfusion service should be a member of the committee but not necessarily its chairman. The transfusion service director already influences blood usage in the hospital on a daily basis, and a committee chairman who directs the transfusion service might be accused of having a conflict of interest if called upon to defend transfusion committee policies. In addition, the chairman is responsible for enforcement aspects of the committee functions. Responsibility for activities viewed as regulatory by staff members may invite resentment and impaired cooperation.[4] Constructive criticism may be more acceptable to staff members when it comes from another clinician.

Functions of the Transfusion Committee

The committee is required to meet at least quarterly and as often as necessary to perform its functions. All committee activities should be documented, usually in the committee minutes. Reports should be made regularly to the hospital staff or its committee responsible for overall quality assurance activities. There are many aspects of hospital transfusion practice suitable for review by the transfusion committee. These include, but are not limited to, use of blood and blood components, the indications for and use of irradiated blood products and the appropriate use of various blood administration devices including filters, warmers, blood pumps and intraoperative autologous transfusion devices. The transfusion committee should monitor the use of cell separators for intraoperative salvage and the collection of plasma or cells from patients undergoing plasmapheresis or cytapheresis procedures. It is appropriate for the transfusion committee to review the use of blood derivatives such as albumin and plasma protein fraction and perhaps immune serum globulins.

Guidelines for evaluating transfusion reactions should be reviewed by the transfusion committee to establish an overall hospital policy. Inservice programs are an important function of hospital transfusion committees and provide a framework for educating all hospital personnel in the appropriate use of blood and blood components. In addition to audits of usage, the transfusion committee may find it useful to evaluate how blood components are ordered, including determination of whether written orders are present in the patient's chart and whether type of component and volume and rate of infusion are specified. These audits also provide the nursing service or the hospital IV team with information on compliance with requirements for recording the times the transfusion was started and stopped, the

performance of appropriate identification checks and the occurrence of any adverse reactions. The committee can also note whether or not transfusion effects are monitored by posttransfusion laboratory tests or notations of clinical conditions.

Outpatient transfusion practices including transfusion, phlebotomy and hemapheresis services should be evaluated by the transfusion committee when necessary. The transfusion committee may wish to review and make recommendations about providing special blood products for segments of the hospital population; for example, the suitability of providing CMV-seronegative blood for low birth weight infants born of CMV-seronegative mothers or the use of cryoprecipitate for hemophiliacs or other individuals who are at high risk of developing AIDS.

In some medical centers the transfusion service director may decide many of these issues. In hospitals where there is no full-time transfusion service director these practices and questions would fall under the jurisdiction of the committee as a whole. Although the transfusion service director may make the decisions, it is appropriate for the transfusion committee to review these issues that affect the entire hospital staff. Valuable input from all sectors of the hospital population can thus be brought to bear on the appropriate use of blood components and transfusion practices in the institution.

A useful formulation of committee functions appeared in the AABB workshop publication on the Transfusion Committee.[5]

These are to:

1. Establish broad policies for blood transfusion therapy.
2. Develop criteria for audits of transfusion practice.
3. Enhance quality of patient care through objective assessment of ongoing blood and blood component therapy.
4. Review and analyze the statistical reports of the transfusion service.

5. Audit blood use, with particular attention to whole blood, components, reactions, hepatitis occurrence and other adverse events. Audits of hemotherapy in specific circumstances are encouraged. The audit will include hospitalized patients, Emergency Room patients, and outpatients, where indicated.
6. Reaudit previously identified problem areas to evaluate improvement.
7. Promote continuing education in transfusion practices for groups of the hospital staff.
8. Assist the hospital or blood center, as appropriate, in blood procurement efforts.
9. Assess adequacy and safety of the blood supply.
10. Ensure that written policies and procedures for the blood transfusion service conform to the American Association of Blood Banks' *Standards* and review these annually.
11. Report to that committee of the hospital charged with the responsibility for overall quality assurance activities and recommend corrective action when indicated.

Monitoring Hospital Transfusion Practice

The need to encourage appropriate blood utilization underlies all these functions of the hospital transfusion committee. How can this be accomplished? There are two broad categories of transfusion practice that can be reviewed by the committee: 1) statistical, or systems, data derived from records of the blood bank and 2) medical practice data generated by analysis of patients' hospital charts.

Statistical Data

Transfusion services will, for inspection and accreditation purposes, record certain statistics, for example: blood component usage; outdate rate for each component; number of each type of transfusion reaction; number of hepatitis cases; crossmatch/transfused ratio; and transfusion service workload and productivity. A more complete list of systems indicators is given in Appendix 22-1.[6] Which variables should be measured and how frequently must be determined by the transfusion committee and the transfusion service director. Computerization of transfusion service recordkeeping makes a greater variety of statistical data available and makes it more current. Manual record-keeping systems are limited in generating such data because of the enormous labor required.

When possible, some critical systems data should be monitored continuously because spot checks are subject to sampling errors, which could prompt a policy change in attempts to correct a nonexistent problem. Once a hospital has accurate statistics on its own transfusion data base, it is possible to measure the effects produced by instituting any new policy or procedure.[6]

Medical Practice Data

In most hospitals these data are extracted by medical audit analysts from reviews of patients' charts. The transfusion committee should draft the audit criteria in an open and participatory manner. All clinical department chairmen should be informed in writing of the purpose and method of the audit process. Most departments will have representation on the transfusion committee. For those that do not, the department chairman may be asked to attend and participate or send a delegate. The committee minutes of the developmental meetings should be distributed to all concerned departments so the staff will be informed that criteria are being drafted.

Development of audit criteria by a group of physicians provides credibility among the clinical staff. It is helpful to have medical records or quality assurance personnel participate in the drafting process because the criteria will be used by nonphysician reviewers to select patient charts for study.

Audit Criteria

Audit criteria are guidelines used by medical audit personnel to select charts that the transfusion committee physicians will review. The criteria serve as a filter that eliminates those charts that reflect acceptable transfusion practice and selects out a few charts that are most likely to reveal practices in need of scrutiny. The criteria should not attempt to define a comprehensive standard of practice. Nonphysician reviewers are not expected to apply complex instructions to the screening process; comprehensive evaluation is the function of the physician reviewers.

Audit criteria have three parts:

1. *Elements* that are the indications for transfusion. Documentation of these exempt a chart from further review.

2. *Exceptions* describe situations that also exempt a chart from further review even though it does not comply with the indications in the Elements. These should be kept to a minimum to facilitate the audit.

3. *Instructions and Definitions* contain detailed directions to records personnel about where to locate information in the chart (in the laboratory report, anesthesia records or doctor's notes, etc.) and information about terminology and intent of the Elements.

Criteria should be developed by the transfusion committee to be appropriate for its own hospital and/or clinical departments. Variable local conditions may make a criterion applicable in one hospital and invalid in another. For example, use of whole blood to treat patients who have suffered acute trauma and massive blood loss may be justified at one hospital, but whole blood may be simply unavailable at another hospital. Some examples of criteria are available in the literature[6,7] and in Appendix 22-2. Some of the criteria in Appendix 22-2 are not appropriate for pediatric patients, newborns, hemodialysis patients, etc. Additional criteria should be formulated for auditing patient records of a particular clinical department; for example, how many trauma service patients receive uncrossmatched blood transfusions.

Performing Audits

Complete charts and thorough documentation are essential for medical audits. Criteria may be debated, but basic criteria appropriate for every audit must include documentation of 1) reason for transfusing and 2) effect of the transfusion. There are other justifications for requiring that such information always be in the chart. If an adverse reaction should occur, the legal position of the physician and the hospital is strengthened. Also, when the ordering physician justifies the transfusion in writing, he or she is likely to think through the decision carefully. Finally, the documentation of effect serves as quality control check both for the decision to transfuse and for the choice of blood components transfused.[8]

Corrective Actions

After criteria have been developed and agreed upon but before any formal audits are conducted, the transfusion committee should agree upon actions that will be taken after chart reviews are completed.[6] There are a number of options:

1. The patient's name and the name of the involved physician can be recorded; or anonymous statistical summary reports can be generated.

2. The committee can send a letter[9] or other written notice of deficient practice to: the responsible physician, the department chairman, the chief of professional services, the hospital risk management office, the hospital credentials committee or a combination of these.

3. The name of the transfusion committee members who reviewed the chart may or may not be made known to the involved clinician.

4. The involved physician may be required to appear before the transfusion com-

mittee or the department chairman to account for inappropriate therapy, or may respond in writing.

These issues should be discussed with the hospital's administration and legal office and decided prior to the first audit. The hospital staff should be informed of the criteria, the audit process and the mechanisms that the committee intends to use for documentation and corrective action.

It is essential to remember at all times that the fundamental concern of the audit is educational and not punitive, because the goal is to improve the practice of blood transfusion.[10,11]

References

1. McCoy KL. The Providence Hospital blood conservation program. Transfusion 1962;2:3–6.

2. Diethrich EB. Evaluation of blood transfusion. Transfusion 1965;5:82–88.

3. Friedman BA. Patterns of blood utilization by physicians: transfusion of non-operated anemic patients. Transfusion 1978;18:193–198.

4. Umiker WO. The pathologist's role: cop or consultant? MLO 1980;12:111–122.

5. Bergin JJ. The composition and function of the hospital transfusion committee: historical perspective. In: Wallas CH and Muller VH, eds. The hospital transfusion committee. Arlington, VA: American Association of Blood Banks, 1982:7–13.

6. Simpson MB. Audit criteria for transfusion practices. In: Wallas CH and Muller VH, eds. The hospital transfusion committee. Arlington, VA: American Association of Blood Banks, 1982:21–60.

7. Editorial Board: In another vein, rationale and criteria for studying blood transfusions. QRB 1977;3:11–16.

8. Myhre BA. Quality control of clinical transfusion practices. In: Myhre BA, ed. Quality control in blood banking. New York: John Wiley & Sons, 1974:175–204.

9. Schmidt PJ. A letter way to improve transfusion practices. MLO 1980;13:95–98.

10. Smith, DE. Utilization review. In: Wallas CH and Muller VH, eds. The hospital transfusion committee. Arlington, VA: American Association of Blood Banks, 1982:61–85.

11. Crosby WH. The hospital transfusion board. Transfusion 1962;2:1–2.

Appendix 22-1. Key Indicators for Systems Audits*

1. UNITS TRANSFUSED—Total number of whole blood, red blood cells, platelet concentrates, apheresis platelets, granulocyte apheresis units, fresh frozen plasma, cryoprecipitate, Factors VIII and IX concentrates, Rh immune globulin, cryopreserved red cells, washed red cells, leukocyte-poor red cells, reconstituted red cells for exchange transfusion.

2. PATIENTS TRANSFUSED—Total number of patients receiving each component or product as listed in item 1 above.

3. UNITS TRANSFUSED PER PATIENT TRANSFUSED—The average number of units of each component or product given to patients receiving that component. In some situations, it may be useful to analyze on the basis of diagnosis or surgical or medical procedure.

4. RELATIVE PERCENT OF WHOLE BLOOD VERSUS RED BLOOD CELLS TRANSFUSED

5. CROSSMATCH TO TRANSFUSED RATIO (C:T)—The number of units requested divided by the number of units transfused. This analysis may be applied to the total operations of the transfusion service, or to the operating room, specific wards, particular surgical procedures, individual physicians, various clinical services or specialties, and emergency versus routine requests.

6. OUTDATE RATE—The total number of units outdated divided by the sum of the units outdated plus the units transfused. This should be monitored for all blood, components and products; in some instances, analysis by ABO and Rh group may prove informative.

(*Reproduced with permission[6])

7. TRANSFUSION REACTIONS— The number and percent of various types of reported transfusion reactions, including posttransfusion hepatitis.

8. WORKLOAD AND PRODUCTIVITY—CAP workload and productivity data may be useful to evaluate the activities and efficiency of the lab; this may be analyzed by day of week and by shift in some situations; workload per unit transfused may be valuable as an efficiency measure.

9. HOURS WORKED PER UNIT TRANSFUSED OR PATIENT TRANSFUSED—In many transfusion services, this variable may be a more valid indicator of the efficiency of operations than that value obtained from traditional workload-productivity figures.

10. UNCROSSMATCHED UNITS— The number and percent of units issued uncrossmatched or with abbreviated pretransfusion testing; analysis by ward, service or physician may be useful.

11. FRESH UNIT REQUESTS—The number and percent of requests for "freshest" or "fresh" units, analyzed by ward, service, physician and diagnosis.

12. TURNAROUND TIME—The total time required between receipt of a transfusion request and availability of the unit for transfusion to the patient. This may be examined for emergency, routine and operative requests.

13. EMERGENCY REQUESTS—The number and percent may be analyzed by ward, service, requesting physician and diagnosis; distribution of requests by day of week, shift and hour may be revealing in some situations; the C:T ratio should be measured for appropriateness of requesting.

14. UNITS RETURNED UNUSED— The number and percent of units that are signed out from the transfusion service and later returned unused; analysis by ward, clincal service and requesting physician may be informative.

15. AGE DISTRIBUTION OF UNITS— Analysis by statistical methods and/or frequency histograms for the age of inventory units and crossmatched units by ABO and Rh; the age at the time of receipt from the supplier; the age at the time of transfusion; the age when returned to supplier.

16. SURGICAL CANCELLATIONS DUE TO UNAVAILABILITY OF BLOOD—The number and percent of cases that were delayed due to unavailability of blood; analysis by number of hours or days delayed, by surgical procedure and by cause, (i.e, antibody versus shortage of particular ABO-Rh group).

17. LATE REQUESTS FOR PREOPERATIVE CROSSMATCHES—The number and percent of preoperative requests that are received by the transfusion service after the deadline for submission of requests; analysis by ward, service and physician may be important.

18. DISTRIBUTION OF REQUESTS— The number of units requested by day of week, shift or hour.

Comments

Unless the transfusion service possesses sophisticated data processing capabilities, many of these indicators are best monitored only when a problem seems apparent. Items 1 through 9 should ideally be monitored by all transfusion services, however, as a continuous audit of basic operational quality. The most appropriate method seems to be compilation on a monthly basis, with quarterly, semiannual and annual summaries; standard statistical methods of mean, range, SEM and SD may be useful for some items. The data are often more meaningful when expressed as percents or rates than simply in total numbers.

Appendix 22-2. Examples of Audit Criteria for Red Cell Transfusion

Elements	Exceptions	Instructions and Definitions
I. Justification for Transfusion		
1. Anemia documented by: hct <30% and/or hemoglobin <10 g/dl	Coronary artery disease Chronic pulmonary disease or cerebral ischemic disease	See admitting notes, MD's progress notes, anesthesia record, laboratory reports

2. Hypovolemia documented by:
    a. Central venous pressure <3 cm H_2O
    b. Systolic pressure <90 mmHg
    c. Hct <30% and falling
    d. Estimated blood loss >1000 ml		

II. Assessment of Utilization		
1. Use of whole blood	Surgical or trauma patient Acute gastrointestinal bleeding	See transfusion record, MD's progress notes
2. Use of platelet concentrates	Pt bleeding and plt. ct ≤50,000/mm³ Plt. ct. ≤20,000/mm³ with no bleeding	See transfusion record, MD's progress notes, laboratory reports
3. Use of fresh frozen plasma	Transfusion of >5 units blood Bleeding disorder (describe)	See transfusion record, MD's progress notes, laboratory reports
III. Assessment of Complications		
1. Mortality	None	
2. Readmission within 6 mos. with hepatitis	None	
3. Hemolytic transfusion reaction	None	Hemolytic reaction = fever, hypotension, bleeding, hemoglobinuria. See transfusion reaction report, nurses' notes, operative note

4. Circulatory overload   None   Circulatory overload =
   during transfusion   Systolic BP increase >50
   characterized by: mmHg
   a. Shortness of breath   Respiratory rate increase
   b. Central venous   >20/min
      pressure >15   See MD's progress notes,
      cmH$_2$O in OR   nurses' notes,
   c. Pulmonary edema   transfusion reaction
   d. Cyanosis   report

IV. Evaluation of Effect

1. Between 24 hrs after   None   See laboratory reports
   transfusion and
   prior to discharge:
   hct<37% or
   hemoglobin <12.5 g/
   dl

(These chart review criteria were developed by the 1979 Transfusion Committee of Memorial Hospital Medical Center of Long Beach, CA)

Blood Inventory Management

Blood from volunteer donors is a precious resource and should be used in the most efficient and effective way. Medical directors of hospital transfusion services, in conjunction with their transfusion committees and regional blood centers, can accomplish this goal by regularly conducting both a systems audit and medical practice audit.

In the systems audit, managerial and operational data are reviewed to determine the efficiency of the hospital transfusion service. Considerations include, but are not limited to, the rate of outdating; the ratio of blood crossmatched to that transfused (C:T ratio); and adequacy of observation and reporting of transfusion reactions.

The medical practice audit is also an important function of the hospital transfusion committee. This committee should monitor whether blood components are used with correct indications and achieve expected results; and whether blood is transfused in accord with accepted medical practice and after consideration of possible complications. See Chapter 22 for more details.

Because hospital transfusion services and regional blood centers face different inventory control problems, they will be considered separately in this chapter. Issues affecting red cell components differ from those affecting platelets and plasma, which

are discussed briefly at the end of the chapter.

Hospital Transfusion Services

Hospital blood inventories have a direct impact on the balance between outdating and shortages. In a hospital with low transfusion activity, the greater the number of units in inventory, the higher the potential for outdating. Conversely, the fewer the units in inventory, the more frequent the shortages and the greater the need for expensive emergency deliveries from the blood supplier. The optimal number of units to be kept in the hospital inventory can be derived by using complex mathematical formulas,[1] can be calculated in a relatively simple computer simulation,[2,3] or can be arrived at empirically as shown below.

Calculation of Optimal Inventory

1. Collect weekly blood usage data over a 6-month period.
2. Arrange by week and ABO and Rh group as shown in Table 23-1. Notice the tremendous week-to-week variation in the amount of blood used in the example given. The amount of O,Rh+ blood used, for example, goes from 0 units to 20 units. Because it is not possible to be prepared for every large volume emergency, the single, unusual

Table 23-1. Whole Blood and Packed Cells Transfused by Week and by Group (Small Hospital Example)

Week	O+	A+	B+	AB+	O−	A−	B−	AB−	Total
1	4	2	—	—	2	—	—	—	8
2	—	6	6	—	—	2	—	—	14
3	10	—	—	—	2	—	1	—	13
4	—	2	—	—	4	2	1	—	9
5	4	2	—	—	9	—	—	—	15
6	—	5	2	—	—	—	—	—	7
7	1	13	—	—	1	2	2	—	19
8	20	9	—	—	5	2	—	—	36
9	2	12	2	—	—	—	—	—	16
10	—	8	—	—	—	—	1	—	9
11	—	—	—	—	—	2	1	—	3
12	4	3	2	—	1	—	—	—	10
13	2	4	—	—	2	—	—	—	8
14	2	9	3	—	—	2	2	—	18
15	7	—	—	—	1	—	—	—	8
16	3	2	—	—	—	—	—	—	5
17	—	2	1	2	1	2	1	—	9
18	11	1	1	2	1	1	1	—	18
19	3	3	4	—	2	—	1	—	13
20	3	3	4	—	—	1	1	—	12
21	2	1	—	—	2	1	—	—	6
22	4	—	1	—	—	—	—	—	5
23	2	5	1	—	—	1	2	—	11
24	4	—	1	—	—	2	—	—	7
25	9	4	1	—	6	8	—	—	28
26	5	—	—	—	4	—	2	—	11
Total	102	96	29	4	43	28	16	0	318

20-unit week should not be used in calculating the average weekly blood usage, which is the next step.

3. Total the number of units of each ABO and Rh group, omitting the highest week in each column.
4. Divide each total by 25 (total number of weeks minus the highest week), as shown in Table 23-2.
5. This is the average weekly blood usage of each ABO and Rh group.

From these figures, an optimal inventory should be established. The choice of how much blood should be kept in inventory depends on many factors, especially those listed below. Additionally, such practical considerations as the amount of refrigerator space must be considered. As an arbitrary starting point, a hospital of less than 150 beds might want to keep a 2-week inventory on hand, while a hospital of 150-500 beds might want to keep a 1-week supply on hand. Large hospitals (over 500 beds) may be limited by refrigerator space and might want to keep only 2 or 3 days' supply in inventory.

These suggestions are only a starting point. Evaluation after a suitable period, eg 6-8 weeks, would have to consider outdating rate versus the frequency of emergency blood shipments, frequency of switching from ABO-specific to ABO-compatible blood, delay in scheduling elective surgery and other practical problems. Following this evaluation, optimal inventory levels can be adjusted up or down. The addition of more beds, of new surgical procedures or of staff members

Table 23-2. Calculating Inventory in a Small Transfusion Service

Blood Group	O+	A+	B+	AB+	O−	A−	B−	AB−
Total used	102	96	29	4	43	28	16	0
Highest week (subtract)	20	13	6	2	9	8	2	0
Subtotal	82	83	23	2	34	20	14	0
Divided by 25 = average weekly blood usage	3.3	3.3	0.9	0	1.4	0.8	0.6	0

in specialties like oncology or hematology would increase blood needs and require reevaluation of the optimal blood inventory.

Considerations in Blood Usage

The outdating rate is affected by factors other than inventory level. These include:

Size of the hospital. A hospital with a large census often receives and uses blood nearing outdate simply because large volumes of blood are transfused daily. Blood centers often preferentially ship short-dated blood to large hospitals because the likelihood of transfusion there is much greater than at a small hospital.[3]

The distance a hospital is from the blood supplier, and the frequency with which shipments are delivered. The hospital that is a great distance from the supplier or that receives infrequent shipments must maintain enough blood to cover most emergencies. The larger the blood inventory compared to the amount of blood actually used, the greater the outdate rate. Proximity to other hospitals that can supply blood in an emergency can reduce the need for large inventories.

Policy of using the oldest blood first. Good inventory management demands transfusing the oldest blood first in order to reduce outdating.

Average dating of products received from blood supplier. In general, the shorter the remaining shelf-life upon receipt, the less likely it is that a unit will be used within the dating period. This varies, of course, with daily usage patterns.

Number of laboratory technologists responsible for ordering blood. If many technologists on all shifts order blood, duplication of orders occurs more frequently than if the responsibility for ordering is centralized.

Services provided by the hospital. Hospitals that perform many surgical procedures may require large inventories of blood to fill requests. Because blood is frequently ordered in amounts adequate to cover potential problems, all units crossmatched may not be used. These units may subsequently outdate.

Presence of a frozen blood program. While costly, frozen blood inventories can decrease outdating by providing an extra margin of safety during emergencies. It should be noted, however, that the length of time needed to thaw and deglycerolize these units limits their use for massively bleeding patients.

Teaching hospitals. Because "better safe than sorry" is a common philosophy, teaching hospitals with inexperienced staff often see larger than usual blood orders, increasing the probability of outdating.

Crossmatch to transfusion ratio. A C:T ratio greater than 2.5:1 usually indicates excessive requests for crossmatches.[4] If units are held in reserve for 24-48 hours for patients who will not use the blood, the available shelf-life of these units diminishes by 24-48 hours each time they are held. Establishing a guideline for transfusion therapy[4,5] or a maximal surgical blood order schedule (MSBOS)[6,7] can decrease the C:T ratio, since data about past blood usage are used to recommend how much blood should be crossmatched for future procedures.

Suggested Ordering Policies

The transfusion guidelines in Table 23-3 are average transfusion levels, derived by tabulating blood usage over a 7 month period for each procedure performed in a large teaching hospital.[5] Data collected included the number of patients for whom blood was requested, number of patients who received blood, number of units crossmatched, number of units transfused, the average number of units transfused per patient crossmatched and the (C:T) ratio. Conclusions could thus be drawn about likelihood of transfusion and probable blood usage for any given sur-

Table 23-3. Transfusion Service Guidelines for Elective Surgical Procedures*

General Surgery			Ear, Nose and Throat Surgery		
Cholecystectomy	T&S[†]		Caldwell-Luc	T&S	
Exploratory laparotomy			Laryngectomy	T&S	
(celiotomy)	T&S		**Plastic Surgery**		
Ileal bypass	T&S		Mammoplasty	T&S	
Hiatal hernia repair	T&S		Thoracoabdominal flap	T&S	
Colectomy and hemicolectomy	2 Units		**Oral Surgery**		
Splenectomy	2 Units		Osteotomy	T&S	
Breast biopsy	T&S		Genioplasty	T&S	
Radical mastectomy	1 Unit		Bilateral subcondylar		
Modified radical mastectomy	1 Unit		osteotomy	T&S	
Simple mastectomy	1 Unit		Vestibuloplasty	T&S	
Gastrectomy	2 Units		LaForte I osteotomy	T&S	
Antrectomy and vagotomy	2 Units		Anterior maxillary osteotomy	T&S	
Inguinal herniorrhaphy	T&S		**Neurosurgery**		
Liver biopsy	T&S		Craniotomy	2 Units	
Vein stripping	T&S		Herniated disk	T&S	
Cardiovascular Surgery			Ventriculoperitoneal shunt	T&S	
Saphenous vein bypass	8 Units		Transsphenoidal		
Open heart surgery (congenital			hypophysectomy	2 Units	
defect)	8 Units		**Orthopedics**		
Valve replacement	8 Units		Open reduction	2 Units	
Pleurodesis	T&S		Scoliosis fusion	3–4 Units	
Aortobifemoral bypass	8 Units		Herniated disk	T&S	
Thoracotomy	3 Units		Arthroplasty	T&S	
Closed mediastinal exploration	T&S		Shoulder reconstruction	T&S	
Resection abdominal aortic			Total hip replacement	2–3 Units	
aneurysm	8 Units		Total knee replacement	T&S	
Carotid endarterectomy	2 Units		**Genitourinary Surgery**		
Obstetric-Gynecologic Surgery			Transurethral resection of		
Total abdominal hysterectomy	T&S		prostate	T&S	
Exploratory laparotomy	T&S		Radical nephrectomy	1 Unit	
Total vaginal hysterectomy	T&S		Renal transplantation	1 Unit	
Vaginal resuspension	T&S		Penile prosthesis insertion	T&S	
Laparoscopy	T&S		Patch graft	T&S	
Repeat C-section	T&S		Prostatectomy	2 Units	
Labor and delivery requests					
(oxytocin drips &					
C-sections)	T&S				

*Modified from Boral, et al.[5]   †T&S = Type and antibody screen.

gical procedure. Use of type and antibody screen (group and screen, page 218) is recommended for procedures for which average usage was 0.5 or below.[8,9]

The guidelines in Table 23-3 are suggestions, reflecting local patterns of surgical practice and patient population. In individual transfusion services, it may be desirable to assemble locally applicable data and calculate guidelines for that locale. A blood order schedule is intended for typical circumstances. The surgeon or anesthesiologist may individualize specific requests to accomodate special needs. For the patient with a positive antibody screen, the antibody should be identified. If the antibody is clinically significant, blood lacking the corresponding antigen should be available; an antiglobulin crossmatch is required before blood is administered to such a patient.

Regional Blood Centers

Recruiting and drawing blood donors are increasingly being concentrated in regional blood centers, which today account for 85% of voluntary blood donations. In hospitals in some areas, donors are still regularly drawn; in others areas, donors are drawn only rarely, in times of acute shortage. When there is a consignment arrangement between a regional blood center and hospital transfusion service, blood remains under the control of the blood center until it is transfused and the hospital is billed for the processing fee only if the unit is transfused. The blood center usually absorbs the cost of outdating blood. If hospitals have a direct reimbursement arrangement with the supplier, the hospital absorbs its own cost for outdating blood and the blood center has little control of the blood after delivery.

To overcome seasonal shortages, blood centers and those transfusion services that draw donors often try to build up inventories in times of plenty. Some convert their excess liquid-stored blood to frozen storage, with a 3-year dating period. With newly licensed blood additives, the shelf-life of red blood cells can be as long as 49 days; and this may increase available blood supplies by decreasing outdating.

During acute shortages, due either to decreased donations or increased usage, regional blood centers may request blood from other blood centers, either directly or through various blood organizations (eg, AABB, CCBC, ARC).

Finally, blood centers depend on the media—TV, radio and newspapers—to make the public aware of the community's low blood inventories.

Managing Platelet Inventories

There are few articles describing platelet inventory management.[10,11] The shelf-life of platelets has increased to as long as 7 days with newly formulated plastic containers and some large users stock an inventory of platelets in anticipation of use. Platelets ordered for one patient and not used can still be used by another patient. Since ABO antigens are expressed only weakly on platelets, platelet concentrates need not be ABO group-specific. The volume of transfused ABO-incompatible plasma can be reduced by pooling concentrates of the same ABO group, centrifuging the pooled product, and subsequently extracting part of the plasma. Both centrifugation and subsequent resuspension of platelets must be done gently and the resulting platelet pool, prepared in an open system and stored at room temperature, has a shelf life of 6 hours.

Communication and cooperation between hospitals and regional blood centers improves management of platelet inventories when platelets are ordered for specific patients; knowing the diagnoses and the expected schedule of platelet transfusions helps the blood center plan how many platelet concentrates to produce daily. Most regional blood centers and hospitals outdated 15-25% of platelet concentrates under 3-day platelet storage.

This figure has decreased with 5-day storage, and can be expected to decrease further with 7-day storage.

Inventory Control of Frozen Plasma Products

Since fresh frozen plasma and cryoprecipitate can be stored for one year, no inventory management policies have been published. Inventories of these products should be derived from the needs of the patient population served.

References

1. Brodheim E, Hirsch R, Prostacos G. Setting inventory levels for hospital blood banks. Transfusion 1976;16:63-70.

2. Friedman BA, Abbott RD, Williams GW. A blood ordering strategy for hospital blood banks derived from a computer simulation. Am J Clin Path 1982;78:154-160.

3. Abbott RD, Friedman BA, Williams GW. Recycling older blood by integration into the inventory of a single large hospital blood bank: a computer simulation application. Transfusion 1978;18:709-715.

4. Mintz PD, Nordine RB, Henry JB, Webb WR. Expected hemotherapy in elective surgery. NY State J Med 1976;76:532-537.

5. Boral LI, Dannemiller FJ, Stanford W, Hill SS, Cornell TA. A guideline for anticipated blood usage during elective surgical procedures. Am J Clin Pathol 1979;71:680-684.

6. Friedman BA, Oberman HA, Chadwick AR, Kingdon KI. The maximum surgical blood order schedule and surgical blood use in the United States. Transfusion 1976;16:380-387.

7. Friedman BA. The maximum surgical blood order schedule. In: Polesky HF, Walker RH, eds. Safety in transfusion practices. Skokie, IL: College of American Pathologists; 1982;169-188.

8. Boral LI, Henry JB. The type and screen: a safe alternative and supplement in selected surgical procedures. Transfusion 1977;17:163-168

9. Boral LI, Hill SS, Apollon CJ, Folland A. The type and antibody screen, revisited. Am J Clin Pathol 1979;71:578-581.

10. Katz AJ, Carter CW, Saxton P, Blutt J, Kakaiya RM. Simulation analysis of platelet production and inventory management. Vox Sang 1983;44:31-36.

11. McCullough J, Undis J, Allen JW Jr. Platelet production and inventory management. In: Platelet physiology and transfusion. Washington, DC: American Association of Blood Banks; 1978:17-38.

Special Methods

SM

General Laboratory Topics

Laboratory Safety

The most hazardous reagent to which laboratory workers are exposed may well be blood itself, specimens from patients or donors. Rules designed to protect against hepatitis exposure are sensible precautions to follow when handling any laboratory material. Workers should avoid undue contact with any reagents used in immunohematology procedures, especially contact with skin, mucous membranes, sores or open cuts. When workers adhere to the following rules for general laboratory safety, there is no reason to believe that the kinds and quantities of reagents appropriate to the techniques described in this manual constitute a health hazard.

1. Do not eat, drink or smoke in the laboratory.
2. Do not pipette by mouth.
3. Do not lick labels, chew pencils or put any objects into the mouth.
4. Wear gloves if there are any breaks in the skin.
5. Wear gloves over intact skin if the procedure is likely to result in spillage.
6. Wash hands when leaving the laboratory area.
7. Maintain ventilation adequate to avoid inhalation of volatile materials.
8. Clean up spills promptly.
9. Obey regulations that protect against fire and explosion hazards.

Shipment of Biomedical Material

Volume Less than 50 ml

Material shall be placed in a securely closed, watertight container (primary container like test tube or vial) which shall be enclosed in a second, durable, container (secondary container). Several primary containers may be enclosed in a single secondary container, if the total volume of all the primary containers so enclosed does not exceed 50 ml. The space at the top, bottom and sides between the primary and secondary containers shall contain sufficient nonparticulate absorbent material to absorb the entire contents of the primary container(s) in case of breakage or leakage. Each set of primary and secondary containers shall then be enclosed in an outer shipping container constructed of corrugated fiberboard, cardboard, wood or other material of equivalent strength.

Volume 50 ml or Greater

Packaging of materials in volumes of 50 ml or more shall include, in addition to the above, a shock-absorbent material, in volume at least equal to that of the absorbent material between the primary and secondary containers, at the top, bottom and sides between the secondary container and the outer shipping container. Single primary containers shall not contain more than 500 ml of material; however, two or more primary containers, the combined volumes of which do not exceed 500 ml, may be placed in a single secondary container. Not more than eight secondary shipping containers may be enclosed in a single outer shipping container. (The maximum amount of etiologic agent that may be enclosed within a single outer shipping container shall not exceed 4000 ml.)

Dry Ice

If dry ice is used as a refrigerant, it must be placed outside the secondary container(s). If dry ice is used between the secondary container and the outer shipping container, the shock-absorbent material shall be so placed that the secondary container does not become loose inside the outer shipping container as the dry ice sublimates.

Labels

The label for Etiologic Agents/Biomedical Material, except for size and color, must be as shown in the figure below.

1. The color of material on which the label is printed must be white and the ink must be red.

2. The label must be a rectangle measuring 51 mm (2 inches) high by 102.5 mm (4 inches) long.
3. The red symbol measuring 38 mm ($1\frac{1}{2}$ inches) in diameter must be centered in a white square measuring 51 mm (2 inches) on each side.
4. Type size of the letters of label shall be as follows:

ETIOLOGIC AGENT	10 point (reverse)
BIOMEDICAL MATERIAL	14 point
IN CASE OF DAMAGE OR LEAKAGE	10 point (reverse)
NOTIFY DIRECTOR CDC, ATLANTA, GEORGIA	8 point (reverse)
404 633-5313	10 point (reverse)

Calculating Probability Levels

Probability levels for antibody identification (see page 226) are calculated by constructing 2 × 2 tables in which the presence and absence of serum reactivity are correlated with the presence and absence of a particular antigen among the red cell

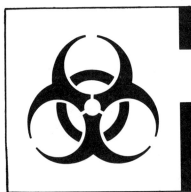

Label for etiologic agents/biomedical material.

samples tested. A 2 × 2 table is constructed as follows:

Serum Reactions	Red Cells		
	Antigen Present	Antigen Absent	Total
Positive	A	B	A + B
Negative	C	D	C + D
Total	A + C	B + D	N

A = number of positive reactions observed with antigen-positive red cell samples

B = number of positive reactions observed with antigen-negative red cell samples

C = number of negative reactions observed with antigen-positive red cell samples

D = number of negative reactions observed with antigen-negative red cell samples

N = total number of red cell samples tested

The formula for calculating probability (p) from a 2 × 2 table is as follows:

$$\frac{(A+B)! \times (C+D)! \times (A+C)! \times (B+D)!}{N! \times A! \times B! \times C! \times D!}$$

Note: ! = the symbol for factorial, the product of all the whole numbers from 1 to the number involved. For example:

6! = 6 × 5 × 4 × 3 × 2 × 1 = 720
3! = 3 × 2 × 1 = 6
1! = 1
0! = 1

Examples

Clearly Defined Results

For a serum reactive with three E+ red cell samples and nonreactive with three E− samples, the 2 × 2 table is:

Serum Reactions	Red Cells		
	E+	E−	Total
Positive	3	0	3
Negative	0	3	3
Total	3	3	6

$$p = \frac{3! \times 3! \times 3! \times 3!}{6! \times 3! \times 0! \times 3! \times 0!} = \frac{36}{720} = \frac{1}{20}$$

This means there is a 1 in 20 likelihood that an antibody other than anti-E could, by chance, have given the observed reactions. This level of probability is the minimum acceptable for statistical significance. Testing the serum against 10 cells, 6 E-negative and 4 E-positive, dramatically improves the probability level of anti-E.

Serum Reactions	Red Cells		
	E+	E−	Total
Positive	4	0	4
Negative	0	6	6
Total	4	6	10

$$p = \frac{4! \times 6! \times 4! \times 6!}{10! \times 4! \times 0! \times 6! \times 0!} = \frac{1}{210}$$

Ambiguous Results

This formula is also useful in determining the significance of discrepant results. For example, a reagent red cell panel has eight e+ samples and two e− samples, and a serum reacts with only seven of the e+ samples:

Serum Reactions	Red Cells		
	e+	e−	Total
Positive	7	0	7
Negative	1	2	3
Total	8	2	10

$$p = \frac{7! \times 3! \times 8! \times 2!}{10! \times 7! \times 0! \times 1! \times 2!} = \frac{1}{15}$$

These results indicate that a serum that does not contain anti-e would, by chance, give these reactions once in 15 trials; this is an unacceptable level for identification. To confirm the presence of anti-e, tests with additional red cell samples are required. The final probability level obtained may be influenced by the phenotypes of the additional red cell samples used. For example, if two additional e+ samples were tested and found to be reactive, the probability level would be improved only modestly:

Serum	Red Cells		
Reactions	e+	e−	Total
Positive	9	0	9
Negative	1	2	3
Total	10	2	12

$$p = \frac{9! \times 3! \times 10! \times 2!}{12! \times 9! \times 1! \times 0! \times 2!} = \frac{1}{22}$$

Greater improvement would have been obtained by testing one additional e+ and one e− sample, if the reactions were as anticipated:

Serum	Red Cells		
Reactions	e+	e−	Total
Positive	8	0	8
Negative	1	3	4
Total	9	3	12

$$p = \frac{8! \times 4! \times 9! \times 3!}{12! \times 8! \times 1! \times 0! \times 3!} = \frac{1}{55}$$

The probability level would be improved still further by using two additional e− samples and finding both nonreactive:

Serum	Red Cells		
Reactions	e+	e−	Total
Positive	7	0	7
Negative	1	4	5
Total	8	4	12

$$p = \frac{7! \times 5! \times 8! \times 4!}{12! \times 7! \times 1! \times 0! \times 4!} = \frac{1}{99}$$

Recommended Reading

1. Moore BPL. Serological and immunological methods of the Canadian Red Cross Blood Transfusion Service. 8th ed. Toronto: The Canadian Red Cross Society; 1980:200-202.

2. Race RR, Sanger R. Blood groups in man. 6th ed. Oxford: Blackwell Scientific Publications; 1975:480-481.

Procedure for Using AABB Rare Donor File

1. Hospital blood bank or transfusion service discovers need for rare blood.
2. Request is referred to nearest AABB-accredited immunohematology reference laboratory.
3. AABB reference laboratory verifies antibody identification and supplies blood if available.
4. If local reference laboratory cannot supply blood, *that reference laboratory* contacts AABB Rare Donor File (612-871-3168, 24-hour telephone). Please see note 1 below.
5. AABB Rare Donor File searches records and informs reference laboratory as to which other AABB reference laboratories may be able to supply appropriate units.
6. Requesting reference laboratory contacts potential supplying reference laboratory and coordinates all shipments of blood. It is the prerogative of the supplying institution to request a patient sample, if deemed necessary. It is strongly recommended that charges be discussed and that the hospital or transfusion service be notified of all costs *before* units are shipped.
7. Supplying institution completes and mails to Rare Donor File a postcard describing the shipment, so that Rare Donor File inventory records can be adjusted.

Notes

1. To prevent confusion that has arisen in the past, *all* requests to the Rare Donor File *must* be made by the local AABB-accredited reference laboratory (or another rare donor file). In the event that requests are received directly from a hospital or transfusion service, the caller will be asked to work through the local AABB-accredited reference laboratory.

2. In the event that no suitable blood is available in the AABB Rare Donor File system, file personnel will contact other rare donor files (American Red Cross, World Health Organization, etc.) and will transmit information to the requesting AABB-accredited reference laboratory as to the procedure to be followed.

Specimens and Reagents

Treatment of Incompletely Clotted Specimens

Serum separated from incompletely clotted blood may continue to evolve fibrin, especially after 37 C incubation. This produces shreds and strands of protein that entrap red cells and make it difficult to evaluate agglutination. Blood from patients who have received heparin may not clot at all, and blood from patients with excessive fibrinolytic activity may reliquify, or contain protein fragments that interfere with examination for agglutination.

To accelerate clotting, either of the following techniques may be used:

1. Add to whole blood or the separated serum the amount of dry thrombin that adheres to the tip of an applicator stick, or one drop of thrombin solution (50 units/ml) per ml of blood.
2. Gently agitate separated serum with small glass beads, at 37 C, for several minutes. Then centrifuge and use supernatant serum.

To neutralize heparin: Add to 4 ml of whole blood one or more drops of 1% saline solution of protamine sulfate (10 mg/ml). Use protamine sparingly because excess protamine can promote rouleaux formation or, in great excess, inhibit clotting.

To inhibit fibrinolytic activity: Add to 4 ml of freshly drawn whole blood 0.1 ml of a solution containing 5 gm epsilon-amino caproic acid in 20 ml saline.

Gentle Elution to Remove Antibody from IgG-Sensitized Red Blood Cells

When cells are heavily coated with IgG antibodies, it is difficult or impossible to interpret results obtained with high-protein antisera or antiglobulin techniques. It is necessary to dissociate antibody from the cell surface without damaging red cell integrity or altering antigenic reactivity. The desired end product is the red cell, not the reactive antibody, so the elution procedure must be somewhat different from those intended to recover active antibody. To demonstrate that elution has not damaged antigenic reactivity, it is desirable to treat in parallel an aliquot of uncoated, normal cells of the appropriate antigenic constitution.

Procedure

1. Place one volume of washed, packed antibody-coated cells and three volumes of normal saline in a test tube of appropriate size. In another tube, place an equal volume of washed, packed cells positive for the antigen thought to be present, usually D.
2. Incubate at approximately 45 C for 30 minutes, with frequent agitation.

3. Centrifuge; discard supernatant.
4. Test for antibody removal by comparing a direct antiglobulin test on the treated cells with the antiglobulin results on untreated cells. If antibody coating is reduced but still present, repeat step 2, incubating for 60 minutes.

Notes

1. If the treated cells are to be tested with high-protein antisera, a diluent control should be run in parallel.
2. If there is no agglutination when the cells are tested with reagent antiserum (eg, anti-D), it is desirable to demonstrate that the treated cells have not lost all antigenic reactivity. Seemingly D-negative cells should be tested with anti-c in parallel with diluent control. If the cells are not agglutinated by anti-c, the negative results on D testing become suspect.
3. An alternative technique is to maintain the cells and saline at 56 C for exactly 3 minutes. Longer incubation will damage antigenic reactivity, but short exposure to higher temperature may more effectively dissociate antibody than longer incubation at moderate heat.

Dissociation of IgG by Chloroquine

Principle and Application

Red cells with a positive direct antiglobulin test due to IgG coating cannot be used directly for blood grouping with antisera, such as anti-Fy^a, that require use of an indirect antiglobulin technique. Under controlled conditions, chloroquine diphosphate dissociates IgG from antibody-coated red cells without damaging integrity of the cell membrane. Use of this procedure facilitates use of antisera reactive only by antiglobulin techniques, for more complete phenotyping of red cells.

Materials

1. Chloroquine diphosphate solution, prepared by dissolving 20 g of chloroquine diphosphate in distilled water. Adjust to pH 5.1 with 1N NaOH, and store at 4 C.
2. Red cells with a positive direct antiglobulin test due to IgG coating
3. Anti-IgG antiglobulin reagent (need not be specific for heavy chains)

Method

1. To 0.2 ml of washed packed IgG-coated red cells add 0.8 ml of chloroquine diphosphate solution.
2. Mix, and incubate at room temperature for 30 minutes.
3. Remove a small aliquot of the treated red cells, and wash for testing with antiglobulin serum.
4. Test the washed red cells with anti-IgG.
5. If nonreactive with anti-IgG, wash the total sample of treated red cells three times in saline, and use for phenotyping with antiglobulin-reactive antisera. Use an anti-IgG reagent when performing these studies.
6. If the treated red cells react with anti-IgG after 30 minutes incubation in chloroquine diphosphate, steps 3 and 4 should be repeated at 30 minute intervals (for a maximum incubation period of two hours), until the red cells are nonreactive with anti-IgG. Then proceed as described in step 5.

Notes

1. Chloroquine diphosphate does not dissociate complement components from red cells. If cells are coated with both IgG and C3 in vivo, tests performed after chloroquine treatment should be performed with anti-IgG.
2. Incubation of red cells in chloroquine diphosphate should not be extended beyond 2 hours. Prolonged incubation may result in hemolysis and loss of red cell antigens.
3. Cells incubated with chloroquine diphosphate give weakened or inconsistent reactions with antisera that cause direct agglutination. Saline-reactive

reagents should not be used on chloroquine-treated cells.

Reference

Edwards JM, Moulds JJ, Judd WJ. Chloroquine diphosphate dissociation of antigen-antibody complexes: a new technique for phenotyping red cells with a positive direct antiglobulin test. Transfusion 1982;22:59-61.

Separation of Transfused from Nontransfused Red Cells by Simple Centrifugation

Principle

Newly formed autologous red cells, having a lower specific gravity than transfused red cells, may be separated from the transfused population by simple centrifugation in microhematocrit tubes without using phthalate esters. The autologous red cells will concentrate at the top of a centrifuged microhematocrit tube. Separation efficiency is reported[1] to be comparable to the phthalate ester technique. Microhematocrit centrifugation provides a simple method for recovering autologous red cells in blood samples from recently transfused patients that can be performed in any clinical laboratory.

Materials

1. Red cells from a recently transfused patient. Blood samples should be collected into EDTA, and used preferably within 24 hours after collection.
2. Microhematocrit equipment: centrifuge, plain (not heparinized) glass hematocrit tubes and a sealant such as Seal-ease®
3. 2-ml syringe and 23-gauge needle

Method

1. Wash the red cells three times in saline, removing as much supernatant as possible without disturbing the buffy coat. For the last wash, centrifuge at 1000 × g for 15 minutes.
2. Fill 10 microhematocrit tubes to the 60-mm mark with packed red cells.
3. Seal the ends of the tubes by heat, or with sealant.
4. Centrifuge all tubes in a microhematocrit centrifuge for 15 minutes.
5. Cut the microhematocrit tubes 5 mm below the top of the centrifuged red cell column.
6. Flush the upper layer of red cells from the cut hematocrit tubes into a clean test tube using a saline-filled syringe and 23-gauge needle.

Notes

1. Separation is better when blood samples are obtained 3 or more days after transfusion, so that substantial numbers of reticulocytes can have accumulated.
2. The packed red cells should be mixed continuously during the filling of microhematocrit tubes.

Reference

Reid ME, Toy P. Simplified method for recovery of autologous red blood cells from transfused patients. Am J Clin Pathol 1983;79:364-366.

Separation by Phthalate Esters of Transfused from Autologous Red Cells

Principle and Application

When red cells are released from the bone marrow they have a specific gravity of approximately 1.078. As the red cells age, this changes to approximately 1.114. In the circulation of a recently transfused patient, donor cells are usually fairly old, whereas the youngest red cells (with the lowest specific gravity) are likely to be the patient's own cells recently released from the marrow. These can be separated from the transfused red cells and the patient's older red cells by exploiting differences in specific gravity. Centrifuging a mixed cell population through water-immiscible solutions of defined specific gravity causes cells with a specific gravity below that of the solution to remain above the column of non-aqueous material, while those with specific gravity greater than that of the non-aqueous solution concentrate below the column. At a certain specific gravity, which varies from patient to patient and must be determined experimentally, only the autologous red cells (essentially the reticulocytes) will remain above the non-aqueous layer. These may be harvested and used to determine the blood group phenotype of the recently transfused patient. The information obtained by such studies can be useful in confirming the specificity of alloantibodies and differentiating autoantibodies from alloantibodies in recently transfused individuals. Mixtures of dimethyl and dibutyl phthalate esters provide non-aqueous solutions of graduated specific gravities.[1]

Materials

1. Phthalate ester mixtures, prepared by weight or volume measurements,[2] as shown in the following tables.
2. Red cells from a recently transfused patient. Blood samples should be collected into EDTA, and used preferably within 24 hours after collection.
3. Microhematocrit equipment: centrifuge, plain (not heparinized) glass hematocrit tubes and a sealant such as Seal-ease®
4. 2-ml syringe and 23-gauge needle

Method

1. Wash the red cells three times in saline. For the last wash, centrifuge at 1000

Preparation of Phthalate Ester Mixtures by Weight

Tube Number	Specific Gravity	Dibutyl Phthalate	Dimethyl Phthalate
1	1.110	6.676 g	5.424 g
2	1.106	5.960 g	5.100 g
3	1.102	6.244 g	4.775 g
4	1.098	6.528 g	4.453 g
5	1.094	6.811 g	4.129 g
6	1.090	7.095 g	3.806 g
7	1.086	7.379 g	3.481 g
8	1.082	7.663 g	3.158 g
9	1.078	7.947 g	2.833 g
10	1.074	8.230 g	2.510 g

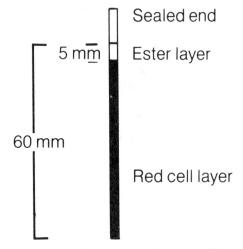

Appearance of microhematocrit tube containing red cells and phthalate ester mixture, before centrifugation.

× g for 15 minutes. Remove as much of the supernatant saline as possible without disturbing the buffy coat. Mix thoroughly.
2. For each ester mixture, fill a microhematocrit tube to the 5-mm mark with ester, and fill to the 60-mm mark with packed red cells (see above figure of single tube).
3. Seal the end of the tubes by heat, or with sealant.
4. Centrifuge all tubes in a microhematocrit centrifuge for 10 minutes.
5. Examine the tubes, and select the phthalate ester mixture which corre-

Preparation of Phthalate Ester Mixtures by Volume

Tube	Specific Gravity	Dibutyl Phthalate	Dimethyl Phthalate
1	1.110	4.8 ml	4.2 ml
2	1.106	5.1 ml	3.9 ml
3	1.102	5.3 ml	3.7 ml
4	1.098	5.6 ml	3.4 ml
5	1.094	5.8 ml	3.2 ml
6	1.090	6.0 ml	3.0 ml
7	1.086	6.3 ml	2.7 ml
8	1.082	6.5 ml	2.5 ml
9	1.078	6.8 ml	2.2 ml
10	1.074	7.0 ml	2.0 ml

1	2	3	4	5	6	7	8	9	10
1.110	1.106	1.102	1.098	1.094	1.090	1.086	1.082	1.078	1.074

Diagrammatic representation of density pattern obtained after centrifuging tubes containing red cells and phthalate ester mixtures of different specific gravities.

sponds to the tube containing approximately 5 mm of red cells above the ester layer (eg, tube #8 in diagrammatic figure shown above).

6. Prepare a number of tubes containing packed red cells and the selected ester mixture. Ten tubes will normally suffice.

7. Centrifuge the tubes in a microhematocrit centrifuge for 10 minutes.

8. Cut the microhematocrit tubes at the interface of the ester layer and the upper layer of packed red cells.

9. Flush the upper layer of red cells from the cut hematocrit tubes into a clean test tube using saline in a syringe with a 23-gauge needle.

10. Wash the separated red cells four times in saline prior to testing.

Notes

1. Accuracy is essential when preparing phthalate ester mixtures. While preparation by weight is preferred, volume measurements will suffice if performed carefully. Use 2-ml conical tubes. Add one ester to all tubes first, and allow to settle. Since the esters are viscous, it may be necessary to adjust the volumes of the first ester before adding the second ester.

2. Phthalate esters should be warmed to room temperature before use.

3. Phthalate esters should be stored in the dark, since they are denatured by light.

4. The packed red cells should be mixed continuously during the filling of microhematocrit tubes.

References

1. Wallas CH, Tanley PC, Gorrell LP. Recovery of autologous erythrocytes in transfused patients. Transfusion 1980;20:332-336.
2. Rolih SD. Personal communication.

General Instructions for Preparing Solutions

Many blood bankers panic when faced with the need to prepare solutions to various specifications. The definitions, calculations and instructions given below should refresh faded memories of elementary chemistry and promote familiarity with these fundamentally simple principles.

Definitions

Mole, gram-molecular weight: Weight, in grams, of a substance so that the number of grams is numerically equal to the molecular weight of the substance

Molar solution: A one molar (1M) solution contains one mole of solute in a liter of solution. The solvent should always be assumed to be distilled or deionized water unless otherwise indicated.

Molal solution: A one molal solution contains 1 mole of solute in 1 kg of solvent. If the solvent is water, there is little practical difference between molar and molal solutions, but the technique of preparation is, theoretically at least, very different. In blood banking, solutions are universally made up to volume and thus are molar, not molal, solutions.

Gram-equivalent weight: Weight, in grams, of a substance, which will produce or react with 1 mole of hydrogen ion.

Normal solution: A one normal (1N) solution contains one gram-equivalent weight of solute in a liter of solution.

Percentage solutions: The percent of a solution gives the weight or volume of solute present in 100 units of total solution. Percent can be expressed as:

Weight/weight (w/w), giving grams of solute in 100 g of solution
Volume/volume (v/v), giving milliliters of solute present in 100 ml of solution
Weight/volume (w/v), giving grams of solute in 100 ml of solution

Most commonly used is weight/volume. Unless otherwise specified, a solution expressed in percentage can be assumed to be w/v.

Water of crystallization, water of hydration: Molecules of water that form an integral part of the crystalline structure of a substance. A given substance may have several crystalline forms, with several different numbers of water molecules intrinsic to the entire molecule. The weight of this water must be included in calculating molecular weight of the hydrated substance.

Anhydrous: The salt form of a substance with no water of crystallization.

Examples

Atomic weights (rounded to whole numbers):

H, 1; O, 16; Na, 23; P, 31; S, 32; Cl, 35; K, 39

Molecular weights:

HCl: $1 + 35 = 36$; NaCl: $23 + 35 = 58$; KCl: $39 + 35 = 74$

H_2O: $(2 \times 1) + 16 = 18$

NaH_2PO_4: $23 + (2 \times 1) + 31 + (4 \times 16) = 120$

$NaH_2PO_4 \cdot H_2O$: $23 + (2 \times 1) + 31 + (4 \times 16) + (2 \times 1) + 16 = 138$

KH_2PO_4: $39 + (2 \times 1) + 31 + (4 \times 16) = 136$

H_2SO_4: $(2 \times 1) + 32 + (4 \times 16) = 98$

Molar solutions:

1M KH_2PO_4 requires 136 g solute made up to 1000 ml

0.15M KH_2PO_4 requires $136 \times 0.15 = 20.4$ g solute made up to 1000 ml

0.5M NaH_2PO_4 requires $120 \times 0.5 = 60$ g solute made up to 1000 ml

Molar solution with hydrated salt:

0.5M $NaH_2PO_4 \cdot H_2O$ requires $138 \times 0.5 = 60$ g of the monohydrate crystals made up to 1000 ml

Normal solutions:

1N HCl requires 36 g solute made up to 1000 ml. One mole HCl dissociates into one mole H^+, so gram-equivalent weight and gram-molecular weight are the same.

12N HCl requires $36 \times 12 = 432$ g solute made up to 1000 ml

1N H_2SO_4 requires $98 \div 2 = 432$ g solute made up to 1000 ml. One mole H_2SO_4 dissociates to give two moles of H^+, so the gram-molecular weight is double the gram-equivalent weight.

Percent solution:

0.9% NaCl requires 0.9 g solute made up to 100 ml solution

Practical Pointers

Accurate results require accurate preparation of reagents. It is important to read all instructions and labels carefully, and to follow instructions meticulously. There should be no variation between individuals in a laboratory, or between performances by the same individual.

1. Know the accuracy of the weighing equipment; the instruction manual includes this in the specifications. Weigh quantities appropriate for the accuracy of the equipment.
2. Prepare the largest volume that is practical, because there is greater accuracy in measuring larger volumes than smaller volumes. If a reagent balance is accurate to $\pm$ 0.01 g, the potential error in weighing 0.05 g (50 mg) will be 20%, whereas the potential error of weighing 0.25 g (250 mg) will be only 4%.

   If the solution retains its activity when stored appropriately, it is usually preferable to prepare a large volume. If the solution deteriorates rapidly, considerations of accuracy must be weighed against cost and convenience.
3. Note whether a substance is in the hydrated or anhydrous form. If the instructions give solute weight for one form, and the available reagent is in another form, be sure to adjust the measurements appropriately. For example, if instructions for 0.5 M NaH_2PO_4 call for 60 g, and the reagent is $NaH_2PO_4 \cdot H_2O$, find the ratio between the weights of the two forms

$$\left(\frac{NaH_2PO_4 \cdot H_2O}{NaH_2PO_4} = \frac{138}{120} = 1.15 \right)$$

   and multiply the designated weight by that figure (60 g $\times$ 1.15 = 69 g).
4. Dissolve the solute completely before making the solution to the final volume. This is especially important for substances, like phosphates, that dissolve slowly. For example, to make 500 ml of 0.15 M KH_2PO_4:

   a. Weigh 10.2 g solute in a weighing boat or glass (0.15 $\times$ 136 $\div$ 2, since only 500 ml will be made).
   b. Place approximately 350 ml water in a 1000-ml beaker on a magnetic stirrer. Add the stirring bar and adjust the speed of stirring.
   c. Add the 10.2 g salt, then rinse the boat with several aliquots of water until no salt remains. Numerous small-volume rinses remove adherent material more effectively than a few larger volumes. Add the rinse water to the material in the beaker and stir until the salt is completely dissolved.
   d. Transfer the solution from the beaker to a 500-ml volumetric flask.
   e. Rinse the beaker and the stirring rod with several aliquots of water, adding the rinse water to the flask. The more concentrated the solution in the beaker, the more thorough the rinsing need be.
   f. Add water to the 500-ml mark and mix by inverting the flask several times.
5. Adjust the pH of the solution before accurately bringing it to final volume so that addition of water (or other solvent) does not markedly change the adjusted pH. For example, to bring 500 ml of 0.1 M glycine to pH 3.0:

   a. Add 3.75 g glycine (H_2NCH_2CCOH: molecular weight, 75) to 400 to 475 ml water in a beaker. Dissolve completely, using magnetic stirrer.
   b. Add drops of concentrated (12N) HCl and measure pH after acid is thoroughly mixed. Continue adding HCl until pH is 3.0.
   c. Transfer the solution to a 500-ml volumetric flask; rinse beaker and stirring bar with aliquots of water, adding the rinse water to the flask. Use the rinses to make to 500 ml.

d. Measure the pH of the solution at final volume.

Recommended Reading

Remson ST, Ackerman PG. Calculations for the medical laboratory. Boston, MA: Little, Brown & Co.; 1977.

Preparation and Use of Phosphate Buffer

1. Prepare acidic stock solution (solution A) by dissolving 22.16 g of $NaH_2PO_4 \cdot H_2O$ in 1 liter of distilled water. This 0.16M solution of the monobasic phosphate salt (monohydrate) has a pH of 5.0.
2. Prepare alkaline stock solution (solution B) by dissolving 17.2 g of Na_2HPO_4 in 1 liter of distilled water. This 0.126M solution of the dibasic phosphate salt (anhydrous) has a pH of 9.0.
3. Prepare working buffer solutions of the desired pH by mixing appropriate volumes of the two solutions. A few examples are:

pH	Solution A	Solution B
5.5	94 ml	6 ml
7.3	16 ml	84 ml
7.7	7 ml	93 ml

4. Check pH of working solution before using it. Add small volumes of acid solution A or alkaline solution B to achieve desired pH.

Phosphate-Buffered Saline

To prepare phosphate-buffered saline (PBS) of a desired pH, add one volume of phosphate buffer at that pH to nine volumes of normal saline.

Reference

Hendry EB. Osmolarity of human serum and of chemical solutions of biologic importance. Clin Chem 1961;7:156-164.

Low Ionic Strength Salt (LISS) Solution

Preparation of Solution

1. Add 1.75 g NaCl and 18 g glycine to a 1-liter volumetric flask.
2. Add 20 ml of phosphate buffer prepared by combining 11.3 ml of 0.15M KH_2PO_4 and 8.7 ml of 0.15M Na_2HPO_4.
3. Add distilled water to the 1000-ml mark.
4. Adjust pH to 6.7 with 1N NaOH.
5. Add 0.5 g sodium azide as a preservative.

Note: Adding sodium azide in this quantity raises the ionic strength from 0.0355 to 0.043. This does not affect the serologic behavior of the solution (Personal communication, Phyllis Morel).

Use in Tests

1. Wash three times in normal saline an adequate volume of the red cells to be used.
2. Completely decant saline.
3. Resuspend the cells to a 2% suspension in LISS.
4. Add 2 drops of serum to properly labeled tube.
5. Add 2 drops of LISS-suspended cells.
6. Mix and incubate 15 minutes at 37 C.
7. Centrifuge, examine supernatant for hemolysis, and examine for agglutination.
8. Wash cells 3 or 4 times with saline and perform an antiglobulin test.

Note: The incubation time and the concentration of cells in the final LISS suspension are those given in the reference cited. Individual laboratories may wish to standardize techniques with somewhat different values.

Reference

Fitzsimmons JM, Morel PA. The effects of red blood cell suspending media on hemagglutination and the antiglobulin test. Transfusion 1979;19:81-85.

Preparation and Use of Enzymes

Principle

Proteolytic enzymes modify red cell antigens in ways that enhance the reactivity of some antigen-antibody systems (notably Rh and Kidd) and abolish antigenic configurations of others (notably M, N, Fy^a and Fy^b). Enzyme modification also alters nonimmune physical properties of the cell suspension and can cause spontaneous aggregation of cells in an immunologically inert system. The preparations used in blood banking differ from lot to lot, so each time a stock enzyme solution is prepared, its reactivity must be tested and incubation periods standardized for optimum effectiveness.

Preparation of Stock Solutions
Ficin

1. Place 1 g powdered ficin in a 100-ml volumetric flask. Handle ficin carefully because it is harmful if inhaled or if it gets in the eyes. Wearing gloves, mask and apron or working under a hood is desirable.
2. Dissolve in phosphate-buffered saline (PBS), pH 7.3 (see page 424), to 100 ml. Agitate vigorously by inversion or on a rotator for 15 minutes, or with a magnetic stirrer for 30-90 minutes. The powder will not dissolve completely.
3. Collect clear fluid, either by filtration or centrifugation, and prepare small aliquots. Store aliquots at -20 C. Do not refreeze thawed solution.

Löw's Activated Papain

1. Grind 0.5 g papain in a mortar with a few milliliters of phosphate buffer, pH 5.5. See page 424 for preparation of buffer.
2. Wash the papain suspension into a 250-ml flask with 190 ml phosphate buffer, pH 5.5.
3. Add 0.6 g L-cysteine hydrochloride dissolved in 10 ml distilled water.

4. Incubate at 37 C for 1 hour. Incubation time should begin when the solution reaches 37 C.
5. Centrifuge the solution. Keep the supernatant fluid and discard undissolved papain.
6. Store activated papain solution at -20 C in small aliquots. Activated papain is not stable at 4 C. Once the solution is thawed, the unused portion must be discarded at the end of the day.

Standardization of Procedure

For a two-stage enzyme procedure, the optimum dilution and incubation conditions must be determined for each new lot of stock solution. The technique given below for ficin can be modified for use with other enzymes.

Materials

1. Stock solution of ficin in phosphate-buffered saline, pH 7.3
2. Several sera that contain no unexpected antibodies
3. Anti-D that agglutinates only enzyme-treated Rh-positive cells and does not agglutinate unmodified Rh-positive cells
4. Anti-Fy^a of moderate or strong reactivity
5. Red blood cells positive for D and Fy^a

Method

1. Dilute 1 volume of stock ficin solution with 9 volumes of phosphate-buffered saline, pH 7.3, to make approximately 0.1%.
2. Label three tubes: 5 minutes, 10 minutes, and 15 minutes.
3. Add equal volumes of washed, packed red cells and 0.1% ficin to each tube.
4. Mix and incubate at 37 C for the time designated. Incubation time is easily controlled if the 15-minute tube is prepared first, followed by the 10- and 5-minute tubes at 5-minute intervals. Incubation will be complete for all three tubes at the same time.
5. Immediately wash the cells 3 times with adequate volumes of saline.

6. Resuspend treated cells to 2-5% in saline.
7. Label four tubes for each serum to be tested: untreated, 5-minutes, 10-minutes, 15-minutes.
8. Add 2 drops of the appropriate serum to each of the four tubes.
9. Add 1 drop of the appropriate cell suspension to the labeled tubes.
10. Mix and incubate at 37 C for 15 minutes.
11. Centrifuge, and examine for agglutination by gently resuspending cell button.
12. Wash cells 3 or 4 times with saline and add antihuman globulin (AHG) serum.

Interpretation

Shown below are hypothetical results with a D-positive, Fy^a-postive cell.

		Inert Serum	Anti-D	Anti-Fy^a
Untreated	37 C inc.	0	0	0
	AHG	0	1+	3+
5 minutes	37 C inc.	0	1+	0
	AHG	0	2+	1+
10 minutes	37 C inc.	0	2+	0
	AHG	0	2+	0
15 minutes	37 C inc.	0	2+	0
	AHG	w+	2+	w+

The optimum incubation time would be 10 minutes. Incubation for only 5 minutes does not completely abolish Fy^a activity or maximally enhance anti-D reactivity. Incubation for 15 minutes causes false-positive antiglobulin reactivity with sera that should not have reacted immunologically.

If incubation for 5 minutes proves to overtreat the cells, it is better to use a more dilute working solution of enzyme than to reduce incubation time, because it is difficult to determine and then to monitor very short incubation times with sufficient accuracy. In additional tests, a single dilution can be selected and studied for different incubation times, or a single time can be selected and the effects of different dilutions studied.

Evaluating Treated Red Cells

After optimum incubation conditions have been determined for a new lot of enzyme solution, treated cells should be evaluated before use to demonstrate that the specific cells are adequately, but not excessively, modified. Satisfactory treatment produces cells that are agglutinable by an antibody that gives only antiglobulin reactions with unmodified cells, and are not agglutinated or aggregated in the presence of inert serum.

1. Select an antibody that agglutinates enzyme-treated cells positive for the antigen but gives only antiglobulin reactions with unmodified cells. Many examples of anti-D in serum from patients behave in this way.
2. Add 2 drops of the selected antibody-containing serum to a tube labeled "positive."
3. Add 2 drops of a serum free of unexpected antibodies to a tube labeled "negative."
4. Add 1 drop of 2-5% suspension of enzyme-treated cells to each tube.
5. Mix and incubate 15 minutes at 37 C.
6. Centrifuge and resuspend the cells by gentle shaking.
7. Examine macroscopically for the presence of agglutination.

There should be agglutination in the "positive" tube and no agglutination in the "negative" tube. If agglutination occurs in the "negative" tube, the cells have been overtreated; if agglutination does not occur in the "positive" tube, treatment has been inadequate.

Use in Testing
One-Stage Technique

Papain or bromelain are suitable for use in one-stage procedures.

1. Add 2 drops of serum to a properly labeled tube.
2. Add 1 drop of a 2-5% saline suspension of red cells.

3. Add 2 drops of enzyme solution. Mix.
4. Incubate at 37 C for 30 minutes.
5. Centrifuge; gently resuspend the cells and observe for agglutination. Record results.

Two-Stage Technique

Ficin should be used only by the two-stage procedure. Other enzymes may also be used in this way.

1. Prepare a diluted ficin solution by adding 9 ml PBS, pH 7.3 to 1 ml of stock ficin.
2. Add one volume of diluted ficin to one volume of packed, washed red blood cells.
3. Incubate at 37 C for the time determined to be optimum for that enzyme solution.
4. Wash treated cells at least 3 times with large volumes of saline.
5. Resuspend cells to 2-5% concentration in saline.
6. Add 2 drops of serum to be tested to properly labeled tube.
7. Add 1 drop of 2-5% suspension of ficin-treated cells.
8. Mix and incubate 15-30 minutes at 37 C.
9. Centrifuge, observe for hemolysis and resuspend cells by gentle shaking.
10. Observe macroscopically for agglutination.
11. Proceed with antiglobulin procedure, if desired.

Note: An alternative method for steps 8 and 9 is to incubate the serum and enzyme-treated cells at 37 C for 60 minutes and then to examine the settled cells for agglutination without centrifugation. This can be useful for serum with strong cold agglutinins and can sometimes prevent problems with false-positive results.

References

1. Issitt PD, Issitt CH. Applied blood group serology. 2nd ed. Oxnard, CA: Spectra Biologicals; 1975;25-26.
2. Löw B. A practical method using papain and incomplete Rh-antibodies in routine Rh blood-grouping. Vox Sang 1955;5:94-98.

Use of Lectins

Saline extracts of seeds make useful typing reagents, and are highly specific at appropriate dilutions. They are easy to prepare and use, but may be difficult to obtain. *Dolichos biflorus* extract agglutinates A_1 cells but not A_2. *Ulex europaeus* extract reacts with H substance; it agglutinates cells that have H antigenic activity in a manner proportional to the amount of H present. Other lectins are useful for special purposes. The volume, proportions and timing of the extraction process are not critical.

1. Grind seeds in a blender until the particles look like coarse sand. Mortar and pestle may be used, or seeds can be used whole.
2. In a large test tube or small beaker, place ground seeds and 3-4 times their volume of saline. (Seeds vary in the quantity of saline they absorb.)
3. Incubate at room temperature for 4-12 hours, stirring occasionally.
4. Transfer supernatant fluid to a centrifuge tube and centrifuge for 1 minute, to obtain clear supernate. Filter the supernatant fluid.
5. Determine activity of extract with appropriate cells.
   For *Dolichos biflorus*:
   a. Add 1 drop of extract to each of 3 tubes, labeled A_1, A_2 and O. Group B, A_1B and A_2B cells may also be included.
   b. Add 1 drop of 2-5% saline suspension of known A_1, A_2 and O cells (and B, A_1B, A_2B if used) to appropriate tubes.
   c. Centrifuge 15 seconds.
   d. Observe for agglutination and record results.
   e. Lectin should agglutinate A_1 and A_1B cells and not A_2, A_2B, B or O. Often, the native extract agglutinates all the cells tested. To make the product useful for reagent purposes, add enough saline to the

extract so that there is 3 or 4+ agglutination of A_1 and A_1B cells, but not of A_2 or other cells.

For *Ulex europaeus*:

a. Add 1 drop of extract to each of 5 tubes, labeled A_1, A_2, A_1B, A_2B and O.

b. Add 1 drop of 2-5% saline suspension of known A_1, A_2, A_1B, A_2B and O cells to appropriate tubes.

c. Centrifuge 15 seconds.

d. Observe for agglutination and record results.

e. Strength of agglutination should be in the order $O > A_2 > B > A_1 > A_1B$. *Ulex* extract tends to be less potent than *Dolichos* extract.

f. Dilute extract with saline if necessary, to a point that O cells show 3 or 4+ agglutination, A_2 cells show less, and A_1 or A_1B cells are not agglutinated.

6. Store extract in refrigerator for several days, or in freezer for longer period (may be stored indefinitely if frozen).

7. To use for testing, include known positive and negative controls each time. Follow the procedure given in step 5.

Reactions of Polyagglutinable Cells with Lectins

	T	Tn	Tk	Cad
Arachis hypogaea	+	0	+	0
Salvia sclarea	0	+	0	0
Salvia horminum	0	+	0	+
Glycine soja	+	+	0	+
Dolichos biflorus*	0	+	0	+

+ = agglutination; 0 = no agglutination

*A_1 cells are positive regardless of the type of polyagglutination.

Elution Procedures

No single elution technique is equally effective in all serologic circumstances. The procedures below employ different techniques for disengaging antibody from antigens on the surface of well-washed red cells. In every procedure, the supernatant saline from the last wash is tested for antibody activity in parallel with the eluate, to determine whether reactivity in the eluate represents recovery of coating antibodies from the red cell or results from residual serum contaminating the suspension of washed cells. Reactivity in the supernatant from the last wash need not indicate inadequate washing; reactivity may occur if the coating antibody has a low affinity for its corresponding antigen and elutes during the washing process.

Heat Elution

Primary Application

Investigation of hemolytic disease of the newborn, particularly ABO hemolytic disease, and the elution of IgM antibodies from red cells.

Materials

1. 6% bovine albumin, prepared by diluting 22% or 30% bovine albumin with saline
2. Packed red cells (2 ml), washed six times in saline
3. Supernatant saline from last wash

Method

1. Mix equal volumes of washed packed red cells and dilute bovine albumin in a 13 × 100-mm test tube.
2. Place the tube at 56 C for 10 minutes. Agitate the tube periodically during this time.
3. Centrifuge the tube at 1000 × g for 2 minutes, preferably in a heated centrifuge.
4. Immediately transfer the supernatant eluate into a clean test tube, and test in parallel with the final wash supernatant.

Reference

Landsteiner K, Miller CP. Serological studies on the blood of primates. II. The blood groups in anthropoid apes. J Exp Med 1925;42:853-862.

Ultrasound Elution

Primary Application

Investigation of ABO hemolytic disease of the newborn

Materials

1. Ultrasound cleaning bath
2. 6% bovine albumin, prepared by diluting 22% or 30% bovine albumin with saline
3. Packed red cells (2 ml), washed six times in saline
4. Supernatant saline from last wash

Method

1. Mix one volume of 6% bovine albumin and two volumes of red cells in a stoppered 13 × 100-mm test tube.
2. Fill the ultrasound cleaning bath with distilled water to within one inch of the top and switch on.
3. Place the tube in the center of the bath, resting the bottom of the tube on the bottom of the cleaning bath.
4. Maintain the tube in this position for approximately 1 minute, until lysis is completed. Mixing the contents of the tube with a pasteur pipette during this time will facilitate hemolysis.
5. Centrifuge the tube at 1000 × g for 5 minutes.
6. Transfer the supernatant eluate into a clean test tube, and test in parallel with the final wash supernatant.

Reference

Jimerfield CA. A rapid and simple method for preparing red cell eluates using ultrasound. Am J Med Technol 1977;43:187-189.

Freeze-Thaw Elution (Lui Elution)

Primary Application

Investigation of ABO hemolytic disease of the newborn

Materials

1. Packed red cells, washed six times in saline
2. Supernatant saline from last wash

Method

1. Dispense 0.5 ml aliquots of washed packed red cells into 13 × 100-mm test tubes. Prepare sufficient tubes to yield the amount of eluate required.
2. Add three drops of saline to each tube of red cells and mix well.
3. Stopper the tubes, and rotate them so as to coat the inner surface of the tubes with red cells.
4. Place the tubes horizontally at a temperature between −20 C and −70 C for 10 minutes.
5. Rapidly thaw the red cells under running warm tap water.
6. Centrifuge all tubes at 1000 × g for 2 minutes.
7. Transfer the supernatant eluates into a clean test tube, and test in parallel with the final wash supernatant.

References

1. Eicher CA, Wallace ME, Frank S, de Jongh DS. The Lui elution: a simple method for antibody elution. Transfusion 1978;18:647.
2. Barnes JM. Evaluation of the Lui easy-freeze elution test. Lab Med 1981;12:227-228.

Ether Elution

Primary Application

Investigation of a positive direct antiglobulin test associated with warm-reactive (IgG) auto- or alloantibodies, and the separation of mixtures of IgG antibodies.

Materials

1. Diethyl ether, reagent or anesthesiologic grade
2. Packed red cells (2 ml), washed six times in saline
3. Supernatant saline from final wash

Method

1. Mix equal volumes of washed packed red cells and ether in a 13 × 100-mm test tube.
2. Stopper the tube with a cork, and agitate the tube vigorously for 1 to 2 minutes.
3. Carefully remove the cork to release pressure slowly and place the tube at 37 C for 15 minutes.
4. Centrifuge the tube at 1000 × g for 5 minutes.
5. Remove and discard the upper layer of ether.
6. Transfer the hemoglobin-stained eluate from below the stromal layer into a clean 13 × 100-mm test tube.

7. Place the tube at 37 C and periodically bubble air through the eluate, using a pasteur pipette, until it no longer smells of ether.
8. Centrifuge the tube at 1000 × g for 5 minutes.
9. Transfer the supernatant eluate into a clean test tube, and test in parallel with the final wash supernatant.

Notes

1. The procedure described by Rubin[2] utilized a 50% red cell suspension in saline, rather than packed red cells.
2. A combined heat-ether technique is reported to yield a more potent eluate than can be obtained by either heat or ether elution alone. (Marsh WL, personal communication) A 50% saline suspension of red cells should be used. At step 3 above, the supernatant ether is removed by suction, and the contents of the tube stirred with an applicator stick. The tube is then placed at 56 C and stirred gently for 5 minutes. The tube should be watched carefully and placed at room temperature if the eluate begins to boil and rise to the top of the test tube, but can be returned to 56 C when boiling ceases. Following centrifugation at 1000 × g for 5 minutes, the procedure is identical to steps 6 through 9 in the preceding method.

References

1. Vos G. The evaluation of specific anti-G (CD) eluates obtained by a double adsorption and elution procedure. Vox Sang 1960;5:472-478.
2. Rubin H. Antibody elution from red blood cells. J Clin Pathol 1963;16:70-73.

Digitonin-Acid Elution

Primary Application

See ether elution technique.

Materials

1. Digitonin (0.5% w/v), prepared by dissolving 0.5 g of digitonin in 100 ml of distilled water. Store at 4 C.
2. Glycine (0.1M, pH 3.0), prepared by dissolving 3.754 g of glycine in 500 ml of distilled water. Adjust pH to 3.0 with 12N HCl. Store at 4 C.
3. Phosphate buffer (0.8M, pH 8.2), prepared by dissolving 109.6 g of Na_2HPO_4 and 3.8 g of KH_2PO_4 in approximately 600 ml of distilled water. Adjust pH, if necessary, with either 1N NaOH or 1N HCl. Dilute to a final volume of 1 liter with distilled water. Store at 4 C.
4. Packed red cells (1 ml), washed six times in saline
5. Supernatant saline from last wash

Method

1. Warm reagents to 37 C before use, and mix well.
2. Mix 1 ml of red cells and 9 ml of saline in a 16 × 100-mm test tube.
3. Add 0.5 ml of digitonin, and mix by inversion until all red cells are hemolyzed (at least one minute).
4. Centrifuge the tube at 1000 × g for 5 minutes, and discard the supernatant.
5. Wash red cell stroma at least five times, or until it appears white. Centrifuge for at least 2 minutes during the washing process.
6. Discard the final supernatant wash solution, and add 2 ml of glycine to the stroma.
7. Mix by inversion for at least 1 minute.
8. Centrifuge the tube at 1000 × g for 5 minutes.
9. Transfer the supernatant eluate into a clean test tube and add 0.2 ml of phosphate buffer.
10. Mix, and centrifuge at 1000 × g for 2 minutes.
11. Transfer the supernatant eluate into a clean test tube and add one-third volume of 30% bovine serum albumin. Test in parallel with the final wash supernatant.

Notes

1. The low pH of the acid buffer enhances elution of antibody from the red cell

stroma. Phosphate buffer is added to restore neutrality to the acidic eluate. Persisting acidity may cause lysis of red cells added to the eluate. Adding bovine albumin to the eluate protects against hemolysis.

2. Ensure digitonin is well mixed and warmed to 37 C before use.
3. Use centrifugation times of at least 2 minutes when washing stroma.
4. Phosphate buffer will crystallize on storage at 4 C. Redissolve at 37 C before use.

Reference

Jenkins DE, Moore WH. A rapid method for the preparation of high-potency auto- and alloantibody eluates. Transfusion 1977;17:110-117.

Cold-Acid Elution

Primary Application

See ether elution technique.

Materials

1. Glycine (0.1M, pH 3.0), prepared by dissolving 3.754 g of glycine and 2.992 g of sodium chloride in 500 ml of distilled water. Adjust pH to 3.0 with 12 N HCl. Store at 4 C.
2. Phosphate buffer (0.8M, pH 8.2), as prepared for the digitonin-acid elution technique
3. Chilled isotonic saline, at 4 C
4. Packed red cells (1 ml), washed six times in saline
5. Supernatant saline from last wash

Method

1. Add 1 ml of chilled saline and 2 ml of glycine to 1 ml of washed packed red cells in a 13 × 100-mm test tube (see note #1).
2. Mix and incubate the tube in an ice bath for one minute.
3. Centrifuge the tube at 1000 × g for 2 minutes.
4. Transfer the supernatant eluate into a clean test tube, and add 0.1 ml of pH

8.2 phosphate buffer for each 1 ml of eluate (see note #2).

5. Mix and centrifuge at 1000 × g for 2 minutes.
6. Transfer the supernatant eluate into a clean test tube, and test in parallel with the final wash supernatant.

Notes

1. Keep glycine at 4 C during use.
2. Phosphate buffer will crystallize on storage at 4 C. Redissolve at 37 C before use.

Reference

Rekvig OP, Hannestad K. Acid elution of blood group antibodies from intact erythrocytes. Vox Sang 1977;33:280-285.

Chloroform Elution

Primary Application

See ether elution technique.

Materials

1. Reagent grade chloroform
2. 6% bovine albumin, prepared by diluting 22% or 30% bovine albumin with saline
3. Packed red cells (1 ml), washed six times in saline
4. Supernatant saline from last wash

Method

1. Add 1 ml of 6% bovine albumin and 2 ml of chloroform to 1 ml of red cells in a 13 × 100-mm test tube.
2. Stopper the tube with a cork, and agitate the tube vigorously for 15 seconds. Mix further by inversion for 1 minute.
3. Remove the cork, and place the tube at 56 C for 5 minutes. Stir the contents of the tube with applicator sticks during this time.
4. Centrifuge the tube at 1000 × g for 5 minutes.
5. Transfer the supernatant eluate into a clean test tube, and test in parallel with the final wash supernatant.

Reference

Branch DR, Hian ALS, Petz LD. A new elution procedure using a nonflammable organic solvent. (abstract) Transfusion 1980;20:635.

Xylene Elution

Primary Application

See ether elution technique.

Materials

1. Reagent grade xylene
2. Packed red cells (2 ml), washed six times in saline
3. Supernatant saline from last wash

Method

1. Mix equal volumes of red cells and xylene in a 13 × 100-mm test tube.
2. Stopper the tube with a cork, and agitate the tube vigorously for 1 to 2 minutes. Remove the cork.
3. Place the tube at 56 C for 10 minutes. Stir the contents of the tube with applicator sticks during this time.
4. Centrifuge the tube at 1000 × g for 10 minutes.
5. Carefully remove and discard the upper layer of xylene and the stroma by vacuum aspiration (see note below).
6. Transfer the eluate into a clean test tube, and test in parallel with the final wash supernatant.

Note

Care should be taken not to contaminate the eluate with stroma. Do not use a pasteur pipette with rubber bulb during step 5. If contamination does occur, recentrifuge the eluate at 1000 × g for 10 minutes.

References

1. Chan-Shu SA, Blair O. A new method of antibody elution from red blood cells. Transfusion 1979;19:182-185.
2. Bueno R, Garratty G, Postoway N. Elution of antibody from red blood cells using xylene—a superior method. Transfusion 1981;21:157-162.

Methylene Chloride Elution

Primary Application

See ether elution technique.

Materials

1. Methylene chloride (dichloromethane)
2. Packed red cells (1 ml), washed six times in saline
3. Supernatant saline from last wash

Method

1. Dilute the red cells with an equal volume of saline in a 13 × 100-mm test tube.
2. Add a volume of methylene chloride equal to the total volume of 50% red cells in saline.
3. Stopper the tube with a cork, and mix by gentle agitation for 1 minute. Remove the cork.
4. Centrifuge the tube at 1000 × g for 10 minutes.
5. Using a pasteur pipette, remove the lower layer of methylene chloride and discard.
6. Place the tube at 56 C for 10 minutes. Stir the contents of the tube with applicator sticks during this time.
7. Centrifuge the tube at 1000 × g for 10 minutes.
8. Transfer the supernatant eluate into a clean test tube, and test in parallel with the final wash supernatant.

Reference

Ellisor SS, Papenfus L, Sugasawara E, Azzi R. Dichloromethane (DCM) elution procedure (abstract). Transfusion 1982;22:409.

Serologic Techniques and Alloantibodies

Microplate Techniques Applied to Routine Blood Bank Procedures

General Principles

Microplate methods were adapted to blood bank use in the late 1960's and have gained popularity for routine blood processing in blood banks too small for cost-effective automation. Advantages of microplate techniques include enhanced sensitivity of reactions; savings in reagents, supplies and equipment; and reduced requirements for laboratory space and technologist time.

Microplate techniques can be used to test either red cells for antigen presence or sera for antibody activity. A microplate can be considered as a matrix of 96 "short" test tubes and principles common to hemagglutination tube tests apply to microwells. Plates may be rigid or flexible, with either U-shaped or V-shaped bottoms. U-bottom plates are more widely used because results can be read either by cell resuspension or "streaming," and agglutination strength can be estimated. Quantities of cells and serum and testing conditions vary with the procedure used.

Comparison with Standard Tube Techniques

1. Equal or greater sensitivity. For example, Rh-positive red cells classified as D^u in tube tests are often unambiguously positive on microplates.
2. Greater speed of testing large numbers of samples
3. Greater economy of reagents because many antisera can be diluted and only small volumes of cells and serum need be used.
4. Greater importance of technical details such as serum:cell ratio, protein concentration of serum-cell suspension, and consistent reproducibility of centrifugation, resuspension and interpretation.

Technical Considerations

1. Protein concentration, antibody strength and viscosity of the reagent system must be monitored. Excessively low or high protein concentrations can impair results. Diluting high-protein anti-D with 3% bovine serum albumin decreases viscosity and often enhances reactivity; other antibodies may perform better with other diluents. If the manufacturer does not certify suitability for microplate testing, antisera marketed for tube testing must be tested for suitability of each lot. Chemically modified reagents may not be used with most diluents.
2. Both volume and concentration of red cell suspensions and antiserum prepa-

435

ration must be carefully standardized. These may be very small, eg, 0.025 ml serum and 0.2% cell suspensions.

3. Centrifugation conditions and resuspension techniques must be carefully standardized. Careless technique leads to cross-contamination of specimens.

4. Use of enzymes enhances reactivity, increasing both sensitivity and likelihood of nonspecific reactions. Suitable controls are essential. Enzyme techniques intended for use with serum are not ordinarily effective if the antibody preparation has a low protein concentration as, for example, in an eluate.

5. Fibrin present in plasma often interferes with interpretations. Most workers prefer serum to plasma.

6. Pretreating new plates improves test conditions. Pretreatment with 0.1% bovine albumin in saline or human serum prevents adsorption of antibody and adherence of cells. Static electricity can be reduced by flaming, by washing or by wiping the bottom of the plate with a wet towel.

7. Evaporation can be a problem if small volumes of fluid are incubated at 37 C or for long periods. Plates can be covered during incubation.

8. Plates may be reused, but must be carefully washed. See page 439.

Potential Problems

1. Accurate sample identification is difficult. Using microplates eliminates labeling a lot of tubes, but in each laboratory there must be a uniform convention for sample placement and all personnel must adhere precisely to this. Consultation with other microplate users is helpful before adopting a protocol.

2. Specimens may spill out of individual wells. The surface of a plate should be considered contaminated, and reagents should be added precisely in the center of wells. There can be cross-contamination of samples without any visible evidence that this has occurred, especially if centrifugation technique has been careless.

3. Antibodies lose stability in solutions with low protein concentration. If the diluents are not sterile, bacterial contamination may cause antibody deterioration. Diluted antisera should be stored at 1-6 C for no more than 7 days. Do not freeze.

FDA Requirements for Microplate Use

Licensed blood banks that institute microplate procedures for required ABO and Rh grouping tests must submit a description of their procedure to the Office of Biologics Research and Review. Unlicensed blood banks do not need FDA approval for microplate use, but the following testing is recommended before adopting the new procedure:

1. The microplate procedure should be run in parallel with the standard procedure for large numbers of specimens, after personnel have had sufficient training. All discrepant results should be recorded, with a summary of the investigations undertaken to resolve each problem.

2. The manual of Standard Operating Procedures (SOP) should describe laboratory procedures used to evaluate each lot of reagent not specifically labeled for microplate use. There should be documentation that each lot of reagent is potent and specific when used according to the SOP. Control testing should include weakly reactive phenotypes wherever possible, eg, D^u examples of Rh-positive cells and A_2B examples of the A antigen. Control samples may be fresh or frozen-thawed cells. If reagents are used at varying dilutions, the protocol should clearly indicate how the correct dilution is selected for use with a new lot.

3. The SOP should describe routine test performance, including daily quality control procedures. At least one positive and one negative control sample

should be used daily to verify that each reagent is giving the expected results.

Reagents and Equipment

Blood grouping sera tested for suitability in microplate procedures and labeled accordingly are now commercially available. The licensed reagents are approved for use in a single, specific protocol. The user who changes the test conditions assumes responsibility for appropriate reagent evaluation. Most Reagent Red Blood Cells licensed for use in tube tests can be used in U-bottom plates without additional preparation.

A hypothetical problem with reagents not specifically prepared for microplate use is that the more sensitive technique might uncover undetected antibodies that could give false-positive results in tests for the expected specificity. The Food and Drug Administration (FDA) requires that blood grouping sera be specific *only* when used according to the manufacturer's directions. Anti-A, anti-B and anti-D very seldom contain extraneous antibodies, and experience to date has demonstrated very few specificity problems when reagents licensed for tube testing are used with microplates. Some reagents, however, give reactions that are very difficult to interpret on the microplate.

Reagent Testing

If a serum is not specifically labeled for microplate use, the FDA requires that each licensed blood bank test each lot of the serum with a panel of reagent red cells. Such testing helps ensure, with a minimum of effort, that the laboratory's routine procedures will provide appropriate positive and negative results. With procedures employing enzymes, appropriate controls to detect nonspecific reactivity are especially important. Such specificity testing does not ensure reactivity with weak examples of the antigen, nor does it exclude antibodies to low-incidence antigens not represented on the test panel.

Daily performance checks are recommended to demonstrate appropriate reactivity and specificity of each serum as well as proper application of the test system. In the ABO system, the serum grouping serves as a control for cell grouping results; additional ABO controls are not required.

Ancillary Equipment

Semi-automated devices are available for dispensing equal volumes to a row of wells. Serial dilution titrations can be automated or performed with the specially calibrated Takatsky loops. Special plate carriers can be purchased to fit common table-top centrifuges or inexpensive, homemade "slings" can be used. Semi-automated cell washers are normally used to wash specimens before adding antiglobulin serum. U-bottom plates are preferred for cell washing because samples resuspend better. An inexpensive plant sprayer combined with a manifold washes cells very effectively.

Automated Detection of Hemagglutination

An automated device is available that reads microplate results with a photometer to measure light absorbance in U-bottom wells. Ninety-six absorbance values can be processed in less than one minute and the results interfaced with a microprocessor. With the automated reader, a light beam passes through the bottoms of the microplate wells. Negative results produce high optical density readings because the cells dispersed over the well bottom absorb more light than the concentrated button of cells in a positive result. The microprocessor interprets the reactions and the blood group results are printed on the laboratory record.

The system requires red cell controls to detect false-positive reactions and serum or plasma controls to prevent falsely high absorbance readings due to bilirubin or hemoglobin. For accurate results, the cell concentrations must be carefully controlled (0.5 to 2% give the best sensitivity)

Storage Requirements for Reagents Used in Microplate Testing

Reagent	Storage Temperature Degrees (C)	Suggested Maximum Storage Time
I. *Antisera*		
Antisera, undiluted	2–8*	as labeled by manufacturer
Antisera, diluted	2–8	1 week
Antiglobulin reagent, undiluted	2–8	as labeled by manufacturer
Antiglobulin reagent, diluted	2–8	1 week
II. *Reagent Red Blood Cells*		
Cells for serum/plasma grouping and antibody screening	2–8	as labeled by manufacturer
Prepared suspensions of Reagent Red Blood Cells	2–8	12 hours
III. *Solutions*		
Stock 1% bromelain	− 18 or colder	1 year
Working dilution of bromelain	on wet ice	12 hours
Phosphate-buffered saline 0.1M stock solution	2–8	6 months
pH 5.5 phosphate-buffered saline	2–8	6 months
0.1% albumin wash solution	2–8	12 hours
Tween 20®	20–25	indefinitely
Saline with Tween 20®	2–8	12 hours
3% bovine albumin	2–8	7 days
2% sodium azide	2–8	indefinitely
Saline	20–25	as labeled by manufacturer

*The FDA-designated temperature range for storage of refrigerated in vitro diagnostic products is 2–8 C.

and centrifugation and resuspension must be performed in a very uniform manner. Therefore, red cells from clotted samples are not suitable for use with the automated microplate reader. The major deficiency of automated microplate readers has been lack of positive sample identification, but this problem is being addressed in newer equipment.

Microplate Techniques
I. Collection of Samples

Samples should be collected in accordance with standard procedures. Red cell grouping may be performed on either anticoagulated or clotted specimens. Either serum or plasma can be used for ABO serum grouping and antibody screening.

II. Supplies, Equipment and Maintenance

A. Supplies and Equipment Requirements

1. Microplates with U- or V-shaped wells
2. Disposable pipettes or reusable pipettes that deliver approximately 0.025 ml
3. Calibrated centrifuge that can accommodate microplate carriers
4. Carriers designed to support microplates in centrifuge
5. 37 ± 1 C dry incubator, a dry block incubator or waterbath
6. Cornwall syringe, micro-drop reagent dispenser with Cornwall syringe apparatus and dispensing

manifold, or a repetitive dispenser equipped with manifold

7. Microplate reader: A support device for microplates with a white translucent surface at an angle of 60 degrees to the bench top. The microplate carrier can also be used as a reading device by placing a white 3 × 5 card on the front of the carrier to support the plate. To facilitate reading, the plate can be illuminated from behind using an agglutination view lamp or any other cool light source.

8. Serologic pipettes for reagent dilutions or manual microdiluters or Multi-Micro diluter handle and loops

9. Agglutination viewer

10. Mechanical mixer

11. Rubber support pad

12. Applicator sticks

B. Microplate Maintenance

1. Soaking overnight in deionized water or distilled water is usually sufficient to eliminate static. If static is apparent when reagents are dropped, the bottom of the plate can be wiped with a damp cloth or passed rapidly over a flame. If static continues to be a problem while adding reagents, the microplate may be placed on a damp paper towel. Microplates may be rinsed before use with 0.1% solution of bovine albumin in saline. Excess wash solution must be removed from the plate before adding reagents.

2. Although disposable, the microplates can be reused after washing, as follows:

a. Invert plate and flick cell and serum residue into sink or a liquid waste receptacle that meets appropriate safety requirements. Sink area should be cleaned daily with disinfectant, eg, 2.5% sodium hypochlorite, which is household bleach diluted with an equal volume of water.

b. Rinse plates in 2.5% sodium hypochlorite. A wash bottle containing 2.5% sodium hypochlorite may be used to accomplish this rinse or the microplates may be immersed in a container of 2.5% sodium hypochlorite.

c. Soak in a soap solution, if desired. The soap used must be one that does not leave any film or residue. Products developed for use with tissue culture plates should be acceptable. Mild household detergents may also be used successfully.

d. Rinse three times with warm tap water and three times with deionized or distilled water after removing plates from the 2.5% sodium hypochlorite, or soap wash if used.

e. Air dry the plates in an inverted position over a drying rack.

3. Inspect plates before use for inadequate washing, irregular wells, or any other defects. Discard any badly scratched or warped plates.

III. Reagents

A. Reagent Requirements

1. Use only licensed anti-A, anti-B, anti-D and anti-human globulin.

2. Reagent Red Blood Cells for ABO grouping. Commercially available cells can be used, or suitable cells can be prepared from anticoagulated donor samples. Cells prepared from tubes or sealed donor segments may be used for up to 5 days after the specimen is first entered.

3. Licensed Reagent Red Blood Cells for antibody screening. To test donor blood samples but not patients' samples, cells may be pooled; the vials of a single lot of screening cells may be pooled or a

commercially prepared cell pool may be used.

4. Diluent for reagent antisera. A suitable diluent is: 3% (± 0.5%) bovine albumin in saline prepared by adding 9 volumes of normal saline to 1 volume of commercially available 30% albumin (or 6.3 volumes of normal saline to 1 volume of 22% albumin). The addition of 0.1% sodium azide is optional.

5. Wash solution. Use either 0.1% albumin prepared by adding 2 ml of 30% albumin to 500 ml of normal saline or use saline with Tween 20® (0.2 ml/liter). These solutions must be prepared fresh daily or purchased ready to use.

6. Enzyme solution. Bromelain solutions may be used for microplate procedures. Appropriate working dilutions must be prepared daily (see Section III, C.1). A 5.5 pH phosphate buffered saline (see page 424) is used as the diluent for preparing the 1% stock bromelain. This diluent ensures stability of the frozen product.

7. Antihuman globulin (AHG). Commercially available reagents may be adapted to microplate procedures, but many AHG reagents licensed for blood bank use cause red cells to adhere to the bottom of wells. Each lot of AHG reagent must be evaluated to determine the dilution that will eliminate prozones and false positives while maintaining a system at least as sensitive as manual tube methods (See Section III, C.3).

8. Sodium azide, used as a 0.1% solution prepared from a 2% stock solution in distilled or deionized water. Add 1 ml of stock solution to 20 ml of 3% bovine albumin in order to achieve a final concentration of 0.1% sodium azide. Take appropriate precautions when using sodium azide.

9. Normal saline (0.9%) with or without sodium azide.

B. Reagent Preparation

1. Because testing is so sensitive in microplates, licensed reagents may be used diluted. For each new lot of reagent, the appropriate dilution must be established before use. Reagents diluted in 3% bovine serum albumin or other suitable diluent may be used for as long as 1 week if stored at 1-6 C when not in use.

2. Records must be maintained of all reagent evaluation for five years. Records should include the following:
   a. Date of testing
   b. Initials of technologist performing procedure
   c. Manufacturer, lot number, expiration date and specificity of reagent tested
   d. Identification number and source of cells tested
   e. Lot number and working dilution of reagent tested
   f. Record of endpoint and working dilution used
   g. Worksheets showing titration format

3. Any containers other than the original reagent vial should be labeled with the following information:
   a. Specificity of reagent
   b. Manufacturer's lot number
   c. Dilution (if applicable)
   d. Date of preparation
   e. Initials of technologist
   f. Date and hour at which diluted reagent expires

4. To establish the appropriate dilution, the serum should be tested against cells with a weak expression of the antigen, eg, A_2B for anti-A, D^u for anti-D. Deglycerolized frozen cells may be used.
   a. Red cell suspensions must be accurately prepared. For V-bottom plates, 0.2% cell suspen-

sions are used; for U-bottom plates, 2-4% suspensions. A 0.2% suspension for use in V plates can be made by diluting 1:10 a 2% suspension made by adding 0.05 ml packed red cells to 1.95 ml of saline. The cell concentration is particularly important if streaming is the end point. If the suspension is too light there may be no streaming when the result is negative; too heavy a suspension may stream when the result is positive.

   b. Comparison standards are useful, especially while personnel are achieving proficiency.

5. If enzymes are used in routine testing, enzyme-treated cells must be used in determining the appropriate reagent dilution according to the testing protocol.

6. Red cells should be mixed with diluted enzyme solutions and allowed to stand at room temperature for at least 10 minutes before use. To avoid overtreatment, these enzyme-suspended red cell samples should be discarded 4 hours after preparation.

7. Once the working dilution of an antiserum lot has been established, daily quality control should include testing the diluted serum against positive and negative controls.

8. The working dilution established for each new lot must be tested against a panel of reagent red cells. If enzymes are used in testing, the panel should be treated in the same manner as routine cell samples. For diluted anti-D to be used in D^u tests, this testing includes an antiglobulin phase using antiglobulin serum at the optimum working dilution. A negative control using 3% bovine albumin must be run in parallel. Use of the red cell panel confirms the specificity of anti-D and the absence of unexpected antibodies in the anti-A, anti-B and anti-A,B reagents under test conditions.

C. Determination of Working Reagent Dilutions

1. If enzymes are used, a diluted enzyme solution is used in this protocol to enhance the reactions of test cells with ABO and D grouping reagents. A commercially available or prepared 1% stock enzyme reagent should be prepared and stored in 1 ml aliquots at temperatures below -20 C. A working dilution of 1:10 (one part stock 1% solution plus nine parts saline) should be prepared daily for use as suspending medium for test cells. A negative control consisting of enzyme-suspended red cells and 3% bovine albumin must be tested in parallel with all tests on enzyme-modified cells. This includes red cell suspensions made for quality control, cell typing, and D^u testing procedures. Red cells treated with the 1:10 dilution of the 1% stock solution should give consistently negative results. If control cells give positive results, a 1:15 (one part stock reagent plus 14 parts saline) working dilution should be prepared and ABO and D reagents should be tested against cells treated with the more dilute enzyme.

2. Dilutions of the reagent are tested against red cell samples to establish the optimal working dilution of the reagent. It is not necessary to use anti-A,B in testing blood from donors or patients.

   a. Anti-A

      1) Select four A_2B red cell samples.

      2) Prepare a suspension, at appropriate concentration, of each cell sample.

      3) Prepare two-fold serial dilutions of the antiserum in 3% bovine albumin. The endpoint usually occurs below

1:128 dilution. Label a series of tubes from 1:1 (undiluted) to 1:128. Place 0.5 ml of diluent into tubes 1:2 through 1:128. Add 0.5 ml of reagent to tubes labeled 1:1 and 1:2. After mixing, transfer 0.5 ml from tube labeled 1:2 to tube labeled 1:4. Mix and continue to transfer 0.5 ml aliquots down the row of tubes. Use a different pipette tip or different serological pipette for each tube. Dilutions can also be made directly in the microplate using a microdiluter system.

4) Add 1 drop of each dilution to separate rows in the microplate using a disposable pipette. Also add 1 drop of the diluent 3% bovine albumin to each of four control wells in the microplate using a disposable pipette.

5) Add 1 drop of each red cell suspension to the wells in a row that contains all the antiserum dilutions.

6) Centrifuge the microplates immediately. Interpret and record results.

7) The endpoint is the last well demonstrating strong agglutination. The maximum working dilution of the antiserum is that of the well preceding the endpoint. Use this dilution to test the serum against the reagent red cell panel (see Section III, B.8).

8) If the several cell samples show different endpoints, choose the lowest dilution that causes agglutination because the working dilution must give strong, clear-cut reactions with all antigen-positive cells.

b. Anti-B
1) Select four A_1B or A_2B red cell samples.
2) Prepare a 1:10 dilution of anti-B (0.1 ml anti-B and 0.9 ml of 3% bovine albumin).
3) Add 1 drop of diluted anti-B to each of 4 wells and 1 drop of 3% bovine albumin as negative control to each of 4 wells.
4) Perform the tests in the manner described above.
5) The 1:10 dilution of the reagent is acceptable if all positive test cells give strong clear-cut positive reactions and all controls are negative. Test the serum at this dilution against a reagent red cell panel. (See Section III, B.8.)
6) If positive test cells do not give strong, clear-cut reactions, reduce the dilution of reagent to 1:5 (0.1 ml of reagent plus 0.4 ml of 3% bovine albumin). Perform the same evaluation as above.

c. Anti-A,B
1) Select four A_2 red cell samples.
2) Anti-A,B reagents demonstrate reactivity against A_2 red cells at high dilutions. It is recommended that a 1:10 dilution (0.1 ml anti-A,B plus 0.9 ml of 3% bovine albumin) be prepared and evaluated as the working dilution.
3) Continue with steps 3 through 6 as detailed in the protocol on testing anti-B.

d. Anti-D
1) Select four D-positive red cell samples and four D^u red cell samples. Ideally, one of these samples should be C and E negative.

2) Continue with steps 2 through 8 as detailed under the protocol for testing anti-A. Use the titration results against D^u red cell samples to establish the optimum dilution.

3) Test serum at this dilution against a reagent red cell panel, using both immediate spin results and an antiglobulin phase with antihuman globulin serum at the optimum working dilution.

3. Antihuman globulin serum
   a. Procedure
      1) Select at least three red cell samples that have negative direct antiglobulin tests.
      2) Prepare three specimens of IgG-coated red cells; two should have weak expressions of the antigen [eg, a heterozygous Jk(a+) red cell sensitized with anti-Jk^a] and one should have strong expression. The IgG-coated cells used to control negative antiglobulin tests may be used as the cell with strong expression. The sensitized cells should be weakly reactive in an antiglobulin test performed by manual tube method with a licensed blood bank reagent.
      3) Prepare two-fold dilutions of antiglobulin serum in 3% bovine albumin, going from 1:1 (undiluted) through 1:16.
      4) Starting with the lowest dilution on the left, add 1 drop of each dilution to separate rows in the microplate, ending with 1 drop of diluent 3% bovine albumin in the last well of the row. Use a separate pipette for each dilution.

5) Add 1 drop of 0.2% suspension of each of the prepared cells to a row in the microplate containing all the antiserum dilutions.

6) Centrifuge the microplate immediately. Interpret and record results after 20-30 minutes.

b. Choosing the optimum working dilution
   1) Note the well in which the least diluted antiglobulin serum gives a negative result (complete streaming) with the unsensitized cells. The optimum working dilution will be the next highest dilution. This dilution must also produce strong agglutination with the sensitized cells. If the reaction with the sensitized cells is not sufficiently strong, use the lowest dilution that gives the negative result (complete streaming).
   2) For commercially available antiglobulin sera, dilutions between 1:2 and 1:5 are usually optimum.
   3) Confirm the presence of a positive result in the well containing the optimum working dilution and the strongly sensitized cell.

c. IgG-sensitized control cells
   1) Add 1 drop of IgG-sensitized control cells to each negative antiglobulin test. Gently mix microplate.
   2) Centrifuge, place on microplate reader and record result after 10-15 minutes.
   3) The wells containing the chosen dilution of antiglobulin serum should show complete agglutination. If the reaction is not strong or if prozone is suspected, adjust the suspension of IgG-sen-

sitized control cells. A pro-zone reaction with strongly sensitized cells may appear to stream (negative reaction) but closer examination with a visual aid will reveal clumping of cells in the stream.

4) Include a control well with the IgG-sensitized cells added to 3% bovine serum albumin. If a positive reaction results, the cells are too heavily sensitized to use. Prepare a new supply and retest.

IV. Protocol for Processing

A. Labeling and Identification

1. On recording sheets for a day's processing, the microplate row number must begin with 1 and continue sequentially, ending with the last whole blood number of the day's processing. Microplate row numbers cannot be repeated within a day's processing unless a color coding system is followed.

2. Microplates must be marked in a way to ensure proper sample identification. Methods suitable for identification include permanently marking a series of microplates with the row position number, or using a combination of the row number and donor number. Use of colored marking pens or colored tape may aid in sample identification.

3. The tubes containing the serum sample and the cell suspension prepared from the blood sample must be labeled to ensure proper identification, including the row number, to relate the samples to their positions in the microplates. It is recommended that the row position number appear on the original laboratory tube.

4. The row number will be the same for each test (ABO cell and serum grouping, D grouping, antibody screening) performed on one sample. If pooled cells are used in antibody screening, the row number may be the actual well number in which the sample is placed.

B. Cell Grouping

1. Twelve or 16 samples can be tested on one plate with anti-A, anti-B, anti-A,B, anti-D and red cell control.

2. The row position numbers can go down the left side or across the top, with wells labeled for antisera and controls going at right angles.

3. Using 8-, 12- or 16-hole test tube supports allows correlation of tube position with plate row position number. A properly labeled tube used for the preparation of a cell suspension can be placed directly in front of the laboratory tube.

C. ABO Serum Grouping

1. It is preferable to perform serum grouping on a separate plate from cell grouping, to permit independent reading and interpretation.

2. The serum grouping procedure should include a group O cell, which functions as a negative control and can also serve as an optional immediate centrifugation phase for antibody screening if the cell is properly selected.

3. Either horizontal or vertical numbering sequence can be used.

D. Antibody Screening, with Antiglobulin Test

1. The antiglobulin phase of the antibody screening requires a third plate.

a. For a two-cell screening test, a total of 32 samples can be tested on one plate by dispensing eight samples in four rows. This arrangement allows for one row of wells separating the specimens. The last vertical row can be used for controls, eg, positive antibody controls.

b. With pooled cells, up to 93 tests may be performed on a microplate, leaving wells available for control samples.

2. The setup formats shown in the figure below are suggestions and may be altered to meet local needs.

E. D" Testing

1. All donor units requiring D" testing can be tested on a limited number of microplates. The original row position number should be written directly to the side of or above the wells used for the D" test and red cell control. Row position numbers can be written on narrow strips of labeling tape placed over rows of empty wells, thus increasing the number of D" tests that can be performed, with controls, on a single microplate.

2. An unused double row of wells on an antibody screening plate may also be used for D" testing.

V. Additional Considerations

A. General Principles

1. Because of the extremely small volume used, the clear fluid (eg, serum or reagent antiserum) should be placed in the wells first, followed by cells. If the cell suspension is added to serum, it is not necessary to mix the cells and serum before incubation or centrifugation.

2. It is extremely important to follow a standardized technique to maintain a reproducible ratio of antigen to antibody. The size of the drops of serum, reagents and cell suspensions being dispensed should be as uniform as possible. Disposable pipettes with regular bore size should be used for microplate work.

3. Appropriate centrifugation conditions must be established for each centrifuge. The following times and relative centrifugal forces, expressed

POOLED SCREENING CELLS

Row position	1	9	17
	O	O	O
	O	O	O
	O	O	O
	O	O	O
	O	O	O
	O	O	O
	O	O	O
	O	O	O
Row position	8	16	24

TWO SCREENING CELLS, USED SEPARATELY

Cell	I	II	I	II
Row position	1	*	9	*
	O O	O O	O O
	O O	O O	O O
	O O	O O	O O
	O O	O O	O O
	O O	O O	O O
	O O	O O	O O
	O O	O O	O O
	O O	O O	O O
Row position	8	*	16	*

*empty row

as *g*, are suggested.

For flexible "U" microplate:

a. 700 *g* for 5 seconds for cell testing, serum grouping and optional immediate-spin phase of antibody screening

b. 700 *g* for 20 seconds for washing the antiglobulin test

c. 700 *g* for 5 seconds after addition of antihuman globulin

For rigid "U" microplate:

a. 400 *g* for 30 seconds for cell testing, serum grouping and optional immediate-spin phase of antibody screening

b. 400 *g* for 3 minutes for washing the antiglobulin test

c. 400 *g* for 30 seconds after addition of antihuman globulin

For flexible "V" microplate:

a. 700 *g* for 10 seconds for cell testing, serum grouping and optional immediate-spin phase of antibody screening

b. 700 *g* for 20 seconds for washing the antiglobulin test

c. 700 *g* for 10 seconds after addition of antihuman globulin

For rigid "V" microplate:

a. 900 *g* for 40 seconds for cell testing, serum grouping and optional immediate-spin phase of antibody screening

b. 900 *g* for 40 seconds for washing the antiglobulin test

c. 900 *g* for 10 seconds after addition of antihuman globulin

B. ABO Cell Grouping

1. Place 1 drop of appropriately diluted antiserum into microplate wells for anti-A, anti-B and anti-A,B, using a disposable pipette.

2. Prepare a suspension of red cells in appropriate diluent. If enzymes are used, it is helpful to perform at least one saline wash on cell samples tested 3 or more days after collection, before suspending in an enzyme preparation.

3. Add one drop of the well-mixed cell suspension to appropriate wells, using a disposable pipette.

4. Centrifuge at appropriate speed and time for centrifuge in use.

5. Interpret and record results (See Section VI.)

C. D Grouping

1. Place one drop of appropriately diluted antiserum into microplate wells for anti-D using a disposable pipette.

2. For each donor sample place one drop of antiserum diluent (3% albumin) into a microplate well to serve as a red cell control.

3. Prepare a suspension of red cells in appropriate diluent.

4. Add one drop of cell suspension to appropriate wells using a disposable pipette.

5. Centrifuge at appropriate speed and time for centrifuge in use.

6. Interpret and record results. (See Section VI.)

D. D^u Testing

1. Use the cell suspension used for the D grouping if the D^u test is performed within 4 hours. After 4 hours a new cell suspension must be prepared. A red cell control must accompany D^u testing.

2. Incubate samples not immediately agglutinated by anti-D with the anti-D reagent at 37 C for 15-30 minutes. Cover trays to prevent evaporation. Trays can be incubated on the top of a dry block incubator, in a 37 $\pm$ 1 C dry incubator, or by supporting the plate on a rack in a 37 $\pm$ 1 C waterbath.

3. After incubation, centrifuge at appropriate speed and time for centrifuge in use. Decant the supernatant with a rapid flicking motion of the wrist over a sink or a properly lined waste receptacle.

4. Resuspend the cells by "riffling," briskly moving the bottom of the tray over the upturned finger tips.

This creates sufficient vibration to resuspend the cells completely. Cells can be resuspended by placing a supported microplate on the vibrating pad of a mechanical mixer. When a mechanical mixer is used, flexible plates must be supported either in a rubber support holder or with several empty plates stacked together beneath the test plate. Flexible plates can also be supported in the microplate carrier used in the centrifuge. A mechanical shaker is available as an alternative method of resuspending cells in U-bottom plates.

5. To each test well, add 0.2 ml of wash solution.

6. Centrifuge at appropriate speed and time for centrifuge in use. Remove the wash liquid between washes. Repeat washing procedure until plates have been washed three or four times.

7. After decanting the last wash, resuspend the cells and add one drop of appropriately diluted antihuman globulin. Gently mix.

8. Centrifuge at appropriate speed and time for centrifuge in use. Place on microplate reader and read after 20-30 minutes (see Section VI, Interpretation of Results).

9. Add 1 drop of IgG-sensitized control cells to each negative test well. Gently mix microplate.

10. Centrifuge at appropriate speed and time for centrifuge in use. Interpret and record results (See Section VI).

E. Serum Grouping

1. Place one drop of serum or plasma into microplate wells for A_1, A_2 and B cells, using a disposable pipette.

2. Add 1 drop of saline-suspended A_1, A_2 and B cells to appropriately labeled wells.

3. Centrifuge at appropriate speed and time for centrifuge in use. Interpret and record results (see Section VI). Note that hemolysis should be recorded as a positive result.

4. If a clear cell pattern is not discernible after initial centrifugation, immediately resuspend and recentrifuge the plates, and reinterpret results. If V-bottom plates are used, tilting the plate in the opposite direction to observe streaming pattern may be sufficient. Ambiguous patterns may result from individual differences in concentration of isoagglutinins or from protein idiosyncracies in individual samples.

F. Antibody Screening, with Antiglobulin Test

1. Add 1 or 2 drops of serum or plasma and 1 drop of the saline suspension of licensed Reagent Red Blood Cells to appropriate microplate wells.

2. Use antibody controls, as described in Section VII, Quality Control.

3. If desired, centrifuge plates and record results before incubation (optional).

4. Incubate at 37 ± 1 C for 30 minutes. Cover plate to prevent evaporation.

5. Centrifuge at appropriate speed and time for centrifuge in use.

6. Remove serum by flicking plate over a sink or proper waste receptacle, and completely resuspend cells.

7. After resuspension, add 0.2 ml of wash solution to each well. Centrifuge plates at appropriate speed and time for centrifuge in use. Remove the wash liquid between washes. Repeat procedure until plates have been washed three or four times.

8. After decanting the last wash, resuspend the cells and add 1 drop of the appropriately diluted antihuman globulin. Mix and resuspend.

9. Centrifuge at appropriate speed and time for centrifuge in use.

Because the procedure is extremely sensitive, avoid over-centrifugation.

10. Interpret and record results.
11. Add 1 drop of IgG-sensitized control cells to each negative test well. Gently mix to resuspend.
12. Centrifuge at appropriate speed and time for centrifuge in use.
13. Interpret and record results.

VI. Interpreting and Recording Results and Resolving Discrepancies

A. Interpreting Results, U-Bottom
   1. Antigen-antibody reactions can be detected in U-bottom microplate systems with several different modes of interpretation.
      a. For cell testing, serum grouping and the optional immediate-spin phase of antibody screening, use either of the following methods: 1) Gently agitate the plate by hand or use a mechanical device to resuspend the cells completely. Examine the pattern of the resuspended cells by using the ceiling lights as a light source or by supporting the microplate over a magnifying mirror. A positive reaction is the presence of small or large agglutinates, comparable to those seen in tube testing. A negative reaction is a smooth cell suspension in the bottom of the well. 2) Observe the streaming pattern of the cell button, as described in b, below.
      b. For D^u testing and the antiglobulin phase of antibody screening, interpret reactions by examining the streaming pattern. Leave the centrifuged microplate on a microplate reader or a support device that is at a 60-degree angle to the bench top for 3 to 5 minutes. A positive reaction is persistence of a red cell button at the bottom

of the well. The margin of the cell button may be smooth or jagged. Negative reactions show streaming of the red cells down the well.
      c. To verify weak reactions in any procedure, interpret the settled red cell pattern, as follows: Gently agitate the microplate to resuspend the cells completely. Place the microplate on a support platform over a magnifying mirror. Allow cell suspensions to settle completely, a minimum of 20-30 minutes. The settled pattern is then read by observing the underside of the well through the magnifying mirror. Negative reactions appear as smooth round cell buttons. Strong positive reactions will appear as jagged clumps of cells. A weak positive reaction appears as a cell button with a "halo" surrounding it.

B. Interpreting Results, V-Bottom
   1. Interpretations on all testing procedures (including antibody screening) are recorded as positive or negative. Because of increased sensitivity, the usual grading scale applied to agglutination reactions cannot be used for reactions in the V-bottom microplate.
   2. Negative reactions = No visible button; a distinct streaming tail is apparent. Positive reaction = Firm button in center of well. Some sera produce positive reactions that are variations of the typical pattern. These are described according to the shape or size of the button and the degree of streaming noted. Several of the forms seen are illustrated on the next page.

C. Recording
   1. All results should be recorded at the time the microplates are examined and interpreted.

TYPICAL REACTIONS

Negative   Positive

Variant appearances of positive reactions

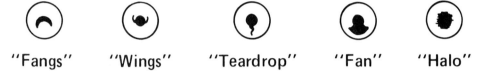

"Fangs"   "Wings"   "Teardrop"   "Fan"   "Halo"

Tests done in V-bottom microplates usually present one of the above appearances.

2. Cell grouping and serum grouping reactions should be interpreted independently. If this is not possible, the results of cell testing should be covered while the plasma or serum results are entered on the recording sheet.

D. Resolution of Discrepancies or Unexpected Results

1. Check to see if results on cell tests and serum or plasma tests are in agreement. All discrepancies must be resolved. Resolve unexpected results by repeating the tests, using microplate and standard tube methods. The repeat tests should be done on the sample originally examined and also, if available, on a segment. Record results and interpretations of repeat testing on a separate laboratory recording sheet.

2. Positive results on the red cell control invalidate the results of the cell grouping.

a. Prepare a new suspension of enzyme-treated, twice-washed donor cells and repeat microplate testing.

b. If microplate testing again gives invalid results, perform cell grouping with standard tube methods.

VII. Daily Quality Control

A. Reagents

1. Setup Protocol. The setup format illustrated in the figure on page 450 is a suggestion and may be altered to meet local needs.

2. Cell Grouping. Positive and negative controls should be tested daily against the established working dilution of each reagent used in the processing protocol (eg, anti-A, -B, -A,B or -D). For this purpose A_2B, D-positive; O, D-negative; and O, D^u cells should be included in the daily quality control protocol.

Cells		Anti-A	Anti-B	Anti-A,B	Anti-D	RBC Cont.
A_2B, D pos	1	O	O	O	O	O
0, D neg	2	O	O	O	O	O
0, D^u	3	O	O	O	O	O
A_1	4	O	O	O	O	O
A_2	5	O	O	O	O	O
B	6	O	O	O	O	O

A format such as this provides suitable quality control testing for cell and antiserum reactivity. The use of A_2 cells for serum grouping and of anti-A,B for cell grouping is not required.

3. Serum Grouping. Reagent red cells for serum grouping should be tested daily to confirm specificity.
4. Antiglobulin Testing
   a. Use samples with known alloantibodies reactive in the antiglobulin phase (and optional immediate-spin phase) as positive controls for antibody screening. Alloantibody samples should be obtained from actual donor specimens. Commercial reagents often contain additives which, once diluted, make results difficult to interpret. Useful antibodies for controls are weak examples of anti-Fy^a, anti-Jk^a, anti-M or anti-Le^a. It is desirable to include a control antibody test with every four microplates, ie, with each centrifuge load.
   b. Include a D-negative cell sample as a negative control with each batch of D^u tests.
   c. Add IgG-sensitized control cells to each antiglobulin test to confirm reactivity of the antiglobulin serum
5. Antihuman Globulin
   a. Commercially available antihuman serum, either polyspecific or monospecific anti-IgG, may be adapted to the U-bottom microplate. Anti-IgG is generally used for V-bottom procedures.
   b. Dilutions. For U-bottom plates it may be necessary to dilute antiglobulin reagent with an equal volume of 3% bovine albumin (a 1:2 dilution), to avoid unclear results due to reagent additives. Test undiluted antiglobulin reagent on serum samples known to lack red cell antibodies, to determine whether a commercial reagent can be used undiluted. If the undiluted or

1:2 preparation of antiglobulin reagent is nonreactive, the dilution selected for routine use (see page 443) should also be nonreactive.

c. Perform routine quality control procedures with the antiglobulin reagents at whatever diluted or undiluted condition has been adopted.

d. The positive controls included in the antiglobulin phase of antibody screening serve as controls for antiglobulin reactivity.

Reference

Adapted with permission from Blood Service Directive 6.44 of the American Red Cross, 1985 revision, Donor Processing Using Microplates.

Capillary Testing for D

Although not as widely used as slide and tube tests for D, the capillary Rh testing method[1] (The Slanted Capillary Method of Rhesus Blood-Grouping) is very convenient when large numbers of bloods are being processed. This procedure utilizes a saline-active anti-D.

Anyone proposing to use this method must: 1) make sure by adequate testing that the antiserum gives satisfactory results in capillaries (most commercially available antisera do not specify use by this technique, and it would usually be necessary to consult the manufacturer); and 2) become familiar with the vagaries of reading test results in capillaries.

The following procedure is given only in brief outline; the interested reader is advised to consult the original literature as well as the more detailed discussion by Moore, Humphreys, and Lovett-Moseley.[2]

1. Use glass capillary tubes, approximately 7.5 cm long and 0.4 cm in diameter.

2. Place the capillary into anti-D serum known to be satisfactory for this method.

Allow a column of serum about 2 cm long to enter the capillary. Wipe the outside of the capillary.

3. Prepare a 20-30% saline suspension of twice-washed red blood cells.

4. Allow about 2 cm of the red blood cell suspension to flow into the capillary at the same end as the serum. Hold the capillary in a vertical position until after the addition of the blood in order to prevent a bubble from forming at the blood-serum interface. Wipe the capillary.

5. Invert the capillary, so that the blood is above the serum, thus enabling the red blood cells to fall into and through the serum. Place the capillary in plasticine in a rack at a 45-degree angle.

6. Observe macroscopically after 5-10 minutes. Agglutination in the form of a rough and beaded thread along the capillary indicates that the blood is Rh-positive. A long smooth line indicates that the blood is Rh-negative.

References

1. Chown B, Lewis M. The slanted capillary method of Rhesus blood-grouping. Clin Pathol 1951;4:464.

2. Moore BPL, Humphreys P, Lovett-Moseley CA. Serological and immunological methods, 6th ed. Toronto: Canadian Red Cross Society; 1968:36-39.

Albumin Layering Technique

This method employs albumin to enhance hemagglutination. It is particularly good for detecting antibodies with Rh specificity, some of which react otherwise only by an enzyme technique. Some examples of anti-Fy^a will directly agglutinate cells if this procedure is used.

1. Add 2 or 3 drops of serum to properly labeled tubes.

2. Add 1 drop of 2-5% cell suspension to each tube.

3. Mix well and incubate at 37 C for 15-30 minutes.

4. Centrifuge for 15 seconds at 3400 rpm. Do not disturb the cell button.
5. Allow 2 drops of albumin (22% or 30%) to run down the side of the tube. Albumin will form a layer on top of the cells. Do not mix.
6. Incubate at 37 C for 5-10 minutes.
7. Read for agglutination by gently dislodging the button. Because there may be nonspecific aggregation of cells, the presence of agglutination should be confirmed by microscopic examination.

Reference

Case J. The albumin layering method for D typing. Vox Sang 1959;4:403-405.

Saline Addition to Demonstrate Alloantibody in Presence of Rouleaux Formation

This technique depends upon the fact that diluted serum frequently retains alloantibody activity, whereas dilution usually eliminates rouleaux-producing conditions. To detect whether alloantibody is present in a serum that causes rouleaux formation, saline is added to the serum before incubation with red cells.

1. Label sets of five tubes for each cell suspension to be tested. One set is for autologous cells; there should be a separate set of tubes for each antibody screening cell employed.
2. Add 2 drops of serum to each tube in each set.
3. Add drops of saline to the tubes as follows:

Tube	1	2	3	4	5
Saline (drops)	0	1	2	3	4

4. Add 1 drop of 2-5% suspension of reagent cells or autologous cells to each tube in the appropriately labeled set. Mix.
5. Incubate at 37 C for 60 minutes, with frequent gentle agitation. With the large volume of diluted serum, antibody

attachment is enhanced by prolonged incubation and mechanical agitation.
6. Wash as usual and add antiglobulin serum.
7. Compare the results obtained with autologous cells and screening cells:

Tube	Screening Cells	Autologous Cells	Interpretation
1	positive	positive	rouleaux formation
2	positive	positive	rouleaux formation
3	positive	negative	alloantibody
4	positive	negative	alloantibody
5	negative	negative	all activity diluted

Manual Polybrene® Test

Principle

Polybrene®, a highly cationic quaternary ammonium polymer, causes reversible aggregation of normal red cells. If red cells sensitized with antibody are brought together by Polybrene®, irreversible agglutination occurs. In the Polybrene® test for antibody activity, the cells are first incubated with serum in a medium of low ionic strength, to facilitate attachment of antibody to cells. Polybrene® is then added to aggregate the cells. After centrifugation the aggregated cells are not manually resuspended; rather the aggregating effect of Polybrene® is neutralized by the addition of sodium citrate. Antibody-mediated agglutination will persist after addition of citrate, but non-agglutinated cells will be dispersed. If the cells are subsequently to be tested with antiglobulin serum, additional citrate is used in the washing process.

Reagents

1. Low ionic medium(LIM):
   To a 500 ml volumetric flask, add 25 g dextrose and 1 g $Na_2EDTA \cdot 2H_2O$. Fill flask to 500-ml mark with distilled water.
2. Polybrene®:
   Stock Solution: Prepare 50 ml 10% Polybrene® by adding 5 g Polybrene to 50 ml normal saline. Store in plastic container. *Working solution:* Make a 0.05%

solution by mixing 0.1 ml of stock solution with 19.9 ml normal saline.

3. Resuspending solution:

0.2M trisodium citrate: Add 5.88 g $Na_3C_6H_5O_7 \cdot 2H_2O$ to a 100-ml volumetric flask; fill to mark with distilled water. *5% dextrose:* Add 5 g dextrose to 100 ml distilled water. *Working solution:* Mix 60 ml trisodium citrate with 40 ml 5% dextrose.

4. Washing solution (for antiglobulin testing)

10 mM sodium citrate: Make a 1:20 dilution of 0.2M trisodium citrate (see above) in normal saline, eg, add 50 ml 0.2M trisodium citrate to 950 ml saline.

Procedure

1. Make a 1% saline suspension of red cells. This can easily be done as follows: Wash 1 drop of a 3-5% suspension. Decant, shake lightly. Resuspend. Decant forcefully.

2. Add 0.1 ml serum to each tube.

3. Add 1.0 ml LIM solution. Mix and incubate for one minute at room temperature.

4. Add 0.1 ml 0.05% Polybrene® to each tube. Mix.

5. Centrifuge for 10 seconds at 3500 rpm and decant supernatant. DO NOT RESUSPEND CELL BUTTON.

6. Add 0.1 ml resuspending solution. Observe for persistence of agglutination after gently shaking. NOTE: If strength of agglutination is weak, compare the test with negative control microscopically. DO NOT RECENTRIFUGE.

7. If desired, the antiglobulin test may be performed as follows:

   a. Add 0.05 ml (50 μl) of resuspending solution to each tube. Mix.

   b. Wash the cells three times with 10 mM sodium citrate solution.

   c. Add 2 drops of anti-IgG to the dry cell button. Mix.

   d. Centrifuge for 15 seconds. Read and record results.

   e. Add IgG-coated cells to each negative tube.

Interpretation

Presence of persisting agglutination after addition of resuspending solution is a positive reaction.

Controls

1. For testing an unknown serum against reagent red cells:

   a. an autologous control should be performed or

   b. an inert serum should be tested against a random panel cell, for comparative purposes.

2. For testing a known antiserum against unknown red cells, a cell sample with heterozygous expression of the antigen and a sample negative for the antigen should be tested.

Reference

Lalezari P, Jiang AF. The manual Polybrene® test: a simple and rapid procedure for detection of red cell antibodies. Transfusion 1980;20:206-211.

AET Treatment of Red Cells

Principle

Red cells incubated with a 6% aqueous solution of 2-aminoethylisothiouronium bromide (AET) lose activity of antigens that are part of, or related to, the Kell blood group system. The Kx antigen (K15) is not inactivated. AET treatment of red cells produces artificial K_0 red cells useful for recognition of antibodies associated with the Kell system.

Materials

1. 6% AET, prepared by dissolving 0.6 g of AET in 10 ml of distilled water. Adjust pH to 8.0 with 5N NaOH. Prepare immediately prior to use.

2. Washed packed red cells to be treated

Method

1. To 1 ml of washed packed red cells add 4 ml of 6% AET.
2. Mix well by inversion, and incubate at 37 C for 20 minutes.
3. Wash the red cells three times in saline and use on the day of preparation.

Notes

1. Red cells treated with AET readily bind complement components in a non-specific manner, similar to the reactivity of cells in paroxysmal nocturnal hemoglobinuria (PNH). Use anti-IgG reagents when performing antiglobulin tests with AET-treated red cells.
2. To determine whether an antibody may have specificity related to a Kell-system antigen, test the serum against both AET-treated and untreated red cells. Loss of reactivity with AET-treated red cells suggests Kell-related specificity. Conversely, reactivity with AET-treated red cells suggests that the antibody does not recognize a product of the Kell gene. Reactions of anti-Kx are enhanced with AET-treated red cells.
3. A panel of AET-treated red cells can be prepared by incubating washed packed red cells from 1 ml of a 5% suspension of reagent red cells and 0.2 ml of 6% AET. These can be used to detect other alloantibodies in the presence of an antibody to a high-incidence Kell-system antigen (eg, anti-k).

Reference

Advani H, Zamor J, Judd WJ, Johnson CL, Marsh WL. Inactivation of Kell blood group antigens by 2-aminoethylisothiouronium bromide. Br J Haematol 1982;51:107-115.

Use of Thiol Reagents to Distinguish IgM from IgG Antibodies

Principle

IgM immunoglobulin molecules consist of five radially arranged subunits linked by disulfide bonds called intersubunit bonds. Each subunit consists of two μ heavy chains and two κ or λ light chains, which are also linked by disulfide bonds known as interchain bonds. Thiol reagents cleave disulfide bonds, but intersubunit bonds are cleaved far more readily by thiol reagents than interchain bonds. The interchain bonds of IgG and IgA monomers, which have a structure similar to that of IgM subunits, are not readily cleaved by thiol reagents.

Treating IgM antibodies with thiol reagents abolishes both agglutinating and complement-binding activities. Thiol treatment is useful in determining the immunoglobulin class of antibodies known to be present in a serum. It can also be used to abolish activity of IgM antibodies so as to permit detection of coexisting IgG antibodies.

Materials

1. Phosphate-buffered saline (PBS) at pH 7.3
2. 0.01M dithiothreitol (DTT), prepared by dissolving 0.154 g of DTT in 100 ml of pH 7.3 PBS. Store at 4 C.
3. 2 ml of serum to be treated

Method

1. Dispense 1 ml of serum into each of two test tubes.
2. To one tube, labeled control, add 1 ml of pH 7.3 PBS.
3. To the other tube, labeled test, add 1 ml of 0.01M DTT.
4. Mix and incubate at 37 C for 2 hours.
5. Test the antibody activity in each sample by titration analysis.

Interpretation

See table on the following page.

Reference

Mollison PL. Blood transfusion in clinical medicine, 7th ed. Oxford: Blackwell Scientific Publications; 1983.

	Dilution					
Test Sample	**1/2**	**1/4**	**1/8**	**1/16**	**1/32**	**Interpretation**
Serum + DTT	3+	2+	2+	1+	0	IgG
Serum + PBS	3+	2+	2+	1+	0	
Serum + DTT	0	0	0	0	0	IgM
Serum + PBS	3+	2+	2+	1+	0	
Serum + DTT	2+	1+	0	0	0	IgG + IgM*
Serum + PBS	3+	2+	2+	1+	0	

Effect of Dithiothreitol on Blood Group Antibodies

*May also indicate only partial inactivation of IgM.

Demonstration of High-Titer, Low-Avidity Antibodies

Principle

Characteristically, high-titer, low avidity (HTLA) antibodies react at high dilutions in antiglobulin tests but the reactions are not strong (2+ or less, even with undiluted serum). In contrast, other undiluted alloantibodies, such as anti-D, anti-Fy^a and anti-K, that react 2+ or less in antiglobulin tests will usually have titers less than 8.

Antibodies of the HTLA group include anti-Kn^a, -McC^a, -Cs^a, -Yk^a, -Ch^a, -Rg^a and -JMH. Occasional examples of anti-Hy^a and antibodies to Lutheran-system antigens may also display characteristics of HTLA antibodies, as do antibodies to leukocyte antigens such as Bg^a.

Materials

1. Reactive red cell samples, selected from previously tested reagent samples. Ideally, three samples should be selected based on the strength of observed reactions (eg, 2+, 1+ and ±).
2. Serum under investigation
3. Polyspecific or anti-IgG antiglobulin reagent

Method

1. Prepare serial two-fold dilutions of test serum in saline. The dilution range should be from 1 in 2 to 1 in 4096 (12 tubes), and the volumes prepared should be not less than 0.6 ml.
2. Place 3 drops of each dilution into each of three appropriately labeled 10 or 12 × 75-mm test tubes.
3. Test each dilution against the three red cells by adding 1 drop of a 2-5% suspension of cells to each suitably labeled series of dilutions.
4. Gently agitate the contents of each tube and incubate at 37 C for 1 hour.
5. Wash the red cells four times in saline and test with polyspecific or anti-IgG antiglobulin reagent.
6. Examine the red cells for agglutination; confirm all nonreactive tests with an optical aid. Grade and record the results.

Interpretation

1. Sera that continue to react at four dilutions beyond that which gives a 1+ reaction can be considered to contain an HTLA antibody.
2. Cells that react at varying strengths with undiluted serum should be tested to determine whether dilution exerts the same effect on all reactions. If some red cells react only or preferentially with low serum dilutions, the serum may also contain non-HTLA antibodies such as anti-E or anti-K.

Plasma Inhibition to Distinguish Anti-Ch^a and Anti-Rg^a from Other HTLA Antibodies

Principle

Anti-Ch^a and anti-Rg^a antibodies, directed against the fourth component of human complement (C4), are inhibited by incubation with plasma containing C4 from Ch(a+), Rg(a+) individuals. Demonstrating such inhibition aids in differentiating anti-Ch^a and anti-Rg^a from other HTLA antibodies.

Materials

1. Reactive red cell samples, similar to those used to demonstrate HTLA antibodies (see preceding procedure)
2. A pool of six or more normal plasma samples
3. Serum under investigation
4. 6% bovine albumin, prepared from stock 22% or 30% bovine albumin by dilution with saline
5. Polyspecific or anti-IgG antiglobulin reagent

Method

1. Prepare serial two-fold dilutions of test serum in saline. The dilution range should be from 1 in 2 to 1 in 4096, or to one tube beyond the known titer as determined above. The volume prepared should be not less than 0.3 ml for each red cell sample to be tested.
2. For each red cell sample to be tested, place 3 drops of diluted serum into each of two appropriately labeled 10 or 12 × 75-mm test tubes.
3. To one tube add 3 drops of pooled plasma.
4. To the other tube add 3 drops of 6% albumin.
5. Gently agitate the contents of each tube and incubate at room temperature for at least 30 minutes.
6. Add 1 drop of a 2-5% suspension of red cells to each tube.

7. Gently agitate the contents of each tube and incubate at 37 C for 1 hour.
8. Wash the red cells four times in saline and test with polyspecific or anti-IgG antiglobulin reagent.
9. Examine the red cells for agglutination; confirm all nonreactive tests with an optical aid. Grade and record the results.

Notes

1. Diluted bovine albumin is used as the negative control because it provides a protein concentration in the incubated serum approximately that in the tube containing serum and pooled plasma.
2. Inhibition of antibody activity by plasma suggests anti-Ch^a or anti-Rg^a specificity. This inhibition is often complete. Partial inhibition may indicate the presence of additional alloantibodies. In such situations, a large volume of inhibited serum can be tested against a reagent red cell panel to see if the non-neutralizable antibodies display specificity.
3. Antibodies to white cell antigens (eg, anti-Bg^a) may also be subject to partial inhibition by plasma.

Coating Red Cells with C4 and Absorption of Anti-Ch^a or Anti-Rg^a

Principle

C4 binds nonimmunologically to red cells when plasma and cells are incubated in a low ionic strength medium. Autologous cells coated with Ch(a+) or Rg(a+) complement can be used to adsorb anti-Ch^a from serum that may contain other alloantibodies.

Materials

1. 2 ml of serum, containing anti-Ch^a or anti-Rg^a, to be absorbed
2. 2 ml of washed packed autologous red cells
3. 20 ml of 10% sucrose in distilled water, 1containing 1.5 mg/ml of K₃EDTA (see note)
4. 2 ml of Ch(a+), Rg(a+) anticoagulated plasma (ACD, CPD or CPDA-1) known to lack unexpected antibodies

Method

Complement Coating

1. Divide the red cells into two 1 ml aliquots, and dispense into 16 × 100-mm test tubes.
2. Add 1 ml of plasma and 10 ml of 10% sucrose to each tube.
3. Mix well, and incubate at 37 C for 15 minutes.
4. Wash the red cells four times in saline. Centrifuge the last wash for five minutes, and completely remove the supernatant fluid. The red cells are now coated with C4.

Absorption

1. To one tube of C4-coated red cells, add 2 ml of serum to be absorbed.
2. Incubate at 37 C for 1 hour.
3. Centrifuge at 1000 × *g* for 2 minutes, and transfer the supernatant serum to the second tube of C4-coated red cells.
4. Incubate at 37 C for 1 hour.
5. Centrifuge at 1000 × *g* for 2 minutes, and transfer the absorbed serum into a clean test tube.
6. Test the absorbed serum for unexpected antibodies using an indirect antiglobulin technique.

Note

The required amount of K₃EDTA to prepare 20 ml of sucrose-EDTA mixture is present in two 16 × 100-mm (10 ml) Vacutainer® tubes (4427/3200 QS, from Becton-Dickinson).

Reference

Ellisor SS, Shoemaker MM, Reid ME. Absorption of anti-Chido from serum using autologous red blood cells coated with homologous C4. Transfusion 1982;22:243-245.

The Donath-Landsteiner Test

Primary Application

Differential diagnosis of immune hemolysis and diagnosis of paroxysmal cold hemoglobinuria (PCH). In particular, this procedure should be considered when high-titer cold-reactive autoantibodies are absent from the serum, C3 alone is present on the red cells, the eluate is nonreactive and the patient has hemoglobinemia or hemoglobinuria, or both.

Materials

1. Serum to be tested, separated from a freshly collected blood sample maintained at 37 C
2. Freshly collected normal serum as a source of complement
3. 50% suspension of washed group O, P-positive red cells (P₁ or P₂ phenotype)

Method

1. Label three sets of three 10 × 75-mm test tubes as follows: A1-A2-A3; B-1-B2-B3; C1-C2-C3.
2. To tubes 1 and 2 of each set, add 10 volumes of patient's serum.
3. To tubes 2 and 3 of each set, add 10 volumes of fresh normal serum.
4. To all tubes, add one volume of the 50% suspension of washed P-positive red cells and mix well.
5. Place the three 'A' tubes first in a bath of melting ice for 30 minutes, and then at 37 C for 1 hour.
6. Place the three 'B' tubes in a bath of melting ice, and keep them in melting ice for 90 minutes.
7. Place the three 'C' tubes at 37 C, and keep them at 37 C for 90 minutes.
8. Centrifuge all tubes, and examine the supernatants for hemolysis.

Interpretation

The Donath-Landsteiner test, indicative of PCH, is considered positive when the patient's serum, with or without added complement, causes hemolysis only in those tubes that have been incubated first in melting ice and then at 37 C (ie, tubes A1 and B1). No hemolysis should be seen in any of the tubes maintained strictly at 37 C or in melting ice, or in which complement alone is present.

Notes

1. To demonstrate the biphasic hemolysin associated with PCH, it is necessary

to incubate the serum with red cells first at or below 4 C, then at 37 C.

2. Complement is essential to demonstrate the antibody. Since patients with PCH often have low levels of serum complement, fresh normal serum should be included in the reaction medium as a source of complement.

3. To avoid loss of antibody by autoabsorption prior to testing, the patient's blood should be allowed to clot at 37 C, and the serum separated from the clot at 37 C.

Reference

Dacie JV, Lewis, SM. Practical hematology, 4th ed. London: Churchill; 1968.

Confirmation of Weak A or B Subgroup by Adsorption and Elution

Principle

Red cells having weak A or B antigen may not be agglutinated by anti-A or anti-B but may adsorb the specific antibody. Removing the adsorbed antibody by elution makes it possible to identify the presence of antigenically active material capable of reacting with antibody of known specificity.

Procedure for Adsorption and Elution

1. Wash 1 ml of the cells to be tested at least three times with saline. Remove supernatant after last wash.

2. Add to the red cells 1 ml of reagent anti-A if a weak variant of A is suspected or 1 ml of anti-B if a weak variant of B is suspected.

3. Mix the red cells with the antiserum and incubate the mixture at room temperature for one hour.

4. Centrifuge the mixture to pack the red cells. Remove the supernatant antiserum.

5. Wash the red cells at least five times with large volumes of saline (10 ml or

more). Save an aliquot of the fifth wash to test for free antibody.

6. Add an equal volume of saline to the washed packed red cells. Mix well.

7. Elute the adsorbed antibody by placing the tube in a 56 C waterbath for ten minutes. Mix the red cell-saline mixture at least once during this period.

8. Centrifuge to pack the red cells.

9. Remove the cherry-colored supernatant eluate. Discard the cells.

Testing the Eluate

1. If anti-A was used, test the eluate against three different examples of A_1 cells and three group O cells at room temperature, at 37 C and with antiglobulin serum.

2. If anti-B was used, test the eluate against three examples of group B and three group O red cells at room temperature, at 37 C and with antiglobulin serum.

3. Test the fifth saline wash (step 5, above) in the same manner to show that washing has removed all antibody not bound to the cells.

Interpretation

If the eluate agglutinates or reacts in antiglobulin testing with specific A or B cells and does not react with O cells, the cells being tested must have active A or B antigen on their surface capable of binding specific antibody. If the eluate also reacts with O cells, it indicates nonspecific reactivity in the eluate, and the results are not valid. If the saline wash material is reactive with A or B cells, the results of tests made on the eluate are not valid, because it indicates that active antibody was present in the medium unattached to the cells being tested.

Reference

Beattie KM. Identifying the causes of weak or "missing" antigens in ABO grouping tests. In: The investigation of typing and compatibility problems caused by red blood cells. Washington, DC: American Association of Blood Banks; 1975.

Saliva Testing for ABH and Lewis

Collection of Saliva

1. Collect 5-10 ml saliva in a small beaker or wide-mouthed test tube. Most people can accumulate this much in several minutes. To encourage salivation, the subject can chew wax, paraffin film or a rubber band, but not gum or anything else that contains sugar or protein.
2. Place beaker or tube of saliva in boiling water bath for 10 minutes to inactivate salivary enzymes.
3. Centrifuge boiled saliva at high speed for 10 minutes.
4. Remove clear or slightly opalescent supernatant. Discard the opaque or semi-solid material.
5. Refrigerate if test is to be done within several hours. If testing will not be done on the day of collection, store the sample in the freezer. Frozen samples retain activity for several years.

Selection of Antiserum Dilution

1. Prepare doubling dilutions of antibody. Use a lectin anti-H to test ABO secretor status and anti-Le^a for Lewis testing.
2. Combine one drop of diluted antibody and one drop of 2-5% saline suspension of cells. Use group O cells for ABO secretor status and Le(a+) cells for Lewis testing.
3. Centrifuge and observe macroscopically for agglutination.
4. Select for testing the highest dilution that gives 2+ agglutination.

Procedure

1. Prepare saliva for positive and negative controls. For ABH secretor status, use saliva from previously tested *Se* and *sese* persons. For Lewis testing, use saliva from a person whose red cells are Le^a-positive and from a Lewis-negative individual. Aliquots of saliva from suitable individuals can be frozen for later use.
2. Add 1 drop of appropriately diluted antiserum to each of four tubes. For ABH secretor, these should be labeled "Secretor," "Nonsecretor," "Saline" and "Unknown." For Lewis, these are "Lewis-positive," "Lewis-negative," "Saline" and "Unknown."
3. Add 1 drop of saliva to the appropriate tubes, and 1 drop of saline to the control tube.

Interpretation of Saliva Testing

| | Testing with anti-H | | | |
Unknown Saliva	Se Saliva (H Substance Present)	Non-Se Saliva (H Substance not Present)	Saline (Dilution Control)	Interpretation
2+	0	2+	2+	Nonsecretor
0	0	2+	2+	Secretor

| | Testing with anti-Le^a | | | |
Unknown Saliva	Le-positive Saliva	Le-negative Saliva	Saline (Dilution Control)	Interpretation
2+	0	2+	2+	Lewis-negative
0	0	2+	2+	Lewis-positive*

*A Lewis-positive person shown to be a secretor of ABH can be assumed to have Le^b as well as Le^a in saliva. A Le(a+) person who is *sese* and does not secrete ABH substance will have only Le^a in saliva.

4. Incubate for 10 minutes at room temperature.
5. Add 1 drop of 2-5% saline suspension of washed indicator cells to each tube.
6. Incubate for 30-60 minutes at room temperature.
7. Centrifuge and observe macroscopically for agglutination.
8. Record results. For interpretation see table on page 459.

Notes

This screening procedure can be adapted for semiquantitation of blood group activity by testing serial saline dilutions of saliva. The higher the dilution needed to remove inhibitory activity, the more salivary blood group substance present. Saliva should be diluted before incubation with antibody.

To detect or to measure salivary A or B substance in addition to H substance, the same procedure can be used with diluted anti-A and anti-B reagents. The appropriate dilution of anti-A or anti-B is obtained by titrating the antiserum against A or B cells, respectively.

Detection of Antibodies to Penicillin or Cephalothin

Primary Application

Investigation of drug-induced positive direct antiglobulin tests associated with penicillin or cephalothin therapy.

Materials

1. Barbital-buffered saline (BBS) at pH 9.6, prepared by dissolving 20.6 g of sodium barbital in 1 liter of saline. Adjust to pH 9.6 with 0.1N HC1. Store at 4 C.
2. Penicillin (approximately 1×10^6 units per 600 mg)
3. Cephalothin sodium (Keflin)
4. Washed, packed group O red cells
5. Serum or eluate to be studied

Method

1. Prepare penicillin-coated red cells by incubating 1 ml of red cells with 600 mg of penicillin in 15 ml BBS for 1 hour at room temperature. Wash three times in saline and store in Alsever's solution at 4 C.
2. Prepare cephalothin-coated red cells by incubating 1 ml of red cells with 400 mg of cephalothin sodium in 10 ml of BBS for 2 hours at 37 C. Wash three times in saline and store in Alsever's solution at 4 C.
3. Mix 2 or 3 drops of serum or eluate with 1 drop of 5% saline suspension of drug-coated red cells; dilute serum 1 in 20 with saline for tests with cephalothin-coated red cells.
4. Test in parallel uncoated red cells from the same donor.
5. Incubate tests at room temperature for 15 minutes. Centrifuge, and examine the red cells macroscopically for agglutination. Grade and record the results.
6. Incubate the tests at 37 C for 30-60 minutes. Centrifuge, and examine the red cells macroscopically for agglutination. Grade and record the results.
7. Wash the red cells four times in saline, and test by an indirect antiglobulin technique using polyspecific or anti-IgG antiglobulin reagent.

Interpretation

Antibodies to penicillin or cephalothin will react with the drug-coated red cells but not with uncoated red cells. Antibodies to either drug may cross-react with red cells coated with the other drug (ie, antipenicillin antibodies crossreact with cephalothin-coated red cells and vice-versa).

Notes

1. Phosphate-buffered saline at pH 7.3 may be substituted for BBS in the preparation of cephalothin-coated red cells.

2. All normal sera react with cephalothin-coated red cells, since such red cells adsorb all proteins nonimmunologically. This reactivity does not occur with incubation times as short as 15 minutes, or if the serum is diluted 1 in 20 with saline before testing.
3. Eluates do not contain enough protein to be adsorbed nonimmunologically by cephalothin-treated red cells. Reactivity of an eluate with cephalothin-coated red cells indicates antibody to cephalosporins, which may crossreact with penicillin-coated red cells.

Reference

Garratty G. Laboratory investigation of drug-induced hemolytic anemia. Supplement, A seminar on laboratory management of hemolysis. Washington, DC: American Association of Blood Banks; 1979.

Demonstration of Immune Complex Formation Involving Drugs

Principle and Application

Immune complexes formed between certain drugs and their respective antibodies attach weakly and in a nonspecific fashion to red cells. The bound immune complex activates complement, which may lead to hemolysis in vivo. The following procedure provides an in vitro means to demonstrate immune-complex formation associated with drug-antidrug interactions.

Materials

1. Drug under investigation, in the same form (tablet, solution, capsules) that the patient is receiving
2. Phosphate-buffered saline (PBS) at pH 7.0-7.4
3. Patient's serum
4. Fresh, normal serum known to lack unexpected antibodies, as a source of complement

5. Group O reagent red cells, both untreated and treated with a proteolytic enzyme (see page 427)

Method

1. Prepare a 1 mg/ml suspension of the drug in PBS. Centrifuge, and adjust the pH of the supernatant to 7.0 with either 1N NaOH or 1N HCl, as required.
2. Prepare the following test mixtures.
   a. patient's serum + drug
   b. patient's serum + complement (normal serum) + drug
   c. patient's serum + complement (normal serum) + PBS
   d. normal serum + drug
   e. normal serum + PBS
   Two sets of these mixtures should be prepared, each containing two to four volumes of each reactant.
3. To one set of test mixtures, add one volume of a 5-10% saline suspenion of group O reagent red cells. To the other set add one volume of a 5-10% saline suspension of enzyme-treated group O reagent red cells.
4. Mix, and incubate at 37 C for 1 to 2 hours, with periodic gentle mixing.
5. Wash the red cells four times in saline, and test with a polyspecific antiglobulin reagent.

Interpretation

Hemolysis, agglutination or coating can occur. Such reactivity in any of the tests containing patient's serum to which the drug was added, and absence of reactivity in the corresponding control tests containing PBS instead of the drug, indicates a drug-antidrug interaction.

Notes

1. The use of a pestle and mortar (if the drug is in tablet form), incubation at 37 C and vigorous shaking of the solution will help dissolve the drug.
2. Most drugs will not dissolve completely, but enough may be dissolved

to react in serologic tests. Other methods, obtained from the manufacturer or other publications, may be needed to dissolve adequate quantities of some drugs.

Reference

Garratty G. Laboratory investigation of drug-induced immune hemolytic anemia. Supplement: A seminar on laboratory management of hemolysis. Washington, DC: American Association of Blood Banks; 1979.

A Code for Scoring Agglutination Reactions

Many workers who assign numerical scores to observed degrees of agglutination use the system of Race and Sanger as adapted by Marsh:

Strength of Agglutination	Score
4+	12
3+	10
2+	8
1+	5
w+	2
0	0

Reference

Marsh WL. Scoring of hemagglutination reactions. Transfusion 1972; 12:352-353.

Autoantibodies

Use of Thiol Reagents to Disperse Autoagglutination

Application

Thiol reagents, which cleave the intersubunit disulfide bonds of pentameric IgM molecules, can be used to disperse agglutination caused by cold-reactive autoantibodies. Treating spontaneously agglutinated red cells with 2-mercaptoethanol (2-ME) or dithiothreitol (DTT) provides a nonagglutinated specimen suitable for use in blood grouping tests.

Materials

1. 0.01M DTT or 0.1M 2-ME
2. Phosphate-buffered saline (PBS) at pH 7.3
3. Packed washed red cells to be treated

Method

1. Dilute red cells to a 50% concentration in PBS.
2. Add an equal quantity of 0.01M DTT in PBS, or 0.1M 2-ME in PBS, to the red cells.
3. Incubate at 37 C for 10 minutes for 2-ME or 15 minutes for DTT.
4. Wash red cells three times.
5. Dilute the treated red cells to a 3-5% concentration in saline, and use in blood grouping tests.

Reference

Reid ME. Autoagglutination dispersal utilizing sulphydryl compounds. Transfusion 1978;18:353-355.

Autologous Absorption of Warm-Reactive Autoantibodies

Application

Detection of clinically significant alloantibodies in the presence of warm-reactive autoantibodies.

Principle

Warm-reactive autoantibodies may mask the presence of concomitant alloantibodies in a serum. Absorbing the serum with autologous red cells can remove autoantibody from the serum, permitting detection of underlying alloantibodies. Circulating autologous cells, however, are already coated with autoantibody.

Autologous absorption of warm-reactive autoantibodies can be achieved most effectively by removing the autoantibody and then pretreating the cells with a proteolytic enzyme. Removal of coating antibody uncovers antigen sites, which are then capable of binding free autoantibody in the serum. Enyzme treatment enhances the absorption process by removing red cell membrane structures that otherwise hinder the association between antigen and antibody.

463

Two procedures are used routinely for autologous absorption of warm-reactive antibodies. One utilizes heat to remove coating antibody, with subsequent enzyme treatment of red cells to increase their absorptive capacity.[1] The other procedure involves the use of ZZAP reagent, a mixture of a proteolytic enzyme and a thiol reagent.[2] Treatment of IgG molecules with a thiol reagent increases their susceptibility to digestion by proteases. When IgG-coated red cells are treated with ZZAP reagent, the immunoglobulin molecules lose their integrity and dissociate from the red cell surface. Simultaneously, the red cells are subjected to the action of a proteolytic enzyme to increase their absorptive capacity.

Autoabsorption should not be performed on cells from a recently transfused patient because the circulating allogeneic cells may adsorb precisely the alloantibodies that are being sought.

Procedure A—Heat and Enzyme Method
Materials

1. 6% bovine albumin, prepared by diluting 22% or 30% bovine albumin with saline
2. 1% ficin or 1% cysteine-activated papain (see pages 425–427)
3. Blood samples containing warm-reactive autoantibodies

Method

1. Wash 2 ml of red cells four times in saline, and discard the final supernatant.
2. Add an equal volume of 6% albumin to the packed red cells. Mix, and incubate at 56 C for 3 to 5 minutes. Gently agitate the mixture during this time.
3. Centrifuge at $1000 \times g$ for 2 minutes, and harvest the supernatant. This may be used as an eluate if the patient's red cells are in short supply.
4. Wash the red cells three times in saline, and discard the final supernatant.

5. Add 1 ml of 1% papain or 1% ficin to the packed red cells. Mix, and incubate at 37 C for 15 minutes.
6. Wash the red cells three times in saline. Centrifuge the last wash for at least 5 minutes at $1000 \times g$. Use suction to remove as much of the supernatant as practical.
7. Divide the red cells into two equal aliquots.
8. To one aliquot, add 2 ml of patient's serum. Mix, and incubate at 37 C for 30 minutes.
9. Centrifuge at $1000 \times g$ for 2 minutes, and transfer the serum to the second aliquot of red cells. Mix, and incubate at 37 C for 30 minutes.
10. Centrifuge at $1000 \times g$ for 2 minutes, and harvest the absorbed serum.
11. Test the absorbed serum for antibody activity using an indirect antiglobulin technique.

Procedure B—ZZAP Method
Materials

1. 1% cysteine-activated papain or 1% ficin (see pages 425–427)
2. Phosphate-buffered saline (PBS) at pH 7.3
3. 0.2M dithiothreitol (DTT) prepared by dissolving 1 g of DTT in 32.4 ml of pH 7.3 PBS. Dispense into 2.5 ml aliquots and store at or below -20 C
4. Blood samples containing warm-reactive autoantibodies

Method

1. Prepare ZZAP reagent by mixing 0.5 ml cysteine-activated papain with 2.5 ml of DTT and 2 ml of pH 7.3 PBS. Alternatively, use 1 ml of ficin, 2.5 ml of DTT and 1.5 ml of pH 7.3 PBS.
2. To two tubes, each containing 1 ml of packed red cells, add 2 ml of ZZAP reagent. Mix, and incubate at 37 C for 30 minutes.
3. Wash the red cells three times in saline. Centrifuge the last wash for at least 5 minutes at $1000 \times g$. Use suction to

remove as much of the supernatant as practical.

4. Proceed as from step 8 in Procedure A, above.

Interpretation

A two-fold autologous absorption ordinarily removes sufficient autoantibody from the serum that alloantibody reactivity is readily apparent, but sometimes two absorptions are insufficient. If the patient's red cells can be shown to have a nonreactive direct antiglobulin test following heat treatment (Procedure A), ZZAP treatment (Procedure B) or after incubation with chloroquine diphosphate (see page 418), such red cells may be used to check the efficacy of the absorption process. For example, if Procedure A was used and the heat-treated red cells obtained after step 4 have a nonreactive direct antiglobulin test, the autoabsorbed serum should be tested against them and against two group O reagent red cell samples.

Results are interpreted as follows:

1. When there is no reactivity against the group O reagent red cells, it is unlikely that alloantibody is present.
2. If there is reactivity against both the patient's heat-treated red cells and the group O reagent red cells, further absorptions of the serum may be necessary.
3. When the absorbed serum reacts with one or both of the group O reagent red cell samples, and not with the autologous red cells, the serum contains alloantibody, and antibody identification studies should be undertaken on the absorbed serum.

Notes

1. Prepare ZZAP reagent immediately prior to use.
2. ZZAP treatment destroys all Kell-system antigens except Kx, in addition to other antigens that are also destroyed by proteases, including M, N, Fy^a, Fy^b and S.

3. There is no need to wash red cells prior to treatment with ZZAP.

References

1. Morel PA, Bergren MO, Frank BA. A simple method for the detection of alloantibody in the presence of autoantibody (abstract). Transfusion 1978;18:388.
2. Branch DR, Petz LD. A new reagent (ZZAP) having multiple applications in immunohematology. Am J Clin Pathol 1982;78:161-167.

Dilution Technique for Investigating Warm-Reactive Autoantibodies

Applications

1. Determining the relative Rh specificity of warm-reactive autoantibodies in serum or eluate
2. Detecting alloantibodies in the presence of warm-reactive autoantibodies. As discussed on page 254 this is not the optimal method to use, and will only be informative if the alloantibody titer is greater than that of the autoantibody.

Materials

1. 2-5% suspensions of group O, R_1R_1, R_2R_2 and rr red cells (see below for additional phenotypes that should be considered when attempting to detect alloantibody)
2. Serum or eluate to be tested
3. Polyspecific or anti-IgG antiglobulin reagent

Method

1. Prepare serial two-fold dilutions of serum or eluate in saline. The dilution range should be from 1 in 2 to 1 in 1024, and the volumes prepared should be not less than 0.5 ml.
2. Place 3 drops of each dilution into each of three appropriately labeled 10 or 12 × 75-mm test tubes.
3. To one tube of each dilution add one drop of R_1R_1 red cells. Similarly test the R_2R_2 and rr red cells.

4. Gently agitate the contents of each tube, and incubate at 37 C for 1 hour.
5. Wash the red cells four times with saline, and test with polyspecific or anti-IgG antiglobulin reagent.
6. Examine the red cells for agglutination. Grade and record the results.
7. Based on the results obtained, select the highest dilution of serum or eluate that gives a 2+ reaction with the most strongly reactive red cell sample.
8. Prepare a sufficient volume of this dilution and test against a panel of reagent red cells by antiglobulin technique.

Notes

1. The relative Rh specificity of warm-reactive autoantibodies may be discerned from the result obtained in step 8. For example, a 1 in 64 dilution of serum or eluate may give a 2+ reaction with R_1R_1 and rr red cells, but R_2R_2 red cells give a 2+ reaction with the 1 in 8 dilution. When a 1 in 64 dilution is tested against a reagent red cell panel, anti-e activity may be observed. In such situations, the autoantibody is said to have relative anti-e specificity.
2. When this method is used to detect alloantibody activity in the presence of warm-reactive autoantibodies, it may be necessary to consider additional phenotypes in selecting red cells for use in the titration study. The three red cell samples used (R_1R_1, R_2R_2, rr) should also be selected to ensure that at least one sample carries and another lacks K, Fy^a, Fy^b, Jk^a and S antigens. This may be modified according to what is known about the phenotype of the patient's red cells; eg, if E+, there will be no need to include R_2R_2 red cells.
3. The presence of alloantibodies may also be discerned from the results obtained in step 8. For example, a serum dilution of 1 in 16 may give a 2+ reaction with Fy(a+) red cells that are rr, but fail to react with R_1R_1 and R_2R_2 red cells that are Fy(a−). When a 1 in 16 dilu-

tion is tested against a reagent red cell panel, anti-Fy^a specificity may be observed.

Cold Autoabsorption

Application

Detection of clinically significant alloantibodies in the presence of cold-reactive autoantibodies.

Materials

1. 1% ficin or 1% papain (see pages 425–427)
2. 2 ml of serum to be absorbed
3. 3 ml of packed autologous red cells

Method

1. Wash the red cells four times in saline and divide into three equal aliquots in 13 × 100-mm test tubes.
2. Add 0.5 ml of 1% ficin or 1% papain to each tube.
3. Mix, and incubate at 37 C for 15 minutes.
4. Wash the red cells three times in saline. Centrifuge the last wash for 5 minutes at 1000 × g, and remove as much of the supernatant saline as possible (see note below).
5. To one tube of enzyme-treated red cells add 2 ml of the autologous serum.
6. Mix, and incubate at 4 C for 30-40 minutes.
7. Centrifuge at 1000 × g for 5 minutes, and transfer the serum into a second tube of enzyme-treated red cells.
8. Mix, and incubate at 4 C for 30-40 minutes.
9. Repeat steps 7 and 8 for the third tube of enzyme-treated red cells.
10. Following the final absorption, test the serum for alloantibody activity.

Note

To avoid dilution of the serum and possible loss of weak alloantibody activity during the absorption process, it is important to remove as much of the residual saline as possible in step 4. Placing a narrow strip of filter paper into the packed red cells helps remove saline that surrounds the packed cells.

Determining the Specificity of Cold-Reactive Autoagglutinins

Primary Application

Determining the specificity of cold-reactive autoantibodies associated with cold hemagglutinin disease

Materials

1. Serum to be studied. Serum should be separated at 37 C from a blood sample allowed to clot at 37 C.
2. Test red cells. The following are required:
   a. Two adult group O, I-positive samples, ordinarily reagent red cells used for alloantibody detection
   b. The patient's own (autologous) red cells
   c. Red cells of the same ABO phenotype as the patient, if the patient is not group O. Use red cells of the same A subtype (ie, A_1 or A_2) if the patient is group A or AB.
   d. Ficin or papain-treated group O, I-positive red cells
   e. Group O, I-negative cord blood or adult I-negative red cells, or both

Method

1. Prepare serial two-fold dilutions of the serum in saline. The dilution range should be from 1 in 2 to 1 in 4096 (12 tubes), and the volumes prepared should not be less than 1 ml.
2. Mix 3 drops of each dilution with 1 drop of a 5% saline suspension of each test red cell sample.
3. Incubate at room temperature for 15 minutes. Centrifuge, and examine the red cells macroscopically for agglutination. Grade and record the results.
4. Transfer the tubes to 4 C, and incubate at this temperature for 1 hour; ideally,

a cold room rather than a household refrigerator should be used. Centrifuge, and examine the red cells for agglutination. Grade and record the results.

Interpretation

The table on page 468 summarizes the reactions of some commonly encountered cold-reactive autoantibodies. Anti-I is seen frequently in cold hemagglutinin disease, but anti-i and anti-Pr specificities may also be encountered. Some examples of anti-I display a preference for red cells that have a strong expression of H antigen (eg, O and A_2); such antibodies are called anti-IH. The reactivity of all autoantibodies with specificity related to the Ii system is enhanced in tests with protease-treated red cells. In contrast, anti-Pr antibodies react weakly if at all with enzyme-treated red cells, and react with all untreated red cells to the same degree regardless of their Ii status.

Notes

1. With potent examples of cold-reactive autoantibodies, specificity may not be apparent when titration studies are performed at room temperature or 4 C. In such circumstances, incubation of tests at 30 to 37 C should be undertaken. Also, speciflicity may be more readily ascertained if incubation times are prolonged and agglutination is evaluated after settling, without centrifugation.
2. Some workers use this procedure for determining both titer and specificity. If multiple readings are taken following incubation at different temperatures, the specificity, titer and thermal amplitude of the autoantibody can be determined with a single set of serum dilutions.

Demonstration of High-Titer Cold-Reactive Autoagglutinins

Primary Application

Demonstrating clinically significant elevation of cold-reactive autoagglutinins

Comparative Reactions to Demonstrate Specificity of Cold-Reactive Autoantibodies

Red Cells	Antibody Specificity				
	Anti-I	Anti-i	Anti-H*	Anti-IH*	Anti-Pr
Oi (adult)	0/ ↓	↑	≡	↓	≡
Oi (cord)	0/ ↓	↑	<	↓	≡
A₁I	≡	≡	↓	↓	≡
OI (enzyme-treated)	↑	↑	↑	↑	0/ ↓
Autologous	≡	≡	↓	↓	≡

0 = nonreactive   ≡ = equal to OI red cells
↑ = stronger than OI red cells   < = equal to or weaker than OI red cells
↓ = weaker than OI red cells
*anti-H and anti-IH antibodies are seen predominantly in A₁ and A₁B individuals

Materials

1. Serum to be tested. Separate serum at 37 C from sample allowed to clot at 37 C.
2. 1% saline suspension of washed group O, I-positive red cells. Red cells should be from sample anticoagulated with ACD or CPD, collected within the preceding 7 days
3. Phosphate-buffered saline (PBS) at pH 7.3 (see page 424)

Method

1. Dilute the serum 1 in 5 with saline.
2. Prepare serial two-fold dilutions of diluted serum in saline. Use 0.5 ml volumes when making these dilutions. The final dilution range should be from 1 in 10 to 1 in 20,480 (12 tubes).
3. Add to each tube 0.5 ml of a 1% saline suspension of washed red cells.
4. Mix, and incubate overnight at 4 C.
5. Do not centrifuge the test mixtures. Examine the red cells macroscopically for agglutination. Grade and record the results.

Interpretation

The reciprocal of the highest dilution of serum at which agglutination is observed is reported as the titer. With this technique, titers above 40 are considered elevated. However, hemolytic anemia due to cold-reactive autoagglutinins is not usually seen unless the titer is above 640. Titers below 640 may be obtained when the autoantibody has anti-i specificity. In this situation, I-negative (i_{cord} or i_{adult}) red cells may be substituted for the I-positive red cells. Alternatively, the previously described technique to determine the specificity of cold-reactive autoantibodies may be used to determine the titer.

Note

It is important to use separate pipettes for each tube when preparing serum dilutions. If a single pipette is used throughout, falsely high titration endpoints may be obtained due to serum carried from one tube to the next. The difference can be as great as an apparent titer of 100,000 using a single pipette, and a true titer of 4000 when separate pipettes are used. Serum dilutions can be prepared more accurately when large volumes (eg, 0.5 ml) are used.

Reference

Rose NR, Friedman H, eds. Manual of clinical immunology. 2nd ed. Washington, DC: American Society for Microbiology; 1980: 735-737

Components

Centrifugation for Component Preparation

Heavy Spin

Packed red cells
Platelet concentrates $\Big\}$ 5000 × g, 5 minutes

Plasmapheresis
Cell-free plasma
Leukocyte-poor red cells $\Big\}$ 5000 × g,
Cryoprecipitate   7 minutes

Light Spin

Platelet-rich plasma   2000 × g, 3 minutes

To calculate relative centrifugal force in g:

$$\text{rcf (in } g) = 28.38\ R* \left(\frac{\text{rpm}}{1000}\right)^2$$

*R = radius of centrifuge rotor in inches

Times include acceleration but not deceleration times. Times given are approximations only. Each individual centrifuge must be evaluated for the preparation of the various components.

Removing Plasma from Platelet Concentrates

Principle

An adequate volume of plasma is necessary for optimum storage of platelets, but the patient receiving the platelets may suffer ill effects if the entire volume is infused. It is permissible to centrifuge stored platelets and remove much of the plasma shortly before transfusion, but appropriate resuspension is necessary. The platelets must remain at room temperature, without agitation, for 20 to 60 minutes and then undergo resuspension into the remaining plasma. Transfusion must take place within 6 hours of the time the platelets were entered. Volume reduction can be performed on individual units of platelets or on a pool of several units.

There is not full agreement on the optimum centrifugation rate. One recent study[1] found 35 to 55% platelet loss in several units centrifuged at 500 × g for 6 minutes compared with 5 to 20% loss in units centrifuged at 5000 × g for 6 minutes or 2000 × g for 10 minutes. The authors recommend the lower centrifugal force to avoid risk of damaging the plastic container. A study by Moroff et al[2] found mean platelet loss to be less than 15% in 42 units centrifuged at 580 × g for 20 minutes.

Procedure

1. Pool platelets into a transfer pack (if desired), using standard technique.
2. Centrifuge at 20-24 C, using one of the following protocols:
   a. 580 × g for 20 minutes
   b. 2000 × g for 10 minutes
   c. 5000 × g for 6 minutes

3. Transfer the bag, without disturbing the contents, to a plasma extractor and remove all but 10-15 ml plasma from single units, somewhat more from a pool or from a concentrate prepared by hemapheresis.
4. Mark expiration time on bag as 6 hours after unit was entered, either the time of pooling or the time the seal on the individual unit was broken.
5. Leave bag at 20-24 C, without agitation, for 20 minutes, if centrifuged at $580 \times g$ or 1 hour if centrifuged at 2000 or $5000 \times g$.
6. Resuspend platelets by either:
   a. gently rubbing and kneading the bag until the platelets are evenly suspended
   b. rotating bag on standard platelet rotator for 1 hour

References

1. Simon TL, Sierra ER. Concentration of platelet units into small volumes. Transfusion 1984;24:173-175.
2. Moroff G, Friedman A, Robkin-Kline L, Gautier G, Luban NLC. Reduction of the volume of stored platelet concentrates for use in neonatal patients. Transfusion 1984;24:144-146.

Removing Plasma from Units of Whole Blood (to Prepare RBCs with Known Hematocrit)

Hematocrit of Segment from Whole Blood Unit	Volume of Plasma to be Removed	Final Hematocrit of Red Blood Cell Unit
40	150	56
39	150	55
38	160	55
37	165	54
36	170	54
35	180	54
34	195	55
33	200	55

Removing Leukocytes from Apheresis Platelet Concentrates

1. Maintain apheresis platelet concentrates in the usual agitation at room temperature until ready for processing to remove leukocytes.
2. Centrifuge at room temperature at 178 g for 3 minutes.
3. Express the leukocyte-poor, platelet-rich supernatant plasma, being careful not to disturb the leukocyte button.
4. Discard the bag containing the leukocyte button.

This procedure removes about 96% of the contaminating white blood cells and about 21% of the platelets. The use of these leukocyte-poor platelet concentrates can diminish undesirable transfusion reactions following incompatible platelet transfusions and may decrease the rate of sensitization to HLA antigens.

References

1. Herzig RH, Herzig GP, Bull MI, et al. Correction of poor platelet transfusion responses with leukocyte-poor HLA-matched platelet concentrates. Blood 1975;46:743-750.
2. Slichter SJ. Controversies in platelet transfusion therapy. Ann Rev Med 1980;31:509-540.

Collecting Specimen to Monitor Hemapheresis Components

1. Strip tubing attached to the component bag four times, to ensure that contents of tubing are representative of component in bag.
2. Seal tubing approximately 45 cm (18 inches) from bag. There should be approximately 2 ml of fluid in the segment. Double seal end of tubing next to component bag and detach segment.
3. Empty contents of segment into a suitably labeled tube, for counting on a device that reports red cells, platelets and leukocytes per mm³. Multiply reported counts by 1000 to obtain cell values per ml; multiply this value by

the volume of the component, in ml, to obtain total cell count in the component.

Procedure for Manual 2-Unit Plasmapheresis

1. *Assembling equipment.* Insert a three-lead recipient set (use spike with integral airway) into a bottle of normal saline for injection and suspend from an upright pole. Remove the sterile cap from the end of the tubing and open the regulator to fill the tubing with saline and eliminate air from the system. Replace the sterile cap. The double bag unit is a closed system designed for the uninterrupted collection of two units of whole blood. Each primary bag is integrally connected to one or two satellite bags for transfer of plasma and possible further component preparation.

2. *Preparing the collection bag.* Tie a loose knot in the tubing of each of the primary blood bags below the "Y" connection.

3. *Setting the scale.* Attach bag No. 1 to a device for regulating volume drawn, either a standard phlebotomy monitor or a dietary scale set to zero, to allow observation of volume drawn. Place the three remaining bags on the donor's chair.

4. *Connecting infusion and phlebotomy lines.* Insert a sterile three-way stopcock to the "Y" connection of the blood bag system and attach the saline to it. At the third junction, attach a sterile 10-ml syringe with the stopcock closed at the syringe. Using the stopcock makes it possible to collect blood samples without opening the closed system.

5. *Preparing the donor.* Review the medical history and physical examination. Confirm the donor's identification. Explain the equipment and the procedure to the donor and have the donor sign the Informed Consent Form with you as a witness. Answer all the donor's questions, getting additional explanation and information from a physician or other knowledgeable personnel, if necessary. Ask the donor to empty his bladder. Help the donor into a comfortable position in the chair. Select the vein to be used and place an inverted blood pressure cuff on the arm approximately four inches above the site of the venipuncture. Prepare the arm, using a standard procedure.

6. *Labeling the bags.* Print the donor's name on each bag. Have the donor sign pressure-sensitive labels and affix one to each bag that will contain components for reinfusion. Before reinfusion of the blood components, ask the donor to identify and initial each bag.

7. *Venipuncture.* Pop the metal bead that occludes the tubing leading from the needle into the first primary bag. Inflate the cuff to 40 mm Hg and have the donor squeeze on a handgrip. Do the venipuncture; secure the needle with tape; and place sterile 2 × 2 gauze squares over the venipuncture site. Instruct the donor to squeeze the handgrip approximately every 5 seconds.

8. *Observing the phlebotomy.* Watch the needle on the dietary scale to ensure that there is continuous blood flow. Gently manipulate the bag approximately each 50 ml to ensure even distribution of the anticoagulant solution.

9. *Ending the phlebotomy.* After 450 ml has been collected, release the pressure in the blood pressure cuff and tell the donor to stop squeezing the handgrip. Clamp the tubing above the "Y" connection. Tighten the knot in the tubing and apply a clamp approximately two inches above the knot. Cut the tubing about an inch above the knot.

10. *Obtaining a laboratory specimen and starting the saline infusion.* Turn the previ-

ously closed stopcock toward the donor to allow blood to enter the syringe. Release the clamp between the donor and the stopcock. Withdraw about 10 ml of blood into syringe. Turn the stopcock to allow the saline infusion and adjust the flow regulator. Replace the blood-filled syringe with another sterile syringe, and place the blood into properly labeled tubes for whatever laboratory tests are indicated.

11. *Handling the whole blood bag.* Remove the bag from the dietary scale. Strip the tubing from the knot to the bag and seal. Cut and discard the excess tubing.

12. *Balancing blood products for centrifugation.* Place the bag of blood in the centrifuge cup and place it on the balance scale. Place a bag filled with saline in another cup on the opposite side of the scale. To adjust balance, add rubber discs to the lighter cup as needed. Having the centrifuge cups properly balanced improves separation of the blood components and reduces wear and tear on the centrifuge.

13. *Centrifugation.* Place cups opposite each other in the centrifuge and secure the lid. The temperature inside the centrifuge should be 4 C. Close the centrifuge and set the speed and time as appropriate for the component being prepared. Observe the centrifuge to be sure that this speed is attained. Properly set, the machine will turn off automatically at the set time. Let the rotor come to a complete stop and open the lid. Do not stop the rotor manually and do not disturb the separation of cells and plasma by handling the bags roughly.

14. *Extracting the plasma.* Remove the cups from the centrifuge and place the blood bag in a plasma extractor. Push the spike into the primary bag; this will release the plasma into the transfer bag. After the desired volume of plasma has been obtained, clamp the tubing between the bags. Remove the primary bag from the extractor and heat-seal or double-clip the tubing above the clamp. Cut the tubing at the seal or between the clips. The primary bag now contains red cells to be returned to the donor.

15. *Transfusing red cells.* Have the donor identify and initial the primary bag. Identify the segment numbers on the primary bag with the segment numbers on the tubing still attached to the donor. Attach the bag to the second lead of the three-way recipient set and suspend from an upright pole. Close off normal saline and open the red blood cell line. Adjust the flow regulator and infuse the red cells rapidly. If the donor experiences tingling around the mouth or in the fingertips, the infusion should be slowed, since this usually arises from citrate-induced hypocalcemia.

16. *Preparing plasma.* Remove the clamp on the plasma tubing and strip from the seal to the bag. Reseal the tubing at the bag. Cut at bag and discard excess tubing. Store the plasma as appropriate for intended use.

17. *Continuing plasmapheresis.* After all erythrocytes are returned to the donor, shut off the infusion flow regulator and begin to withdraw the second bag of whole blood. Repeat steps 8 through 16 for the completion of the second unit.

18. *Discontinuing plasmapheresis.* Clamp the tubing above the "Y" connector and remove the blood pressure cuff, tape and needle. Apply pressure on the bandage over venipuncture site and have the donor raise the arm straight up and maintain pressure for three minutes or long enough to achieve hemostasis. After the allotted time, inspect the area for hemostasis and allow the donor to lower the arm if there is no bleeding.

19. *Postplasmapheresis instructions.* Apply a sterile bandage over the phlebotomy site. Have the donor leave the dress-

ing exposed while he remains at the blood center, so that bleeding will be easily noticed. Observe the donor for any untoward reactions. Inform the donor of possible postphlebotomy complications, as for any other blood donor.

Washing Red Blood Cells Without Special Equipment

1. Centrifuge the blood in a refrigerated centrifuge at 1-6 C using a light spin.
2. Express the plasma and buffy coat into the satellite bag. Seal the tubing and salvage the plasma, if desired.
3. Place a temporary clamp on a plasma-transfer set. Insert one end of the set into the injection site of a 250-ml container of sterile cold (1-6 C) isotonic saline (Sodium Chloride Injection USP 0.9%). Insert the other end into one of the outlet sites of the primary bag.
4. Drain the saline into the bag. Place a temporary clamp on the tubing. Remove the cannula from the saline container; replace the cannula's original plastic cover. Cover the exposed site of the saline container with sterile gauze. Bind the transfer set tubing to the outside of the primary bag with tape; be sure the cannula is in a vertical position at the top of the bag to prevent leakage or damage to the bag.
5. Resuspend the red cells in the saline and mix thoroughly. Centrifuge again at 1-6 C, this time using a heavy spin.
6. Place the blood bag on the expressor, and carefully release the taped tubing-covered cannula. Reenter the injection site of the empty saline bottle with the transfer tubing cannula, and express the saline and residual buffy coat into the empty saline container. Keep the saline container inverted and below the level of the blood bag outlet site during the procedure.
7. When only red blood cells remain in the blood bag, transfer the cannula from the discard container into another 250-ml container of cold, sterile saline.
8. Repeat steps 3 through 7 until the red blood cells have been washed a total of three times. Do not remove the cannula after the last washing.
9. Seal the tubing close to the blood bag, separate and discard.
10. Note that the expiration date is 24 hours from the time the unit is entered.

Equipment

Calibrating Serologic Centrifuges

Each centrifuge is to be calibrated upon receipt and after adjustments or repairs. Calibrating the centrifuge evaluates the behavior of cells in solutions of different viscosity; it does not test the reactivity of different antibodies.

For Immediate Agglutination

1. Use serum containing an antibody that produces 1+ agglutination macroscopically.
2. Select one sample of red cells positive for the appropriate antigen and one negative sample. Prepare a fresh suspension of red blood cells in the concentration routinely used in the laboratory (eg, 2-5%).
   a. For saline-active antibodies: Serum from group A person (anti-B) diluted with 6% albumin to give 1+ mac-

roscopic agglutination (3 ml 22% bovine albumin + 1 ml normal saline = 6% bovine albumin)
      Positive control: Group B red blood cells in a 2-5% saline suspension
      Negative control: Group A red blood cells in a 2-5% saline suspension
   b. For high-protein antibodies: 1 part anti-D diluted with 25-30 parts of 22% or 30% albumin to give 1+ macroscopic agglutination
      Postive control: D-positive red blood cells in a 2-5% saline suspension
      Negative control: D-negative red blood cells in a 2-5% saline suspension
3. For each set of tests, saline and albumin, prepare five 10 × 75 mm or 12 × 75 mm tubes for positive reactions and a duplicate set of tubes for negative reactions. Add the serum and test cells to each tube just before centrifugation.
4. In pairs, one positive and one negative, centrifuge the tubes for different times

Criteria	Time in Seconds				
	10	15	20	30	45
Supernatant fluid clear	No	No	Yes	Yes	Yes
Cell button clearly delineated	No	No	No	Yes	Yes
Cells easily resuspended	Yes	Yes	Yes	Yes	Yes
Agglutination	±	±	1+	1+	1+
Negative tube is negative	Yes	Yes	Yes	Yes	Resuspends roughly

(eg, 10 seconds, 20 seconds, 30 seconds). Observe each tube for agglutination and record observations. (See example on page 475.)

5. The optimum time of centrifugation is the *least* time required to fulfill these criteria:

   a. Agglutination in the positive tubes is as strong as determined in preparing reagents.
   b. There is no agglutination or ambiguity in the negative tubes.
   c. The red cell button is clearly delineated and the periphery is sharply defined, not fuzzy.
   d. The supernatant fluid is clear.
   e. The red cell button is easily resuspended.

   Since, in the example shown in the table, the 30-second and the 45-second spins fulfill these criteria, the optimum time for this centrifuge is 30 seconds.

For Washing and Antiglobulin Testing

The addition of antihuman globulin (AHG) serum to cells may require centrifugation conditions different from those for immediate agglutination because AHG is added to a dry cell button. The only fluid in the tube is the AHG serum itself. Centrifugation conditions appropriate for both washing and AHG reactions can be determined in one procedure. Note that this procedure does not monitor the completeness of washing; use of globulin-coated cells to control negative AHG reactions provides this check. The procedure described below addresses only the mechanics of centrifugation.

Materials
1. Antiglobulin serum, unmodified
2. Positive control: A 2-5% saline suspension of D-positive cells incubated for 15 minutes at 37 C with anti-D diluted to give 1+ macroscopic agglutination after addition of antiglobulin serum
3. Negative control: A 2-5% suspension of the same D-positive cells, incubated

for 15 minutes at 37 C with 6% albumin.
4. Saline, large volumes

Method
1. Prepare 5 pairs of tubes with positive and negative controls.
2. Fill tubes with saline and centrifuge pairs for different times, eg, 30, 45, 60, 90 and 120 seconds. The red cells should form a clearly delineated button, with no cells trailing up the side of the tube. After the saline has been decanted, the cell button should be easily resuspended in the residual fluid. The least time that accomplishes these goals is the optimum time for washing.
3. Repeat washing process on all pairs two more times, using time determined to be optimum.
4. Decant supernatant saline thoroughly and blot rims dry.
5. Add AHG to each of the pairs and centrifuge for different times, eg, 10, 15, 20, 30 and 45 seconds.
6. Select optimum time according to criteria described in step 5 of previous procedure.

Calibrating Centrifuges for Platelet Separation

Each centrifuge should be calibrated upon receipt and after adjustment or repair.
1. Collect from the donor an EDTA tube in addition to the specimen drawn for routine processing.
2. Perform a platelet count on the EDTA specimen. If the donor has a platelet count below 133,000/mm^3, this unit of blood should not be used for calibration.
3. Calculate the number of platelets in the unit of whole blood (WB): platelets per mm^3 $\times$ 1000 $\times$ volume of WB = number of platelets in WB.
4. Prepare platelet-rich plasma (PRP) at a selected speed and time (see Chapter 3, Preparation of Blood Components).
5. Place a temporary clamp on the tubing so that one satellite bag is closed off.

Express platelet-rich plasma into the other satellite bag. Seal close to primary bag and disconnect the two satellite bags. Do not remove the temporary clamp to the satellite bag until the next step.

6. Strip the tubing several times so the tubing contains a representative sample of platelet-rich plasma.

7. Seal off a segment of the tubing and disconnect so the bag of platelet-rich plasma remains sterile.

8. Perform a platelet count on the sample of platelet-rich plasma in the segment and calculate the number of platelets in the bag of platelet-rich plasma:

platelet count/mm^3 × 1000 × volume of PRP = number of platelets in PRP

9. Calculate % yield:

$$\frac{\text{number of platelets in PRP}}{\text{number of platelets in WB}} = \% \text{ yield}$$

10. Repeat the above process three or four times with different donors, using different centrifuges, different speeds and times of centrifugation.

11. Compare the yields for each set of centrifuge conditions.

12. Select the shortest time and lowest speed that results in the highest % yield of platelets in platelet-rich plasma without unacceptable red cell contamination.

13. Centrifuge the platelet-rich plasma at a selected time and speed to prepare platelet concentrate (PC).

14. Express the platelet-poor plasma into the second attached satellite bag and seal the tubing, leaving a long section of tubing attached to the platelet concentrate bag.

15. Place the platelet product on an agitator and leave for at least 1 hour to ensure that the platelets are evenly resuspended. Platelet counts cannot be performed accurately on a product immediately after centrifugation.

16. Strip the tubing several times, mixing its contents well with the contents of the platelet concentrate bag. Let the concentrate flow back into the tubing. Seal off a segment of the tubing so that the platelet concentrate bag remains sterile.

17. Perform a platelet count on the platelet concentrate. Calculate the number of platelets in the platelet concentrate:

platelet count/mm^3 × 1000 × volume of PC = number of platelets in PC

18. Calculate % yield:

$$\frac{\text{number of platelets in PC}}{\text{number of platelets in PRP}} = \% \text{ yield}$$

19. Repeat steps 13 through 18 using different centrifuges, different speeds and times of centrifugation.

20. Compare the yields for each set of centrifuge conditions.

21. Select the shortest time and lowest speed that results in the highest % yield of platelets in the platelet concentrate.

Once each centrifuge has been calibrated, it is not necessary to recalibrate unless there is a problem with the mechanical functions of the centrifuge.

Calibrating Vacuum-Assist Devices for Collecting Donor Blood

Equipment and Supplies

1. Vacuum-assist device
2. Vacuum source
3. Graduated cylinder capable of measuring 500 ml
4. Water
5. Blood bag with one attached satellite bag
6. Hemostat

Procedure

1. Weigh the empty primary bag containing anticoagulant-preservative solution and associated tubing.

2. Use 500 ml of water or saline, in a container that can be penetrated by the needle of the collecting system.
3. Add the 500 ml of water to the anti-coagulant-preservative solution present in the bag. Seal needle end of tubing to prevent leakage; remove needle and discard properly.
4. Penetrate the closure to primary bag and express into the satellite bag as much water as it will hold. It is not necessary for the primary bag to be completely empty. Apply a hemostat or other temporary closure to the integral tubing close to the satellite pack. The satellite pack is now the "donor."
5. Place the primary pack, label side down, in the vacuum-assist device, with the bottom of the bag barely touching the end of the cylinder. The blood bag must be centered on the stainless steel plate. Thread the connecting tubing through the donor tube slot. Turn on vacuum source, close lid of the cylinder and start cylinder agitating. Release the clamp or closure on the satellite pack and allow the contents of the satellite pack to fill the primary pack. When the door of the cylinder opens and the shut-off clamp closes, remove the bag and clamp tubing to satellite pack.
6. Weigh filled blood bag to determine volume of water.
7. If volume aspirated is not 450 ml, adjust the device appropriately. It is more practical to start with excess fluid than to start with less volume and increase by increments.

Notes

1. The volume collected is determined by the distance of the vacuum port from the stainless steel shelf of the cylinder. If the door of the cylinder opens when volume is inadequate, the port is too low. If the door of the cylinder fails to open when the satellite pack is empty, the port is too high.
2. One complete turn of the vacuum port will adjust the volume drawn by 6-8 ml.

Turn the vacuum port clockwise to decrease the volume and counterclockwise to increase it.
3. This same bag may be reused many times. Between uses, it should be stored in the refrigerator and brought to room temperature just before use.

Testing Refrigerator Alarms

The alarm on each blood-storage refrigerator should be checked periodically to be sure that it functions properly. Monthly intervals are appropriate if there have been no special problems. Some alarm systems have a push button to check that the electrical circuits are intact and that the alarm rings. The high and low temperatures of activation must be checked and the results recorded.

General Considerations

1. The thermocouple for the alarm should be easily accessible, and equipped with a cord long enough so that it can easily be manipulated.
2. The thermocouple for the recording thermometer need not be in the same container as that of the alarm.
3. When the temperatures of activation are checked, the change in temperature should be allowed to occur slowly enough that slowly responding thermocouples can respond. Too rapid a change in temperature may give the false impression that the alarm does not sound until a higher or lower temperature is registered.
4. The low temperature of activation should be no lower than 1 C; the high temperature of activation no higher than 6 C. Low activation above 1 C and high activation below 6 C are acceptable within the AABB *Standards*.
5. The amount of fluid in which the thermocouple is immersed must be no larger than the volume of the smallest component stored in that refrigerator. The thermocouple may be immersed in a smaller volume, but this makes the alarm

go off with smaller temperature changes than those registered in a larger volume of fluid. Excessive sensitivity may create a nuisance.

Technique

1. Be sure the alarm circuits are operating and the alarm is switched on. Immerse an easy-to-read mercury thermometer in the container with the alarm thermocouple, and be sure the temperature is between 1-6 C.
2. For low activation: Place the container with the thermocouple and thermometer in a pan containing a slush of ice and water colder than 0 C. To achieve this temperature, add several spoonfuls of table salt along with the ice. The temperature should be − 4 C or lower.
3. Close the refrigerator door so that the temperature of the interior is not significantly affected.
4. Allow the container to remain in the pan of cold slush, with periodic gentle agitation, until the alarm sounds. Record this temperature as the low-activation temperature.
5. Remove the container from the slush bath. Allow the fluid to return to normal temperature, and note temperature at which audible or visible alarm signal stops.
6. For high activation: Place the container with thermocouple and thermometer in a pan containing water at 12-15 C. Keep refrigerator door closed. Allow the fluid in the container to warm slowly with occasional agitation. Record temperature at which alarm sounds as high temperature of activation.
7. Remove container from warm pan, and note temperature at which audible or visible alarm signal ceases.
8. Record the date, the identity of the refrigerator, the low temperature of activation, the high temperature of activation and the name or initials of the person performing the test.
9. Take appropriate corrective actions if temperatures of activation are too low

or too high, and record the nature of the correction.

Testing Freezer Alarms

Freezer Malfunction

Freezer temperatures may rise to unacceptable levels for a variety of reasons, some fairly common. It is essential to have a functioning alarm and to have, in a conspicuous place, directions for protective measures to take if the freezer temperature cannot rapidly be corrected. Common causes of rising temperature include:

1. Freezer door or lid not properly shut
2. Low level of refrigerant
3. Compressor failure
4. Dirty heat exchanger
5. Loss of electrical power

General Considerations

Freezers must be equipped with a recorder for continuous temperature monitoring, and an audible alarm that sounds at such a temperature that appropriate action can be taken to prevent stored components from reaching undesirable temperatures. The diversity of available freezers makes it impossible to give specific instructions applicable to all storage conditions. The procedures manual for each facility must include a detailed description of the methods in local use. If suitable directions for devising a test method are not available in the owner's manual for the freezer/alarm system, the manufacturer should be consulted.

1. Test alarms at regular intervals, frequently enough so that personnel are proficient in handling the alarm, and so that malfunctions, should they develop, are likely to be detected.
2. Protect frozen components from exposure to elevated temperatures during the test.
3. Use an independent thermometer of suitable type to record the temperature

of alarm activation as well as noting the temperature registered on the recorder.

4. Warm the alarm probe and thermometer slowly. It is difficult to note the specific temperature of activation during very rapid warming, and the apparent temperature of activation will be too high.

5. Record the temperature at which the alarm sounds, the date of the test, the identity of the person testing and any observations that might suggest impaired activity.

6. Return the freezer and the alarm system to their normal conditions.

7. Take appropriate corrective actions if the alarm sounds at too high a temperature and record the nature of the correction.

Notes

1. Test battery function, electrical circuits and power-off alarms, if these indicators are present, more frequently than testing the temperature of activation.

Record function, date and identity of person testing.

2. For units with the sensor installed in the wall, apply local warmth to the site, while protecting the contents of the freezer from rising temperature while the door is open.

3. For units with the sensor in the wall or in air, allow the temperature of the entire compartment to rise to the point at which the alarm sounds; remove the contents or protect frozen contents with insulation during this process.

4. For units with thermocouple located in antifreeze solution, pull the container and the cables outside the freezer chest for testing, leaving the door shut and the contents protected.

5. For units with a tracking alarm that sounds whenever the temperature reaches a constant interval above the setting on the temperature controller, set the controller to a lower setting and note the temperature interval at which the alarm sounds.

Hemolytic Disease of the Newborn

Indicator Cell Rosette Test for Fetal-Maternal Hemorrhage

Principle

This test detects D-positive cells in the blood of a D-negative woman who has given birth to a D-positive infant. The small amount of D-positive fetal blood present is never enough to undergo direct agglutination when anti-D is added to the mother's blood sample. The D-positive cells do, however, become coated with anti-D when the blood is incubated with reagent antibody. Mixed-field agglutination occurs when antiglobulin serum is used to demonstrate coating antibody, but the mixed-field positive result may be difficult to detect. This test uses D-positive cells as the indicator to demonstrate antibody coating. The indicator cells combine with the anti-D present on the coated cells, and form easily visible rosettes of several cells clustered around each antibody-coated D-positive cell in the mixed population.

Although the number of rosettes is roughly proportional to the number of D-positive cells present in the mixture, this test provides only qualitative information about fetal-maternal admixture. Specimens giving a positive result should be tested with an acid-elution procedure to quantify the number of fetal cells present.

Materials

1. 3-4% saline suspension of washed cells from mother's postdelivery blood sample
2. Negative control: 3-4% saline suspension of washed cells known to be D-negative
3. Positive control: 3-4% saline suspension of a mixture of cells containing approximately 0.6% D-positive cells and 99.4% D-negative cells (see note)
4. Indicator cells: 0.2-0.5% saline suspension of group O, R_2R_2 cells. Either enzyme-treated or untreated cells in an enhancing medium can be used.
5. Chemically modified reagent anti-D serum

Method

1. To each of three 12 × 75 mm test tubes, add 1 drop (or follow manufacturer's instructions) of reagent anti-D.
2. Add 1 drop of maternal cells, negative control cells or positive control cells to the appropriately labeled tubes.
3. Incubate at 37 C for 15 to 30 minutes, or as specified by manufacturer's instructions.
4. Wash cell suspensions at least four times with large volumes of saline. Decant saline completely after last wash.
5. To the dry cell button left after the last wash, add 1 drop of indicator cells and

mix thoroughly to resuspend. Add enhancing medium if appropriate.

6. Centrifuge tubes for 15 seconds at approximately 1000 g.
7. Resuspend cell button and examine cell suspension microscopically at 100-150 × magnification.
8. Examine at least 10 fields and count the number of cell rosettes in each field.

Interpretation

Absence of rosettes is a negative result. With enzyme-treated indicator cells, up to 1 rosette per 3 fields may be seen as a negative result; with a system that enhances agglutination, there may be up to 6 rosettes per 5 fields in a negative test. The presence of more rosettes than the allowable minimum constitutes a positive result and the specimen should be examined with a quantitative test for the amount of fetal blood present.

The presence of rosettes or agglutination in the negative control tube indicates inadequate washing after incubation, such that residual anti-D is present to agglutinate the D-positive indicator cells.

Blood from a woman whose Rh phenotype is D^u rather than D-negative will give a strongly positive result. A massive fetal-maternal hemorrhage may produce an appearance difficult to distinguish from results seen on D^u blood. Evaluating the clinical status of the infant, the mother's total Rh phenotype and the appearance of the positive test will help in deciding whether or not to perform a quantitative test for fetal cells in the mother's blood.

Note

A control mixture containing 0.6% D-positive cells can be prepared from 3% saline suspensions of washed D-positive and D-negative cells as follows:

1. Add 1 drop of 3% suspension of D-positive cells to 15 drops of 3% suspension of D-negative cells. Mix well.
2. Add 1 drop of the suspension from step 1 to 9 drops of the 3% suspension of D-negative cells. Mix well.

Reference

Sebring ES, Polesky HF. Detection of fetal maternal hemorrhage in Rh immune globulin candidates. Transfusion 1982;22:468-471.

Acid Elution Stain (Modified Kleihauer-Betke)

This procedure exploits the fact that fetal hemoglobin is resistant to acid elution, whereas adult hemoglobin is not. When a thin blood smear is exposed to an acid buffer, the adult red blood cells lose their hemoglobin into the buffer so that only the stroma remains. Fetal red blood cells are unaffected and retain their hemoglobin. The percentage of fetal cells in the maternal blood film is used to calculate the approximate volume of fetal-maternal hemorrhage. Either clotted blood or anticoagulated blood may be used.

Reagents

Buffer. McIlvaine's buffer, pH 3.2, prepared by adding 75 ml stock solution A to 21 ml stock solution B. Prepare fresh mixture for each test. The temperature of this final buffer mixture should be approximately 25 C (room temperature).

Stock Solution A. 0.1M citric acid, F.W. 210. (21.0 g $C_6H_8O_7 \cdot H_2O$ diluted to 1 liter with distilled water). Keep in refrigerator.

Stock Solution B. 0.2M sodium phosphate, F.W. 268. (53.6 g $Na_2HPO_4 \cdot 7H_2O$ diluted to 1 liter with distilled water). Keep in refrigerator.

Stains. Erythrosin B—0.5% in water
Harris hematoxylin (filtered)

Fixative. 80% ethyl alcohol

Controls

Positive. 1. Mixture of 10 parts of an adult's blood with 1 part of cord blood (ABO-compatible)
2. Cord blood

Negative. Adult blood

Procedure

1. Prepare very thin blood smears, diluting blood with equal volume of saline. Air-dry.
2. Fix smears in 80% ethyl alcohol for 5 minutes.
3. Wash smears with distilled water.
4. Immerse smears in McIlvaine's buffer, pH 3.2, for 11 minutes.
5. Wash smears in distilled water.
6. Immerse smears in Erythrosin B for 5 minutes.
7. Wash smears completely in distilled water.
8. Immerse smears in Harris hematoxylin for 5 minutes.
9. Wash smears in running tap water for 1 minute.
10. Observe, using 40 × magnification.
11. Count 2000 adult cells and record the number of fetal cells observed during this count.
12. Calculate percent fetal cells in the total counted.

Interpretation

Normal adult cells appear as very pale ghosts. Fetal cells appear as bright pink refractile bodies.

Volume of fetomaternal hemorrhage in ml of whole blood = percent fetal cells × 50.

Reference

Clayton EM Jr, Foster EB, Clayton EP. New stain for fetal erythrocytes in peripheral blood smears. Obstet Gynecol 1970;35:642-645.

Spectrophotometric Analysis of Amniotic Fluid

Scanning normal amniotic fluid with a continuous-recording spectrophotometer between 350-700 nm of the visible-light wavelength spectrum gives a smooth curvilinear tracing with higher absorbance at the shorter wavelengths. Bilirubin has a characteristic absorption peak at 450-455 nm.

Scanning clarified undiluted amniotic fluid in this visible range reveals bilirubin as a peak at 450 nm above a baseline drawn to simulate a normal curve. This height of the bilirubin peak is expressed as the ΔOD 450.

Equipment

1. DU spectrophotometer (or other suitable high-accuracy spectrophotometer)
2. Square quartz cuvettes with 1-cm light path
3. No. 42 Whatman filter paper
4. Suitable filtering apparatus

Specimen Requirements

Ample volume of amniotic fluid. Keep specimen away from light; ie, wrap aluminum foil around sample tube. Exposure to light will invalidate readings.

Procedure

1. Centrifuge the amniotic fluid at 3000 rpm for 10 minutes.
2. Filter through Whatman No. 42 filter paper using millipore apparatus.
3. If specimen is turbid, dilute with distilled water until OD readings can be obtained. Diagnostic curves are based on deviations of the optical density from the normal linear curve and not on absolute values.
4. Place 2.5 ml water in one cuvette for the blank. Place 2.5 ml amniotic fluid in the other cuvette for the test.
5. Take OD readings of the amniotic fluid against water at the following wavelengths: (Use the tungsten lamp for all readings) 700, 650, 600, 550, 500, 480, 470, 460, 450, 440, 430, 420, 415, 410, 400, 390, 380, 370, 365, 360 and 350.

Note: Be sure to zero the blank with the slit control and set absorbance scale at zero each time the wavelength is changed. Nelson and Talledo[1] give an excellent discussion of spectrophotometers, recorders and chart paper for amniocentesis.

Calculations

1. Using semilog paper, plot OD readings obtained against the wavelength settings used. Use vertical axis for OD and horizontal axis for nm. Start the 700 nm at lower right corner of paper at same point as the zero OD.

2. Draw a straight line from the 550-nm plot to the 365-nm plot on the graph paper, as shown on the figure below.

3. To determine the rise in OD at 450 nm, read the OD reading at 450 nm where the drawn straight line crosses it. Subtract this value from the plotted value at 450 nm.

4. A hemoglobin peak at 415 nm may add to the absorption at 450 nm. This error can be corrected by subtracting 5% of the specific rise in OD at 415 nm from the rise in OD at 450 nm.

5. Place a point at the Liley graph[3] (see figure on next page) relating to the ΔOD 450 logarithmic scale on the vertical axis and the weeks of gestation on the horizontal axis.

Comments

1. If the fluid cannot be analyzed immediately after collection, it may be held for later analysis up to 24 hours at room temperature if protected from light. Sunlight causes pigment to disappear. Storage at room temperature for three days may result in losses of 20% or more of the pigment.[1] This is an important consideration in mailing samples.

2. Samples may be preserved in the frozen state with little or no change in the ΔOD 450.

References

1. Nelson GH, Talledo OE. Amniotic fluid spectral analysis in the management of patients with rhesus sensitization. Am J Clin Pathol 1961;52:363-369.

2. Alperin WM. Spectrophotometric analysis of amniotic fluid. In: Charles AG, Friedman EA, eds. Rh isoimmunization and erythroblastosis fetalis. New York: Appleton-Century-Crofts; 1969;118.

3. Liley AW. Liquor amnii analysis in the management of the pregnancy complicated by rhesus sensitization. Am J Obstet Gynecol 1961;82:1359-1370.

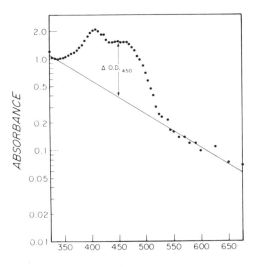

Visible absorption spectrums of amniotic fluid—absorbance plotted against wavelength. A tangent drawn to each curve corrects for background absorbance. The peak at 450 millimicrons above background (ΔOD$_{450}$) is directly related to the severity of the disease of the fetus in utero.

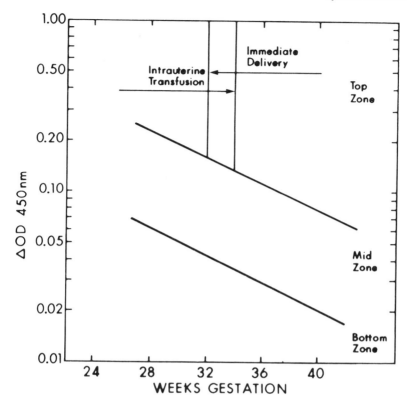

Liley graph for collecting data from amniotic fluid studies. Intrauterine transfusion should be done if the OD value is in the top zone prior to 32 weeks' gestation. After 34 weeks, top zone values indicate immediate delivery. Either intrauterine transfusion or immediate delivery may be indicated for top zone OD between 32 and 34 weeks depending on studies of fetal maturity. Modified from Liley.[3]

Miscellaneous

In Vivo Crossmatch with ^{51}Cr Tagging

If all donor units are incompatible in a patient whose antibody(ies) cannot be characterized and transfusion is urgently needed, it may be desirable to observe the in vivo survival of red cells incompatible in vitro. Donor red cells are tagged with ^{51}Cr and their short-term survival measured by counting residual radioactivity in the patient's circulating red cells. Chromium tagging is also used to measure long-term survival of autologous or transfused red cells, but a transfusion service faced with a problem patient ordinarily derives enough clinically important information from observing survival in the first minutes or hours after transfusion. It is customary to select for in vivo crossmatching the donor unit least compatible on in vitro tesing; if these cells survive satisfactorily, it is assumed that other units can safely be transfused.

There are many variations on this basic technique employing different doses of ^{51}Cr, different methods of tagging the cells and different schedules at which blood is drawn for testing. The technique given below is simple and permits rapid approximate assessment of short-term survival. As a control for the technical problems that often surround radioisotope techniques, this procedure uses an in vitro dilution of tagged red cells that simulates the distribution of radiolabeled red cells in the patient's circulation.

Tagging and Injecting Donor Cells

1. Select the least compatible unit of donor blood. Use red blood cells, not whole blood. This unit will be entered and must, therefore, be transfused within 24 hours, either to the patient under study or to another patient. Use sterile techniques throughout.
2. Place 25 μCi of ^{51}Cr in a sterile 10-ml vial. This must be done with a sterile preparation of isotope, and all precautions involving radioisotopes must be followed.
3. Withdraw 7 ml red cells from the donor unit, and inject the cells into the vial. Mix well and place in 37 C waterbath for 30 minutes. Agitate mixture frequently during incubation.
4. Calculate the patient's total blood volume, using figures for height, weight, age and sex from a standard hematology text.
5. Draw a preinfusion sample of patient's blood into EDTA.
6. Inject 5 ml of radiolabeled red cells into the patient's vein, being sure that the needle is securely in the vein and that there is no extravasation of injected cells.
7. Calculate the dilution that 5 ml of injected cells will undergo in the patient's

circulation. If the patient's blood volume is 5300 ml, the dilution is 5 in 5300.

8. Make a dilution of radiolabeled red cells in saline equal to the dilution in the patient. Use 0.2 ml of the labeled cells remaining in the vial and calculate as follows:

$$5/5300 = 0.2/x$$
$$5x = 1060$$
$$x = 212$$

In this example, add 0.2 ml labeled red cells to 212 ml saline, and mix thoroughly. This is the "control" dilution.

Measuring Survival

1. Draw a postinfusion sample into EDTA after 30 minutes. Mix thoroughly and then place half the specimen into a separate tube for centrifugation. Separate plasma from cells in this aliquot and save plasma.
2. Label four counting vials and transfer 1 ml of the following specimens:
   a. preinfusion whole blood
   b. 30-minute whole blood
   c. 30-minute plasma
   d. control dilution
   Be sure all samples are well mixed before transferring an accurately measured aliquot.
3. Count each specimen, using a gamma counter and standard technique. Record counts per minute (CPM) for each specimen.
4. Calculate survival of infused labeled cells by comparing CPM in whole blood with CPM in the control dilution.

$$\% \text{ survival} = \frac{\text{CPM of 30-min. whole blood}}{\text{CPM of control dilution}} \times 100$$

Interpretation

If the infused red cells have 80% survival or better at 30 minutes, it is probable that the transfusion will not cause severe adverse effects. The radioactivity in the 30-minute plasma should be compared with that of whole blood. If there has been rapid intra-vascular hemolysis, significant radioactivity will be found in the plasma. If red cell destruction is extravascular, the radioactivity will have been cleared from the circulating blood by liver or spleen. If survival is less than 70% or if there is substantial radioactivity in the plasma, the blood should not be used for transfusion.

If the results are equivocal, falling between 70 and 80% survival, or if longer-term observation is desired, samples can be drawn at additional intervals. When the 30-minute survival is between 70 and 80%, testing a 90-minute specimen usually resolves the issue of safe transfusion. If there has been little further drop in percent survival, and the 90-minute specimen continues to show survival above 70%, the unit can probably be considered safe. If there has been continuing decline in survival, the unit should not be given.

The International Committee for Standardization in Haematology has published a reference method for ^{51}Cr-tagged red cell survival studies. This material includes cautions and considerations applicable to the above technique, as well as giving a detailed method for short- and long-term survival studies. The method given above is intended only for predicting survival of a specific donor unit in a specific patient.

Reference

International committee for standardization in haematology: recommended method for radioisotope red-cell survival studies. Br J Haematol 1980;45:659-666.

Lymphocyte Cytotoxicity Test

This technique permits the performance of 1000 tests using 1 ml of antiserum. Also, 1 ml of blood yields sufficient numbers of lymphocytes to run 500 to 1000 separate tests.

Lymphocyte Preparation

It is essential that pure lymphocyte suspensions without granulocytes and red blood cells are used for the test.

1. Place 2 ml of fresh, heparinized blood into two 1-ml centrifuge tubes.
2. Centrifuge for 2 minutes at 3500 × *g*.
3. Remove the buffy coat and place in a centrifuge tube containing 0.3 ml of anti-A,B or anti-H, depending on ABO type.
4. Agglutinate red blood cells by turning slowly on a vertical wheel at approximately 8 rpm for 2-5 minutes.
5. Pack the agglutinated red blood cells by centrifuging for 7 seconds at 1000 × *g*.
6. Remove the supernatant and gently layer it over 0.3 ml of Ficoll-metrizoate mixture. (Ficoll-metrizoate is prepared by adding 9 g of Ficoll to 100 ml of distilled water. Then add 20 ml of 75% sodium metrizoate to 24 ml of distilled water to make a 33.9% solution. Mix 24 parts Ficoll solution with 10 parts metrizoate solution.) When layering the supernatant, it is critical not to mix the Ficoll-metrizoate and lymphocyte suspension.
7. Centrifuge at 3500 × *g* for 3 minutes. (Ficoll-metrizoate acts as a density gradient. Residual agglutinated red cells and granulocytes are packed in the bottom, lymphocytes remain at the interface and platelets remain in the anti-A,B or -H supernatant.)
8. Take out white interface and resuspend in 1-ml centrifuge tube containing 0.4 ml Modified Collins medium with 0.5% fetal calf serum. (Critical to pull all of the interface but minimum of Ficoll and supernatant. Excess Ficoll causes granulocyte contamination; excess supernatant results in platelet contamination.)
9. Remove platelets by a 1-minute centrifugation at 1000 × *g*. Discard the supernatant and resuspend the lymphocyte pellet in 1 ml of Modified Collins medium with 0.5% fetal calf serum.

10. Centrifuge for 1 minute at 5000 × *g*, to agglutinate excess granulocytes. Resuspend pellet.

Setting Up Test
Preparation of Antiserum Trays

All antisera are dispensed into microdroplet testing trays.

1. To prevent evaporation, add 0.005 ml mineral oil to each well with a multiple needle dispenser attached to a multiple pipetting device.
2. Add 0.001 ml serum to each well with a 50-λ multiple repeating dispenser.
3. Store trays in a −70 C freezer.

Test Incubation

1. Thaw antiserum trays immediately before using.
2. Thoroughly mix the lymphocyte suspension. With a 50-λ multiple repeating dispenser, add 0.001 ml of cell suspension to each well, being careful not to touch antiserum with needles.
3. Make certain that cells and antisera are mixed.
4. Incubate for 30 minutes at room temperature.
5. With a 250-λ multiple repeating dispenser, add by "soft drop" technique 0.005 ml of rabbit complement (stored in liquid nitrogen) to cell-serum mixture. Only 1 microdroplet per well should exist; mix if necessary. ("Soft drop" technique is a gentle layering of reagent onto cell-serum mixture so that the cells are not stirred up.)
6. Incubate for 60 minutes at room temperature.
7. Using a multiple needle dispenser, by "soft drop" technique, add 0.003 ml of 5% aqueous eosin to each well; mix if necessary.
8. After 2 minutes, by "soft drop" technique, add 0.008 ml of formaldehyde to each well using a multiple needle dispenser and jet pipette; mix if necessary.

9. Lower a 50 × 75-mm microscope slide onto the wells in order to flatten the top of the droplet.
10. Add heated petroleum jelly around the rim of the slide to prevent evaporation and siphoning of fluid from individual wells.

Reading Tests

Read reactions with an inverted phase-contrast microscope using a 10× objective. Living lymphocytes are small and refractile, whereas the dead lymphocytes are larger and stained with eosin. It is essential that red cells and granulocytes do not contaminate the lymphocyte suspension, for at this magnification they are difficult to distinguish from lymphocytes. Good phase contrast is necessary for clear definition of viable and nonviable cells.

Results are graded as shown below. Basically, the principle is to fix the proportion of viable cells in control wells as the baseline, and read other wells according to whether a detectably larger fraction of cells is killed. This rapid-judgment method has been found to be of considerable accuracy among different readers, and extremely rapid. With some training one can read 60 wells in 1.5 minutes.

Code

1 = Negative reaction in which the viability is the same as in controls
2 = Doubtful negative reaction with a perceptible increase in barely dead cells over the control level
4 = Doubtful positive reaction with a slight detectable change in viability
6 = Positive reaction, clearly different from controls (10-90% of cells killed)
8 = Strong positive reaction with essentially all cells killed (90-100%)
0 = No reading can be made.

Urine Hemosiderin

Principle

Hemosiderin is an iron-containing degradation product of hemoglobin. Hemoglobin that accumulates in the renal tubular cells following intravascular hemolysis is converted to hemosiderin. When tubular cells are sloughed into the urine, hemosiderin can be detected in the urine. Hemosiderinuria is thus indicative of a recent intravascular hemolytic episode. Adding Prussian Blue reagent to the centrifuged urothelial cells causes hemosiderin to turn blue, and microscopic examination of the treated sediment reveals stained urothelial cells.

Procedure

For best results, a fresh first-voided morning specimen should be collected directly into an iron-free container. Centrifuge and scan the sedimented urine for the presence of epithelial cells. If present, proceed with hemosiderin test. If no epithelial cells are seen, obtain another specimen.

Reagents

Prussian Blue reagent (mix fresh each time from stock solutions)
  0.1 ml 20% $K_4Fe(CN)_6 \cdot 3H_2O$
  0.9 ml demineralized H_2O
  1.0 ml 2 % HCl
Positive control
  0.75 cc demineralized H_2O
  iron filings

Technique

1. Collect urine and centrifuge at 2000 × g for 5 min.
2. Add 1 ml of Prussian Blue reagent to urine sediment and 1 ml to the positive control.
3. Cap tubes and mix.
4. Incubate at room temperature for 30 min.
5. Centrifuge 2000 × g for 5 min.
6. Discard supernatant.

7. Examine sediment microscopically for blue granules.
8. Report: negative (no granules seen) or positive (intracellular granules seen).

Interpretation

A positive result implies recent intravascular hemolysis, either acute or chronic. A negative result implies either that no hemolysis has occurred or that the hemolytic episode occurred in the past and the iron-containing epithelial cells have already been sloughed.

Differentiation of Hemoglobin and Myoglobin in Urine

Principle

Hemoglobin and myoglobin both give positive results on testing with the o-tolidine or benzidine indicators used to detect occult blood with reagent dipsticks such as CHEMSTRIP® or HEMASTIX®. It can be useful to distinguish between hemoglobinuria and myoglobinuria when investigating possible transfusion-related hemolysis. Myoglobin will oxidize in urine to a dark brown color that can be confused with hemoglobin. Myoglobin has a lower molecular weight (17,000 daltons) and is therefore more soluble than hemoglobin (molecular weight 68,000). In an 80% saturated ammomium sulfate solution, hemoglobin is completely precipitated whereas undenatured myoglobin remains in the supernatant. Since denatured myoglobin may be precipitated in 80% ammonium sulfate, a freshly voided urine sample should be tested. If the urine is to be stored, the pH should be adjusted to 7.0.

Procedure

1. Centrifuge fresh urine to remove intact red blood cells; test with indicator strip for a positive occult blood reaction.
2. If occult blood is positive:
   a. adjust pH of urine to pH 9 with 5% NaOH
   b. put 2.5 ml urine into a glass tube with 1.4g of ammonium sulfate
   c. mix well, filter (use 8-15 nm millipore filter) to obtain a clear supernatant
   d. recheck supernatant with urine indicator strip

Interpretation

If occult blood reaction is positive on the filtered supernatant, the specimen contains myoglobin. The presence or absence of hemoglobin is not confirmed. If the occult blood reaction is negative on the filtered supernatant, when the untreated specimen was positive, the specimen contains hemoglobin and no myoglobin. Results may be confirmed with cellulose acetate eletrophoretic screening.

Reference

Brodine CE, Vertress KM. Differentiation of myoglobinuria from hemoglobinuria. In: Sunderman FW, Sunderman FW Jr., eds. Hemoglobin: its precursors and metabolites. Philadelphia: Lippincott; 1964.

Normal Values

Normal Hematology Values in Adults*

Determination	Normal Range (Conventional Units)	Normal Range (SI Units)
Hematocrit		
Males	40–54%	0.40–0.54
Females	38–47%	0.38–0.47
Hemoglobin		
Males	13.5–18.0 g/dl	2.09–2.79 mmol/l
Females	12.0–16.0 g/dl	1.86–2.48 mmol/l
Red blood cells		
Males	$4.6–6.2 \times 10^6/\mu l$	$4.6–6.2 \times 10^{12}/l$
Females	$4.2–5.4 \times 10^6/\mu l$	$4.2–5.4 \times 10^{12}/l$
Mean corpuscular volume (MCV)	$80–96\ \mu^3$	80–96 fl
Mean corpuscular hemoglobin (MCH)	27–31 pg	27–31 pg
Mean corpuscular hemoglobin concentration (MCHC)	32–36%	0.32–0.36
White blood cells	$4.5–11.0 \times 10^3/\mu l$	$4.5–11.0 \times 10^9/l$
Reticulocyte count	0.5–1.5%	0.005–0.015
	$25–75 \times 10^3/\mu l$	$25–75 \times 10^9/l$
Platelet count	$150–400 \times 10^3/\mu l$	$15–40 \times 10^{10}/l$
Red cell volume		
Males	20–36 ml/kg	0.020–0.036 l/kg
Females	19–31 ml/kg	0.019–0.031 l/kg
Plasma volume		
Males	25–43 ml/kg	0.025–0.043 l/kg
Females	28–45 ml/kg	0.028–0.045 l/kg
Hemoglobin A_2	1.5–3.5% total hgb	0.015–0.035 total hgb
Hemoglobin F	<1% total hgb	0–0.01 total hgb
Methemoglobin	<1% total hgb	0–0.01 total hgb

*Henry JB, ed. Todd-Sanford-Davidsohn clinical diagnosis and management by laboratory methods. 17 ed. Philadelphia: WB Saunders; 1984.

Coagulation Factors*

International Designation	Common Name	% of Normal Needed for Hemostasis	Stability in Stored Blood	Biologic Half-Life
Factor I	Fibrinogen	(70–100 mg/dl)	Stable	3–5 days
Factor II	Prothrombin	?20–40	Stable	3 days
Factor V	Proaccelerin	15–25	Labile	?12–36 hours
Factor VII	Proconvertin	5–10	Stable	4–6 hours
Factor VIII	Antihemophilic factor	25–30	Labile	11–14 hours
Factor IX	Christmas factor	?15–25	Stable	24 hours
Factor X	Stuart factor	10–20	Stable	24–60 hours
Factor XI	PTA	?10	?Stable	48–84 hours
Factor XIII	Fibrin stabilizing factor	2–3	Stable	50–60 hours

*Wintrobe MM, Lee GR, Boggs DR, et al., Clinical hematology. 8th ed. Philadelphia: Lea & Febiger; 1981.

Normal Values* in Tests of Hemostasis and Coagulation (Adults)

Bleeding time	
Ivy	1–9 minutes
Template	1.5–7.5 minutes
Clotting time	8–18 minutes
Prothrombin time	11–15 seconds
Partial thromboplastin time	
Standard	68–82 seconds
Activated	32–46 seconds
Plasma thrombin time	13–17 seconds
Fibrinogen	160–415 mg/dl
Fibrin degradation products	<8 μ/ml

*Wintrobe MM, Lee GR, Boggs DR, et al. Clinical hematology. 8th ed. Philadelphia: Lea & Febiger: 1981

Nomogram for Calculating the Body Surface Area of Adults*

Height	Surface area	Weight

*From the formula of DuBois and DuBois, Arch Intern Med, 1916; 17:863. $S = W^{0.425} \times H^{0.725} \times 71.84$, or $\log S = 0.425 \log W + 0.725 \log H + 1.8564$, where S = body surface area in square centimeters, W = weight in kilograms, H = height in centimeters.

Nomogram for Calculating the Body Surface Area of Children*

Height	Surface area	Weight

*From the formula of DuBois and DuBois, Arch Intern Med, 1916;17:863. $S = W^{0.425} \times H^{0.725} \times 71.84$, or log $S = 0.425$ log $W + 0.725$ log $H + 1.8564$, where S = body surface area in square centimeters, W = weight in kilograms, H = height in centimeters.

Index

Index

Anti-Le^c, 166
Anti-Le^d, 166
Antilymphocyte globulin, effect of on DAT, 244
Anti-M, 155-156, 227-229
Anti-M^g, 156-157
Anti-N, 156
    reactivity of, with MN cells, 156
Anti-P$_1$, 160
Anti-penicillin antibodies, 257-258
    detection of, 460-461
Anti-platelet antibodies, in neonatal thrombocytopenia, 317
Antipyretics, in treating transfusion reactions, 333
Anti-Rg^a
    autoabsorption of, 456-457
    distinction from other HTLA antibodies, 456
Anti-S, 157
Anti-s, 157
Antisera
    chemically modified, 146
    contaminating antibodies in, 140
    for slide or rapid tube test, 120-121, 141-143
    high-protein, 141, 148
    quality assurance of, 374-375
    saline-reactive, 145-146
Antispecies antibody, contaminating AHG reagents, 98
Antithrombin III, 281
Antithymocyte globulin, effect of on DAT, 244
Anti-"total Rh", 139
Anti-U, 157
Anti-Ve, 173-174
Aspirin
    effect of on platelets, 46
    in donors, 4
    in hemapheresis donors, 20
AT III, see Antithrombin III
ATP, effect of on red cell shelf-life, 35
Audits, 399-400, 400-403
    criteria for, 399-400, 402-403
    statistics for evaluation during, 398, 400-401
Autoabsorption, cold, 466-467
Autoagglutination, thiol reagents to disperse, 232, 253, 463
Autoagglutinins, cold-reactive, determining titer of, 467-468
Autoantibodies, 247-248
    drug-induced, 259-260
    effects of on pretransfusion testing, 212
    management of patients with, 252-256
    serologic investigation of, 248-251
Autoantibodies, cold-reactive
    autoabsorption of, 466-467
    effects of in pretransfusion testing, 211-212
    in cold hemagglutinin disease, 247-248
    in Donath-Landsteiner test, 249
    in paroxysmal cold hemoglobinuria, 248
    specificities of, 248, 252, 467-468
Autoantibodies, warm-reactive, 246-247
    autologous absorption of, 463-465
    investigation of by dilution, 465-466
    specificity of, 251

Autoanti-I, 125, 171
Autoanti-i, 171
Autoimmune hemolytic anemia, 245-256
    cold-antibody type, see Cold Hemagglutinin Disease (CHD)
    transfusion therapy for, 255, 256, 284-285
    warm-antibody type (WAIHA), 246-247
Autologous antigens, usefulness of determining, 226, 228, 229, 253-254
Autologous control, 200-201, 211, 215-216, 222-223
Autologous red cells, separation from transfused cells, 419-421
Autologous transfusion, 359-368
    of bone marrow, 367
    of platelets, 273, 366-367
    of red cell products, 359-366
Autosomes, defined, 103
A$_x$, see A antigen, subgroups

B

B antigen
    acquired, 123-124
    biochemistry of, 118-120
    subgroups, 115
    tests for, 120-121
    weak, confirmation by adsorption and elution, 458
B lymphocytes, 77
Bacteria
    as immune stimulus in ABO system, 115
    cold-growing, 334
    culturing donor blood for, 49, 328, 334
Basophils, binding of IgE, 74
Bg antigens, 177
Bilirubin
    elevated levels of in newborns, 312-313
    excretion of, in HDN, 301
    in investigating hemolysis, 329
Biomedical material, shipment of, 411-412
Biphasic cold autohemolysin, 160
    Donath-Landsteiner test for, 249, 457-458
Bleeding tendency in donors, 6
"Blocked D", 148, 304-305
Blood bag, return of to blood bank, 290
    examination of, in evaluating suspected hemolytic transfusion reaction, 325
Blood groups
    ABO, 113-126
    chromosomal assignments of, 107
    HLA, 181-194
    other than ABO and Rh, 155-178
    Rh, 127-153
        terminology of, numerical, 128, 130
Blood group substances, soluble, 232-233
Blood pressure
    in donors, 7, 14
    medications for, 4
Blood sample
    for antibody identification, 221
    for investigating positive DAT, 245
    for pretransfusion testing, 196-197

frequency of, 363
iron supplement and, 363
pregnancy and, 363
use of blood for homologous transfusion, 365
Donors, deferral of,
acceptable rate, 2
for AIDS contact, 5-6
for hepatitis contact, 4-5
for previous surgery, 3
in prisons, 5
medications and, 3-4
Dopamine, in treating hemolytic transfusion reaction, 332
Dosage effect, 103
with Fy antibodies, 167
with Jk antibodies, 168
with MN antibodies, 156
2,3-DPG, see 2,3-diphosphoglycerate
DR antigens, 182
Drugs
abusers of, as prospective donors, 7
as cause of
positive DAT, 256-262
thrombocytopenia, 272
effect of, on DAT, 244
history of, in prospective donors, 3-4
Dry ice, use of
forbidden in shipping red cells, 50
necessary for shipping frozen components, 51
D^u phenotype, 132-135
significance of
in donors, 134
in obstetrical patients, 302, 319
in patients, 135, 146
D^u testing, 144-145
as screen for fetomaternal hemorrhage, 321
in evaluating RhIG candidates, 319
on donor blood, 16, 134
on pretransfusion blood specimens, 198
suitability of reagents for, 146
Duffy blood group system, 167-168
Dye exclusion test, in HLA, 188

E

e antigen in Rh system, variants in blacks, 136-137, 148
e antigen of hepatitis B, 345
EACA (epsilon-amino caproic acid) for inhibiting fibrinolysis, 417
ELISA, see Enzyme-linked immunoassay
Eluate
findings in, in autoimmune hemolytic conditions, 250
use of in crossmatching for hemolytic disease of the newborn, 311
Elution
as cause of false-negative antiglobulin test, 96
in evaluating delayed hemolytic reactions, 337-338
results of in
autoimmune conditions, 247-248, 250
hemolytic disease of the newborn, 305
techniques of and problems with, 235-236
Elution techniques, 429-433
chloroform, 432-433

cold-acid, 432
digitonin-acid, 431-432
ether, 430-431
freeze-thaw, 430
gentle, to obtain Ig-free cells, 417-418
heat, 429
Lui, 430
methylene chloride, 433
ultrasound, 429-430
xylene, 433
Emergency transfusion
issue of blood for, 216-217, 282
records of, 392
selection of blood for, 217
Enhancement procedures, for antibody identification, 231-232
Enzyme-linked immunoassay
as endpoint of antigen-antibody reactions, 83
in HBsAg testing, 351-352
Enzyme-treated cells, enhanced reactivity of with anti-species antibody, 98
Enzymes, proteolytic
effect of on
agglutination, 85
immunoglobulin molecules, 75, 76
preparation of for serologic testing, 425-427
use of in
antibody identification, 222, 228, 231
autologous absorption, 464
pretransfusion testing, 207
Errors, records of, 392-393
Erythrocyte sedimentation rate, in calculating concentration of hydroxyethyl starch (HES), 21
Erythropoiesis,
in hemolytic disease of the newborn, 301
in normal fetus and newborn, 297-299
ESR, see Erythrocyte sedimentation rate
Ether elution, 430-431
Exchange transfusion
efficiency of, 23-25, 313
in neonates, 310-316
complications of, 311
indications for, 312-315
techniques of, 315-316
plasma, see Therapeutic hemapheresis

F

$F(ab')_2$ fragment, 75, 76
Fab fragment, 75, 76
Factor B, in alternative pathway, 81
Factor H, as complement inhibitor, 81
Factor I, 81, 99
Factor II, VII, IX and X, deficiency, 279-280
Factor VIII
calculating dosage of, 277-278
composition of, 277
concentrates
heat treatment of, 279
preparation of, 44